Oxford Specialty Training:
Training in Surgery

Oxford Specialty Training: Training in Surgery

The Essential Curriculum

Edited by

Matthew D. Gardiner

Research Fellow in Plastic and Reconstructive Surgery
Kennedy Institute of Rheumatology
Imperial College London
London

Neil R. Borley

Consultant Colorectal Surgeon
Cheltenham General Hospital
Cheltenham

Editorial advisor

Ashok I. Handa
Consultant Vascular Surgeon and Clinical Tutor in Surgery
Nuffield Department of Surgery
John Radcliffe Hospital
Oxford

Foreword by

Bernard Ribeiro CBE
Former President of the Royal College of Surgeons of England

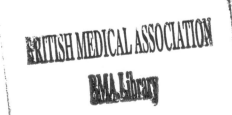

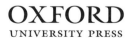

OXFORD
UNIVERSITY PRESS

OXFORD
UNIVERSITY PRESS

Great Clarendon Street, Oxford OX2 6DP

Oxford University Press is a department of the University of Oxford.
It furthers the University's objective of excellence in research, scholarship,
and education by publishing worldwide in

Oxford New York

Auckland Cape Town Dar es Salaam Hong Kong Karachi
Kuala Lumpur Madrid Melbourne Mexico City Nairobi
New Delhi Shanghai Taipei Toronto

With offices in

Argentina Austria Brazil Chile Czech Republic France Greece
Guatemala Hungary Italy Japan Poland Portugal Singapore
South Korea Switzerland Thailand Turkey Ukraine Vietnam

Oxford is a registered trade mark of Oxford University Press
in the UK and in certain other countries

Published in the United States
by Oxford University Press Inc., New York

British Library Cataloguing in Publication Data

Data available

Library of Congress Cataloging in Publication Data

Data available

Typeset by Cepha Imaging Private Ltd, Bangalore, India
Printed in Italy
on acid-free paper by
LEGO SpA – Lavis, TN

ISBN 978-0-19-920475-5

1 3 5 7 9 10 8 6 4 2

Foreword

Each generation of surgeons has a special textbook that defined their early learning and provided the basis for passing College examinations. In my case it was Bailey and Love's *Textbook of Surgery*, a heavy tome, but an excellent reference book. The development of the web-based Intercollegiate Surgical Curriculum Programme (ISCP) in 2007, has seen the introduction of a structured curriculum, approved by the Postgraduate Medical Education and Training Board (PMETB) for all surgical trainees. It identifies a shift away from textbooks as the only source of learning and signposts the use of e-learning and other means of accessing knowledge. Given the commitment by the surgical royal colleges to take responsibility for the management and oversight of training in the early years of surgery (ST1 and ST2) it behoves us to ensure that the right learning tools are available to assist our trainees. A textbook that has as many contributions from trainees as consultants is likely to find credibility amongst young trainees, who will appreciate the experience of those who have gone before. The ISCP requires trainees to define learning objectives with their educational supervisor in order that progress can be assessed. Case-based discussions form part of this process and I am delighted that this book is liberally sprinkled with examples at the end of each chapter. I was particularly pleased to see the section on core skills and knowledge, for in this age of specialisation it is important that future surgeons have a sound basis in the core principles of surgery. I do not believe we want technical surgeons, but rather doctors who as surgeons can deal with uncertainty and retain the skills to assess conditions outside their normal sphere of influence. This excellent textbook goes a long way to fulfil these principles. It follows the pattern familiar to those using the STEP course and will in the future gain the same affection from a new generation of surgeons as my well-thumbed copy of Bailey and Love.

Bernard Ribeiro

Preface

'All is flux; nothing stays still'

Heraclitus of Ephesus, c.500 BC

Although Heraclitus was referring to the universe he might well have been talking about surgical training. The recent introduction of Modernizing Medical Careers and the Postgraduate Education and Training Board (PMETB) has been responsible for much of the current flux in surgical education.

From a trainee's perspective the Intercollegiate Surgical Curriculum Project® (ISCP) has been one of the most visible consequences of this change. Initially designed by the surgical Royal Colleges to guide educational and training goals, it will become an integral part of delivering online content and assessment.

'So there is a new website, why do I need a new textbook?' The ISCP® is more than just window dressing. It has fundamentally restructured the curriculum and now clearly states the key topics for each specialty and level. It also outlines clinical, technical, and generic skills that will be needed to progress through surgical training.

This brand new textbook directly maps the initial stages (CT1/CT2) of the curriculum and delivers the core information that will be needed to get ahead in a surgical career. As if that wasn't enough, it doesn't need to be plugged in, won't give you a headache, and is compact enough to take to bed!

We hope you enjoy the book and welcome any feedback on how it might be improved in the future.

How to use this book

The book is divided by specialty. It has a simple layout, with the chapters containing a double page spread for each of their key topics. Core clinical and technical skills have been placed in separate boxes. These are clearly labelled and listed in the overview at the start of each chapter.

We would welcome your feedback on the book. If you have any comments or suggestions, please email us at ost@oup.com.

M.D.G
N.B

Acknowledgements

First, we must acknowledge Oxford University Press for commissioning this book. In particular we would like to thank Fiona Goodgame and Christopher Reid for their hard work and support during the production of this manuscript.

We would also like to thank the contributors for their hard work and those friends and colleagues who have commented on the manuscript during its production, including Stephen Barrett, Bill Flemming, Sarah Miller, Albert Pace-Balzan, Sankhya Sen, and Jessica Wilson.

The book is illustrated with some excellent radiological and clinical images. Many come courtesy of the radiology and clinical photography departments at Charing Cross Hospital, the John Radcliffe Hospital, Broomfield Hospital, and University College Hospital. We should also like to thank Dominic Blunt, Sally Barbrook, Jackie Kelly, Ramesh Pydiah, Etienne Cassar Delia, Sean Marven, Sarah Ridgwell, Elizabeth Higgins, Philippa Hutton, and Nikki Webster for their help with the images. In addition, William E. Svensson supplied the breast imaging and John Martin the gastrointestinal endoscopic images.

On behalf of the editors and OUP we should also like to thank the many reviewers who gave us valuable feedback and guidance which has helped to shape the final book.

Finally, this project would not have been possible without the unstinting support and encouragement of our families (Judith, Mark, Rhiannon, and family—M.D.G) to whom we dedicate this book.

Contents

Detailed contents

Contributors

Tipu Aziz BSc MD FRCS FRCS(SN)
Professor of Neurosurgery
Nuffield Department of Surgery
John Radcliffe Hospital
Oxford

Dominic Blunt MRCP FRCR
Consultant Radiologist
Charing Cross Hospital
London

Neil R. Borley MS FRCS FRCS(Ed)
Consultant Colorectal Surgeon
Cheltenham General Hospital
Cheltenham

Joanna Chikwe MPhil FRCS(CTh)
Specialist Training Registrar in Cardiothoracic Surgery
Royal Brompton Hospital
London

Nicholas de Pennington MA MRCS
Research Fellow in Neurosurgery
Nuffield Department of Surgery
John Radcliffe Hospital
Oxford

Peter Dziewulski FRCS FRCS (Plast)
Consultant Plastic and Reconstructive Surgeon
St Andrew's Centre for Plastic Surgery and Burns
Chelmsford

Matthew D. Gardiner MA MRCS
Research Fellow in Plastic and Reconstructive Surgery
Kennedy Institute of Rheumatology
Imperial College London
London

Elizabeth H. Gemmill MRCS
Clinical Research Fellow in Upper GI Surgery
Nuffield Department of Surgery
John Radcliffe Hospital
Oxford

Ashok I. Handa FRCS FRCS(Ed)
Consultant Vascular Surgeon and Clinical Tutor in Surgery
Nuffield Department of Surgery
John Radcliffe Hospital
Oxford

Georgina M. Howard-Alpe FRCA
Research Fellow in Anaesthesia
Nuffield Department of Anaesthesia
John Radcliffe Hospital
Oxford

Joseph K. C. Huang FRCS(Gen)
Consultant Colorectal and General Surgeon
Queen's Hospital
Romford

Adam Jones FRCS(Uro)
Consultant Urologist
Royal Berkshire Hospital
Reading

Pablo Martinez-Devesa FRCS(Ed) FRCS(ORL-HNS)
Specialist Training Registrar in Otolaryngology
John Radcliffe Hospital
Oxford

Radu Mihai MD PhD FRCS
Clinical Fellow in Endocrine Surgery
John Radcliffe Hospital
Oxford

David Mitchell BSc MD MRCS
Specialist Training Registrar in General Surgery
Northampton General Hospital
Northampton

Jeremy E. Newman MRCS
Research Fellow in Vascular Surgery
Nuffield Department of Surgery
John Radcliffe Hospital
Oxford

Paul Sauven MS FRCS
Professor of Surgical Oncology
Broomfield Hospital
Chelmsford

Warwick J. Teague DPhil MRCS
Research Fellow in Paediatric Surgery
Nuffield Department of Surgery
John Radcliffe Hospital
Oxford

William W. Williams FRCS
Consultant Trauma and Orthopaedic Surgeon
Broomfield Hospital
Chelmsford

Mark Woodward MD FRCS (Paed)
Consultant Paediatric Surgeon
Bristol Royal Infirmary
Bristol

Abbreviations

AAA	abdominal aortic aneurysm
ABC	airway, breathing, circulation
ABG	arterial blood gas
ABPI	ankle:brachial pressure index
ACE	angiotensin-converting enzyme
ACL	anterior cruciate ligament
ACS	acute coronary syndrome
ACTH	adrenocorticotrophic hormone
ADH	antidiuretic hormone
ADL	activities of daily living
ADM	abductor digiti minimi
ADP	adenosine diphosphate
AIDS	acquired immunodeficiency syndrome
AJCC	American Joint Comittee on Cancer
AKA	above-knee amputation
ALT	alanine aminotransferase
AMTS	abbreviated mental test score
ANCA	anti-neutrophil cytoplasmic antibody
AP	adductor pollicis
APB	abductor pollicis brevis
APC	antigen-presenting cell
APD	automated peritoneal dialysis
APL	abductor pollicis longus
APTT	activated partial thromboplastin time
AR	aortic regurgitation
ARDS	acute respiratory distress syndrome
ARF	acute renal failure
AS	aortic stenosis
ASA	American Society of Anesthesiologists
ASCA	anti-*Saccharomyces cerevisiae* antibodies
ASD	atrial septal defect
ASIA	American Spinal Injuries Association
AST	aspartate aminotransferase
ATG	antithymocyte globulin
ATLS	advanced trauma life support
ATN	acute tubular necrosis
ATP	adenosine triphosphate
AV	aortic valve
AVM	arteriovenous malformation
AVN	avascular necrosis
AVR	aortic valve repair
BCC	basal cell carcinoma
bd	*bis die* (twice a day)
BIPAP	biphasic positive airway pressure
BKA	below-knee amputation
BMI	body mass index
BNP	B-type natriuretic peptide

BP	blood pressure
BPM	beats per minute
BPPV	benign paroxysmal positional vertigo
BSA	body surface area
BT	bleeding time
CABG	coronary artery bypass grafting
CAD	coronary artery disease
CAPD	continuous ambulatory peritoneal dialysis
CCF	congestive cardiac failure
CCU	coronary care unit
CI	cardiac index
CMV	cytomegalovirus
CO	cardiac output
COPD	chronic obstructive pulmonary disease
CRF	chronic renal failure
CRP	C-reactive protein
CRPS	chronic regional pain syndrome
CSF	cerebrospinal fluid
CT	computed tomography
CVA	cerebrovascular accident
CVC	central venous catheter
CVP	continuous venous pressure
CXR	plain chest radiograph
dB	decibel
DIC	disseminated intravascular coagulation
DNA	deoxyribonucleic acid
DPG	diphosphoglycerate
DPL	diagnostic peritoneal lavage
DRE	digital rectal examination
DSA	digital subtraction angiogram
DVT	deep vein thrombosis
EAM	external auditory meatus
EBV	Epstein–Barr virus
ECG	electrocardiogram
ECRB	extensor carpi radialis brevis
ECRL	extensor carpi radialis longus
ECU	extensor carpi ulnaris
EDC	extensor digitorum communis
EDM	extensor digiti minimi
EDV	end-diastolic volume
EI	extensor indicis
EMG	electromyography
EMLA	eutectic mixture of local anaesthetic
EPB	extensor pollicis brevis
EPL	extensor pollicis longus
ERCP	endoscopic retrograde cholangiopancreatography

ESLF	end-stage liver failure
ESRF	end-stage renal failure
ESV	end-systolic volume
ET	endotracheal
EUA	examination under anaesthesia
EVAR	endovascular aneurysm repair
EWS	early warning score
FBC	full blood count
FCR	flexor carpi radialis
FCU	flexor carpi ulnaris
FDM	flexor digiti minimi
FDP	flexor digitorum profundus
FDS	flexor digitorum superficialis
Fe	iron
FEV_1	forced expiratory volume in 1 second
FFP	fresh frozen plasma
FiO_2	fractional concentration of oxygen in inspired gas
FNAB	fine needle aspiration biopsy
FPB	flexor pollicis brevis
FPL	flexor pollicis longus
FTSG	full-thickness skin graft
GCS	Glasgow Coma Scale
GFR	glomerular filtration rate
GI	gastrointestinal
GMC	General Medical Council
GOS	Glasgow Outcome Score
GTN	glyceryl trinitrate
HAS	human albumin solution
HBV	hepatitis B virus
HCV	hepatitis C virus
HDU	high dependency unit
HIV	human immunodeficiency virus
HLA	human leucocyte antigen
H_2O	water
HR	heart rate
Hz	Hertz
IABP	intra-aortic balloon pump
iaDSA	intra-arterial digital subtraction angiography
ICU	intensive care unit
Ig	immunoglobulin
IHD	ischaemic heart disease
IL	interleukin
IM	intramuscular
INOS	inducible nitric oxide synthase
INR	international normalized ratio
IPPV	intermittent positive pressure ventilation
ISCP	Intercollegiate Surgical Curriculum Project
IV	intravenous
IVC	inferior vena cava
IVU	intravenous urography
JVP	jugular venous pressure
LA	left atrium
LAD	left anterior descending coronary artery

LBBB	left bundle branch block
LFT	liver function tests
LMWH	low molecular weight heparin
LOC	loss of consciousness
LRTI	lower respiratory tract infection
LSV	long saphenous vein
LV	left ventricle
MAP	mean arterial pressure
MC+S	microscopy, culture and sensitivities
MCV	mean corpuscular volume
MELD	model for end-stage liver disease
MEN	multiple endocrine neoplasia
MHC	major histocompatibility complex
MI	myocardial infarction
MMF	mycophenolate mofetil
MODS	multiorgan dysfunction syndrome
MPH	miles per hour
MR	mitral regurgitation
MRA	magnetic resonance angiography
MRI	magnetic resonance imaging
MRCP	magnetic resonance cholangiopancreatography
MRSA	methicillin-resistant *Staphylococcus aureus*
MSU	midstream urine
NBM	nil by mouth
NCS	nerve conduction studies
NICE	National Institute for Health and Clinical Excellence
NIPPV	non-invasive positive pressure ventilation
nocte	at night
NOHL	non-organic hearing loss
NSAID	non-steroidal anti-inflammatory drug
NSGC	non-seminomatous germ-cell
NYHA	New York Heart Association
OCP	oral contraceptive pill
od	omni die (once a day)
ODM	opponens digiti minimi
OP	opponens pollicis
ORIF	open reduction internal fixation
$PaCO_2$	partial pressure of carbon dioxide in arterial blood
PAF	platelet-activating factor
PaO_2	partial pressure of oxygen in arterial blood
PAOD	peripheral arterial occlusive disease
PAOP	pulmonary artery occlusion pressure
PAR	patient at risk score
PAWP	pulmonary arterial wedge pressure
PB	palmaris brevis
PCA	patient-controlled anaesthesia
PCI	percutaneous coronary intervention
PDA	patent ductus arteriosus
PE	pulmonary embolus
PEEP	positive end-expiratory pressure
PEG	percutaneous endoscopic gastrostomy

PEJ	percutaneous endoscopic jejunostomy
PET	positron emission tomography
PICC	peripherally inserted central catheter
PL	palmaris longus
Plts	platelets
po	*per os* (by mouth)
PONV	postoperative nausea and vomiting
PPI	proton-pump inhibitors
PQ	pronator quadratus
pr	*per rectum* (by rectum)
PRC	packed red cells
prn	*pro re nata* (as required)
PT	prothrombin time
PT	pronator teres
PTCA	percutaneous transluminal coronary angioplasty
PTS	permanent threshold shift
pv	*per vagina* (by vagina)
qds	*quater die sumendum* (four times a day)
RA	right atrium
RAST	radio allergosorbent test
RBBB	right bundle branch block
RNA	ribonucleic acid
RSTL	resting skin tension lines
RTC	road traffic collision
rt-PA	recombinant tissue plasminogen activator
RV	right ventricle
SALT	speech and language therapy
sc	subcutaneous
SIADH	syndrome of inappropriate antidiuretic hormone secretion
SIRS	systemic inflammatory response syndrome
SLE	systemic lupus erythematosus
SMR	submucous resection
SSG	split-thickness skin graft
SSI	surgical site infection
SSV	short saphenous vein
SV	stroke volume
SVC	superior vena cava
SVR	systemic vascular resistance
TAA	thoracoabdominal aneurysm
Tc	technetium
TCR	T cell receptor
tds	*ter die sumendum* (three times a day)
TEDS	thromboembolic deterrent stockings
TFT	thyroid function tests
TGF	transforming growth factor
TIA	transient ischaemic attack
TNF	tissue necrosis factor
TNM	tumour, nodes, metastasis
TOE	transoesophageal echocardiography
TPA	tissue polypeptide antigen
TPN	total parenteral nutrition

TR	tricuspid regurgitation
TTE	transthoracic echocardiography
TTS	transient threshold shift
TURBT	transurethral resection of bladder tumour
TURP	transurethral resection of the prostate
U+E	urea and electrolytes
UICC	Union Internationale Centre le Cancer
UKT	United Kingdom Transplant
URTI	upper respiratory tract infection
USS	ultrasound scan
UTI	urinary tract infection
VDRL	venereal disease research laboratory
VF	ventricular fibrillation
VRE	vancomycin-resistant enterococci
VSD	ventral septal defect
VT	ventricular tachycardia
VTE	venous thromboembolism
WCC	white cell count
WHO	World Health Organization

Chapter 1

Professional skills and behaviour

1

1.1 Good surgical practice

Good Surgical Practice (2008) is a document published by The Royal College of Surgeons of England. It complements *Good Medical Practice* (2006), published by the General Medical Council (GMC).

Good Surgical Practice outlines the standards that all surgeons should strive to uphold in their clinical practice. It is based on seven key areas which are summarized below.

1. Good clinical care

- Good surgical practice should deliver high quality patient care according to priority and in a timely, safe, and competent manner
- Emergency care should be provided promptly in an appropriate setting. Patient transfer to another unit should be considered, and unfamiliar operations only performed if there is no clinical alternative
- Working with children should be confined to those with appropriate training and ongoing experience
- Organ and tissue transplantation should be carried out within the law and on the basis of clinical priority. Fully informed consent must be acquired from the donor
- Be aware of your limitations and use others' expertise
- Medical records should be accurate and contemporaneous

2. Maintaining good surgical practice

- Surgeons must maintain knowledge and expertise in their chosen field. This can be achieved through personal development, attending conferences, courses, and keeping up to date with the relevant literature
- Clinical audit and appraisal are mechanisms for assessing and improving performance
- Use of innovations in practice is encouraged but there must be the relevant regulatory and ethical approval. Patient safety is paramount. Adverse events should be identified and reported

3. Teaching, training, and supervising

- Learning continues throughout a surgeon's career. During this time he or she will be expected to create an environment in which students and trainees can learn and be trained
- Consultant surgeons should take responsibility for their trainees, including teaching, supervision, and assessment

4. Relationships with patients

- The doctor–patient relationship is based on trust. Good communication, informed consent, and awareness of particular cultural needs of patients are part of developing and maintaining this relationship
- Consent should be sought for all procedures and should follow the Department of Health guidelines (📖 Topic 1.6)
- Communication (📖 Topic 1.2) should involve active listening with respect for the patients' and their supporters' views. Enough time should be made available to inform the patient of their diagnosis and treatment fully. Surgeons must also recognize the varying needs of patients for information and explanation

5. Working with colleagues

- Effective team working improves patient care and is built on good communication and leadership
- Surgeons should actively participate in delivering multi-disciplinary care where appropriate

6. Probity in professional practice

- Probity is 'complete and confirmed integrity; uprightness'. It can be achieved by following the tenets of *Good Medical Practice* and maintaining an honest and objective view of oneself and one's colleagues
- Probity should be carried through into any private practice and research

7. Health

- Surgeons have a duty of care to their patients that not only covers their clinical practice but their own health and well-being
- Surgeons must be fit to practise and not be compromised by ill health, fatigue, drugs, or alcohol
- Exposure-prone procedures put surgeons at risk of acquiring or transmitting serious communicable diseases. In the event of a needlestick injury surgeons must follow the relevant local guidelines. The relevant authority must be informed if they suspect they may be carrying a communicable disease

Duties of a doctor registered with the GMC

Patients must be able to trust doctors with their lives and health. To justify that trust, respect must be shown for human life and the surgeon must:

1. make the care of the patient the primary concern
2. protect and promote the health of patients and the public
3. provide a good standard of practice and care, which involves:
   —maintaining professional knowledge and keeping skills up to date
   —recognizing and working within the limits of competence
   —working with colleagues in the ways that best serve patients' interests
4. treat patients as individuals and respect their dignity; treat patients with manners and consideration; respect patients' right to confidentiality
5. work in partnership with patients:
   —listen to patients and respond to their concerns and preferences
   —give patients the information they want or need in a way they can understand
   —respect patients' right to reach decisions with you about their treatment and care
   —support patients in caring for themselves to improve and maintain their health
6. be honest and open, and act with integrity
   — act without delay if you have good reason to believe that you or a colleague may be putting patients at risk
   — never discriminate unfairly against patients or colleagues
   — never abuse your patients' trust in you or the public's trust in the profession

1.2 Communication

Good professional–patient and healthcare team communication results in increased patient satisfaction and improved delivery of healthcare. In contrast, poor communication is frequently cited as the reason for complaints and litigation.

Importance of effective communication

In many situations, healthcare provision has a safety-critical element to it, much like the airline industry and other high reliability organizations (HRO). This is especially true of surgery, where safety-critical communications are commonplace and so poor communication is dangerous!

ABC of clear communication

- **A**ccurate
- **B**rief
- **C**lear

Safety-critical communications

- Speak up if you feel something is going wrong. Many errors are a result of communication never happening
- Address the correct person
- Time the communication so that you have the full attention of the receiver and do not interrupt a critical activity (unless an absolute emergency)
- Use correct grammar, avoid pronouns, and do not confuse verb tenses
- Read back the message or paraphrase it to confirm you received the correct message
- Summarize the message to confirm your understanding and double check the required course of action

Doctor–patient relationship

The doctor–patient relationship is different to normal social interactions. Within a short space of time, doctors have to gain a patient's trust and develop an effective rapport.

- *A good interpersonal relationship* is the foundation for what follows. It should be patient-centred, open, and involve active listening
- *Exchange of information* is a two-way activity. The doctor needs to gather diagnostic information and the patients need to be kept informed to enable joint decision-making
- *Decision-making* has traditionally been paternalistic. The doctor led and the patient followed. This has moved towards shared decision-making in which active discussion and patient participation in the process is encouraged

Doctor–patient communication

Doctor–patient communication can be complex. Values that create a solid foundation from which to base any consultation include understanding, truth, respect, empathy, and confidentiality.

Doctors should be aware of, and try to overcome, any barriers to effective communications. These difficulties may include sensory or speech impairment, language barriers, and the cultural needs of patients from different ethnic backgrounds.

Documentation and record-keeping

Accurate documentation and record-keeping is important for both clinical and legal reasons. Records provide a means of communication and a record of events.

- Patient records should be factual, consistent, and accurate
- Write during or as soon as possible after the event, with date and timings
- Write clearly, legibly, and preferably with a black ink pen which will be readable on a photocopy and will not degrade with time
- Avoid personal slurs and value-judgements
- Sign and clearly identify the author

◉ Breaking bad news

Breaking bad news is difficult for everyone concerned. However, doing it badly makes a bad situation worse. Below are some factors to consider when breaking bad news.

- Environment: quiet, private area with no interruptions. Include relatives and supporters if appropriate. Involve nursing staff and choose an area which is free for the patient to stay in for as long as is needed
- Establish the patient's current understanding of the situation and their desire for further information
- Share the bad news and start to inform the patient of the consequences from his or her starting point
- Take time, speak clearly, and avoid jargon
- Recognize the patient's feelings and respond to any questions or concerns
- Plan the future care and follow-up

◉ Writing an operation note

General details
- Date and time
- Patient details (name, date of birth, hospital number)
- Medical personnel involved (i.e. lead surgeon, assistants and anaesthetists)
- Emergency/elective and type of anaesthetic

Operation
- Name of operative procedure and indications
- Incision
- Operative findings
- Operative procedure actually performed
- Details of tissue samples removed or altered and implanted material used (i.e. serial number)
- Closure, including suture material used

Postoperative care
- Any special instructions related to procedure
- Analgesia or any other drugs that need to be administered
- Postoperative observations
- Eating and drinking status
- Plan for review, discharge, and follow-up if appropriate
Finally sign, print name, and leave contact details.

1.3 Judgement and decision-making

Good judgement and decision-making are cornerstones of surgical practice and make significant contributions to clinical performance. Most surgeons have little formal training in judgement and decision-making but acquire these skills during their career. The Royal College of Surgeons of England runs a course on judgement and decision-making for surgical trainees.

Judgement

Judgement is defined as 'the ability to judge, make a decision, or form an opinion objectively, authoritatively, and wisely especially in matters affecting action.' Attributes of good surgical judgement include:

1. accurate risk assessment
2. managing probabilities
3. managing uncertainty
4. integration of the above with patient preferences
5. reaching good decisions

Decision-making

'Experience is making the same mistake over and over again with increasing confidence'

Good decision-making is not innate but improves with experience but not as the quote suggests!

Surgeons, like other professionals in high-risk organizations, are called upon to make potentially important decisions with uncertain outcomes under pressure. The pressured environment is a result of limited information, lack of time, and distractions.

Novice versus expert

There is a transition seen from novice to expert decision-making. Novices have a tendency towards in-depth analysis. They will consider and attempt to weigh the possible pros and cons of a decision, all of which takes time.

Experienced decision-makers are more intuitive. They appear to have a more 'subconscious' approach, with the individual steps in the thought process skipped, so shortening the time to a final decision.

Top-down versus bottom-up

Clinical decision-making is driven by top-down processing (such as pattern recognition and goal-directed strategies) or bottom-up processing (which tends to be data-driven). Cognitive factors (See heuristics and biases below) influence these processes to shape the final decision.

Decision-making strategies

Below are some of the decision-making strategies that apply to clinical practice (Croskerry 2002).

Pattern recognition

A combination of patient-derived information is combined with clinical experience of similar circumstances to reach a decision. This is a good example of both bottom-up and top-down information being combined.

As with other strategies, pattern recognition is open to biases, including the clinician's previous experience, and misleading clinical signs.

Worst case scenarios

Ruling out worst case scenarios is a strategy to exclude critical diagnoses that must not be missed. Although it is a 'safe' strategy, it is much more resource-intensive and may bias towards overdiagnosis.

Clinical guidelines attempt to streamline this process to make the most efficient use of resources.

Goal-directed

Goal-directed diagnosis involves establishing a differential list early on during the clinical assessment and then attempting to eliminate or refine the order in response to further assessment and investigation.

Exhaustive review

Novice decision-makers tend to take an exhaustive ('no stone unturned') approach to collecting clinical information before making a decision. More experienced clinicians are able to elicit focused data that is directly relevant to the decision in hand.

Heuristics and biases

Heuristics are a set of rules learned 'on the job.' They provide short cuts in decision-making that are usually successful but can go wrong. When this occurs they are referred to as biases. Over 20 heuristics have been described; some of the more common ones are described below.

- *Availability* is the tendency to favour more common diagnoses or those that 'come to mind'. The opposite is the 'zebra retreat'. A rare diagnosis (zebra) may be a differential but the clinician lacks courage of conviction to pursue it, leading to a delay in diagnosis
- *Confirmation bias* is the tendency to accept information that confirms a hypothesis but ignore that which refutes it. This is done to avoid going 'back to square one'
- *Hindsight bias* ('retrospectoscope') distorts the perception of the previous decision-making and may underestimate or overestimate its success
- *Overconfidence* places too much belief in one's own opinions, with decisions made on insufficient information and instead relying on 'inherent ability' and hunch
- *Omission bias* (watchful waiting) is the general preference for inaction rather than active treatment. This fits with the maxim 'do no harm', and may avoid blame which is often assigned to the last person to touch the patient
- *Representativeness:* 'If it looks like a duck, walks like a duck, and quacks like a duck, it's a duck'—or is it? In this heuristic, clinicians rely too much on identifying clinical features that represent a condition. It mainly affects cases which present with atypical features that do not fit the surgeon's mental template of a condition

Improving decision-making

Attempts have been made to improve and support clinical decision-making. Strategies include:

- decision-making tools such as PROACT (Hammond et al. 1999)
- computerized decision support
- de-biasing is training that aims to overcome the cognitive biases discussed above

> **Extra**

- Croskerry P. Achieving quality in clinical decision-making: cognitive strategies and detection of bias. Acad Emerg Med 2002; 9: 1184–204
- Hammond et al. The hidden traps in decision-making. Clin Lab Manage Rev 1999; 13(1): 39–47

1.4 Clinical governance and patient safety

Clinical governance

'A system through which NHS organisations are accountable for continuously improving the quality of their services and safeguarding high standards of care by creating an environment in which excellence in clinical care will flourish'

Scally and Donaldson 1998

The fundamental aim of clinical governance is to improve the quality of healthcare continually by generating effective change.

Clinical governance encompasses a number of themes including

- Patient, public and carer involvement
- Risk management
- Education, training and professional development
- Clinical effectiveness-research and audit
- Information management
- Communication
- Leadership and team working

Patient safety

Patient safety encompasses identifying, reporting, analysing, and preventing adverse events in healthcare. It is estimated that 10% of hospital patients in the UK will be subject to an adverse event during their stay. Fifty per cent of these errors are probably avoidable.

Patient safety has only recently been identified as an area in which significant gains can be made in preventing morbidity and mortality of patients. It is estimated that, annually, almost 100 000 deaths in the USA are the result of medical error.

Sources of error
There are often multiple factors involved in medical error, with examples including:

- human factors: poor training, lack of experience, and fatigue
- medical factors: complex procedures and drug errors
- systems failures: poor communication, cost cutting, and lack of safety culture

Improving patient safety
Patient safety is becoming a major priority in the delivery of healthcare. In the UK there are a number of organizations involved, including the National Patient Safety Agency (NPSA) and the Medicines and Healthcare Products Regulatory Agency (MHRA). Strategies to improve safety have included:

- learning from other high-risk organizations, such as the airline industry
- encouraging incident and near-miss reporting
- fostering a safety culture through education and training
- technological innovations such as electronic health records and electronic prescribing and dispensing
- standard operating procedures and guidelines (encompassing evidence-based medicine)
- clinical governance

National Patient Safety Agency
The aim of the NPSA is to identify problems relating to patient safety and implement appropriate solutions. It oversees a number of confidential enquires into particular aspects of clinical care and also runs campaigns to improve safety such as the 'clean your hands campaign.'

Medicines and Healthcare Products Regulatory Agency
The MHRA is a government body which was set up to regulate medicines and medical devices and equipment in healthcare. It also collates and investigates incidents related to these products and has the power to prosecute.

> **→ Extra**
>
> - Scally G, Donaldson LJ, Clinical governance and the drive for quality improvement in the new NHS in England. BMJ 1998; 317: 61–65.
> - Safety first. A report for patients, clinicians and healthcare managers. London: Department of Health, 2006
> - National Patient Safety Agency. www.npsa.nhs.uk
> - Medicines and Healthcare Products Regulatory Agency. www.mhra.gov.uk

1.5 Audit, appraisal, and revalidation

Clinical audit

'Clinical audit is a quality improvement process that seeks to improve patient care and outcomes through systematic review of care against explicit criteria and the implementation of change. Aspects of the structure, processes, and outcomes of care are selected and systematically evaluated against explicit criteria. Where indicated, changes are implemented at an individual, team, or service level and further monitoring is used to confirm improvement in healthcare *delivery.'*

Principles for best practice in clinical audit

The audit cycle

Clinical audit is a continuous process, often described as a cycle or spiral.

1. Identify question

The audit question is often in response to a particular problem encountered during clinical practice or where current clinical practice can be compared with accepted guidelines.

2. Select criteria

The outcomes that are going to be measured have to be clearly defined.

A criterion can be defined as a 'systematically developed statement that can be used to assess the appropriateness of specific healthcare decisions, services, and outcomes' (Institute of Medicine 1999[1]).

3. Measure performance

Data collection needs to be accurate and as complete as possible. The sample group and data items should be clearly defined. Ethical and confidentiality issues surrounding audit should be considered.

4. Compare performance with standards

The data is compared with the predefined criteria and performance outcomes. This identifies areas for improvement and helps to guide the implementation.

5. Make improvements

Implementation of change is often hard work. There are many potential barriers, including staff behaviour, lack of resources and/or expertise, poor communication, and organizational issues. A working environment with a positive attitude towards audit and change, coupled with strong leadership, help implementation.

6. Sustain improvement

Once the changes have been implemented the cycle starts again. The intervention needs to be evaluated and, if successful, should be sustained. Demonstration of the improvements and the benefits they provide help to reinforce the audit environment and continuing cycle of improvement.

Appraisal

Appraisal aims to provide feedback on doctors' performance, record their continuing professional development, and identify future educational and developmental goals. It is based around the core headings in *Good Medical Practice*[2] published by the GMC (📖 Topic 1.1) and is tailored to an individual doctor's area of practice and the needs of the organization for which they work.

All doctors in training must maintain a portfolio of evidence related to these core topics. This may include:

- educational achievements related to the Intercollegiate Surgical Curriculum Project (ISCP) and examinations
- clinical assessments (e.g. mini-CEX)
- personal development plans
- evidence of reflective learning
- team working and 360° appraisal
- publications and presentations
- attendance at courses and educational meetings
- employment history
- occupational health

Revalidation

Revalidation is a process to 'quality-assure' the medical profession. Revalidation occurs every 5 years and is mandatory for all fully trained doctors. It examines their fitness to practise, with reference to *Good Medical Practice*[2]. Annual appraisal and evidence of continuing professional development will usually be sufficient evidence for revalidation. It does not currently involve any further examinations or practical assessments of clinical competence

➲ Extra

1. To err is human: building a safer health system. Institute of Medicine, 1999. Washington: National Academy Press 1999
2. General Medical Council. *Good Medical Practice*. London: GMC, 2006
3. A first class service: quality in the new NHS. London: Department of Health, 1998
4. *Trust, Assurance and Safety—The Regulation of Health Professionals in the 21st Century*. London: HMSO, 2007
5. Principles for best practice in clinical audit. NICE, London 2002

1.6 Consent and confidentiality

Consent

Valid consent should always be obtained before treatment or examination of a patient.

Consent should be performed by a clinician suitably trained and qualified. It is good practice for this to be the clinician providing the treatment, but it can be delegated to someone with appropriate experience.

Valid consent

Ask the following questions when deciding whether consent is valid.

1. Does the patient have capacity?

For a patient to have sufficient capacity they must be able to comprehend and retain information relevant to making the decision.

2. Is the consent given voluntarily?

The decision to consent has to be made voluntarily and freely by the patient. Relatives, friends, and healthcare professionals must not unduly influence or coerce the patient into making a decision.

3. Is the patient sufficiently informed?

Patients need to be informed of the nature and purpose of the procedure or examination, and any other relevant information such as the possible risks and adverse outcomes. This enables the patient to make a balanced judgement.

The legal standard for deciding what is sufficient information is based on what would be considered appropriate by a responsible body of medical opinion (Bolam test) used in medical negligence cases. The Sidaway case challenged this and stated that it would be negligent not to provide information about a significant risk even if a responsible body of medical opinion might not think it necessary. Clinicians are therefore guided to include any 'significant risk which would affect the judgement of a reasonable patient'.

Consent in different patient groups

Competent adults (over 18 years old)

- Competent adults may refuse treatment. The only exception is when the patient is detained under the Mental Health Act 1983
- A competent pregnant woman may refuse any treatment even if detrimental to the fetus

Incompetent adults

- Incompetent patients must be treated in their best interests; this may not necessarily equate to their best *medical* interests. Nobody can give or withhold consent on their behalf. The professional judgement should stand up to the Bolam test (reasonable body of medical opinion)
- Patients with fluctuating competence should have their views assessed when competent. If the incapacity is temporary, then non-urgent treatments should be delayed until capacity is regained
- Advanced care directives and living wills are legally binding and should be followed

Children and young people (under 18 years old)

- Competent children over 16 years can give consent but can have a decision to refuse treatment overruled if they are at risk of suffering 'grave and irreversible mental or physical harm.' Children under 16 years can technically give consent if competent ('Gillick' competence). They may have this competence for some procedures but not others
- Children under 16 years or those that are 16–17 years old, but incompetent, generally need a parent or guardian to give consent

- Refusal of treatment by a competent child under 16 years of age does not necessarily overrule parental consent to proceed. This is a rare situation
- Refusal of treatment by the parents of a child which is deemed in the child's best interest may need a second opinion and referral to the courts

The Mental Health Act 1983

There are some circumstances in which patients held under the Mental Health Act can have their mental disorder treated without their consent. It does not apply to any physical disorders they may have, for which the usual rules of consent apply.

Confidentiality

Doctors are entrusted with sensitive information by patients. Disclosure of such information by the patient confers a duty of confidence which is a legal obligation and part of the professional code of conduct.

Confidential information covers any patient identifiable information such as name, address, date of birth, clinical photographs, and identifiable NHS codes.

Caldicott and the Data Protection Act 1998

The Caldicott Report 1997 referred specifically to patient-identifiable information. It made a number of recommendations, including the appointment of a Caldicott Guardian for each NHS organization to oversee the use of confidential information.

The Data Protection Act 1998 lays out a framework for processing identifiable information. This includes holding, obtaining, recording, using, and disclosing information. It covers all forms of media such as paper and images.

It is good practice for all those processing confidential information to notify the Information Commissioner[6].

Using or disclosing confidential information

Case law has established that information given in confidence cannot be used or disclosed beyond the original understanding of the confider or without further permission (bar exceptional circumstances).

When do I have to ask for consent for use or disclosure?

Use of confidential information that contributes directly to audit or the patient's care carries implied consent, although every effort should be taken to inform the patient of this. Generally, any other uses require explicit consent.

When is disclosure allowed without consent?

Statute law requires or permits the disclosure of confidential information in some circumstances. Disclosure is permitted if it is 'in the public interest' or to protect the public. This most often applies to serious crime or to prevent abuse or serious harm.

> ### ➲ Extra
>
> 1. Reference guide to consent for examination or treatment. London: DoH, 2001
> 2. *Bolam v Friern Hospital Management Committee*, 1957
> 3. *Sidaway v Board of Governors of the Bethlem Royal Hospital*, 1985
> 4. *Gillick v West Norfolk and Wisbech AHA*, 1986
> 5. Confidentiality NHS Code of Practice, London: DoH, 2003
> 6. Information Commissioner's Office www.ico.gov.uk

1.7 Education, training, and research

Education and training

Surgical training is often thought of as an apprenticeship. In the past, trainees acquired knowledge and skills on the job with no formal framework. Modern surgical education has formalized this structure. Trainees are now required to form 'learning partnerships' with their teachers and follow a defined curriculum. They are also required to record their achievements as they progress through the scheme.

Learning opportunities

The College broadly divides learning opportunities into three areas:

1. Learning from practice is probably the most significant and includes almost all clinical situations. Initially, trainees will be 'watching', but will progress to 'doing' as they become more proficient
2. Formal situations include teaching sessions, courses, and the increasing use of surgical simulators
3. Self-directed learning requires some self-motivation! The Intercollegiate Surgical Curriculum Project will help to guide learning objectives

Assessment

Formal selection and assessment of surgeons has been based on in-training assessment and exams. Considerable effort is being put into developing methods of objectively assessing the craft element of surgery. Other new assessment tools such as mini-clinical evaluation exercises are attempting to assess trainees objectively.

Intercollegiate Surgical Curriculum Project

The Intercollegiate Surgical Curriculum Project (ISCP) is a comprehensive web-based training system that lays out the knowledge and skills that trainees should acquire at each stage of their training.

It also enables trainees and their supervising trainer to agree learning objectives during their placement and add to a portfolio that records the trainee's achievements.

Postgraduate Medical Education and Training Board

The Postgraduate Medical Education and Training Board (PMETB) is an independent regulatory body responsible for postgraduate medical education and training in the UK.

It approves specialist training curricula, such as the ISCP, ensures that the quality of training programmes is maintained, and certifies trainees so that they can be added to the specialist register held by the GMC.

Continuing professional development

One of the defining aspects of a profession is the acquisition and maintenance of a body of knowledge. Continuing professional development (CPD) formalizes this concept and sets the standards for doctors to continue their learning and adapt to change following their formal period of postgraduate education. CPD should include all areas of good medical practice and contributes to the process of revalidation.

Research

Medical research makes significant contributions to improvement in human health. The focus is increasingly on 'translational' research in which discoveries at the laboratory bench are converted into effective treatments at the bedside.

The UK has a strong track record in biomedical research. However, the career of a clinical academic has often been difficult, with a lack of structure and support. The new career structure aims to address these issues by identifying potential clinical academics early in their careers and enabling them to follow an explicit academic training pathway.

Funding and support

There are many sources of funding and support in the UK. Further information can be found on the MMC website. Other organizations directly involved in fostering UK biomedical research include the UK Clinical Research Collaboration, National Coordinating Centre for Research Capacity Development (NCCRCD), and the Academy of Medical Sciences.

Research funding comes from many different sources, including the Medical Research Council (government body), charitable organizations (e.g. The Wellcome Trust), and industry.

Ten steps in the research process

The general steps involved in developing and performing research are outlined below. See www.rdfunding.org.uk for further information.

1. Develop a research question
2. Review the literature
3. Design the study and methodology
4. Write the research proposal
5. Apply for funding
6. Obtain ethical and local R&D approval
7. Collect data (see consent and confidentiality)
8. Analyse data
9. Determine impact of data
10. Report and disseminate findings

National Research Ethics Service

It is likely that you will be involved with some form of research or investigation during your career. It is important that this is done ethically and with patients' best interests at heart. The National Research Ethics Service (NRES) maintains the framework for research ethical review in the UK.

Ethical considerations

There are six values commonly applied to medical ethics.

1. Beneficence: always act in the patient's best interest
2. Non-maleficence: 'first, do no harm' (primum non nocere)
3. Autonomy: respect the patient's right to refuse or choose their treatment
4. Justice: limited healthcare resources should be distributed fairly
5. Dignity: both patients and doctors have the right to dignity
6. Truthfulness and honesty: encompasses the concept of informed consent and patient education

> ### ➲ Extra
> - Modernising Medical Careers. www.mmc.nhs.uk
> - PMETB. www.pmetb.org.uk
> - Academy of Medical Sciences. www.acmedsci.ac.uk
> - UK Clinical Research Collaboration. www.ukcrc.org
> - NCCRCD. www.nccrcd.nhs.uk
> - Medical Research Council. www.mrc.ac.uk
> - The Wellcome Trust. www.wellcome.ac.uk

1.8 Child protection

A number of high profile child abuse cases and subsequent inquiries have reinforced the importance of having systems in place to detect and manage suspected child abuse.

The annual incidence is approximately 3 in 1000 children (UK), with over 80 deaths a year related to child abuse.

Types of abuse
There can be overlap, with a child being subjected to more than one type of abuse.

- **Physical** abuse includes hitting, shaking, throwing, poisoning causing either physical harm or illness
- **Sexual** abuse includes inappropriate physical contact, involvement in viewing adult material, or encouraging sexually inappropriate behaviour
- **Neglect** is a failure of the child's carer to meet the child's physical and/or psychological needs, resulting in poor health and/or development. This may include inadequate shelter, food, clothing, and access to medical care
- **Emotional** abuse involves the persistent denigration of a child's emotional state through psychological ill treatment. It is always present to a certain degree in the other forms of abuse

Risk factors
These can be child- or adult-related. Preterm babies and infants under 1 year old are at greatest risk. Teenage mothers, single parent families, mental health problems, drug and alcohol misuse, and domestic violence are all factors that increase the risk of an adult committing child abuse.

Clinical assessment
General
- Identify adult accompanying the child and their relationship to the child
- Identify who has parental responsibility
- Check details of GP, school, and health visitor or social worker
- Check child protection register

History
- Try to take the history directly from the child without influence from the carers. Children may disclose information suggesting they have been subject to abuse
- Delayed presentation or failure to seek healthcare following injury, multiple presentations with different injuries
- Poor explanation for an injury
- History not consistent with the injuries sustained

Examination
- Poor personal hygiene and dress
- Physical signs of abuse, include slap marks, unusual bruising
- Injury patterns inconsistent with the history
- Unusual behaviour or interaction with carers and other adults

Investigations
In most cases investigations are not routinely indicated other than for the suspected underlying condition or injury

- Urinalysis to exclude UTI
- FBC, U+E, clotting in cases with bruising
- Plain radiographs to exclude fractures. A skeletal survey may be indicated in exceptional circumstances
- CT brain if intracranial haemorrhage suspected

Management
Doctors with child patients have a duty to act 'single-mindedly in the interests of the child' and not the parents (House of Lords).

Generally, concerns should be discussed with the responsible adult only if this will not put the child at a greater risk of significant harm.

Keep good notes of the initial assessment and all subsequent communications with the parents and healthcare professionals involved in the case.

Any suspicion of child abuse should be brought to the attention of the local named healthcare professionals for child protection issues (paediatrician and paediatric nurse). They will be able to offer advice with regard to the Local Safeguarding Children Board child protection procedures.

> ### ⊃ Extra
> - The Victoria Climbié inquiry: report of an inquiry by Lord Laming. London, 2002
> - What to do if you're worried a child is being abused. London, 2003
> - Child protection—every nurse's responsibility. London, 2005

1.9 End-of-life care

End-of-life care is not just for 'old people with cancer' but should be available to anyone with incurable disease.

Definitions
- Palliative care is synonymous with end-of-life care and is the active care of patients with incurable disease, often involving the input of trained specialists
- Terminal care is the active care of patients in the final days or weeks of their life and marks the end stage of palliative care
- Euthanasia and assisted suicide are active steps to hasten a patient's death and are illegal. They are distinct from withholding life-sustaining treatment

Ethical and legal aspects
Towards the end-of-life, decision-making capacity is often lost. Where possible, decisions on end-of-life care should be made before this occurs. Withholding and/or withdrawal of life-prolonging treatment may be indicated in the dying patient

Advanced care directives and living wills
Advanced care directives and living wills are made voluntarily by an informed patient whilst they have capacity. They give guidance for specific clinical situations in the event of them losing capacity. However, they cannot force a clinician to carry out a procedure that they think is clinically inappropriate.

Withdrawal or withholding life-prolonging treatment
Adults with capacity can decide to refuse life-prolonging treatment. A child with capacity may have a similar decision overruled.

Aims of end-of-life care
NICE defines palliative care as 'the active holistic care of patients with advanced progressive illness. Management of pain and other symptoms and provision of psychological, social and spiritual support is paramount. The goal of palliative care is achievement of the best quality of life for patients and their families. Many aspects of palliative care are also applicable earlier in the course of the illness in conjunction with other treatments.'

Aims include:
- relief of pain and other symptoms
- addressing the patient's psychological and spiritual needs
- helping the patient to lead an active live for as long as possible
- helping the family cope with their relative's illness and subsequent death

Liverpool Care Pathway
The Liverpool Care Pathway (LCP) for the dying patient was developed to transfer good practice from the hospice model to other care settings such as hospitals. Key aims are to:
- discontinue or alter delivery of medications
- discontinue interventions
- document cardiopulmonary resuscitation status
- deactivate implanted cardiac defibrillators
- discontinue inappropriate nursing interventions
- communicate with the patient and assess their insight into the condition
- assess and meet religious and spiritual needs
- liaise with the family to keep them informed
- be aware of hospital procedures following death and bereavement advice for relatives

Symptom control
Symptom control is one of the core aims of end-of-life care. It needs to be regularly reviewed and have rapid implementation. Issues include the following.
- Pain: the WHO analgesic ladder guides initial management. Where possible, also treat the underlying cause. If strong opioids are required, remember to prescribe laxatives to prevent constipation. Also consider the most effective route of delivery
- Nausea and vomiting: there are a number of different anti-emetics used for different situations. In terminal care they are often delivered via a syringe pump in combination with opioid analgesia and sedation
- Malignant spinal cord compression is usually diagnosed on an urgent MRI. Dexamethasone is the initial therapy. Surgical decompression may be indicated; however, radiotherapy is the treatment of choice for malignant spinal cord compression. See NICE guidance
- Disease-specific: many conditions have particular symptoms that will need to be addressed, e.g. dysphagia caused by inoperable oesophageal carcinoma

> ### ➲ Extra
> - Marie Curie. www.mariecurie.org.uk
> - The National Council for Palliative Care. www.ncpc.org.uk

---

> ### ☉ No cardiopulmonary resuscitation orders
>
> Cardiopulmonary resuscitation (CPR) is a form of treatment. Withholding resuscitation or 'inaction' goes against the professional duty to save life. Therefore, like interventions, omissions also have to be justified.
>
> #### No CPR orders
> When consenting patients or making a 'No CPR' decision the chance of success, quality of life following resuscitation and their views need to be considered.
> - A No CPR order means that no attempt at resuscitation will be made (i.e. no BLS or ALS) and that the crash team will not be called
> - A No CPR order has no implications for other clinical decisions such as use of fluids and antibiotics
> - Following a cardiopulmonary arrest, if there is no pre-existing No CPR order then resuscitation should be attempted
>
> #### Consent
> - The standard rules of consent apply. It should be discussed with competent patients so that they are fully informed of what CPR involves and the potential outcomes. Advanced directive and living wills should be followed
> - Clinicians make the decision 'in the best interests' of incompetent patients. The views of relatives should be sought but they cannot give or withhold consent
>
> #### Procedure
> - Following patient consent or a senior clinical decision the No CPR order is completed and signed
> - No CPR orders should also be clearly documented in the notes and communicated to the healthcare professionals involved in the patient's care
> - A review date should be set. This is dependent on the patient's clinical state and prognosis

Chapter 2

Cardiothoracic surgery

Basic principles

Knowledge

Covered elsewhere

- Ischaemic heart disease (15.3)
- Cardiothoracic trauma (6.9)
- Emphysema and bullae (15.1)

✚ Technical skills and procedures

- Cardiopulmonary bypass
- Coronary artery bypass grafting
- Heart valve surgery
- Repair of thoracic aortic dissection
- Repair of thoracic aortic aneurysm
- Lung resection
- Chest drain insertion
- Video-assisted thoracoscopic surgery

Cardiac muscle

The heart comprises three types of muscle fibre: (1) atrial, (2) ventricular, and (3) specialized excitation and conductive fibres.

Like all muscle, cardiac muscle is striated and made from myofibrils containing actin and myosin filaments. Unlike skeletal muscle fibres, it has intercalated discs between cells, allowing them to act as a syncytium ('one unit'). With the neural connections from the sinoatrial (SA) and atrioventricular (AV) nodes and conduction bundles linked to rate changes from sympathetic and vagal input among others, the regular coordinated beat of the heart reflects the cellular 'one-unit design.'

In the normal heart, the atrial and ventricular muscles are separated by fibrous tissue and so act as separate syncytia. Conduction between the two is normally restricted to the AV node. Aberrant conduction pathways lead to arrhythmias.

Excitation–contraction coupling refers to the method by which the cardiac action potential causes contraction of cardiac muscle. The mechanism is largely the same as in skeletal muscle (📖 Topic 9.1).

Cardiac action potential

The majority of cardiac cells are non-nodal and require an external electrical stimulus to depolarize (Fig 2.1). Nodal cells have a different type of action potential and depolarize without external stimulus (automaticity).

Cardiac cycle

A normal cardiac cycle starts with one heartbeat to the next and describes a sequence of contraction and relaxation (Fig 2.2). The duration at rest is ~0.8 s (75 beats per min). During exercise each phase shortens but with disproportionate shortening of ventricular relaxation (diastole). This is the phase when the coronary arteries themselves receive most blood flow, hence its importance to heart function.

Cardiac output and regulation of function

Cardiac output (CO) is the volume of blood ejected by the heart each minute. It depends on preload, afterload and contractility (see below).

In a young healthy man, CO is approximately 5 L/min. It is the product of heart rate (HR) and stroke volume (SV), which is the volume of blood ejected by the heart each beat. CO varies with body size and so the cardiac index (CI) is used to give a more accurate reflection of cardiac function.

$$CO = HR \times SV$$

$$CI = CO/BSA$$

(BSA body surface area.)

Preload

Preload is equivalent to the volume of blood in the ventricle at the end of diastole (EDV). It is affected by circulating volume, ventricular compliance, length of diastole, and strength of atrial contraction.

Afterload

Afterload is the resistance to ventricular ejection. It is determined in part by the preload, which determines the maximum 'stretch', and by the resistance against which the heart must eject, which is a function of systemic vascular resistance (SVR), vascular compliance, mean arterial pressure, and any left ventricular outflow tract pressure gradient, e.g. obstruction.

Contractility and compliance

Contractility is a measure of the strength of myocardial contraction at a given preload and afterload. Mean arterial pressure and CO are commonly used as indirect measures of contractility.

Compliance is a measure of the distensibility of the left ventricle (LV) in diastole. Cardiac catheterization or echocardiography can be used to estimate LVEDV as a surrogate measure of compliance.

Venous return

Venous return is the rate of blood flow returning to the right atrium each minute and is the total of all of the returns from individual peripheral tissues. It is the most important factor in regulating normal cardiac function.

The Frank–Starling mechanism (Fig 2.3) describes the intrinsic ability of the heart, under normal physiological conditions, to pump all of the venous return without causing congestion.

Increasing venous return to the left ventricle leads to increased left ventricular end-diastolic pressure (LVEDP), which causes greater heart muscle stretch. This increased preload results in greater force of contraction and increased SV. The plateau is where increasing preload no longer results in increased force of contraction. In the clinical setting, this represents fluid overload.

The arterial pressure against which the heart pumps has no influence on cardiac function under normal physiological conditions; this has a molecular and structural basis determined by the crosslinking of actin and myosin. When an organ such as the heart is distended by too much volume, the effect at the molecular level is to prevent the molecular crosslinking thus preventing the myofibril from contracting.

Nervous system

The autonomic nervous system plays an important role in regulation of both cardiac function directly, and the circulation by altering vessel diameter (altering resistance).

Sympathetic stimulation of the heart causes increased heart rate and force of contraction. Parasympathetic stimulation causes a decrease in heart rate and slightly reduced force of contraction.

Blood supply of the normal heart

The arterial blood supply is provided by the left coronary distribution and right coronary artery (Fig 2.4). Both arise from the sinuses of Valsalva above the aortic valve.

At rest, coronary blood flow in the adult is 225 mL/min (5% of CO). During exercise this can rise to 1 L/min. Unlike the flow in all other vascular beds the coronary artery flow is maximal during diastole when the ventricles are relaxed. The rate of flow is controlled by locally-produced metabolic products (e.g. H^+, lactate, CO_2) which induce vasodilatation; sympathetic β_2-adrenoceptor stimulation can also cause vasodilatation, as can endothelial nitric oxide.

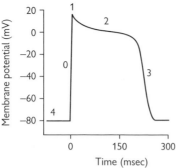

Fig 2.1 Cardiac action potential of non-nodal cardiac cells
(e.g. Purkinje cells of the conduction system or muscle cells)

0 Rapid depolarization phase is caused by opening of fast Na^+ channels and rapid inflow of Na^+ ions into the cell

1 Fast Na^+ channels close. The small downward deflection is caused by continuing outflow of K^+ and Cl^- ions

2 Plateau phase balancing inflow of Ca^{2+} through slow Ca^{2+} channels and outflow of K^+ through the slow delayed rectifying K^+ channels

3 Slow Ca^{2+} channels close while the slow delayed rectifying K^+ channels stay open. The net outward current leads to a negative change in membrane potential and the opening of rapid delayed rectifying K^+ channels. This repolarization returns the cell to its resting state

4 Resting membrane potential is restored and remains until the cell is stimulated by an external electrical source, i.e. the adjacent cell. It is maintained by the difference between the K^+ ion concentrations inside and outside the cell.

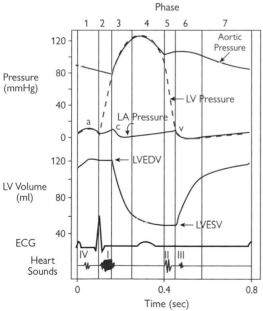

Fig 2.2 Cardiac cycle divided into seven phases

1 Atrial contraction contributes about 10% of LV filling at rest but up to 40% during exercise ('atrial kick')

2 Isovolumetric contraction, which is initiated by the QRS complex, leads to a rapid increase in ventricular pressure but no change in volume as ejection has not occurred

3 Rapid ejection occurs when the ventricular pressures exceed those in the pulmonary artery and aorta

4 Reduced ejection occurs as ventricular repolarization occurs (T wave)

5 Isovolumetric relaxation leads to a drop in ventricular pressure and the abrupt closure of the aortic and pulmonary valves (S2). The volume stays the same as the valves are all closed

6 Rapid filling begins as the ventricular pressure falls below that of the atria, and tricuspid and mitral valves open

7 Reduced filling occurs as the ventricles become less compliant and the intraventricular pressure increases.

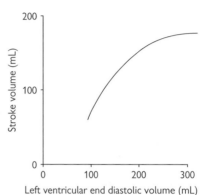

Fig 2.3 Frank–Starling mechanism (Starling's Law of the heart).

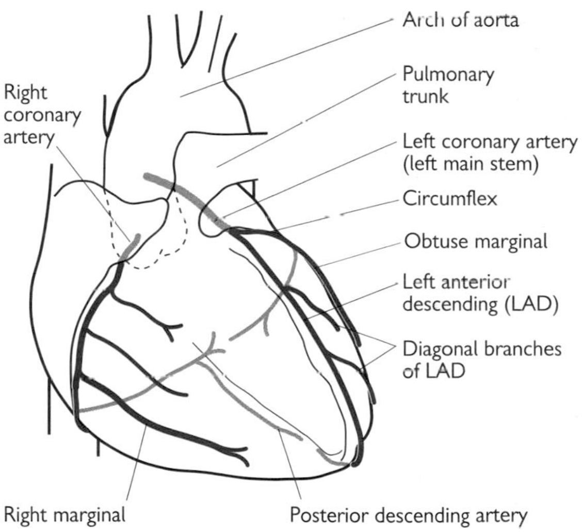

Fig 2.4 Coronary arteries. The anatomy described above does vary but is right-dominant in >90% of hearts. The right coronary artery reaches the crux of the heart where it turns through 90° to form the posterior descending artery (PDA), which runs towards the apex in the posterior interventricular groove (as above). In left-dominant hearts the Cx turns 90° into the posterior interventricular groove to form the PDA. About 3% of hearts are co-dominant.

2.2 Respiratory physiology

The purpose of respiration is to deliver oxygen and remove carbon dioxide from the circulation and thus regulate acid–base balance. The lungs also provide a complex filtering mechanism for particulate matter entering from the air and various metabolites from the blood, akin to a similar function provided by the liver which immediately precedes it in the circulatory system.

Pulmonary ventilation

The expansion and contraction of the lungs during normal breathing is almost exclusively caused by movement of the diaphragm, which contracts during inspiration and relaxes during expiration owing to the intrinsic elastic recoil of the lungs and chest wall.

During times of increased ventilation, movement of the rib cage and use of accessory muscles (sternocleidomastoid and scalenes) can increase the expansion and contraction of the lungs by up to 20%.

Compliance

Lung compliance is a static measure of lung and chest recoil. It is expressed as the change in lung volume for each unit increase in transpulmonary pressure (L/cmH$_2$O).

Lung compliance is greater during expiration than inspiration. This phenomenon is called hysteresis.

Lung volumes and capacities

There are four volumes which, when added together, are equivalent to the maximal lung volume at full expansion (Fig 2.5).

- **Residual volume** (RV) is the volume remaining following forceful expiration of air
- **Tidal volume** (TV) is the volume of air inspired or expired during normal breathing
- **Inspiratory reserve volume** (IRV) is the extra volume of air that can be inspired following normal inspiration
- **Expiratory reserve volume** (ERV) is the extra volume of air that can be expired following normal expiration

There are four lung capacities that describe the combination of two or more lung volumes.

- **Vital capacity (VC)** (ERV + TV + IRV) is the maximum quantity of air that can be expelled following maximal expansion of the lungs
- **Inspiratory capacity** (TV + IRV) is the quantity of air from the normal expiratory level to maximal expansion of the lungs
- **Functional residual capacity** (RV + ERV) is the quantity of air that remains in the lungs at the end of normal expiration
- **Total lung capacity** (RV + VC) is the total quantity of air that the lungs can hold following maximal inspiratory effort

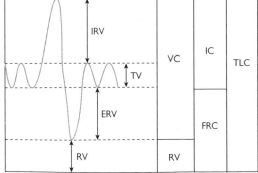

Fig 2.5 Diagram showing the lung volumes and capacities achieved during normal breathing and during maximal inspiration and expiration.

Alveolar ventilation

Alveolar ventilation is the rate at which fresh air reaches the gas exchanging areas of the lung (alveoli and respiratory bronchioles). It is the most accurate measure of ventilation.

During normal quiet respiration air from each tidal volume only reaches the terminal bronchioles and travels the final distance by diffusion.

Dead space is the volume of each tidal volume that fills the respiratory passages but never reaches the gas exchanging areas. In a young healthy man this is 150 mL.

- Anatomical dead space includes all respiratory passages not involved in gas exchange
- Physiological dead space is the anatomical dead space plus the alveoli not taking part in gas exchange, i.e. those that are not perfused

At any given metabolic rate, doubling the alveolar ventilation halves the alveolar PaCO$_2$, and vice versa, whereas the relationship between ventilation and PaO$_2$ is more complicated: hypoventilation and hyperventilation are therefore defined in terms of PaCO$_2$.

Gas exchange

The gas concentrations of alveolar air are not the same as atmospheric air. The concentration of oxygen drops from that in the atmosphere (PO$_2$ = 21 kPa) to that in the alveoli (PO$_2$ = 14 kPa) and again in arterial blood (PO$_2$ = 13.3 kPa). The alveolar concentrations of oxygen and carbon dioxide are dependent on the rate of gas absorption or production and level of alveolar ventilation. These differentially affect O$_2$ and CO$_2$ in diseased states owing to the relatively highly diffusible status of CO$_2$ compared to O$_2$.

Gas diffusion

The respiratory membrane is very thin and has a very large surface area (70 m^2). The factors that influence gas exchange across the membrane include: thickness, surface area, and the pressure gradient across it.

Gas transport

Oxygen

Over 99% of oxygen is transported bound to haemoglobin inside red blood cells; an insignificant amount is dissolved in solution. Under normal physiological parameters, in 100 mL of blood there is 20 mL of oxygen bound to haemoglobin and only 0.3 mL dissolved.

Haemoglobin

Haemoglobin A, the commonest type of haemoglobin molecule in the adult human, is a tetramer of four globular subunits, (two alpha and two beta chains). Each chain is tightly bound around a haem group consisting of an iron atom (Fe^{2+}) held in a heterocyclic porphyrin ring. The iron atom is the site of non-covalent oxygen binding, enabling a total of four oxygen molecules (eight atoms) to bind one haemoglobin molecule. In CO poisoning, covalent bonding permanently occupies the O$_2$-binding site, thus reducing the number of O$_2$ molecules that can be carried. Hence in this process once a certain number of molecules are covalently bound, the decrease in O$_2$-carrying capacity is permanent and cannot be reversed by increasing O$_2$ saturations but only by changing the number of haemoglobin molecules not covalently bound.

Oxygen saturation

The oxygen saturation of blood (SaO$_2$) is the percentage of arterial haemoglobin-binding sites actually bound to oxygen.

The relationship between PaO_2 and SaO_2 is described by the oxygen–haemoglobin dissociation curve (Fig 2.6).

The sigmoid shape of the curve is a result of the cooperative binding characteristics of haemoglobin. In response to an oxygen molecule binding to it, it undergoes a conformational change in its structure which increases its affinity for the next molecule. As the partial pressure increases, i.e. in the lungs, the haemoglobin rapidly becomes saturated, accounting for the steep part of the curve. It then flattens once the partial pressure rises above 8 kPa as there are few oxygen binding sites left.

Bohr effect

The Bohr effect describes a reduction in affinity of haemoglobin for oxygen in metabolically active tissues in response to a drop in pH caused by increased CO_2 production. As a result, oxygen is readily offloaded.

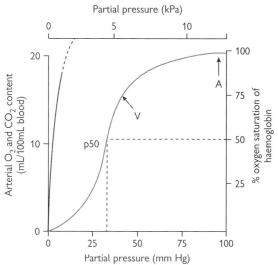

Partial pressure (kPa)

Fig 2.6 Oxygen-haemoglobin dissociation curve (blue) and carbon dioxide dissociation curve (red). Normal PaO_2 of arterial blood (A) is 13.3 kPa which corresponds to a saturation of 97%. Mixed venous blood (v) has a saturation of ~75%. The p50 is the PaO_2 at which 50% of haemoglobin is saturated (26.8 mmHg). Various factors can 'shift' the O_2 dissociation curve:
Left shift: ↓ $PaCO_2$, ↑ pH, ↓ temperature, ↓ 2,3 DPG
Right shift: ↑ $PaCO_2$, ↓ pH, ↑ temperature, ↑ 2,3 DPG

Carbon dioxide

Carbon dioxide (CO_2) is carried in blood by three mechanisms:
1. bicarbonate ions (85%)
2. bound to proteins, such as haemoglobin, to form carbamino compounds (10%)
3. Dissolved in solution (5%). Carbon dioxide is 24 times more water-soluble than oxygen

Bicarbonate

Red blood cells contain carbonic anhydrase, which accelerates the hydration of carbon dioxide (Fig 12.7).

Haldane effect

The Haldane effect describes the increased CO_2-carrying capacity of deoxygenated blood. This means that, for any given $PaCO_2$, the CO_2 content of deoxygenated blood is greater than that of oxygenated blood. This enhances the removal of CO_2 from respiring deoxygenated tissues and its release in the oxygenated blood of the lungs.

Regulation of respiration

Involuntary control of ventilation by the nervous system keeps arterial PO_2 and PCO_2 unaltered during most types of respiratory stress.

Control of respiration

There are three main groups of neurons in the brainstem that control normal breathing. Cortical centres allow voluntary control of ventilation when required.
- **Medullary respiratory centre** has inspiratory and expiratory areas which control the rhythm of breathing
- **Pneumotaxic centre** in the upper pons controls the duration of inspiration
- **Apneustic centre** in the lower pons prolongs the inspiratory phase

Sensors

Rises in arterial PCO_2 or H^+ are the usual controllers of respiration. Hypoxia stimulates the peripheral chemoreceptors and in comparison plays a minor role.

Chemoreceptors

- **Central chemoreceptors** are located on the ventral surface of the medulla surrounded by cerebral extracellular fluid. CO_2 readily crosses the blood–brain barrier so, as $PaCO_2$ rises so does the PCO_2 of cerebrospinal fluid, liberating H^+. This drop in pH stimulates the central chemoreceptors and causes an increase in ventilation
- **Peripheral chemoreceptors** are located in the carotid bodies at the carotid bifurcation. They respond to decreased PaO_2, decreased pH, and increased $PaCO_2$

Other receptors

Respiratory tract receptors are found both in the lungs and respiratory tract. They comprise:
- mechanical stretch receptors
- irritant receptors
- chest wall receptors

Effectors

The diaphragm and other muscles of respiration are under central control, and their coordinated response enables ventilation to continue under extreme conditions.

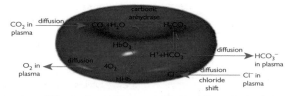

Fig 2.7 Diagram outlining CO_2 carriage by red blood cells and the inward chloride shift required to balance the outflow of HCO_3

2.3 Congenital heart disease

Congenital heart disease (CHD) is relatively common and is seen in ~1% live births.

Overview of cardiac embryology

The development of the four-chambered heart follows a complex sequence of events.

Day	Events
19	Migration and differentiation of cardiogenic mesenchyme. The vascular plate forms four simple tubes which coalesce
21	Paired anterior tubes fuse to form a single-chambered heart. Paired posterior tubes become two dorsal aortae. Constrictions (sulci) and expansions subdivide the primary heart tube into the sinus venosus, bulbus cordis, and conus truncus
22	Heart starts to beat and by day 24 blood starts circulating around the embryo
23	Heart tube begins to elongate, loop, and fold. It bends to the right (d-looping) and the caudal portion (sinus venosus) folds behind
27	Endocardial cushion growth and fusion partition the atrioventricular tract to create canals in which the valves develop
28	Septum primum extends down to divide the atria and, along with the septum secundum, forms an interatrial septum. The foramen ovale maintains a right-to-left shunt until birth
30	Interventricular septum formation, along with division of the truncus arteriosus into the aorta and pulmonary trunk finally separate the aortic and pulmonary systems

Changes in circulation at birth

The left and right sides of the fetal circulation are closed off from one another by a combination of circulatory changes, e.g. decrease in pulmonary artery pressures, and mechanical changes, e.g. foramen closure and ductal fibrosis.

1. **Gas exchange changes from placental to pulmonary**
   Inspiration causes decreased pulmonary artery pressures, increasing pulmonary artery blood flow
2. **Closure of foramen ovale** occurs as the pulmonary venous return increases left atrial pressure and forces the septum primum to close against the foramen ovale
3. **Closure of fetal vessels**. The ductus arteriosus closes immediately, the umbilical arteries close shortly after birth, and are followed by the umbilical veins and ductus venosus. The delay allows placental blood to return to the neonatal circulation until division of the umbilical cord

Aetiology

The underlying cause is unknown in most cases. A number of genetic conditions are known to cause CHD and maternal infection (Rubella), drugs (anti-epilepsy), and lifestyle (excess alcohol) increase risk. CHD includes abnormalities of both anatomy and physiology of the heart, and often forms part of congenital syndromes (e.g. Down's and Turner syndromes).

Haemodynamics
Acyanotic
- Left-to-right shunts are caused by a defect connecting the systemic circulation to the pulmonary circulation. The clinical features are dependent on its size

- Obstructive lesions can be minor (mild aortic stenosis, adult coarctation) or major (neonatal coarctation, critical aortic stenosis

Cyanotic
Cyanosis occurs in conditions with a right-to-left shunt that allows desaturated systemic venous blood to bypass the lungs and directly enter the systemic arterial circulation.

Nomenclature and classification

CHD can be classified in terms of clinical presentation (cyanotic, non-cyanotic), anatomy (intracardiac or extracardiac), physiology, or outcome (Aristotle index). The conventional order for describing a lesion is outlined below.

- Syndrome
- Cardiac position
- Connections of atria, ventricles, and great vessels
- Chamber, valve, and vessel abnormalities, including coronary arteries
- Physiological diagnoses, including arrhythmias
- Surgical corrections and persistent problems

Intracardiac defects

Atrial septal defect
A communication between the right and left atria creates a shunt. The degree of left-to-right shunt is dependent on ventricular compliance and the size of the defect. There are four main types:

1. **Ostium secundum defect** (70%) is a widely patent foramen ovale after failure of the septum primum to close against it. This is not to be confused with a patent foramen ovale where the tissue of the septum primum covers the foramen but fails to fuse with the sides, leading to 'probe patency' during cardiac catheterization
2. **Ostium primum defect** (20%) is a failure of the atrial septum to fuse with endocardial cushions, leaving a defect above the AV valves
3. **Sinus venosus defect** (10%) is high in the atrial septum and is associated with partial right-sided anomalous pulmonary venous drainage to the SVC and RA
4. **Coronary sinus defect** (<1%) is low in the atrial septum and results from the failure of development of the wall between the RA and coronary sinus

Ventricular septal defects
Ventricular septal defects (VSD) are the most common CHD. Their classification is based around the division of the septum into membranous and muscular components, with further division of the muscular septum into three areas (inlet, trabecular, and outlet).

Perimembranous defects are the most common (70%) and are situated between the inlet and outlet portions of the septum. VSD size rather than location has the greatest bearing on outcome. Defects similar in size to the aortic annulus are described as large and result in a significant left-to-right shunt.

Atrioventricular septal defects
Atrioventricular septal defects (endocardial cushion defects) are a spectrum of defects in the AV septum above and below the

AV valves. They commonly result in a left-to-right shunt which can be at an atrial level, ventricular level, or both, depending on how complete is the defect.

Hypoplastic left heart syndrome

The anatomical anomalies vary in severity. Generally there is mitral valve atresia with an absent or hypoplastic left ventricle. The aortic valve is stenosed and there is hypoplasia of the ascending aorta. Blood passes through the right side of the heart and lungs normally but does not enter the systemic circulation which relies on a patent ductus arteriosus for supply. It is a common cause of cardiac death in the newborn.

Extracardiac defects

Patent ductus arteriosus

PDA is the persistence of a functioning lumen in the fetal ductus arteriosus which connects the proximal descending aorta to the left pulmonary artery.

A normal neonatal ductus arteriosus is closed by smooth muscle contraction within hours of birth. Over the subsequent weeks this is made permanent by fibrosis of the lumen to leave the ligamentum arteriosus.

Coarctation of the aorta

Coarctation is a narrowing of the proximal descending thoracic aorta. It is often associated with conditions that reduce aortic flow early in fetal life.

The coarctation is usually juxtaductal (i.e. opposite the ductus arteriosus) but can be pre- or post-ductal. It is a form of left ventricular outflow obstruction and the pressure overload on the left ventricle eventually leads to left ventricular hypertrophy and congestive cardiac failure (CCF).

Tetralogy of Fallot

The anatomy is variable but is characterized by four lesions. A right-to-left shunt typically results from right atrial outflow obstruction caused by the pulmonary stenosis.

1. Pulmonary stenosis (level of outflow tract, valve or pulmonary artery)
2. Right ventricular hypertrophy
3. Overriding aorta
4. VSD

Truncus arteriosus

A single great artery arises from the ventricular outflow tracts via a single semilunar valve. There is an associated VSD. Patients develop severe CCF and pulmonary hypertension.

Transposition of the great arteries

The aorta arises from the right ventricle and the pulmonary trunk from the left ventricle. This condition often coexists with other cardiac anomalies such as coarctation of the aorta and PDA. Mixture of blood between the two systems is crucial for survival.

Clinical assessment

Most patients present within a few years of birth, although some remain asymptomatic into adult life.

History

- Birth history and family history of cardiac anomalies
- Decreased exercise tolerance and dyspnoea
- 'Squatting' as a right-to-left shunt develops on exercise
- Haemoptysis

Examination

- Dysmorphic or syndromic features
- Presence or absence of cyanosis
- Irregular pulse
- Heart failure
- Heart murmurs

Investigations

- ECG may show ventricular hypertrophy and arrhythmias
- Chest radiograph often shows cardiomegaly
- Echocardiography (TTE or TOE) is usually diagnostic
- Cardiac catheterization is now mainly therapeutic rather than diagnostic. It may help to establish the degree of shunt and presence of pulmonary hypertension

Management

Conservative

This can be expectant, with regular reviews or drug therapy.

Percutaneous intervention

This is typically used to close a PDA or manage a coarctation with either dilatation or stenting.

Operative

Generally, surgery is either palliative or corrective. Palliative procedures include cardiopulmonary shunting. Corrective procedures aim to improve anatomy or physiology.

Complications and prognosis

Patent defects may remain asymptomatic until later in life when pulmonary vascular changes lead to irreversible pulmonary hypertension and reversal of the left-to-right shunt (Eisenmenger's syndrome). The management of adult CHD poses different challenges to that in childhood.

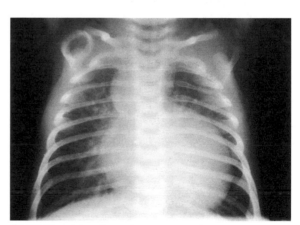

Fig 2.8 Neonatal cardiomegaly

2.4 Coronary artery bypass grafting

Stenotic coronary artery disease refers to the atherosclerotic narrowing of the coronary arteries. Its clinical manifestation is ischaemic heart disease (📖 Topic 15.13). This topic concentrates on the interventional and surgical management of IHD.

Luminal diameter narrowing by atherosclerotic plaques reduces flow delivery, particularly on exercise. The greater the reduction in vessel diameter the greater is the mechanical effect.

Acute thrombosis related to plaque fissure is a different process, and is usually related to instability at the shoulder region of a young atheromatous plaque which may have an insignificant effect on luminal diameter. The effect of this process is sudden platelet deposition, leading to thrombosis.

The overall effect clinically is governed principally by the site of thrombosis as well as its extent, thus a tiny end-arterial thrombosis will be insignificant whereas the same process in the left main or left anterior descending (LAD) coronary artery is likely to result in death.

Clinical assessment

Patients referred for operative management need the severity of their symptoms and co-morbidities fully assessed. The New York Health Association classification (Table 2.1) is used to assess the impact on activities of daily living.

History
- Cardiac symptoms—angina pectoris, dyspnoea, syncope, palpitations, and fatigue
- Previous management (drug history, percutaneous coronary intervention (PCI), coronary artery bypass grafting (CABG))
- Co-morbidities (CVA, COPD, CRF, PAOD)
- Risk factors: smoking, diabetes, hyperlipidaemia, family history, hypertension

Examination
Assess fitness for surgery and suitable conduit.
- General—obesity, chest wall deformity
- Cardiovascular—arrhythmias, valvular heart disease, heart failure, hypertension, carotid artery disease, PAOD
- Respiratory—COPD, asthma
- Conduit selection—varicose veins, Allen's test for radial artery

Table 2.1 NYHA classification	
Class 0	No angina under any circumstances
Class I	Angina only with prolonged or strenuous exertion
Class II	Angina causing slight limitation of ordinary activity
Class III	Angina with marked limitation of ordinary activity
Class IV	Angina occurring even with mild activity, or at rest
Deterioration in angina, or angina at rest is 'unstable' angina	

Investigations
- Bloods—FBC, U+E, LFT, TFT, CRP, fasting lipid profile
- 12-lead ECG
- Chest radiograph
- Treadmill ECG stress test
- Coronary angiography is the gold standard for defining flow-limiting stenoses requiring intervention
- Carotid duplex in patients >65 years or with TIA/CVA or carotid bruit

- Echocardiography in patients with valvular lesions
- Myocardial perfusion scanning with Thallium-201 or sestamibi identifies akinetic regions that will not benefit from revascularization.

Management
Conservative management of patients with IHD is discussed elsewhere. Some patients go on to have revascularization by PCI or CABG.

Percutaneous coronary intervention
The ratio of PCI to CABG is 3:1 in the UK, which is less than that in several other European countries. Stenting with bare metal or drug-eluting stents has largely superseded plain old balloon angioplasty (POBA).

Coronary artery bypass grafting
There are many more clinical trials which have validated the role of CABG as compared to PCI. Direct comparisons between the two techniques are fraught with difficulties of interpretation and meaning. However, it is clear on present evidence that PCI for prognostically significant disease, i.e. two- and three-vessel disease or in the presence of moderate to poor LV function has a much less secure evidence base than CABG.

In selected patients surgery is associated with longer survival without death, myocardial infarction, stroke or re-intervention than PCI or medical therapy. Indications include:
- disabling angina despite maximal medical therapy
- significant left main stem disease (LMS, LAD, Cx)
- significant (>70%) stenosis proximal LAD and Cx
- three-vessel disease
- failed PCI with ongoing ischaemia
- patients with less significant coronary disease having other cardiac surgery, e.g. aortic valve replacement

Complications and prognosis
Complications are more likely with advanced age, poor LV function, renal failure, and COPD. Ninety per cent of patients achieve either complete resolution or significant improvement in their quality of life. As time passes, re-stenosis occurs and angina recurs in 20% at 5 years and 40% at 10 years.

> ### ➜ Extra
>
> #### Cardiopulmonary bypass ('on-pump') versus 'off-pump'
> Off-pump coronary artery bypass (OPCAB) surgery aims to provide multi-vessel arterial or venous bypass grafting without the use of cardiopulmonary bypass (CPB), thereby attempting to reduce or mitigate the established deleterious aspects of CPB for individual patients.
>
> In high-risk patients evidence suggests that OPCAB may have lower morbidity and mortality rates by reducing the incidence of atrial fibrillation, renal failure, and urological effects
>
> #### Minimally invasive surgery
> The standard sternotomy provides excellent access but results in trauma to the chest wall. Minimally invasive direct coronary artery bypass (MIDCAB) involves a left anterior small thoracotomy (LAST) incision and allows access to LAD and diagonal territories.

Keyhole techniques for conduit harvest and vessel anastomosis are currently being extended to other areas in the heart by innovative use of CAB keyhold retractors, stabilizers, and suction devices. Along with advances in thoracoscopic anastomoses it may soon be possible to perform multi-vessel revascularization thoracoscopically. This opens the door for the potential for almost day case cardiac revascularization surgery.

➕ Cardiopulmonary bypass

CPB provides circulatory support to the rest of the body in operations that require the heart, lungs, and great vessels to be operated upon.

Indications
- CABG ('on-pump')
- Valve surgery
- Repair of septal defects
- Ascending and arch aortic dissection and aneurysm surgery; resection of tumours invading the great vessels
- Resection of renal cell carcinoma extension into the IVC

Procedure
1. Access gained to the heart
2. Patient is fully heparinized to prevent coagulation in the CPB circuit
3. Cannula placed in the ascending aorta (24F) and venous cannula (32F) in the right atrium, SVC, IVC or femoral vein or complex access via axillary and other arteries. Both cannulas are then connected to the bypass circuit
4. The venous blood is oxygenated, filtered, and can be cooled or warmed, and is pumped back to the patient via the aortic cannula
5. Once finished, the heparin is reversed with protamine

Complications
- Coagulopathy from activation of coagulation and complement cascades is usually prevented by heparinization
- Emboli from aortic cannulation can cause stroke and peripheral limb and end-organ ischaemia
- Peripheral oedema owing to increased capillary permeability and haemodilution
- Renal, pulmonary, hepatic, and pancreatic dysfunction

Myocardial protection
During CPB the heart is arrested and is not perfused. It therefore needs to be protected from ischaemic damage.
- **Cardioplegia** is the intentional and temporary cessation of myocardial contraction. Infusion of a potassium-rich solution causes the heart to arrest in diastole, reducing its oxygen consumption to near zero. It can be cold or warm, delivered antegrade and/or retrograde, and continuous or intermittent. Usually a cold blood-based solution is used as this is better for oxygen delivery and biochemical buffer capacity

- **Intermittent fibrillation** is the deliberate fibrillation of the heart for up to 20 min at a time. It is then possible to perform the distal anastomosis of coronary artery bypass grafts, before removing the cross-clamp and allowing the heart to beat so that it is perfused again. Myocardial oxygen consumption during fibrillation on bypass is almost as low as it is during cardioplegic arrest
- **Deep circulatory hypothermic arrest** involves cooling the patient to below 20°C. This reduces global tissue metabolism and allows circulatory arrest for 30 min. It is most commonly used during surgery to the distal ascending or arch of the aorta

➕ Coronary artery bypass grafting

Conduit selection
Conduit selection is tailored to the patient. The highest patency rates are achieved with the internal mammary arteries (90% at 10 years). Patency rates for other arterial grafts (e.g. radial artery) are less well established but superior to those for venous conduits in any direct comparative studies.

Long saphenous and other vein grafts have good early patency rates (90% at 1 year) but lower late patency rates (<50% at 10 years), and are usually reserved for non-LAD territories.

Procedure
- Median sternotomy
- CPB and application of aortic cross-clamp. Heart arrested in diastole with cardioplegia
- The distal anastomoses are usually made first and then the aortic cross-clamp is removed and the heart re-perfused before finishing with the proximal aortic anastomoses
- The left internal mammary artery is usually anastomosed to the LAD as this combination has the best evidence for prolonged patency. The LAD is also the most important stenosis to treat
- Once the anastomoses are complete, ventilation is restarted and the CPB discontinued

Complications
The primary elective CABG mortality rate is 2% but varies according to the risk associated with patient groups. It is always higher in the acute or emergency scenario.

Intraoperative and early	Intermediate and late
- Haemorrhage	- Wound infection
- Myocardial ischaemia	- Graft occlusion
- Myocardial infarction	- Myocardial failure
- Cardiac arrhythmias	- CVA
- CVA	- Recurrent angina
- Pericarditis	
- Acute renal failure	
- Pneumonia	
- DVT/PE	

2.5 Heart valve disease

Four valves regulate blood flow through the heart. Congenital or acquired conditions can make them insufficient (regurgitant), stenotic or both.

Aetiology

- Congenital heart valve conditions
- Degenerative changes with age
- Post-MI traumatic rupture of chordae or papillary muscles
- Infective endocarditis is an infection of the endocardial surface of the heart. It is most prevalent in mitral valve prolapse, prosthetic valves, and intravenous drug users
- Rheumatic fever is the most prevalent cause in Africa. It is an immune-mediated acute inflammatory reaction of the heart valves secondary to cross-reaction of group A beta-haemolytic streptococci and cardiac proteins. Following this trauma there is progressive valve fibrosis and calcification

Pathophysiology

Insufficient valves lead to regurgitation of blood back into the preceding chamber. This increased volume load leads to dilatation and some degree of hypertrophy.

Stenotic valves cause outflow obstruction of the preceding chamber. The increased pressure required to eject the blood through the valve causes hypertrophy of the chamber wall. The associated back pressure can sequentially affect the preceding chambers and organs, i.e. lungs and liver.

Clinical assessment

The general assessment before surgery is similar to that for CABG. Each condition is discussed below.

Investigations

- Bloods—FBC, U+E, lipid profile
- 12-lead ECG—arrhythmias, axis deviation, ventricular hypertrophy, and ischaemia
- Chest radiograph—heart size, pulmonary hypertension, pulmonary oedema, valve calcification
- Echocardiography is diagnostic. TTE quantifies valve lesions and LV function. TOE has better resolution; it is used to diagnose endocarditis, and to obtain more accurate information before surgery
- Coronary angiography is performed in patients >40 years with suspected coronary artery disease

Mitral stenosis

Mitral stenosis is narrowing of the mitral valve area leading to restriction of blood flow from the left atrium to the left ventricle. It is almost always rheumatic in origin.

The valve leaflets undergo progressive fibrosis and calcification, leading to fusion of the cusps. The resultant outflow obstruction leads to dilatation and hypertrophy of the left atrium and pulmonary hypertension.

Clinical assessment

Patients are asymptomatic for many years. The first presentation is often of dyspnoea precipitated by tachycardia (exercise, infection, sexual intercourse, pregnancy, fast atrial fibrillation).

Examination

- Malar flush (dusky pink discoloration of the cheeks owing to arteriovenous anastomosis and vascular stasis)
- Low volume pulse with a tapping, undisplaced apex beat

- Atrial fibrillation is common in late disease
- Auscultation: opening snap followed by rumbling mid-diastolic murmur loudest at the apex

Management

Mild symptoms are managed conservatively. Diuretics reduce left atrial pressure and pulmonary congestion. Beta-blockers and rate-limiting calcium antagonists slow the heart rate and improve left ventricular filling. Atrial fibrillation is treated with digoxin and anticoagulation.

Balloon valvuloplasty, open or closed valvotomy, or valve replacement is considered in patients with more severe symptoms (mitral valve area <1 cm^2, normal valve 3–4 cm^2). Prognosis is poor following the onset of heart failure.

Mitral regurgitation

The mitral valve apparatus is complex. Disease involving one or more of its components can lead to prolapse and regurgitation of blood from the left ventricle to the left atrium.

Acute MR is caused by ruptured chordae or papillary muscle following an acute MI or acute failure of a prosthetic valve. Chronic MR is more common, and is caused by a primary defect of the mitral valve or rheumatic heart disease (50%), LV dilatation, and CAD.

Clinical assessment

Chronic MR remains asymptomatic for many years. Gradual left ventricular impairment causes reduced exercise tolerance and fatigue.

Examination

- Laterally displaced, hyperdynamic apex beat with a systolic thrill
- Auscultation: pansystolic murmur loudest at the apex
- Atrial fibrillation, pulmonary hypertension, left and then right heart failure develop late

Management

Mild MR can be managed conservatively. Mitral valve repair or replacement is indicated in acute MR or chronic severe MR. The operative mortality rate is 2–3% for low-risk cases. The mortality rate of untreated severe MR is 5% per year.

Aortic stenosis

Aortic stenosis is narrowing of the aortic valve area, reducing the flow from the left ventricle into the ascending aorta. It may be caused by progressive calcification of a congenitally bicuspid valve, presenting in middle age, or senile calcification of a normal tricuspid valve which presents later in life.

The pathogenesis seems to be similar to atherosclerosis and 50% of patients have associated CAD.

The obstructed emptying of the left ventricle leads to increased left ventricular pressure and hypertrophy. Progressive deterioration leads to myocardial ischaemia, left ventricular failure, and arrhythmias.

Clinical assessment

There is a prolonged latent period where patients are largely asymptomatic. The valve area must reduce to ~25% of normal before symptoms develop, at which point there is a rapid deterioration with mean survival <3 years. Symptoms include angina, syncope, heart failure, and sudden death.

Examination
- Slow rising, low volume pulse with a heaving apex beat
- Auscultation: reversed split S2, ejection systolic murmur loudest in the aortic area and radiating to carotids

Management
Symptomatic aortic stenosis requires surgical intervention and is the commonest indication for valve replacement in the UK. Conservative therapy and percutaneous aortic valve repair (AVR) are reserved for patients unfit for surgery.

Aortic valve repair
The main indication is symptomatic aortic stenosis. LV dysfunction is an indication in asymptomatic aortic stenosis. CABG is performed at the same time if there is CAD. Operative mortality rates are <5%. Balloon valvuloplasty has been superseded by percutaneous AVR, which is currently an experimental procedure.

Without surgery, 50% of patients with angina die within 5 years, 50% with syncope die within 3 years, and 50% with dyspnoea are dead in 2 years.

Aortic regurgitation

Insufficiency of the aortic valve has many causes, including idiopathic dilatation, congenital abnormalities, calcific degeneration, and rheumatic heart disease.

Clinical assessment
Acute AR (infective endocarditis, aortic dissection, trauma) presents with acute LVF. Chronic AR is initially asymptomatic but orthopnoea, fatigue, and dyspnoea develop late.

Examination
- Wide pulse pressure with collapsing water-hammer pulse
- Hyperdynamic circulation (Quinke's sign—nail bed pulsation; Corrigan's sign—visible neck pulsation; De Musset's sign—head nodding; Durozier's sign—femoral diastolic murmur; pistol shot femorals—sharp bang with every beat heard over the femoral arteries
- Laterally displaced apex beat
- Auscultation: early diastolic murmur loudest at the left sternal edge in the fourth intercostal space. Austin Flint mid-diastolic murmur owing to regurgitant stream hitting anterior MV cusp

Management
Aortic valve surgery (replacement or repair) is guided by haemodynamic assessment of the heart and should be performed before symptoms progress. Conservative management with diuretics and vasodilators is reserved for patients unsuitable for surgery.

Acute AR is a surgical emergency. Chronic AR is operated on before the ejection fraction <55%, or LV dilates >5.5 cm in systole.

Acute AR has a poor prognosis. Chronic AR has a good prognosis until heart failure develops (50% 2 year mortality rate).

Tricuspid valve disease

Tricuspid valve disease is usually associated with mitral valve disease (functional) and is rare in isolation.

Pulmonary valve disease

Acquired pulmonary valve disease is rare. Pulmonary stenosis is usually congenital and may be associated with a ventricular septal defect (e.g. Fallot's tetralogy). Pulmonary regurgitation results from dilatation of the valve ring and is usually asymptomatic.

✚ Heart valve surgery

Ideally, valves would be repaired rather than replaced. However, this is usually only possible with the mitral and, occasionally, the tricuspid valve. Repair is technically more demanding than replacement, and may be impossible if the valve is very heavily calcified or destroyed by endocarditis Replacement valves are either biological or prosthetic.

Biological heart valves
Tissue valves are either homografts (cadaveric) or xenografts, which are pig valves or pericardium from cow or horse suspended on a metal frame covered by a cloth sewing ring (bioprosthetic valve). The main advantage is that patients do not need anticoagulation, but the disadvantage is the limited life span: 10–15 years in the aortic position and 6–10 years in the mitral position.

Prosthetic heart valves
Mechanical valves can be mono- or bi-leaflet and are now made from pyrolytic carbon. Ball and cage valves, such as the Starr Edwards, are no longer used. The main disadvantage is the need for lifelong anticoagulation with warfarin. This excludes some patient groups from having a mechanical replacement, e.g. women of childbearing age and professional sportsmen. Patients must always have prophylactic antibiotics during interventional procedures, including dentistry.

Procedure
- Median sternotomy incision. The mitral valve may be approached via right thoracotomy
- CPB with cardioplegia
- Valve is inspected and removed via an aortotomy for the aortic valve, and via a left atriotomy for the mitral valve
- Once the valve is sewn into place, these incisions are closed. Air is then removed from the heart, which is then weaned from bypass
- TOE assesses the valve, particularly in mitral valve repair. If there is any MR further surgery is required

Complications

Intraoperative and early	Late
Myocardial infarction	Prosthetic valve endocarditis
CVA	Myocardial failure
Paravalvular leak	CVA
Intrathoracic bleeding 5%	Structural valve failure
Thrombosis	
Cardiac arrhythmias (AF)	
Pacemaker	
Chest infection	
Death	

2.6 Thoracic aortic dissection

An aortic dissection occurs when blood leaves the aortic lumen via an intimal tear and enters the space between the intima and media of the aortic wall.

The incidence is 5–30 per million per year, and increases with age (peak >60 years). It is more common in men (M:F ratio 2:1).

Aetiology

The pathogenesis of aortic dissection is incompletely understood. Several theories have been proposed to explain the intimal tear, such as cystic medial degeneration as a mechanism of initial tearing. This is detected in a minority of patients with acute aortic dissection.

Atherosclerotic ulceration penetrating to the media as the source of the intimal tear is also uncommonly detected.

Finally, intramural haematoma resulting from bleeding of the vasa vasorum into the media is thought to account for sufficient stress to cause an intimal tear.

Traumatic aortic dissection is discussed in the emergency surgery chapter (☐ Topic 8.9).

Risk factors

- Advanced age
- Hypertension
- Atherosclerosis
- Hypervolaemia and high cardiac output states, e.g. pregnancy
- Connective tissue disorders (Ehlers–Danlos syndrome, Marfan syndrome, Turner syndrome)
- Congenital aortic stenosis or bicuspid aortic valve
- Iatrogenic (aortic catheterization, cross-clamping, IABP)

Pathophysiology

The human aorta is exposed to a limited range of blood pressure. Mechanical damage and aneurysm formation can occur outside these limits.

An intimal tear allows arterial blood at high pressure to penetrate the aortic intima and create a space between the intima and media. A distal exit tear creates a false lumen. Blood flow is slower in the false lumen, which often becomes aneurysmal and thrombotic.

Clinical assessment

Most cases are acute (<48 h) but some present later as subacute (2 days–2 months) or chronic (>2 months).

Initial approach follows ABC guidelines. Assessment and management runs concurrently if the patient is unwell.

History

Only occasionally painless, the dissection classically presents with sudden severe 'tearing' chest pain radiating through to the back and sometimes the neck and arms. Acute coronary syndrome is caused by a dissection flap occluding the coronary ostia in ~20% of type A dissections.

Examination

- Difference between right and left brachial blood pressure if dissection involves left subclavian artery
- Hypotension resulting from haemopericardium with cardiac tamponade occurs in ~25% of type A dissections. Loss of circulatory volume into the false lumen also contributes to the clinical finding
- Diastolic murmur and pulmonary oedema with acute severe aortic regurgitation caused by disruption of the aortic annulus

- End-organ ischaemia as a result of vessel occlusion. Paraplegia develops in 2–5% of type B dissections as a result of spinal artery occlusion. Stroke is caused by aortic arch vessel occlusion in 5% of type A dissections
- Peripheral vascular examination is abnormal in 20%

Investigations

The primary aim is to image the aorta to differentiate a type A dissection from a type B dissection.

- Bloods are usually normal. Troponin (involvement coronary arteries), creatinine (involvement of renal arteries)
- ECG usually normal (exclude acute MI)
- Plain chest radiograph
- Contrast-enhanced CT chest is used in stable patients
- Echocardiography (TOE better than TTE) is as sensitive and specific as CT/MRI and can be used in unstable cases
- MRA is the gold standard but is expensive and often unavailable. It has superseded aortography

Classification of thoracic aortic dissection

The Stanford classification is the only one used in clinical practice.

Stanford classification

Type A	Ascending aorta ± other region
Type B	Ascending aorta not involved

Debakey classification

Type I	Ascending aorta extending into descending aorta
Type II	Ascending aorta only
Type III	Descending aorta distal to left subclavian artery
	A No extension below diaphragm
	B Extends below diaphragm

Management

Management is based on the Stanford classification.

Type A

An acute type A dissection is an indication for emergency surgery. Subacute and chronic dissections can be managed on an urgent and elective basis, respectively.

Contraindications include advanced age, recent MI, CVA, coagulopathy, terminal illness, and dementia. Medical management of acute type A dissection is essentially palliative.

Type B

Generally, type B dissections are managed medically. The aims are good analgesia, reduction of mean arterial pressure, and reduction of the force of ventricular ejection. This is achieved using aggressive antihypertensive therapy. Surgery is considered if there is acute rupture or malperfusion of end organs, causing ischaemia.

Complications and prognosis

About 30–40% of patients with type A dissection die immediately; 50% die within 48 h. The cause of death includes aortic rupture, cardiac tamponade, MI, CVA, and cardiogenic shock from acute severe AR. Medical management has a 90% in-hospital mortality rate.

✚ Repair of thoracic aortic dissection

Aortic repair aims to relieve symptoms and reduce complications such as intrapericardial aortic rupture, severe aortic regurgitation, and myocardial ischaemia. Recent advances in CPB and graft design have reduced complications and mortality rates.

Procedure

Type A
- Median sternotomy
- CPB and cardioplegia
- Resection of dissected ascending aorta and replacement with interposition graft. The aortic valve is resuspended if it is normal or replaced if diseased

Type B
- Left thoracotomy, left heart bypass
- Resection of dissected aorta
- Replacement with interposition graft, preserving intercostals and spinal arteries

Complications

The operative mortality rate of acute type A dissection is 10–20%, with 66% surviving 1 year.

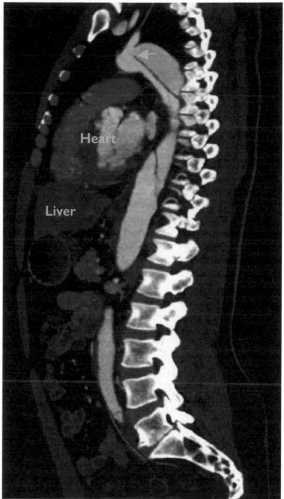

Fig 2.9 CT scan (sagittal section) showing an aortic dissection (arrows) that begins at the origin of the left subclavian artery and extends the entire length of the thoracic and abdominal aorta. This is a Stanford type B dissection as the ascending aorta is not involved.

2.7 Thoracic aortic aneurysm

An aneurysm [Gr. *aneurysma*, a widening] is a permanent localized dilatation of an artery (≥50% the expected normal diameter). Over 95% of aortic aneurysms occur in the infrarenal aorta (📖 Topic 7.7).

Thoracic aneurysms are subdivided by location into ascending aorta, arch of the aorta, or descending aorta. Twenty-five per cent are associated with abdominal aortic aneurysms.

The incidence is 6 per 100 000 per year (USA) and increases with age. It is more common in men (M:F ratio is 5:1).

Aetiology

The aetiology is multifactorial. Advanced age leads to degenerative changes in elastin and collagen, which weaken the wall and predispose to dilatation.

Genetic factors are also important, as demonstrated by Marfan syndrome and Ehlers–Danlos Type IV.

Risk factors

- Advanced age, except in Marfans and Ehlers–Danlos
- Family history of aneurysms
- Smoking
- Hypertension
- Bicuspid aortic valve

Pathophysiology

Originally, atherosclerosis was thought to play a role in the pathogenesis of aneurysms. Recent research suggests that the overproduction of matrix metalloproteinases contributes to the loss of medial elastin and smooth muscle cells, and the excess deposition of adventitial collagen (cystic medial degeneration).

Normal elastin content is highest in the ascending aorta and the media becomes thinner distally. The ascending aorta expands and recoils with systole and diastole, respectively, maximizing forward flow. When elasticity is lost, the aorta begins to dilate.

These extracellular matrix abnormalities lead to a loss in tensile strength of the arterial wall, causing it to dilate. Larger aneurysms (>6 cm) expand faster than smaller aneurysms, as predicted by Laplace's Law.

Marfan syndrome is a rare autosomal dominant connective tissue disorder caused by a defect on chromosome 15 which results in abnormal fibrillin, a structural protein found in the aorta. Patients develop cystic medial degeneration at a young age. Genetic counselling of the associated family members is important.

Ehlers–Danlos syndrome is a rare inherited connective tissue disorder with several subtypes. Type IV results in abnormal production of type III collagen.

Clinical assessment

Most patients are asymptomatic and the aneurysm is an incidental finding on a chest radiograph, TTE, or coronary angiography.

History

- Anterior chest pain can be acute and severe, which suggests dissection or impending rupture. Chronic pain results from compression or distension. Arch aneurysms cause the pain to radiate through to the back, and interscapular pain suggests a descending aneurysm
- Hoarse voice results from arch aneurysms stretching the recurrent laryngeal nerve

- Stridor, wheeze or cough may result from compression of the trachea or bronchus by a large descending aneurysm
- Acute lower limb or bowel ischaemia caused by thromboemboli
- Rarely, haemoptysis or haematemesis from an aortic fistula

Examination

Examination is usually normal. Acute rupture or dissection can present as hypovolaemic shock, cardiac tamponade, myocardial infarction or acute aortic insufficiency. Erosion into the vertebral column may cause neurological signs.

Investigations

- Bloods—FBC, clotting (DIC in acute rupture), U+Es (renal function helps to stratify risk), cross-match
- 12-lead ECG to exclude ACS or acute MI
- Plain chest radiograph may demonstrate aortic calcification outlining the aneurysm or abnormal peri-aortic shadowing
- Chest CT scan quickly establishes the size and extent of the aneurysm and presence of complications
- Echocardiography assesses the aortic valve and root to detect aortic insufficiency
- Aortic MRA may help further define anatomy
- Coronary angiography to identify treatable CAD in elective cases

Management

Conservative

Patients with small asymptomatic aneurysms are offered lifestyle advice and strict control of hypertension. They have yearly CT scans to assess progression.

Operative

The type of repair depends on anatomical location and extent of the aneurysm. Indications include:

- acute dissection (emergency)
- symptomatic or rapidly enlarging aneurysms (>1 cm/year)
- asymptomatic aneurysms >5.5 cm
- aneurysms >5 cm and known connective tissue disorder

Complications and prognosis

The 5-year survival rate of patients with thoracic aortic aneurysms is ~40%. The size of aneurysm at presentation is the most important predictor of risk of rupture. Median size of rupture or dissection of ascending aneurysms is 5.9 cm. Once symptoms develop, the mean time to rupture is ~2 years.

The elective operative mortality rate is 2–10% for repair of aneurysms of the ascending aorta, with a 5-year survival of ~85%.

⊕ Repair of thoracic aortic aneurysm

Contraindications to surgery include advanced age (>85 years), malignancy, and end-organ failure.

Procedure

Ascending aneurysm
- Median sternotomy, CPB
- Resection of dissected ascending aorta
- Replacement with graft ± AVR or root replacement

Arch repair
- Normally requires hypothermic circulatory arrest for cerebral protection

Descending aneurysm
- Left thoracotomy, left heart bypass
- Resection of dissected aorta
- Replacement with graft, preserving intercostals and spinal arteries
- Some are amenable to endovascular repair

Complications

Intraoperative and early
- Intrathoracic haemorrhage
- CVA
- Paraplegia (descending)
- Acute MI
- Cardiac arrhythmias
- Respiratory failure
- Renal failure
- Sepsis

Late
- Dissection
- Aortoenteric fistula

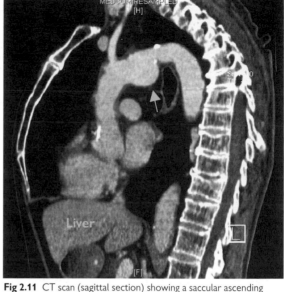

Fig 2.11 CT scan (sagittal section) showing a saccular ascending aortic aneurysm (arrow).

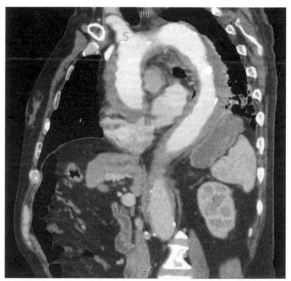

Fig 2.12 CT scan (sagittal section) showing aneurysmal dilatation of the thoracic aorta from the supravalvular part of the root of the aorta (arrow) extending down to the level of the suprarenal segment of the abdominal aorta (AA). The aneurysm also involves the origin of the left subclavian artery (LS). (A separate infrarenal abdominal aortic aneurysm is not seen in this section.)

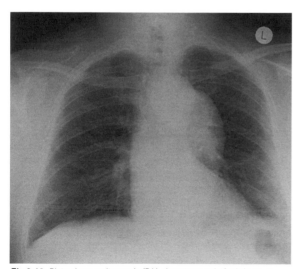

Fig 2.10 Plain chest radiograph (PA) showing a calcified thoracic aortic aneurysm.

2.8 Miscellaneous cardiac and mediastinal conditions

Pericarditis

Pericarditis is inflammation of the pericardium leading to restriction of the heart. It may be acute or chronic. The majority of cases are idiopathic. Other causes include viral infection, TB, and neoplasia.

Clinical assessment

- Acute pericarditis causes tearing chest pain in the left anterior chest which is exacerbated by deep breathing and lying flat but relieved by sitting up and leaning forward. On examination there might be a pericardial friction rub
- Chronic constrictive pericarditis may be asymptomatic for years before presenting with fatigue, exertional dyspnoea, and peripheral oedema

Investigations

- Bloods—FBC (raised WCC), raised CRP
- 12-lead ECG shows diffuse concave upward ST elevation
- Plain chest radiograph may show a flask-shaped enlarged cardiac shadow with a large pericardial effusion
- Echocardiography shows a pericardial effusion

Management

Simple acute pericarditis is managed with analgesia and NSAIDs. Significant effusions require drainage by percutaneous pericardiocentesis or surgical drainage.

Pericardial effusion

A pericardial effusion is an abnormal volume of fluid (>20 mL) in the pericardial space between the visceral and parietal pericardium.

Aetiology

Acute

- Infection
- Trauma
- Surgery

Chronic

- Pericarditis
- Congestive cardiac failure
- Metastatic spread to pericardium (lung or breast)
- End-stage hepatic and renal failure
- Infection (HIV)
- Collagen vascular disorders

Pathophysiology

Increase in pericardial fluid and pressure reduces venous return. Reduced venous filling leads to decreased preload, stroke volume, and cardiac output. The fall in arterial blood pressure triggers baroreceptors in the carotid sinus, which leads to an increase in sympathetic activity. This results in increased heart rate, contractility, and vasoconstriction.

Continued increases in the volume of pericardial fluid eventually lead to near complete reduction in venous return and RV diastolic filling, finally resulting in cardiac arrest (usually Pulseless electrical activity (PEA)).

Clinical assessment

Clinical presentation is dependent on the time course. Acute accumulation of a small amount of fluid can cause life-threatening cardiac tamponade, but slow accumulations of large volumes of fluid may be well tolerated.

Chronic pericardial effusion may present with decreased exercise tolerance, atypical chest pain, orthopnoea, and congestive cardiac failure and eventually cardiac tamponade.

Management

Conservative management includes diuretics and pericardiocentesis. Operative management using either an open technique or video-assisted thoracoscopic surgery (VATS) aims to create a hole in the pericardium or a pericardial window so that fluid can drain away.

Myxoma and rare cardiac tumours

Myxomas [L. *myxo*, mucus] are rare sporadic neoplasms of the endocardium. Although typically benign, metastatic spread has been reported. There is a female preponderance.

The majority are solitary and 80% are found in the left atrial cavity. They are smooth, firm or gelatinous masses that can be polypoid, round or oval in shape.

Clinical presentation is usually related to mechanical interference of cardiac function by obstruction, or systemic embolization of tumour.

- Intracardiac obstruction: atrial outflow obstruction and reduced ventricular filling leads to pulmonary oedema and right ventricular failure
- Embolization
- Constitutional symptoms: fatigue, fever, arthralgia, myalgia, anaemia, and weight loss
- Infection: infected myxoma and septic emboli

Chest radiograph may show left atrial enlargement, pulmonary oedema, and occasionally eccentric calcification. TOE is usually diagnostic and can detect very small masses (1–3 mm in diameter). MRI is used to define the anatomy further.

Following diagnosis myxomas are urgently excised owing to the high risk of sudden death. Operative mortality rates are <5% for atrial myxomas and 10% for ventricular myxomas.

Thymoma

The thymus is a bi-lobed lymphoid structure located in the anterior mediastinum and is the site of T cell maturation in early life.

A thymoma is a rare neoplasm of the thymus gland that may be benign or malignant. Seventy-five per cent of patients develop myasthenia gravis. Children often present with thoracic outlet or airway obstruction whereas adults tend to be asymptomatic.

Clinical features of myasthenia gravis are related to muscle weakness, which affects phonation, facial muscles, shoulder girdle, and the limbs. It is clinically important in thymic carcinoma not to breach the capsule of the tumour in an attempt to make a tissue diagnosis. *En bloc* resection which is encapsulated remains the best prospect of cure in these patients. Malignant tumours require adjuvant radiotherapy.

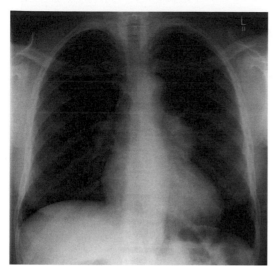

Fig 2.13 Plain chest radiograph showing a thymoma. It appears as an anterior mediastinal mass projected over the hilum with the pulmonary artery visible through it. The heart is at the upper limit of normal size.

2.9 Lung cancer

Primary bronchial carcinoma is the commonest cause of cancer death in both men and women in the UK and the leading cause of death from cancer worldwide. It remains most common in men. The incidence in women has dramatically increased in the past decade. It remains the case that ultimate outcome has not changed over many years. This is most likely related to late presentation and lack of early detection.

- Incidence—1 per 1000 per year in UK
- Age—50–70 years
- Sex ratio (male:female)—>5:1
- Geography—global

Aetiology

Ninety per cent of lung cancer is associated with cigarette smoking. Sir Richard Doll first established the statistical basis for this link.

Risk factors

- Cigarette smoking (polycyclic aromatic hydrocarbons and nicotine-related carcinogens)
- Occupational (asbestos, arsenic, nickel, silica, coal tar, aluminium production, coal gasification, paints, chromium compounds)
- Environmental radon exposure

Pathophysiology

Bronchial carcinoma is classified as **non-small cell** (NSCLC) or **small cell** (SCC). Squamous metaplasia and dysplasia precedes carcinoma formation and there is evidence for a field change effect which provides the rationale for lobar rather than limited or wedge lung resection.

Non-small cell lung cancers (75%)

- **Squamous cell carcinoma** (50%) is the most common histological type in Europe. It is found centrally in large airways as an endobronchial mass. It is relatively slow-growing and metastasizes late
- **Adenocarcinoma** (15%) is found peripherally, grows moderately quickly, and metastasizes early
- **Large cell undifferentiated carcinoma** (10%) is relatively aggressive and locally destructive. It is usually peripheral. It has two subtypes: clear cell carcinoma and giant cell carcinoma. Giant cell tumours are uncommon and have a poor prognosis
- **Adenosquamous carcinoma** (<10%)

Small (oat) cell lung cancer (25%)

These have a significant neuroendocrine element and are regarded as the malignant end of a spectrum beginning with benign carcinoid.

Clinical assessment

Approximately 10% of patients are asymptomatic at diagnosis. Most present with symptoms of the tumour, locoregional spread, or metastatic disease.

- **Proximal tumours** tend to produce symptoms of major airway irritation (haemoptysis, dyspnoea, cough, wheezing, stridor). Hoarseness suggests recurrent laryngeal nerve involvement
- **Peripheral tumours** are often asymptomatic or present with features of local invasion or pleural effusion
- **Metastatic spread** can present with headache, blurred vision, nausea, diplopia, altered consciousness, ataxia, bony pain and pathological fracture, liver and abdominal pain, anorexia, jaundice, ascites, liver failure, hepatomegaly, and symptoms of Addison's disease

- **Paraneoplastic syndromes** result from the secretion of hormones by the tumour, e.g. Cushing's, SIADH, and hypercalcaemia (parathyroid hormone secretion by SCC)

Examination

- Cachexia
- Localized chest wall pain
- Pleural effusion (squamous and large cell)
- Lymphadenopathy
- Finger clubbing, cutaneous lesions, SVC obstruction
- Pain, upper limb weakness, and Horner's syndrome may indicate a **Pancoast tumour**. This is an apical tumour that may involve the brachial plexus, sympathetic ganglia, and vertebral bodies
- Horner's syndrome: ipsilateral miosis (small pupil), ptosis, enophthalmos, and decreased sweating on affected side of face
- Signs of metastatic spread

Investigations

- Sputum and pleural fluid for cytology
- Bloods—FBC (anaemia), LFT
- Chest radiograph localizes tumour and related pathology
- Bronchoscopy identifies endobronchial involvement and obtains cytology from bronchoalveolar lavage and tissue biopsy. Useful for assessing extent of required resection
- Chest CT ± percutaneous-guided needle biopsy allows assessment of the tumour, lymph nodes, and metastasis
- PET scan is used to assess metastatic spread in candidates for aggressive therapy. It is important to note that the negative PET is more sensitive and more specific than a positive PET, hence the current requirement for tissue confirmation where the PET is positive
- Bone scan is not routinely performed. Metastatic spread is assessed with CT chest, liver, adrenals

Staging

TNM classification of NSCLC

Primary tumour

TX	Positive malignant cytology results, no lesion seen
Tis	Carcinoma *in situ*
T1	Diameter ≤3 cm
T2	Diameter >3 cm
T3	Extension to pleura, chest wall, diaphragm, pericardium, within 2 cm of carina, or total atelectasis
T4	Invasion of mediastinal organs (e.g. oesophagus, trachea, great vessels, heart), malignant pleural effusion, or satellite nodules within the primary lobe

Regional lymph nodes

NX	Regional lymph nodes cannot be assessed
N0	No regional lymph node metastases
N1	Ipsilateral bronchopulmonary or hilar nodes involved
N2	Ipsilateral mediastinal or subcarinal nodes involved
N3	Contralateral mediastinal, hilar, any supraclavicular nodes involved

Distant metastasis

MX	Presence of distant metastasis cannot be assessed
M0	No distant metastasis
M1	Distant metastasis

Management

There are many advances in modern management of lung cancer which are likely to result in significant gains. These are occurring in the areas of early diagnosis, improved staging, improved fitness for radical therapy, and palliation.

Curative resection offers the best chance of long-term survival for patients with stage I, II, and III disease. However, only 30–35% of patients with NSCLC present with sufficiently localized disease to attempt resection or are fit enough to proceed with surgery or radical radiotherapy.

Conservative
- Chemotherapy cures have been reported but its major setting is in prolongation of survival and palliation or as an adjunct to radical therapies
- Radiotherapy can be used as a radical treatment option
- Combined chemoradiotherapy is used in patients with locally advanced NSCLC and offers better survival rates compared with monotherapy
- Biological therapy is still experimental. Overexpression of epidermal growth factor receptors (EGFR) appears to be associated with more aggressive tumour growth and metastasis. Therapeutic agents that inhibit the EGFR pathway may have potential

Operative
Surgical resection in patients with stage I and II disease is potentially curative. Adjuvant chemotherapy and radiotherapy do not appear to improve overall survival rates.

Palliation
Supportive and palliative care should be delivered in accordance with NICE cancer guidance. External beam radiotherapy is effective in treating cough, haemoptysis chest pain, hoarseness, and bone metastasis. Intrinsic airway obstruction can be relieved by endobronchial de-bulking and extrinsic obstruction by stenting. Pleural effusions can be aspirated.

Complications and prognosis
Complications are often related to metastatic spread (spinal cord compression) and the chemotherapy (neutropenic sepsis and renal failure). Prognosis is generally poor. Values for 5-year survival follow:
- stage I—75%
- stage II—40%
- stage III—30%
- stage IV—0%

Metastatic lung cancer

Any neoplasm can metastasize to the lungs: this includes thyroid cancer, malignant melanoma, breast cancer, and colorectal cancer. The spread is usually haematogenous rather than direct spread. Pulmonary metastases are often asymptomatic and are only discovered on screening (chest radiograph). This is followed by a chest CT scan to better define the disease.

The presence of lung metastases is a sign of advanced disease for most cancers. Surgical resection is therefore only considered in fit patients with no other extrapulmonary metastases and an adequately controlled primary tumour. The majority receive palliative chemotherapy.

➔ Extra

Sir Richard Doll
Sir Richard Doll [1912–2005, British epidemiologist] pioneered research into the epidemiology of cancer and helped to identify the causes of lung cancer in industry (asbestos, nickel, and coal tar workers) and in relation to cigarette smoking. He also investigated leukaemia and its relationship to radiation.

Smoking cessation and prevention
In recent years there has been a concerted effort to reduce the prevalence of cigarette smoking. Legislation banning tobacco advertising and smoking in public places has been complemented by public health campaigns.

Further reading
1. Doll R, Bradford Hill A. The mortality of doctors in relation to their smoking habits: a preliminary report. *Br Med J* 1954; **ii**: 1451–5
2. NICE guideline for lung cancer (CG24). London: NICE
3. NHS campaign (www.gosmokefree.co.uk)

⊕ Lung resection
Patients require preoperative assessment to determine fitness. The options are lobectomy or pneumonectomy depending on tumour location. Segmental resection is avoided as there is a higher risk of recurrence owing to the field change effect, but can be an option where lung function is borderline.

If staging procedures can accurately determine N2 disease, then, technically, keyhole lobectomy (which can be performed in many centres) has the potential to provide better recovery and shorter hospital stay by avoiding anaesthetic and wound-related complications.

Procedure
- Posterolateral thoracotomy incision or VATS
- No spillage of cells from primary tumour during resection
- Entire tumour must be resected along with intrapulmonary lymph nodes: lesser resections are proven to have worse outcome and are only considered in high-risk patients
- All accessible mediastinal lymph nodes should be excised or biopsied to allow complete staging and plan for any adjuvant therapy
- Frozen section analysis of resection margins if there is doubt about complete resection to confirm complete excision of primary tumour

Complications

Intraoperative and early	Intermediate and late
- Chest infection	- Bronchopleural fistula
- Wound infection	- Recurrence
- Atrial fibrillation	
- Death: lobectomy 2%, pneumonectomy 7%	

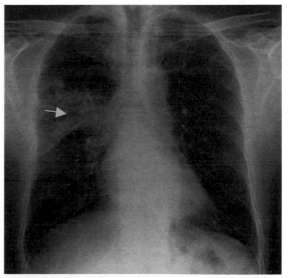

Fig 2.14 Plain chest radiograph (PA) showing a mass centred on the right hilum (arrow).

2.10 Miscellaneous thoracic conditions I

Pleural effusion

A pleural effusion is the presence of an abnormal amount of fluid within the pleural space. Pleural effusions can be divided into transudates and exudates according to Light's criteria, but the divide is not always clear.

Aetiology

Transudates
- Trauma and surgery
- Congestive cardiac failure
- Liver cirrhosis
- Nephrotic syndrome and glomerulonephritis
- Myxoedema
- Sarcoidosis
- Multiple pulmonary emboli

Exudates (protein >2.9 g/dL or lactate dehydrogenase >60% of serum)
- Malignant neoplasia (metastatic disease, mesothelioma)
- Pulmonary emboli
- Infection (pneumonia)
- Gastrointestinal disease—pancreatitis, subphrenic abscess, intrahepatic abscess, perforated oesophagus
- Post-myocardial infarction syndrome

Clinical assessment

Small effusions are often asymptomatic. Larger effusions cause cough, chest pain, and dyspnoea. On examination there is decreased ipsilateral chest expansion, dullness to percussion, decreased breath sounds, and crepitations over the effusion.

Investigations
- Chest radiograph: effusions >400 mL cause blunting of the costodiaphragmatic angles; larger effusions produce a fluid level with a meniscus
- Thoracocentesis (needle aspiration) for cytology, biochemistry (protein, lactate dehydrogenase, albumin, amylase, and glucose) and Gram stain and culture
- Chest ultrasound is used to guide aspiration and pigtail or tube thoracostomy
- Chest CT assesses the lung parenchyma and pleura

Management

If possible treat the underlying cause.
- Thoracocentesis
- Pigtail or tube thoracostomy
- Pleurodesis using chemicals (tetracycline, talc, blood) or surgical abrasion
- Open or VATS pleurectomy
- Pleuroperitoneal shunt

Empyema

An empyema is a purulent pleural effusion.

Aetiology

Post-pneumonic empyema owing to bacterial infection of pleural fluid is most common. Postoperative empyema accounts for 20%. Other sources of infection include:
- lung parenchyma (pneumonia, lung abscess)
- chest wall (surgery, trauma, chest drain)
- mediastinum (perforated oesophagus)
- abdominal disease (subphrenic collection)

Pathophysiology

Common organisms include *Staphylococcus aureus*, *Haemophilus influenzae*, Gram-negative rods, *Streptococcus pyogenes*, and TB. In a third of cases no organism is isolated. The development of an empyema is divided into three stages:
- stage I: acute exudative stage. The fluid has low cellular content and viscosity
- stage II: fibrinopurulent stage. The fluid becomes turbid or purulent with heavy fibrin deposits
- stage III: chronic organizing phase. There is lung trapping by collagen with ingrowth of fibroblasts and capillaries

Clinical assessment

There is usually a history of pulmonary infection or sepsis. Symptoms include dyspnoea, cough, chest pain, fever, and sweats. Examination findings are similar to that of a pleural effusion.

Investigations
- Bloods—FBC (WCC), U+Es, CRP
- Chest radiograph shows an effusion, air fluid levels, and pleural thickening
- Chest CT scan or ultrasound is used to localize loculated collections and guide insertion of pigtail catheter for drainage

Management

The underlying cause needs to be treated and sepsis controlled with antibiotics. The next aim is to obliterate the pleural space.
- Stage I empyema may be treated with chest drain
- Stage II empyema may be treated with VATS
- Stage III empyema needs open surgery

Complications and prognosis

Complications include empyema necessitans (spontaneous drainage through chest wall), bronchopleural fistula (drainage into bronchial tree), pulmonary fibrosis, chest wall contraction, osteomyelitis, pericarditis, and abscess (mediastinal or subphrenic).

Chylothorax

Chylothorax is the abnormal accumulation of lymphatic fluid in the pleural space.

Aetiology
- Congenital (atresia or fistula of the thoracic duct, trauma)
- Trauma (blunt or penetrating)
- Iatrogenic (surgery or diagnostic procedures)
- Neoplasia, e.g. lymphoma

Clinical assessment

Slow accumulation is associated with an insidious onset of shortness of breath. Rapid accumulation may result in respiratory distress. The clinical findings are similar to those of a pleural effusion.

Management

The underlying cause and extent of nutritional depletion guides the management. Traumatic chylothorax is managed conservatively initially with tube thoracotomy to drain the pleural cavity and total parental nutrition. However, continuing excessive fluid loss (>500 mL/day for 2 weeks) is an indication for surgical ligation of the supradiaphragmatic thoracic duct. This can be achieved through VATS or open techniques in the chest or the abdomen.

➕ Chest drain insertion

A chest drain (tube thoracostomy) is used to drain air and/or fluid from the pleural cavity. Premedication should be considered to reduce patient discomfort. See the latest British Thoracic Society guidelines.

Indications

- Pneumothorax (ventilated patient, following needle decompression of tension pneumothorax)
- Traumatic haemopneumothorax
- Following elective surgery (e.g. thoracotomy, oesophagectomy)
- Empyema and complicated pleural effusions

Procedure

- Collect all the equipment needed and an assistant
- Maintain an aseptic technique. Prep and drape the insertion area between the mid-axillary and anterior axillary lines and between the fourth and seventh intercostal spaces
- Infiltrate local anaesthetic into soft tissues down to the rib
- Make a 2 cm transverse incision in the insertion area over the fifth intercostal space and bluntly dissect above the rib to reduce risk of damage to the neurovascular bundle
- Use artery forceps to puncture the parietal pleura and use a finger to enlarge the hole and sweep away any pleural adhesions
- Use a clamp to hold the end of the tube and advance it so that the most proximal hole is in the pleural cavity
- Connect the tube to the underwater seal apparatus, secure the tube with a heavy suture, and place an air-tight dressing around the entry point. Leave a pursestring suture untied in place for closing the wound when the tube is removed
- The underwater seal apparatus allows air to escape via the drain but not to re-enter the pleural cavity. Always keep the collection chamber below the level of the patient, otherwise its contents will syphon back into the pleural cavity
- Persistent bubbling of air through the water indicates a persistent air leak from the lung into the pleural cavity. Never clamp a chest tube as there is a risk of developing a tension pneumothorax
- If indicated, the air outlet of the collection chamber may be connected to suction (~20 cmH$_2$O). This assists lung re-expansion (i.e. if an air leak is present)
- Obtain a chest radiograph to check the drain position

Complications

Up to 10% of patients have complications from chest drain insertion. Injury to almost every thoracoabdominal organ has been described!

Intra-procedure and early	Late
• Bleeding (haemothorax)	• Recurrent pneumothorax
• Incorrectly positioned tube	• Intercostal neuralgia
• Subcutaneous emphysema	
• Persistent pneumothorax	
• Infection (empyema)	
• Injury to organs	

Removal

- The chest tube can be removed once the drainage has stopped and any air leak has resolved
- Maintain aseptic technique
- Remove the tube at either the end of expiration or at peak inspiration to avoid further air being entrained into the pleural cavity
- Following removal, the wound is closed with the purse-string suture already present or an occlusive dressing
- Request and check a plain chest radiograph

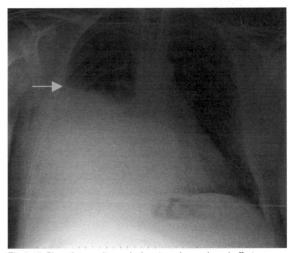

Fig 2.15 Plain chest radiograph showing a large pleural effusion on the right side. The trachea is not deviated and the mediastinum appears normal. A meniscus (arrow) is visible.

Pneumothorax

A pneumothorax is the presence of air or gas in the pleural space preventing the lung from occupying its normal space.

Aetiology

Spontaneous pneumothorax

Primary spontaneous pneumothorax is idiopathic and commonly seen in tall thin young male smokers. It is occasionally associated with specific conditions such as an alpha anti-1 trypsin deficiency.

Secondary spontaneous pneumothorax occurs in the presence of an underlying lung condition.

- COPD, asthma, cystic fibrosis
- Interstitial lung disease
- Infection: cavitating lesions rupture into the pleural space
- Malignancy: primary or metastatic lung cancer
- Connective tissue disorders (Ehlers–Danlos syndrome, histiocytosis X, scleroderma, Marfan's syndrome)
- Rupture of the oesophagus

Secondary pneumothorax

Secondary pneumothorax is caused by trauma or iatrogenic injury to the pleura (□ Topic 8.9).

Pathophysiology

Spontaneous pneumothoraces are closed, which means that air enters the pleural space from the lung. This usually follows the rupture of an apical bleb (<5 mm^3) or bullae (larger air-filled spaces).

Secondary pneumothoraces are usually open, which means that air enters from the outside via a traumatic hole in the chest wall.

Clinical assessment

History

- Sharp chest pain worse on inspiration (pleuritic). The chest wall is often splinted to reduce pain
- Dyspnoea and cough

Examination

- Tachycardia and pulsus paradoxus
- Tachypnoea
- Ipsilateral decreased chest wall movement
- Hyper-resonance on percussion
- Absent or quiet breath sounds on auscultation

Investigations

- ABG if there is persistent hypoxia
- Chest radiograph is usually diagnostic
- Chest CT scan is not routinely performed. It can accurately assess the pneumothorax and lung parenchyma

Management

Conservative

- Observation (small, less than 20% pneumothorax), stop smoking, and no flying
- Needle aspiration
- Tube thoracostomy

Operative

Surgery is indicated if there is a prolonged air leak, bilateral pneumothoraces or residual collapsed lung. Access is via a mini-thoracotomy, axillary incision or VATS. Blebs and bullae are resected and the pleural space obliterated using chemical or abrasion pleurodesis, or parietal pleurectomy.

Complications and prognosis

Untreated or persistent pneumothorax can lead to tension pneumothorax, pneumomediastinum, and haemopneumothorax. The recurrence rate is 30% in the first 6 months for conservatively treated primary spontaneous pneumothorax and is <5% following VATS.

Mesothelioma

Mesothelioma is a rare cancer of the pleura which is most prevalent in men owing to its association with asbestos exposure and other mineral fibres. Its incidence is rapidly rising worldwide.

Pathophysiology

Mesothelium is derived from embryonic mesoderm that lines the body cavity in the embryo and becomes the epithelial layer of the pleura, pericardium, and peritoneum.

The inhaled asbestos fibres are deposited in the lung parenchyma and are eventually carried to the visceral pleura where they both initiate and promote the development of mesothelioma. Blue asbestos fibres are more potent carcinogens than white fibres.

Clinical assessment

The mesothelioma can be asymptomatic for years. There appears to be a time delay between exposure and development of malignancy which is poorly understood. This can range from 5 to 20 years but would appear to be accelerated in those who smoke as they have a fourfold increase in incidence compared to non-smokers.

Symptoms include chest pain, cough, dyspnoea, anorexia, and weight loss. On examination there may be signs of pleural effusion and reduced lung expansion. A chest wall mass and supraclavicular lymph nodes are occasionally palpable.

Investigations

- Chest radiograph shows pleural thickening and effusion
- Pleural fluid cytology is positive in 50% of patients
- Chest CT is used to stage disease
- Pleural biopsy gives histological diagnosis

Management

Management is mainly palliative. Chemotherapy, radiation therapy, immunotherapy, and surgery have limited effect. VATS pleurodesis gives symptomatic relief of effusions. Median survival is 12–18 months.

Congenital chest wall conditions

Pectus excavatum

Pectus excavatum (funnel chest) is depression of the sternum and lower costal cartilages. It occurs in approximately 1 in 400 live births, with a male preponderance. It is of unknown aetiology.

It is usually diagnosed in the first year of life and remains asymptomatic until adolescence when it may cause pain, palpitations, and syncope.

Asymptomatic cases are usually managed conservatively. Silicon implants can be used to improve cosmesis in mild-to-moderate deformities, but more severe cases require operative correction. There are several options:

- Ravitch technique uses an open approach via a large inframammary incision to gain access to the chest wall. A sternal wedge osteotomy is performed and the ribcage is elevated with one or more metal bars which can be removed at a later stage
- Nuss technique uses a closed approach to place metal bars across the chest wall to elevate the ribcage

Pectus carinatum

Pectus carinatum ('pigeon chest') is the protrusion of the sternum and is less common than pectus excavatum. The deformity is usually symmetrical. Surgical correction is with a sternal osteotomy and costal cartilage resection via an inframammary incision.

Poland's syndrome

Sir Alfred Poland first described the syndrome in 1841. There is unilateral hypoplasia of the skin and soft tissues, musculature, and bones of the upper limb and chest wall. The cause is likely to be a vascular event during embryological development known as subclavian artery supply disruption sequence.

The clinical manifestations are usually mild with minimal functional deficit. Patients, especially women, present with concerns regarding cosmesis.

Surgery aims to reconstruct the chest deformity and in women the hypoplastic breast is augmented with a tissue expander implant.

⊕ Video-assisted thoracoscopic surgery

VATS is a minimally invasive approach to the chest cavity. One or more 5-mm or 1-cm port sites are used to introduce a range of endoscopic instruments into the chest cavity. Advantages include less postoperative pain, faster mobilization, and early discharge. Disadvantages include higher recurrence rates for pneumothorax and longer procedure times.

Indications
- Spontaneous primary pneumothorax
- Bullectomy and lung reduction in emphysema
- Lymph node sampling, pleural biopsy, lung biopsy
- Pleurodesis and pleurectomy
- Evacuation of loculated pleural effusion

Complications
- Fever
- Pleural tear
- Subcutaneous emphysema
- Rare: haemorrhage, lung perforation, gas embolism

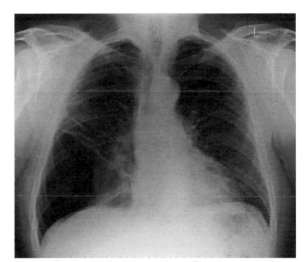

Fig 2.16 Simple right-sided pneumothorax. There is no tracheal or mediastinal deviation.

2.12 Case-based discussions

Case 1

You are fast-bleeped to the emergency department to see a 76-year-old man who collapsed at home with severe central chest pain.

- What is your initial approach?
- What is the differential diagnosis of central chest pain?

He is sitting up in bed, alert, and oriented. You take a history and examine him. The observation chart shows HR 106 regular, BP 120/70 mmHg, SaO$_2$ 98% on 6 L O$_2$.

- For what particular signs are you looking?

Blood pressure in the right arm is 62/30 mmHg. Following an ECG and chest radiograph you arrange a transthoracic echo which shows no evidence of pericardial effusion but there is aortic regurgitation.

- What might the ECG show?
- What might you see on a chest radiograph?
- Given your suspected diagnosis, what further investigations would you arrange?
- What are the management options?

Discussion

He has a Stanford type A dissection. This is causing acute aortic regurgitation, which results in pulmonary oedema. The right and left coronary artery and right subclavian artery are being supplied by the false lumen, which explains the global ischaemia on the ECG, and lower BP in the right arm. He needs either a CT or TOE to confirm the diagnosis which should be followed by emergency surgical repair.

- What other complications are associated with a Stanford type A dissection?
- How would you prepare this patient for surgery?

Case 2

You are asked to help out in a busy cardiothoracic clinic. You pick the thinnest set of notes which belong to a 77-year-old woman. She had a left VATS pleural biopsy and talc pleurodesis 2 weeks ago for a recurrent pleural effusion.

- What is VATS talc pleurodesis?
- What symptoms do you ask her about?
- What results must you look for in the notes?

She is in a lot of pain. On examination she looks dehydrated. There is decreased chest expansion, reduced air entry, and decreased breath sounds on the left side. Two of the port sites look well healed. The third is covered in a dressing soaked with purulent fluid. The surrounding skin is cellulitic. The port site oozes when the patient coughs.

- Write a problem list for this patient
- What is your differential diagnosis?

The pleural biopsy from theatre shows reactive cells only with no evidence of malignancy. However, the cytology sent at the same time shows adenocarcinoma cells, suggesting metastatic disease from an unknown primary. Microbiology was negative but the preoperative screening swabs were MRSA-positive.

- What other investigations would you request to aid your management decision?
- What are the principles of treating an empyema?
- What would you tell this patient about her prognosis?

Discussion

This elderly woman has an empyema which is complicating a malignant pleural effusion for which she needs a referral to oncology. However, the most pressing problem is the infection. She needs admission for intravenous antibiotics, further imaging, and drainage of the empyema.

Chapter 3

Breast and endocrine surgery

◎ Clinical skills

- Breast cancer screening
- Thyroid axis
- Hypothyroidism versus hyperthyroidism
- Hypercalcaemic crisis
- Calcium homeostasis
- Glucocorticoid axis
- Renin–angiotensin–aldosterone axis

➕ Technical skills and procedures

- Pathological examination of breast tissue
- Wide local excision of breast lump and axillary clearance
- Total thyroidectomy

35

3.1 Oncology

Cancer [L. *cancer*, crab] is a general term used to describe a malignant neoplasm. It is an important cause of morbidity and mortality worldwide. The incidence is generally rising although there are large geographic differences related to cultural and environmental factors.

Cancer has superseded cardiovascular disease as the leading cause of death in developed countries. It is rare in children and increases with age (70% diagnosed >65 years).

Oncogenesis

Oncogenesis (carcinogenesis) is the process by which a normal cell becomes neoplastic. The multistep hypothesis suggests that a cell has to go through a number of mutations before becoming neoplastic.

Host predisposition

Various host factors such as age, race, nutritional status, immune status, and hormone environment influence the chance of developing cancer. There are also hereditary forms of some tumours where loss of function of certain genes leads to cancer (e.g. familial retinoblastoma and familial adenomatous polyposis).

Carcinogens

Carcinogens are agents that stimulate cells to become neoplastic. The process involves initiation (exposure to carcinogen), promotion (alteration of cell genes controlling growth and survival), persistence (irreversible change in cell growth), and finally, neoplasm formation.

Chemical

- Polycyclic aromatic hydrocarbons are found in cigarette smoke. They are pro-carcinogens and so require hydroxylation before becoming carcinogenic. They have a direct effect on laryngeal and bronchial epithelium
- Aromatic amines such as β-naphthylamine used in the rubber industry are converted to 1-hydroxy-2-naphthylamine in the liver and then excreted in the urine. The prolonged exposure to these products can cause squamous cell carcinoma of the bladder

Physical

- Ultraviolet light increases the risk of skin cancer
- Ionizing radiation is linked with leukaemia, bone, breast, and thyroid cancer

Biological

- Viruses—HIV (lymphoma, leukaemia, Kaposi sarcoma), hepatitis B virus (hepatocellular carcinoma), human papilloma virus (cervical carcinoma)
- Bacteria—*Helicobacter pylori* (gastric carcinoma)
- Protozoa—schistosoma (bladder squamous cell carcinoma)

Cancer biology

There are three main disturbances in cell behaviour that lead to cancer. These are the control of cell proliferation, cell differentiation, and the relationship of proliferating cells with the surrounding tissue.

Three classes of gene have been identified that play a role in these processes. Abnormalities in them can lead to loss of the dynamic equilibrium of growth promotion and growth suppression and ultimately lead to neoplastic change.

Oncogenes

Proto-oncogenes are normal genes that encode for proteins that are involved in *normal* cell proliferation. They are expressed at certain stages of embryogenesis and healing or repair of normal tissue.

They are termed oncogenes when their encoded proteins are overexpressed, truncated or mutated so that they are no longer regulated and controlled, resulting in oncogenesis.

Tumour suppressor genes (anti-oncogenes)

The products of tumour suppressor genes normally inhibit excessive cell proliferation. Mutation or loss of these genes leads to loss of their ability to inhibit oncogenesis.

Products of tumour suppressor genes include nuclear proteins (p53, Rb), cytoplasmic proteins (nf-1), and membrane proteins.

The p53 oncoprotein is a normal suppressor of cell division, preventing cells from entering the S-phase of the cell cycle. A mutated form of p53 exists in over 50% of breast, colon, lung, and bladder cancers, making it the commonest tumour suppressor abnormality seen in human cancers.

DNA repair genes

The products of these genes are important in DNA repair. They were first discovered during investigation of hereditary non-polyposis coli which is associated with msh-2.

Tumour progression

1. Initiation

The cell or tissue is exposed to a carcinogen that initiates the carcinogenic process.

2. Promotion

The carcinogens cause alterations in the genes controlling cell proliferation and survival to promote the neoplastic cells. These changes are irreversible and the tumour persists.

3. Uncontrolled proliferation

Removal of the growth stimulus from a normal population of cells stops them proliferating. This mechanism is lost in neoplastic cells, and they undergo autonomous cell proliferation.

4. Angiogenesis

Angiogenesis within the primary tumour permits increased cell proliferation. A high density of microvessels is associated with a greater risk of metastatic spread.

5. Invasion

The ability to invade local tissues and spread to a distant site defines a malignant neoplasm. Malignant cells break through the basement membrane around the structure in which they have arisen and spread into surrounding tissues. This process requires:

- loss of adhesion between tumour cells but increased adhesion to the basement membrane
- proteolysis of the basement membrane and extracellular matrix
- active movement of tumour cells through the basement membrane

6. Metastasis

A metastasis (secondary deposit) is an established colony of malignant cells surviving at a location away from and with no connection to the primary tumour. It is essentially an embolic process with tumour first invading blood vessels and lymphatics before cells are carried away to a distant site. Here they migrate from the vessels and establish a secondary colony.

- **Lymphatic** spread is particularly characteristic of carcinomas which, unlike sarcomas, have a tendency for haematogenous spread. Malignant cells can grow in cords along the lymphatics which can cause local lymphoedema (e.g. peau d'orange skin changes in breast carcinoma).

  Malignant cells in the lymphatics can also cross into the bloodstream via lymph node blood vessels and the thoracic duct

- **Haematogenous** spread follows invasion of blood vessels within the tumour or close by. Sometimes cells extend as a solid mass along the vessels (e.g. renal adenocarcinoma along the renal vein)

- **Transcoelomic** spread occurs when malignant cells become incorporated in the serosal surface of an organ in a body cavity. They get carried away in the exudate and 'seed' the walls or other organs (e.g. Krukenburg tumour of the ovary following transcoelomic spread from a gastric tumour)

- Other methods of spread include perineural invasion and via the CSF. Iatrogenic spread can follow medical interventions such as a FNA biopsy or surgery

7. Evasion

The cancer cells resist killing by host macrophages, natural killer cells, and activated T cells.

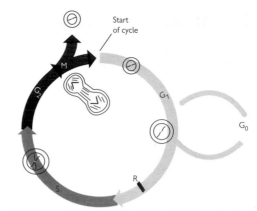

Fig 3.1 Diagram of the cell cycle which is divided into the M phase and interphase (G1, S, and G2). Cyclins and cyclin-dependent kinases (CDKs) are the two main classes of molecules involved in regulating the cycle.

Stages

- Gap 0—A resting phase of variable duration. It is permanent for terminally differentiated cells (e.g. neuron)
- Gap 1—High rate of biosynthetic activity. At the restriction point (R) the cell decides whether to complete the cycle
- Synthesis—DNA synthesis occurs
- Gap 2—Further cell growth and differentiation before division
- Mitosis—Cell division occurs, including both nuclear division (mitosis) and cytoplasmic division (cytokinesis)

Table 3.1 Definitions
Apoptosis is the deliberate death of an individual cell. The signal for this may be internal or external. It leads to cell shrinkage and fragmentation, allowing phagocytosis to occur without releasing potentially harmful intracellular substances into the surrounding tissue
Atrophy is the decrease of both cell size and numbers. It can be physiological or pathological and is often mediated by apoptosis
Differentiation occurs when a cell develops an overt specialized function and morphology which distinguishes it from its parent cells
Dysplasia is a premalignant condition. There is increased cell growth, atypical morphology and altered differentiation. Carcinoma *in situ* is the final step for a dysplastic cell before it becomes a cancer
Growth is the process of increase in size
Hamartoma is the abnormal overgrowth of mature cells
Hyperplasia is the increase in cell numbers by mitoses
Hypertrophy is the increase in cell size
Metaplasia is the reversible replacement of one terminally differentiated cell type with another. It is not synonymous with dysplasia and does not necessarily lead to neoplasia. A good example is Barrett's oesophagus in which squamous epithelium of the oesophagus exposed to excessive acid reflux is replaced by columnar glandular epithelium
Neoplasia is abnormal, uncoordinated and excessive cell growth that persists after the initiating stimulus has been withdrawn. A neoplasm (tumour) can be benign or malignant depending on its potential for local invasion and metastasis
Regeneration is the replacement of injured or dead cells. The ability of cells to regenerate varies.
Labile cells have a short life span, rapid turnover, and are highly susceptible to the effects of radiation and drugs (e.g. haematopoietic cells and epithelial cells).
Stable cells are conditional renewal cells. They divide infrequently in normal circumstances but respond to injury (e.g. liver, bone, and renal tubules).
Permanent cells have no regeneration potential (e.g. neurons, cardiac, and skeletal muscle).

3.2 Cancer diagnosis and classification

Screening

Cancers often present at a late stage in their natural progression. Early detection and treatment should theoretically improve prognosis. This is the basis of population screening.

The disease

- Important health problem
- Common in the population
- Long pre-morbid period which is asymptomatic
- Reliable detection at an early stage
- Treatable at the time of detection

The test

- High sensitivity (i.e. it detects most cases, with few false-negative results)
- High specificity (i.e. it detects only patients with cancer, with few false-positive results)
- Cost-effective so that it can be made available to the entire population at risk
- Safe, non-invasive, and acceptable to patients

Limitations of screening

- **Lead time bias**: detecting tumours early may not change the final prognosis. Early diagnosis of cancer might give false reassurance that patients live longer only because their disease is observed for a longer period of time
- **Length bias**: aggressive screening identifies slow-growing tumours that may not have become clinically apparent during the patient's life. This leads to diagnosis and treatment of disease that would otherwise have remained occult
- **Selection bias**: screening programmes tend to attract the educated 'worried-well' rather than patient populations that have most to gain from the early detection of disease

Tumour diagnosis

Both benign and malignant tumours can cause a wide range of symptoms and signs related to local, metastatic or systemic effects.

Local

- Visible or palpable mass
- Pain
- Bleeding
- Compression or obstruction of local structures
- Destruction of local structures (e.g. ulceration)
- Abnormal function (e.g. liver dysfunction in hepatic carcinoma)

Metastatic

The symptoms and signs depend on the site of the secondary tumour. For instance, bone metastases may cause pain and pathological fractures.

Systemic

- Fever is common in patients with malignant neoplasia, especially if lymphoid in origin. It is mediated by release of cytokines (IL-1, TNF-α) by either the tumour cells or associated macrophages
- Weight loss and muscle wasting is often associated with advanced disease. Some tumours are known to cause anorexia and malabsorption, resulting in cachexia

- Immunosuppression
- Paraneoplastic syndromes may be associated with a tumour but are not directly caused by it. They may be caused by humoral secretions, immunological attack or an unknown process
- Anaemia and other haematological conditions

Tumour biopsy

There are many different ways of obtaining cells or tissue for cytological or histological diagnosis. In addition to diagnostic information, techniques such as immunohistochemistry give important prognostic information.

Cytology

The specimen is usually taken by FNA biopsy but can be a fluid sample. Cytology is fast and cheap. It gives information about cell morphology but the tissue architecture is lost.

Histology

A histological specimen is a piece of tissue with its gross structural architecture intact. The tissue needs to be processed before being examined which can be time-consuming. It also only examines a small field. The various biopsy techniques are discussed later in the chapter.

Tumour markers

Some tumours release specific products into the systemic circulation that can be measured by sensitive assays. Changes in plasma concentration of these products can be used to assess the response to treatment or to detect recurrence/progression of the tumour.

Hormones

- β-human chorionic gonadotrophin (β-hCG)—choriocarcinoma and non-seminomatous germ cell tumours of the testis (NSGCT)
- ACTH—small cell lung carcinoma
- Calcitonin—medullary thyroid carcinoma

Proteins

- Thyroglobulin—thyroid carcinoma
- Paraproteins—multiple myeloma
- CA 15-3—occasionally elevated in breast carcinoma
- CA 19-9—pancreatic and advanced colorectal carcinoma
- CA 125—non-mucinous ovarian carcinomas

Enzymes

- Prostatic acid phosphatase (PSA)—prostate carcinoma
- Placental alkaline phosphatise—germ cell tumours, bronchus, pancreas, and colon

Oncofetal antigens

- Alpha-fetoprotein (AFP)—germ cell tumours and hepatocellular carcinoma
- Carcinoembryonic antigen (CEA)—colorectal carcinoma

Imaging

Plain radiographs

A plain chest radiograph is necessary at presentation for most malignant lesions to identify possible pulmonary metastases. Otherwise plain radiographs have a limited role.

Ultrasound

Ultrasound is used in diagnosis and staging. It is often used to guide FNAC. Endoscopic US has become a very accurate imaging technique for staging the local invasiveness of oesophageal and rectal tumours by demonstrating the extension of the tumour through the mucosa and muscular layers, and the presence/absence of involvement of local lymph nodes.

Cross-sectional imaging (CT and MRI scans)

Cross-sectional imaging enables localization of primary and metastatic disease. The size and anatomical relationships of the tumour can be determined as well as the presence of local invasion and metastatic spread. CT can also be used to guide tissue biopsies.

Functional imaging

Positron emission tomography (PET) scanning uses a fluorinated derivative of glucose (FDG) to show areas of increased cellular metabolism. It allows the most accurate assessment of small metastatic deposits and can provide information on the response to chemotherapy.

Nuclear medicine

- **Octreoscan scintigraphy** using a radioactive labelled derivative of somatostatin. It shows the presence of somatostatin receptors and predicts the response to somatostatin analogues (e.g. carcinoid tumours)
- **MIBG scans**—uptake of meta-iodobenzylguanetidine is characteristic for neuroendocrine tumours (phaeochromocytomas, medullary thyroid cancer)
- **Bone scintigraphy** demonstrates areas of increased bone metabolism such as osteolytic bone metastases. It is used for staging of patients with advanced breast or prostate cancer
- **Radiolabelled lymphoscintigraphy**. Identifying sentinel nodes in the lymphatic drainage of a particular tumour (e.g. melanoma, breast cancer) is greatly facilitated by the local injection of a radiolabelled compound that drains preferentially in the local lymphatic system. The use of a hand-held gamma probe during operation allows identification of the 'hot' lymph nodes previously demonstrated on a scintigraphic lymphogram.

Tumour stage and grade

Cancer staging describes the extent to which a malignant tumour has spread. Clinical staging is based on information obtained from clinical assessment, imaging, and endoscopy before surgery. Additional pathological stage is obtained by microscopic examination of the excised tumour.

Staging aims to improve patient selection for appropriate therapy, provide an informed prognosis, and helps to evaluate new forms of therapy by enabling comparison of different treatments applied to similar patients.

TNM staging

Some cancers have multiple staging systems and some have none. The TNM staging system is one of the most commonly used. It was developed and is maintained by the American Joint Committee on Cancer (AJCC) and the Union Internationale Contre le Cancer (UICC).

The TNM staging system is based on the extent of the tumour (T), the extent of spread to the regional lymph nodes (N), and the presence of metastasis (M). TNM classifications are then placed in overall group stages (0, I, II, III, IV).

Tumour grade

Tumour grade is the degree of differentiation of a tumour according to well-defined histological criteria (e.g. degree of nuclear pleomorphism, capacity to resemble the original tissue architecture, number of mitoses). It is generally reported as well, moderately or poorly differentiated. Most tumours have mixed elements of this grading system.

◎ Breast cancer screening

In 1985 the Forrest report recommended the introduction of a national breast cancer screening programme based on evidence from early trials in Scandinavia. All women aged between 50 and 70 years are invited for 3-yearly screening. The two standard mammography views are craniocaudal (CC) and mediolateral oblique (MLO).

Proponents argue that there is evidence to support a 25% reduction in breast cancer mortality in women screened. Others consider that the patient cost in terms of anxiety, unnecessary biopsies, and overdiagnosis of small tumours with very good prognosis in the elderly, reduce the beneficial impact.

Standards for the screening programme

- >70% response rate
- <10% of patients called for further assessment
- Operation within 2 weeks to confirm histological diagnosis in >90% of patients and operation within 3 weeks for treatment in >90% of patients

False-positive mammograms

Some 10% of screening mammograms are read as abnormal, but only 3% of abnormal mammograms are due to breast cancer. After 10 mammograms, 50% of women will have had a false-positive mammogram. This risk is increased in young women, those with dense breasts, on HRT or with a positive family history.

3.3 Cancer treatment

The aim of treatment is to cure or relieve the symptoms of a cancer. The delivery of cancer treatment is based on local and national guidelines, and is often run by a multidisciplinary team of healthcare professionals.

Multidisciplinary team

Multidisciplinary teams (MDT) are often used to deliver cancer care. Guidelines vary but generally all new referrals are discussed and then follow-up arranged for cases that are more complicated.

Team members
- Lead clinician (surgeon or physician)
- Radiologist
- Histopathologist
- Oncologist (medical or clinical)
- Clinical nurse specialist
- Palliative care nurse
- MDT coordinator

Pros
- Team approach to delivering care
- Maintain standards set by guidelines
- Disseminate good practice
- Data collection for audit purposes
- Potential for more patients to be recruited to clinical trials

Cons
- Lack of leadership and poor team working can be a problem
- Logistic difficulties with team members working in different centres
- Potential for delay in treatment—'got to wait for MDT'

Performance status

The performance status of a patient is a measure of their general level of activity and quality of life. It is important to consider this when deciding treatment options.

There are a number of scoring systems, of which the Karnofsky (Table 3.2) is most commonly used.

Treatment options

Treatment decisions are based on tumour characteristics (stage, grade, and location), patient factors (performance status), and the limitations of the treatment options.

Operative
- Curative surgery aims to excise the tumour completely
- Surgical staging of disease is important as a prognostic indicator as well as a guide for further management
- Palliative surgery controls symptoms caused by the tumour (e.g. relieving spinal cord compression)

Radiation therapy
Radiation therapy is the use of ionizing radiation to kill malignant cells by damaging the DNA in dividing cells. It can be used as therapeutic, adjuvant, neoadjuvant, or palliative treatment.

The amount of radiation required is measured in Grays (Gy). The total dose is usually fractionated into small doses which are delivered over a set period of time.

Tumours may be radiosensitive (e.g. head and neck tumours and lymphoma) or radioresistant (e.g. renal cell carcinoma).

Route of administration
- Conventional external beam
- Radioisotopes are delivered orally or intravenously. An antibody, with specificity for a tumour-associated antigen, is labelled with a radionucleotide. It delivers a lethal dose of radiation targeted more accurately to the tumour rather than normal tissues
- Brachytherapy is the use of an implantable radioactive source

Side effects
Early
- Damage to epithelial tissues
- Oedema of local tissues
- Infertility

Long term
- Fibrosis and scarring of irradiated tissues
- Hair loss is most pronounced in patients receiving brain irradiation. More likely to be permanent than following chemotherapy
- Dryness of mucosal surfaces in local tissues
- Secondary cancer

Chemotherapy
Chemotherapy refers to the use of cytotoxic drugs to treat cancer (Table 3.3). They are either effective throughout the cell cycle (cycle-specific) or during part of the cycle (phase-specific) and capitalize on the rapid cell division of cancer cells. Chemotherapy is used in a number of ways:
- combined therapy with surgery or radiation therapy
- neoadjuvant (preoperative) to try and down-stage a tumour to make it locally operable
- Adjuvant therapy (postoperative) to reduce the risk of recurrence even though the tumour has been resected
- Palliative chemotherapy is used to control symptoms and prolong survival without the intent to cure

Route of administration
The majority of chemotherapy agents are delivered intravenously via a long-term venous catheter (Hickmann line, Port-a-Cath®, PICC line).

Side effects
Early
- Fatigue and lethargy (80% of patients)
- Hair loss
- Nausea and vomiting ($5\text{-}HT_3$ inhibitors are the most effective antiemetics)
- Immunosuppression and neutropaenic sepsis

Late
- Anaemia
- Secondary cancers (e.g. leukaemia in 3% at 15 years)
- Organ toxicity (cardiac, hepatic, renal, ototoxicity)
- Early menopause

Hormone therapy

Altering the hormone environment can be used to treat a minority of tumours successfully. Examples include the use of finasteride in the treatment of prostate cancer and the use of aromatase inhibitors and tamoxifen in women with oestrogen and/or progesterone receptor-positive breast cancer. These are discussed in more detail in the relevant topics.

Monoclonal antibody therapy

Monoclonal antibodies bind to an antigen to disrupt its function. An example is trastuzumab (Herceptin), which is a humanized monoclonal antibody used in the treatment of HER2/neu (erbB2) receptor-positive breast cancer patients. It binds to this receptor, resulting in tyrosine kinase blockade and arrest of the cell cycle.

Palliative care

Palliative care (end-of-life care) takes a holistic approach to the patient's needs. It includes control of symptoms (e.g. pain, nausea, vomiting, pruritis), as well as psychological support (📖 Topic 1.9).

Table 3.2 Karnofsky scale	
100	Normal, no complaint, no signs or symptoms of disease
90	Able to carry on normal activity, minor signs and symptoms of disease
80	Normal activity with effort, some signs or symptoms of disease
70	Cares for self, unable to carry out normal activities or continue active life
60	Requires occasional assistance, but is able to care for most of his or her needs
50	Requires considerable assistance and frequent medical care
40	Disabled, requires special care and assistance
30	Severely disabled, hospitalization is indicated, although death not imminent
20	Very sick, hospitalization necessary, active supportive treatment necessary
10	Moribund, fatal processes progressing rapidly
0	Dead

Table 3.3 Chemotherapy agents

Alkylating agents

Alkylating agents covalently bond alkyl groups to DNA, preventing it from uncoiling and separating
Examples: cisplatin, carboplatin, cyclophosphamide

Antimetabolites

Antimetabolites are purine, pyrimidine or folic acid analogues. Folic acid is vital in the synthesis of purines and pyrimidines, which are both the building blocks of DNA. The drugs prevent these substances becoming incorporated in DNA during the S-phase of the cell cycle
Examples: folic acid—methotrexate; purine—azathioprine; pyrimidine—fluorouracil

Anthracyclines

Anthracyclines inhibit DNA and RNA synthesis by including themselves in the space between two adjacent base pairs to prevent replication
Examples: daunorubicin, doxorubicin

Plant alkaloids

Plant-derived alkaloids prevent microtubule function which is critical for cell division. The two main classes are vinca alkaloids and taxanes
Examples: vinca—vinblastine, vincristine; taxane—docetaxel

Topoisomerase inhibitors

Topoisomerases are enzymes that maintain DNA structure. Inhibitors interfere with the transcription and replication of DNA and its subsequent coiling

The normal life cycle of the breast commences with early development prior to the menarche. It continues through monthly, cyclical changes throughout the reproductive life with additional marked changes in differentiation of terminal duct lobular units during any pregnancy. Finally, following the menopause the breast involutes. Most benign breast conditions seen in clinical practice are considered to be aberrations occurring during this normal life cycle. Their incidence varies with age (Table 3.4).

Breast embryology

The breasts are modified apocrine glands. They begin their development during the fifth week of gestation when paired epidermal thickenings ('milk lines') form along either side of the body from the future axilla to the medial thigh. During the sixth week most of the ridges regress apart from in the pectoral region where they become the primary breast buds.

Secondary buds branch from the primary buds and continue to branch and elongate so that by full term there are 15–20 lactiferous ducts opening on to the mammary pit. Following birth, further growth leads to eversion of the nipple and development of the areola.

Congenital breast anomalies

- Amastia—complete failure of breast development
- Hypoplasia—deficient development (e.g. Poland's syndrome)
- Athelia—complete failure of nipple development
- Supernumerary nipple development along milk line
- Axillary breast tissue (usually bilateral)

Aberrations of breast development

Juvenile hypertrophy

Prepubertal uncontrolled breast enlargement in adolescent girls may occur because of overgrowth of the interlobular stroma. There is proliferation and branching of the ducts without lobule formation.

The large breasts cause neck and back pain as well as social embarrassment. The enlargement is usually bilateral but can be asymmetrical. Reduction mammoplasty may improve quality of life.

Fibroadenoma

Fibroadenomas are aberrations of normal lobule development and are very common in young women.

Presentation is usually as a smooth, rubbery, non-tender, mobile lump ('breast mouse'), showing no changes in size with menstruation. Triple assessment with clinical examination, ultrasound examination, and fine needle biopsy or core biopsy should be undertaken to exclude malignancy.

After reassuring the patient, small tumours (<4 cm) can be left alone. The majority reduce in size within a year and some may disappear completely. Those enlarging, creating significant pressure symptoms or causing undue anxiety should be excised.

Giant fibroadenoma

Giant fibroadenomas measure over 5 cm in maximum diameter. They are common in young women of African descent. They require a core biopsy for diagnosis and then excision.

Phyllodes tumour

Phyllodes tumour is a tumour of the interlobular stroma (i.e. non-epithelial) of the breast. It tends to present in pre-menopausal women aged between 40 and 50 years of age as a large firm well-circumscribed mass which occasionally grows rapidly. They are rarely malignant.

Diagnosis is by clinical assessment, ultrasound and mammography, and then core biopsy. The pathologist will state the number of mitoses per high power field (<5 benign, 5–10 borderline, >10 malignant). Malignant lesions metastasize by haematogenous spread to lungs, not by lymphatic spread.

Management is normally by wide local excision with a large margin, but recurrences may be multifocal if treated inadequately and require a mastectomy. Regional spread is rare and so axillary dissection is not indicated. There is a high risk of local recurrence, particularly for large tumours.

Aberrations of mature reproductive life

Mastalgia

Breast pain is a common symptom and accounts for >50% of breast clinic referrals. The aetiology is unknown, although there are a number of theories with little scientific basis, including water retention, psychological factors and a disturbed hormone environment. Mastalgia does not occur before the menarche and is rare after the menopause.

The pain is termed non-cyclical or cyclical depending on its relationship to the menstrual cycle. In 15% of patients the pain is significant enough to impact on activities of daily living. Breast examination often reveals diffuse tenderness in one or both breasts and should exclude any breast lumps which would need triple assessment. In the absence of any other symptom most breast units do not offer women a mammogram. Other conditions causing anterior chest wall pain, such as costochondritis (Tietze's syndrome), should be excluded.

Simple measures, including the use of a well-fitting firm bra and regular exercise, have been shown to reduce the severity of mastalgia. Mastalgia is rarely a symptom of breast cancer. Women with a normal clinical assessment and mammogram can be reassured and discharged from clinic.

In those patients with severe cyclical mastalgia the first line therapy is gamma linoleic acid (Evening Primrose oil) which improves the symptoms in 50% of women. In severe mastalgia either danazol or bromocriptine may be used though they have significant side effects. Tamoxifen is not licenced for mastalgia. Non-cyclical mastalgia is treated with NSAIDS and/or injection of local anaesthetic or steroids.

Benign duct papilloma

Duct papillomas are caused by benign epithelial hyperplasia within large mammary or lactiferous ducts. Patients present with nipple bleeding or blood-stained discharge from a single duct. A sample should be sent for cytology.

Breast carcinoma needs to be excluded and so a mammogram is usually carried out. The affected duct is excised (microdochectomy).

Table 3.4 Aberrations of normal development and involution (ANDI)

	Normal process	Common aberrations	Uncommon aberrations
Development	Ductal	Nipple inversion Single duct obstruction	Mammary duct fistula
	Lobular Stromal	Fibroadenoma Juvenile hypertrophy	Giant fibroadenoma Prepubertal breast enlargement
Cyclical change	Hormonal activity Epithelial activity	Cyclical mastalgia Cyclical nodularity (focal or diffuse) Benign duct papilloma	
Pregnancy and lactation	Epithelial hyperplasia Lactation	Blood-stained nipple discharge Galactocoele and inappropriate lactation	
Involution	Ductal Lobular Micropapillomatosis	Nipple retraction and duct ectasia Cysts and sclerosing adenosis Simple hyperplasia	Periductal mastitis Hyperplasia with atypia

Terminal Ductal Lobular Unit (TDLU)

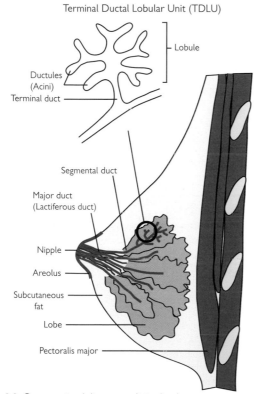

Fig 3.2 Cross-sectional diagram outlining key breast anatomy.

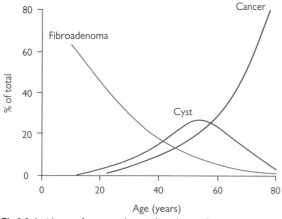

Fig 3.3 Incidence of common breast disorders with age.

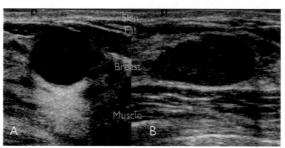

Fig 3.4 Breast ultrasound scans showing: (A) well-circumscribed cyst with no signal within it suggesting it is fluid-filled; (B) well-circumscribed fibroadenoma which is echogenic, suggesting it is a solid lesion.

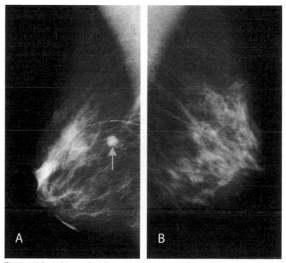

Fig 3.5 Medial lateral oblique mammograms from different women. (A) Fibroadenoma. (B) Malignant changes suggested by distortion of the breast tissue and microcalcification.

Characteristics of breast lesions on mammography:

Benign	**Malignant**
● Smooth round mass	● Irregular spiculated mass
● Calcifications >1 mm	● Microcalcifications <0.5 mm
● Normal breast architecture	● Distorted breast architecture

3.5 Disorders of breast development and involution II

Aberrations of breast involution

Involution is the decrease in size and decline of normal physiological function of the breast seen with ageing. It occurs following pregnancy or after the age of 30 years in nulliparous women.

Cysts

Up to 10% of women develop symptomatic cysts at some point during their reproductive years. Cysts may be single or multiple, unilateral or bilateral. Most are found on self-examination in women 30–50 years of age and cause severe anxiety.

Women require triple assessment. Aspiration yields a yellow–green clear or turbid fluid. Only blood-stained fluid should be sent for cytology unless the ultrasound suggests an intramural lesion (commonly an intracystic papilloma), in which case a core is required. Some cysts recur and need further aspiration.

Table 3.5 Benign versus malignant breast lumps

Benign	Malignant
• Firm and rubbery	• Hard
• Painful	• Painless
• Smooth shape	• Irregular shape
• Mobile	• Fixed to skin or chest wall
• No skin dimpling	• Skin dimpling
• No nipple retraction or discharge	• Nipple retraction and bloody discharge

Periductal mastitis

Periductal mastitis presents with non-cyclical mastalgia, nipple discharge, and periareolar inflammation. It may develop a mammary fistula and non-lactating breast abscess.

Duct ectasia

Duct ectasia (dilatation) can occur with periductal mastitis. It affects the subareolar breast ducts, which dilate and shorten with age. Women with excessive changes present with slit-like nipple retraction or inversion and cheesy discharge.

Acute episodes are managed with antibiotics (need anaerobic cover). Chronic disease may need major duct excision.

Other conditions

Nipple discharge

Nipple discharge may be spontaneous or induced, unilateral or bilateral, have different colours and textures, and be from one or many ducts.

Physiological discharge of small amount of serous white–yellow or green fluid can be expressed in up to two-thirds of non-lactating pre-menopausal women.

Nipple discharge is considered significant only if it occurs spontaneously or is associated with one or more suspicious features (Table 3.6). In these cases, clinical assessment should include cytology and mammography (>35 years old).

If the volume is small and discharge occurs only when the nipple is expressed, reassurance is sufficient. If the volume is large and localized to one duct, consider microdochectomy and major duct excision with segmental resections if multiple ducts are involved.

Table 3.6 Characteristics of nipple discharge

Benign	Malignant
• Bilateral	• Unilateral
• Spontaneous or induced	• Spontaneous
• Multiple duct orifices	• One duct orifice
• Thick green or yellow, induced and bilateral (duct ectasia)	• Bloody, serosanguineous, or serous (clear)

Nipple eczema

Eczema of the nipple when it affects the breast always involves the areola and only secondarily affects the nipple (Fig 3.6). Removal of the sensitizing agent can result in rapid resolution. A short course of topical steroids can be tried.

The main differential is Paget's disease of the nipple, which always involves the nipple first and requires urgent referral. A skin punch biopsy and mammogram is performed.

Fat necrosis

Trauma to the breast can trigger local inflammation of the glandular tissue and subsequent fat necrosis. The mechanism of injury may be minimal (e.g. seat-belt injury) and may go unnoticed. The presentation is often similar to that of a malignant lump and so triple assessment is required.

Gynaecomastia

Gynaecomastia is benign hypertrophy of glandular tissue in the male breast. It results from a physiological or pathological alteration in the body's oestrogen/androgen balance.

Gynaecomastia (Fig 3.7) should not be confused with adipomastia which is excessive fat deposition in obesity.

Physiological gynaecomastia occurs in neonates, pubescent teenagers, and elderly men. Pathological gynaecomastia has a number of causes related to:

- decreased production or action of testosterone (hypogonadism)—hypopituitarism, renal failure, androgen insensitivity syndrome, and drugs (finasteride, spironolactone)
- increased production or action of oestrogen—secretion of oestrogen by testicular tumours or ectopic human chorionic gonadotrophin secretion by lung, kidney, or GI tumours
- increased production of oestrogen in liver disease, malnutrition, hyperthyroidism, and familial gynaecomastia
- drugs: this is the commonest cause in men over 50 years and is caused by a large number of drugs, including oestrogen-containing drugs or analogues and drugs that increase synthesis, such as anabolic steroids and phenytoin

Clinical assessment

Exclude the presence of an isolated breast lump suggestive of male breast cancer. Clinical assessment is complemented by USS/mammography and FNAB or a core biopsy if suspicious.

Management

Patients should be reassured that it is a benign condition. Conservative management is rarely successful except when a cause is established and the stimulus stopped.

The standard operative management is the removal of breast tissue through a periareolar or inframammary incision. Liposuction or reduction mastopexy may be performed for cosmetic reasons.

⊕ Pathological examination of breast tissue

The choice of diagnostic procedure is dependent on whether the lesion is palpable or non-palpable.

Non-palpable lesions usually require either needle localization and open biopsy or image-guided core needle biopsy using ultrasound or stereotactic mammography.

Fine needle aspiration biopsy

Fine needle aspiration cytology (FNAC) allows a minimally invasive, rapid diagnosis of tissue based on cytological appearance. It is highly accurate when used as part of triple assessment (sensitivity ~90%, specificity ~100%).

Procedure

- A narrow gauge (21G) needle is attached to a 10 mL syringe and held in a 'gun' to improve manipulation
- Under aseptic technique the needle is advanced to the lesion
- Once the tip of the needle reaches the tumour, a negative pressure is created by withdrawing the syringe plunger 2–3 cm. The needle is passed across the tumour four or five times. The suction is released before withdrawing the needle from the tissue
- The aspirate is expressed on glass cover slips and fixed according to the local protocol (air-dried or fixed with alcohol-based solution)
- Rapid interpretation by a cytologist enables results to be available at the same clinic visit (one-stop clinic)
- The degree of cellularity and nuclear polymorphism is used to grade the overall appearance on a five-point scale: C1—insufficient breast epithelial cells to reach a diagnosis; C2—benign cells (e.g. fibroadenoma); C3—atypical cells, probably benign; C4—atypical cells, probably malignant; C5—malignant cells
- C1 samples should be repeated. C3 and C4 samples should be further investigated with a core biopsy

Core biopsy

Local anaesthetic is infiltrated around the biopsy site. An automated biopsy gun is used to fire a 14G needle across the lesion. It delivers a core of tissue with its structure intact, allowing histological assessment. Large-bore suction cores may also be performed by a mammotome.

Histological findings are classified into the following: B1—normal breast tissue; B2—benign breast disease; B3—indeterminate, most likely benign; B4—indeterminate, most likely malignant; B5a—ductal carcinoma *in situ;* and B5b—infiltrating carcinoma.

Open biopsy

Open surgical biopsy for histological diagnosis of breast abnormalities is rarely performed nowadays, since the diagnosis is usually established using triple assessment, including needle biopsy. However, in inconclusive cases, the lesion can be excised for definitive histological diagnosis and, if this is impalpable, then localization, using imaging guidance, is necessary for accurate excision.

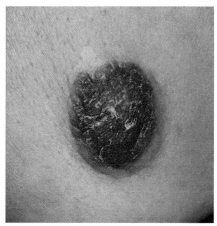

Fig 3.6 Nipple eczema. In Paget's disease of the nipple there is a unilateral erythematous, eczematous lesion affecting the nipple and areola, with a tendency to ulceration. Within the epidermis of the nipple there is infiltration with malignant cells derived from an adjacent breast cancer.

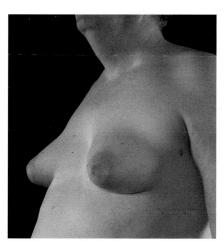

Fig 3.7 Gynaecomatia.

Table 3.7 Comparison of breast imaging techniques				
	Ultrasound	**Mammography**	**MRI**	**PET**
Pros	Imaging of choice in women <35 years Very useful in clinic for guiding cytology or core biopsy Distinguishes between cystic and solid masses Assessment of elderly women on endocrine therapy	Cost advantage Increased sensitivity with increasing age Films may be read by multiple observers Digital mammography allows image manipulation but is expensive	Assessing mammographically occult cancers Assessing neoadjuvant chemotherapy response Assessing invasive lobular cancers Screening in women	May be useful in determining recurrence (unproven)
Cons	Not suitable for screening Operator-dependent	Not suitable in women under 35 years or with strong family history	Expensive and time-consuming. Not suitable for ductal carcinoma *in situ*	Cost and limited availablity

3.6 Breast cancer I—assessment

Breast cancer is the most common cancer affecting women. It has recently been superseded by lung cancer as the most common cause of cancer death in women. In the UK, over 40 000 new cases are diagnosed each year and there are 12 000 deaths.

The female lifetime risk of having breast cancer is 1 in 9 (UK). It is rare in those under 35 years, but the incidence rises rapidly until 50 years and then slows (F:M 100:1). It is most prevalent in North America and Northern Europe.

Aetiology

The aetiology of breast cancer is multifactorial and involves the interaction of both environmental and genetic factors. Protective factors include early first childbirth, late menarche, prolonged breastfeeding, diet high in monounsaturated fat, and physical exercise.

Risk factors

Many risk factors are thought to act by increasing lifetime exposure to oestrogen.

High

- Increasing age (median 65 years)
- Family history (see below)

Medium

- High socioeconomic status
- Late first pregnancy (>30 years)
- Past history of breast cancer
- Breast irradiation <20 years (typically for lymphoma treatment)

Low

- Early menarche (<11 years)
- Nulliparity
- Late menopause (>55 years)
- Oral contraceptive pill and postmenopausal use of hormone replacement therapy
- Obesity and alcohol

Family history increasing risk of breast cancer

- First-degree relative diagnosed at <40 years
- Two close relatives diagnosed at <50 years
- Three close relatives diagnosed at <60 years
- First- or second-degree relative with bilateral breast cancer
- Male relative with breast cancer
- Family history of breast and ovarian cancer

Inherited genetic factors

Five per cent of breast cancers are familial, although more have inherited factors influencing their development. Genes commonly involved in familial breast cancer are *BRCA1*, *BRCA2*, and *p53*. *BRCA1* mutations are associated with ovarian cancer and *BRCA2* mutations are also associated with cancers of the prostate, pancreas, and bladder.

Li–Fraumeni syndrome is an inherited autosomal dominant disorder characterized by a mutation in *p53*. Patients are more susceptible to certain cancers, including breast, brain, and soft tissue cancers. Li–Fraumeni syndrome is identified in 1% of women with early onset breast cancer. Bilateral breast cancer is noted in up to 25% of patients.

Pathophysiology

As with all cancers, acquired or inherited, genetic mutation results in tumour formation. Invasive breast cancer is increasingly seen as a micrometastatic disease from inception.

In situ carcinoma

An *in situ* carcinoma is contained within the epithelium with an intact basement membrane and no signs of invasion.

Ductal carcinoma in situ (DCIS)

DCIS is a clonal proliferation of ductal luminal cells that accumulate into the lumen of the mammary duct. It originates in a single gland but may spread through the breast ductal system. Two-thirds of patients have multifocal disease, characterized by discontinuous intraductal growth, with gaps of up to 1 cm between tumour foci.

The pathological classification of DCIS is based on nuclear grade (low, intermediate or high), architectural pattern of tumour growth (solid, papillary, cribriform), and the presence or absence of comedonecrosis.

Comedonecrosis refers to the pathological appearance of the necrotic ductal cells that can be expressed out, just like a skin comedo (blackhead), and which are seen as microcalcifications on mammography.

Lobular carcinoma in situ (LCIS)

LCIS accounts for ~5% of all breast cancers and predominates in premenopausal women. It is not thought to be a precursor of invasive cancer but a risk factor indicating an increased lifetime risk of 20–30%. It is often multifocal and may be bilateral. It rarely presents as a mass but is found incidentally in biopsies performed for a palpable benign lesion. It is normally mammographically occult.

Within the breast acini the normal cells are replaced by relatively uniform cells and appear loose and non-cohesive. The size of the acini increases but the lobular shape is maintained and, unlike DCIS, necrosis is not a feature.

Invasive carcinoma

Invasive ductal carcinoma (IDC) develops in ~50% of patients with untreated DCIS within 10 years of diagnosis and is the most common form of invasive breast cancer.

Invasive lobular carcinoma (ILC) represents 10% of all breast cancers. Only ~30% of patients with LCIS go on to develop ILC. It is often multifocal and may be bilateral. A majority of tumours express oestrogen and progesterone receptors, but *HER2/neu* or *p53* overexpression is rare.

Other types of invasive breast cancer are rare. They include medullary, mucinous, and tubular carcinomas.

Clinical assessment

The commonest presentation is a breast lump. About 1% of single duct bloody nipple discharges may also be due to cancer. The diagnosis of a malignant breast lump is based on triple assessment: clinical, pathological, and radiological.

History

- Symptoms related to breast lump
- Associated nipple discharge and mastalgia
- Identify risk factors
- Metastatic symptoms: bone pain, weight loss

Examination

- Breast shape: altered profile or asymmetry between breasts
- Breast skin changes: peau d'orange, ulceration
- Nipple: inversion, bloody discharge, Paget's disease
- Lymph nodes: axilla and supraclavicular fossa
- Metastatic signs: cachexia, bone pain, palpable liver

Investigations
- Radiological assessment: breast ultrasound and mammography (>35 years)
- Pathological assessment: core biopsy is increasingly used in the preoperative assessment of all malignant tumours. It can be used for both histological diagnosis of invasive and pre-invasive cancers and immunohistochemistry (IHC) studies
- IHC studies determine oestrogen and progesterone receptor status. Oestrogen receptors are nuclear transcription factors present in the normal breast and in 60–70% of breast cancers. Receptor status guides the use of adjuvant hormone therapy
- HER2/neu status is also undertaken from the core biopsy. This is initially done by IHC and defined as negative, borderline or positive. Borderline cases require substitute for detailed FISH estimation of HER2 status
- Routine bloods: FBC (anaemia), LFT (raised alkaline phosphatase, gamma-glutamyl transpeptidase, and calcium suggest bone or liver metastasis). Ca 15-3 tumour marker is raised in some early breast cancers and almost all advanced cancer but is not routinely measured
- Chest radiograph is not done routinely
- CT scans, liver ultrasound, and isotope bone scan are only requested to assess metastatic disease

Staging
Pathological grading, tumour size, and lymph node status give the most useful prognostic information in breast cancer.

TNM classification
Primary tumour

TX	Cannot be assessed
T0	No evidence of primary tumour
Tis	Carcinoma *in situ,* intraductal carcinoma, LCIS, or Paget's disease of the nipple with no associated tumour
T1	Tumour ≤2 cm in greatest dimension
T2	Tumour >2 cm but ≤5 cm in greatest dimension
T3	Tumour >5 cm in greatest dimension
T4	Tumour of any size with direct extension to: (a) chest wall; or (b) skin. (Note: chest wall includes ribs, intercostal muscles, and serratus anterior muscle, but not pectoral muscle)

Regional lymph nodes

NX	Cannot be assessed (e.g. previously removed)
N0	No regional lymph node metastasis
N1	Metastasis to moveable ipsilateral axillary lymph node(s)
N2	Metastasis to ipsilateral axillary lymph node(s) fixed to each other or to other structures
N3	Metastasis to ipsilateral internal mammary lymph node(s)

Distant metastasis

MX	Cannot be assessed
M0	No distant metastasis
M1	Distant metastasis present (includes metastasis to ipsilateral supraclavicular lymph nodes)

Overall stage grouping

Stage 0	Tis	N0	M0
Stage I	T1	N0	M0
Stage II	T0	N1	M0
Stage III	T0	N2	M0
Stage IV	Any T	Any N	M1

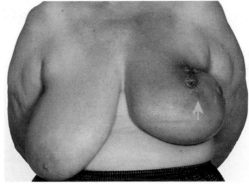

Fig 3.8 Locally advanced cancer of the left breast. The breast is tethered and the tumour is fungating through the skin. The nipple is not involved (arrow).

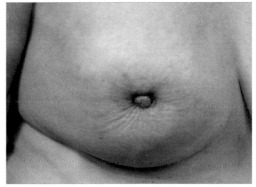

Fig 3.9 Right breast with locally advanced breast cancer. There is tethering of the nipple and surrounding peau d'orange skin changes. This is because of cutaneous oedema following obstruction of the dermal lymphatics.

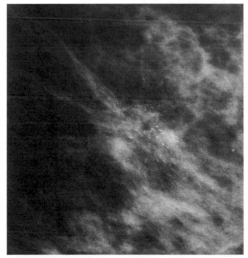

Fig 3.10 Mediolateral oblique view (close-up of Fig 3.5b) showing an irregular and spiculated mass, associated with distortion of breast architecture and microcalcification. This is characteristic of breast cancer. Up to 10% of palpable cancers may be missed on mammography.

3.7 Breast cancer II—management

Management overview

Ductal carcinoma *in situ*

The goal of treating DCIS is prevention of local recurrence and, progression to invasive breast cancer.

The options include mastectomy or breast-conserving surgery (BCS). No randomized trials have compared these surgical options in the way that has been done for invasive breast cancer. Following BCS for DCIS there is a risk of local ipsilateral recurrence; half of these are invasive tumours.

The predictors of recurrent tumour include young age (<45 years), close margins (<1 mm), positive margins, high grade, and comedonecrosis. The risk of local recurrence is reduced by 40–60% by the addition of breast radiotherapy after BCS, but the benefit of radiotherapy to women with small, well-differentiated DCIS is unknown, and trials are ongoing. The role of endocrine therapy in oestrogen receptor (ER)-positive tumours needs further clarification as early studies suggest a benefit, but further trials are ongoing.

Lobular carcinoma *in situ*

The appropriate management of LCIS is unclear. It is potentially both a precursor lesion and also a marker of risk, but the rate of transformation into invasive cancer is very low. The risk of invasive cancer is also equal in both breasts and may be either lobular or ductal. If LCIS is found with invasive cancer this should guide management. Isolated LCIS on a biopsy is used to inform women of their estimated future risk. The majority of surgeons would recommend continued screening, although it has to be explained that LCIS, unlike DCIS, is frequently radiologically occult.

Invasive carcinoma

The management of patients with invasive breast cancer is dependent upon the stage at presentation with treatment being divided into:

- early or operable (stage I–II)
- locally advanced (stage III)
- metastatic (stage IV)

Neoadjuvant therapy

Preoperative chemotherapy

Neoadjuvant chemotherapy (NACT) is used to downstage locally advanced, but non-metastatic, cancer in patients who would prefer BCS rather than mastectomy. Approximately 40–50% are downstaged sufficiently.

Note that there is no evidence from prospective randomized trials to suggest that NACT improves survival. The other indication for NACT is inflammatory breast cancer.

Neoadjuvant hormone therapy

Neoadjuvant hormone therapy (NAHT) is used in a similar manner. More elderly patients presenting with large but ER-positive tumours may benefit from initial hormonal therapy using aromatase inhibitors prior to surgery.

Operative

Surgical excision remains the mainstay of locoregional control of breast cancer. BCS followed by radiotherapy is equivalent to mastectomy in terms of local recurrence and long-term survival.

Conservation breast surgery—wide local excision

The surgical management of breast cancer requires a discussion with the patient to ensure that, whilst the patient's wishes are met wherever possible, this must result in oncologically sound surgical practice. The advance of oncoplastic surgery has meant that a greater proportion of patients can be treated by breast conservation.

Conservation surgery is followed by adjuvant radiotherapy. The local recurrence rate should be less than 5% at 5 years.

Mastectomy

Possible contraindications to conservation surgery are below. Patients with these conditions may require simple mastectomy.

- Locally advanced tumours (stage III)
- Large tumour relative to breast size
- Large high-grade invasive cancer in the presence of vascular invasion or extensive DCIS
- Multifocal tumours
- Widespread DCIS (often high grade)
- Tumours arising during pregnancy
- Recurrence following conservative breast surgery
- Radiotherapy contraindicated

Axillary surgery

The most important prognostic indicators in breast cancer are tumour size, nodal status, and histological grade. Axillary surgery may thus be considered both therapeutic and prognostic.

The axilla is defined anatomically into three levels:

- level 1—inferior to pectoralis minor
- level 2—posterior to pectoralis minor
- level 3—superior to pectoralis minor

Axillary sampling is defined as a dissection of a minimum of four nodes, usually from levels 1 and 2. Axillary clearance is defined as the complete removal of nodes within levels 1 and 2, and occasionally from level 3 also. The majority of patients with invasive cancer (with the possible exception of the elderly and those with very small grade I tumours <5 mm) should have an assessment of their axillary status. An axillary clearance is contraindicated in the presence of DCIS alone, which is managed by conservation surgery. Patients treated with a sampling that results in positive nodes require either a clearance or axillary radiotherapy. Radiotherapy is contraindicated in patients following clearance. Patients receiving axillary radiotherapy have an increased risk of shoulder immobility, but clearance is associated with a long-term risk of lymphoedema. Sentinel lymph node techniques may reduce unnecessary morbidity.

Sentinel lymph node biopsy

Sentinel lymph nodes were first used in penile cancer surgery and are now widely used for melanoma and breast surgery. The sentinel node, or nodes, are the initial nodes draining the tumour; they are normally located in level 1 but may be found at any level or the intramammary chain. The sentinel nodes are identified by using either dye or a radioactive isotope, or both. Patent blue dye is injected either peritumorally or by subdermal injection in the areola within the same quadrant as the tumour. The isotope is generally injected peritumorally. A lymphoscintigram may be performed preoperatively, and a gamma probe is used during the operation to identify the sentinel node, or nodes. A sentinel node is thus ideally identified as being both 'hot' and blue although may only be either 'hot' or blue.

If on subsequent pathological examination there is no evidence of tumour then no further axillary surgery is carried out. If positive the patient will require either axillary radiotherapy or a clearance. Screen-detected cancers have an approximate 25% chance of involved nodes and thus 75% of patients can avoid the morbidity of more radical surgery.

Adjuvant therapy

Chemotherapy
Use of adjuvant chemotherapy is based on a patient's risk of recurrence, age, tumour hormonal status, menopausal status, and fitness. The assessment of risk may be undertaken using web-based software (e.g. Adjuvant online), or evidence-based guidelines. Patients who are under 40 years of age or who have either large, poorly differentiated, ER-negative or involved nodes are likely to benefit most from chemotherapy. The regimens are based on clinical trials and generally include an anthracycline. Patients with poor prognosis may also be given Taxol.

Radiotherapy
Radiotherapy is indicated following BCS for invasive tumours or high-grade DCIS. Its role after surgery for small or low-grade DCIS is uncertain. It is recommended following mastectomy for patients at high risk of local recurrence (large size, high grade, node-positive or presence of vascular invasion).

Hormone therapy
All patients with ER-positive tumours should receive postoperative hormone therapy for 5 years.

- Tamoxifen is a selective ER modulator. It inhibits the expression of oestrogen-regulated genes, including growth factors and angiogenetic factors, resulting in a block in the G1 phase of the cell cycle and a slowing of tumour cell proliferation. Tumours may then regress because of this altered balance between cell proliferation and ongoing cell loss. Tamoxifen treatment results in a 50% annual reduction in the recurrence rate and a 28% annual reduction in death rate. There is similar reduction in the recurrence and death rates in women with positive and negative nodes. Tamoxifen may be used in women before or after menopause
- Aromatase inhibitors (AI) inhibit the conversion of androstenedione into oestrogen and hence reduce the levels of circulating oestrogen. In postmenopausal women they are effective in suppressing extra-ovarian oestrogen production in adipose tissue, muscle, and liver

Historically, ovarian ablation in premenopausal women has been achieved by either surgery or radiotherapy. More recently, luteinizing hormone-releasing hormone (LHRH) agonists have been used to block the pituitary secretion of FSH and LH, producing a reversible chemical oophorectomy.

Premenopausal women should receive tamoxifen, with those at higher risk benefiting from an LHRH agonist in addition. In postmenopausal women several large trials have shown that tamoxifen followed by an AI, to complete 5 years, is superior to tamoxifen alone. The ATAC study showed an AI alone (Arimidex) to be superior to tamoxifen for 5 years. A further study showed that women with a poorer prognosis may benefit from extended AI therapy (letrozole) following an initial 5 years of tamoxifen therapy.

Herceptin
About 25% of breast cancers overexpress receptors for epidermal growth factors (EGF-R) encoded by the *HER2* gene. These cancers carry an overall poor prognosis. Herceptin is a humanized monoclonal antibody against EGF-R and can be used in any patient with a tumour overexpressing *HER2*. Initial trials in both advanced and early breast cancer suggest an overall survival benefit.

Breast reconstruction
Mastectomy is still a commonly performed procedure and is associated with significant cosmetic and psychological morbidity. Breast reconstruction can be immediate or delayed, and aims to provide breast symmetry of volume and shape (projection and ptosis) with a comfortable breast mound. A contralateral procedure on the normal breast may also be needed. Reconstructive options include:

- **tissue expansion** with subpectoral tissue expanders (e.g. Becker's prosthesis) is relatively simple but can only match a small-to-medium-sized contralateral breast
- **pedicled flap** using a latissimus dorsi flap (+/- implant) is reliable with very low incidence of failure. It is also difficult to match a large contralateral breast and is unable to recreate the same degree of ptosis
- **free flap** options include a transverse rectus abdominus myocutaneous (TRAM) flap, a deep inferior epigastric perforator (DIEP) flap or a transverse myocutaneous gracilis (TMG) flap

Prognosis
Survival of breast cancer is dependent on tumour size, histological grade, nodal status, and age. Overall 20-year survival regardless of age, stage or treatment is over 78%. Five-year survival for women in the USA is 98% for localized breast disease. This decreased to 81% with nodal involvement and 25% with distant metastasis.

⊕ Wide local excision of breast lump and axillary clearance

Procedure
- Mark the side and position of the breast lump
- Position the patient supine, with the arm in abduction (take care to avoid brachial plexus injury)
- Inject Patent blue (2 mL under the ipsilateral nipple) if the patient is due to have sentinel node biopsy
- Place an incision along the skin crease, lift the cutaneous flaps, and dissect through breast tissue some 1 cm away from the tumour down to fascia surrounding the pectoralis major
- Make a second transverse incision in the axilla. Dissect through subcutaneous fat and clavipectoral fascia. Outline the lateral border of pectoralis major, identify the axillary vein and thoracodorsal pedicle. Try to protect the intercostobrachial nerves (although they could be divided if needed to ensure complete excision of the lymph nodes)
- The use of drains varies between centres

Complications

Intraoperative and early	Intermediate and late
- Haematoma,	- Local recurrence
- poor cosmesis,	- Lymphoedema
- arm numbness (division of intercostobrachial nerves)	

3.8 Goitre

The term goitre refers to an enlarged thyroid gland that is easily visible or palpable with the neck in a neutral position.

It is rare before puberty and declines with advancing age. It is more common in women (female:male 4:1). The condition is found worldwide, with endemic goitre in areas of iodine deficiency (e.g. mountainous regions).

Aetiology

Physiological

- Puberty and pregnancy are both periods of increased stress, requiring higher levels of thyroxine

Pathological

- Primary iodine deficiency ('endemic goitre')
- Secondary iodine deficiency owing to dyshormonogenesis or goitrogens (drugs—sulphonylureas; food stuffs—vegetables of the *Brassica* family, e.g. cabbage)
- Autoimmune (Grave's disease)
- Autoimmune thyroiditis (Hashimoto's disease, de Quervain's, and Reidel's thyroiditis)
- Inflammatory
- Neoplastic

Pathophysiology

Goitres result from follicular cell hyperplasia at one or more sites within the thyroid gland.

Non-toxic

- **Diffuse goitre** can be physiological or caused by primary (endemic) or secondary iodine deficiency
- **Multinodular non-toxic goitres** occur sporadically. They may develop from diffuse goitres. The diffuse hyperplasia becomes localized in areas of disorganized thyroid metabolism. The hyperplastic acini undergo a number of processes, including colloid involution, haemorrhage, cystic degeneration or necrosis. Longstanding goitres will become fibrosed and calcified
- **Solitary nodular non-toxic goitre** often turns out to be multinodular on USS or histological examination. The differential diagnosis includes benign adenoma, degenerative nodule, colloid cyst, carcinoma or secondary to thyroiditis

Toxic

- **Diffuse toxic goitre** occurs in Graves' disease and is a result of antibodies directed against the thyroid-stimulating hormone (TSH) receptor on the thyroid membrane
- **Toxic multinodular goitre** (Plummer's disease) is a result of tissue within a longstanding multinodular goitre producing excessive thyroid hormones leading to thyrotoxicosis
- **Toxic solitary nodular goitre** is a result of a single hyperplastic nodule. The size of the nodule correlates with the degree of hormone overproduction

Other conditions

- **Autoimmune thyroiditis** can lead to enlargement owing to lymphocytic infiltration
- **Acute suppurative thyroiditis** is rare. It usually results from *Staphylococcus aureus* or *Streptococcus pyogenes* infection. There is no thyroid dysfunction and it usually resolves with antibiotics
- **Primary thyroid carcinoma** or, very rarely, metastatic deposits can result in goitre.

Clinical assessment

Assessment should establish the underlying aetiology and the patient's thyroid status. Generally, goitres are asymptomatic although patients are often concerned about their poor aesthetic appearance.

History

- Growth pattern of goitre
- Obstructive symptoms include dysphagia, stridor, dyspnoea, voice change, and facial congestion
- Dietary intake of iodine
- Altered thyroid state (hypothyroidism or hyperthyroidism)
- Family history

Examination

- Neck examination, including the thyroid gland. General features (size, shape, asymmetry, consistency); mobility and relationship to swallowing; thyroid bruit
- Obstruction: retrosternal extension of the goitre may lead to narrowing of the thoracic inlet when the patient raises their arms above their head. A positive Pemberton sign is when this results in distended neck veins, facial plethora and, stridor
- Cervical lymphadenopathy
- Altered thyroid state: the majority of patients are euthyroid but signs of hyperthyroidism or hypothyroidism must be assessed

Investigations

- Bloods—normal TFTs (TSH, T_3, free T_4,) usually confirm a euthyroid state
- FNAC is highly accurate and cost-effective for investigating a solitary thyroid nodule
- Radionuclide thyroid imaging with [123]iodine or technetium-99m pertechnetate (^{99m}Tc) is used to assess a solitary toxic nodule or toxic multinodular goitre
- Chest radiograph may show retrosternal extension or tracheal deviation in large multinodular goitres (Fig 3.11)
- Neck USS is able to identify nodules as small as 0.3 mm in diameter and is useful in assessing multinodular goitres
- Chest CT or MRI define the anatomy in patients with possible intrathoracic extension and obstruction

Management

Conservative

Addition of iodine to the diet prevents endemic goitre. Thyroxine therapy has minimal efficacy in reducing the size of goitres in patients with iodine deficiency or subclinical hypothyroidism (i.e. when a raised TSH stimulates the enlargement of the thyroid gland).

Radioactive iodine for non-toxic goitres is used on mainland Europe but has not found favour in the UK or the USA. It induces a gradual destruction of thyroid tissue, with a decrease in goitre volume of up to 50% in 2 years.

Operative

Total thyroidectomy is the standard treatment. It offers immediate improvement of obstructive symptoms. Thyroid lobectomy is feasible if there is asymmetric enlargement, with only the one lobe creating the obstructive symptoms. Long-term thyroxine replacement is still needed in 30% of cases.

Table 3.8 WHO goitre grading system

Grade	Size of goitre
0	No goitre palpable or visible
1A	Goitre palpable but not visible
1B	Goitre palpable and visible but only with neck extended
2	Goitre visible with neck in normal position
3	Very large goitre visible from a distance

Indications for total thyroidectomy in patients with a goitre

- Suspicion of malignancy on clinical assessment or FNAC
- Compression of structures (e.g. trachea). Bleeding into an intrathoracic nodule can lead to a sudden increase in goitre size and airway obstruction
- Toxicity (hyperthyroidism)
- Anxiety and depression associated with poor cosmesis

Complications and prognosis

Many patients with simple goitres are happy to live with them once reassured that they are benign. Patients are advised about the symptoms of an altered thyroid state and malignancy.

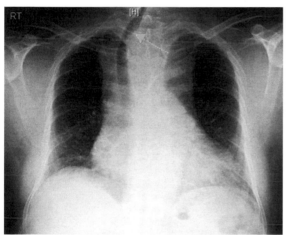

Fig 3.11 Chest radiograph (PA) showing a large retrosternal goitre arising from the left thyroid gland. The trachea is deviated to the right and slightly narrowed (arrow). The superior mediastinum is widened and the heart is enlarged.

⊚ Thyroid axis

Thyroid hormones play an important role in regulating the metabolic rate of most tissues. They are controlled by the hypothalamic–pituitary–thyroid axis.

Thyroid gland

Embryologically, the thyroid gland develops in the floor of the pharynx at the base of the tongue before descending along the thyroglossal duct to its usual position in the neck. Failure of the thyroid to migrate may lead to a lingual thyroid at the base of the adult tongue.

In the adult the thyroid gland is a bi-lobed structure lying in the anterior neck. The two lateral lobes are connected by the isthmus which may have an associated pyramidal lobe extending cephalad towards the base of the tongue.

The gland is tightly bound to the upper tracheal rings through Berry's ligament and this explains the upward movement of the thyroid during swallowing.

Biochemistry

The thyroid hormones T_3 (triiodothyronine) and T_4 (thyroxine) are synthesized in the thyroid gland by iodination of tyrosine. An excess of T_4 is produced which is converted in some peripheral tissues (kidney, liver, and muscle) to T_3 by monodeiodination. Over 99% of all T_3 and T_4 is bound to plasma proteins (thyroxine-binding globulin, TBG; thyroid-binding prealbumin, TBPA, albumin).

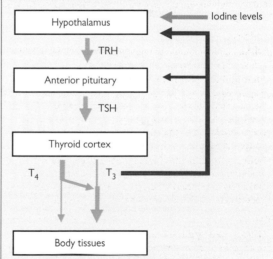

Fig 3.12 Hypothalamic–pituitary–thyroid axis.

1. Thyrotropin-releasing hormone (TRH) is released by the hypothalamus into the hypophysial portal circulation. This triggers the anterior pituitary thyrotroph cells to release thyroid-stimulating hormone (TSH)
2. TSH binds to specific G protein-coupled receptors on the membrane of thyroid cells to increase the synthesis of thyroid hormones and release stored hormones
3. Most circulating T_4 is converted to T_3 which is the active hormone. Unbound T_3 acts on the cell membrane, mitochondria, and cell nucleus
4. Negative feedback, predominantly by T_3 on the hypothalamic–pituitary–thyroid axis, inhibits secretion of TSH. Other factors, such as iodine availability and autoantibodies, play a role in regulation of thyroid function

51

3.9 Altered thyroid state

Hypothyroidism

Hypothyroidism is underactivity of the thyroid gland, leading to insufficient production or release of thyroid hormones. It is common and has a female preponderance (female:male 6:1).

Spontaneous primary atrophic autoimmune hypothyroidism is the most common cause. Other causes include:

- post-thyroidectomy or radioactive iodine ablation
- drug-induced: amiodarone, lithium
- iodine deficiency
- dyshormonogenesis
- rare: congenital (cretinism); secondary hypothyroidism due to pituitary insufficiency; tertiary hypothyroidism due to hypothalamic tumour

Clinical assessment

The symptoms and signs often have an insidious onset and are quite subtle (see box). Investigations include a FBC (normochromic macrocytic anaemia), TFT (high TSH, low free T_4), high triglycerides and cholesterol, antibodies to thyroid peroxidase, and antithyroglobulin in Hashimoto's thyroiditis.

Management

Low-dose levothyroxine (T_4) replacement therapy is slowly titrated to clinical state. The aim is to restore TSH to within normal range but not to cause suppression.

Hyperthyroidism

Hyperthyroidism (thyrotoxicosis) is caused by overactivity of the thyroid gland, leading to raised serum T_3 and T_4. The incidence is 30 per 1000 per year (UK), with peak incidence at 30–50 years old, with a female preponderance (female:male 3:1).

Aetiology

- Diffuse toxic goitre (Graves' disease) is most common
- Solitary toxic nodule
- Toxic multinodular goitre (Plummer's syndrome)
- Thyroiditis
- Rare causes: exogenous intake of thyroid hormones (factitious thyrotoxicosis), drugs (amiodarone), and TSH-secreting pituitary tumours

Pathophysiology

In Graves' disease, thyroid-stimulating IgG antibodies bind to TSH receptors and stimulate the thyroid cells to produce and secrete excessive amounts of thyroid hormones. The autoimmune process can also lead to mucopolysaccharide infiltration of the extraocular muscles.

Clinical assessment

Excess circulating thyroid hormones lead to hypermetabolism and heat production. Cardiac symptoms are caused by beta-adrenergic sympathetic stimulation (see box).

Investigations

- Bloods—TFTs (low TSH, high free T_4 and free T_3)
- Thyroid autoantibodies are positive in Graves' disease
- Radionuclide thyroid imaging (iodine or technetium) helps in distinguishing the diagnosis of Graves' disease (bilateral uptake), thyroiditis (no uptake), toxic nodule (unilateral uptake) or toxic multinodular goitre (uneven bilateral uptake).

Management

Antithyroid drugs block hormone synthesis. Carbimazole is favoured in the UK. Propylthiouracil, favoured in the USA, has the additional benefit of blocking the peripheral conversion of T_4 to T_3. Beta-blockers (e.g. propranolol) are used to control tachycardia and tremor.

Radioactive iodine (^{131}I) can be used to control thyrotoxicosis by destruction of thyroid tissue. Patients who are not candidates for ^{131}I therapy include those with severe eye disease, which could worsen after ^{131}I treatment; young women likely to be pregnant in the near future; patients who are the main carers of small children.

Operative

Total thyroidectomy for Graves' disease is indicated in patients who are not candidates for ^{131}I therapy and in those with persistent disease despite adequate medical therapy.

Surgical options include bilateral subtotal thyroidectomy or total thyroidectomy.

Complications and prognosis

Recurrence of hyperthyroidism may occur if drugs are discontinued in the treatment of toxic multinodular goitre. Patients require follow-up after thyroidectomy to detect hypothyroidism.

Thyrotoxic crisis

This is a rare presentation of extreme signs of thyrotoxicosis and severe metabolic disturbances. Precipitating causes can be non-thyroid surgery, major trauma, infection, or imaging studies with iodinated contrast medium in patients with unrecognized thyrotoxicosis.

Patients present with insomnia, anorexia, vomiting, diarrhoea, fever, and sweating. Early diagnosis and management is essential. Patients may require ITU admission.

Thyroiditis

A number of conditions cause local or diffuse inflammation of the thyroid which may result in thyroid dysfunction.

Subacute thyroiditis (de Quervain's)

Subacute or granulomatous thyroiditis is a self-limiting inflammation of the thyroid. It is probably viral in origin and is characterized by localized destruction of thyroid epithelium.

Approximately 60% of patients are symptomatic and present with a tender and enlarged thyroid associated with low-grade fever and myalgia. This usually follows an episode of sore throat or upper respiratory tract infection. They can have transitory signs of hyperthyroidism owing to release of hormones by destruction of thyroid follicles.

NSAIDs provide symptomatic relief. Antithyroid drugs are of no value as they do not prevent the destruction of follicles and release of excess thyroid hormones.

Autoimmune thyroiditis (Hashimoto's)

In autoimmune thyroiditis, 95% of patients have circulating autoantibodies against thyroglobulin and thyroid peroxidase.

The classical presentation is with a diffuse goitre although there may be nodularity and signs suggestive of hypothyroidism. Diagnosis is confirmed by measuring serum autoantibodies. FNAC is performed to exclude malignancy in patients with dominant nodules.

Thyroxine is prescribed for hypothyroid patients and leads to reduction in size of the goitre. This usually relieves pressure symptoms and avoids the need for surgery.

Acute suppurative thyroiditis
Acute infection of the thyroid causes an acute inflammatory response. It is most common in developing countries. The gland becomes painful, enlarged, and tender on palpation. FNA for microbiology confirms the diagnosis and guides antibiotic therapy.

Reidel's thyroiditis
This extremely rare condition is characterized by dense fibrosis of the thyroid and invasion of adjacent tissues. It may be associated with other idiopathic fibroses (e.g. retroperitoneal fibrosis). Patients present with a stony-hard enlargement or induration of the thyroid. Thyroid carcinoma needs to be excluded. FNAC is unhelpful and a biopsy is often needed instead.

⊙ Hypothyroidism versus hyperthyroidism	
Hypothyroidism	Hyperthyroidism
Symptoms	
• Cold intolerance	• Heat intolerance
• Weight gain	• Weight loss
• Tiredness and malaise	• Sweating
• Anorexia	• Tiredness and lethargy
• Constipation	• Diarrhoea and vomiting
• Menorrhagia, hoarse voice	• Irritability and emotionally labile
Signs	
• Mental slowness	• Warm, sweaty skin and hands
• 'Peaches and cream' complexion	• Tachycardia and arrhythmias
• Coarse skin and dry hair, oedema	• Goitre (>80%)
• Bradycardia	• Pretibial myxoedema
• Pericardial effusion	• Thyroid acropachy (clubbing seen with Graves')

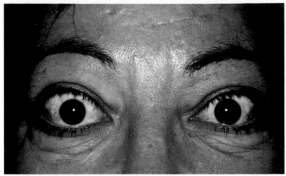

Fig 3.13 Middle-aged woman with thyroid eye disease. There is lid retraction as a result of the proptosis.

Grading of ophthalmic Graves' disease

Grade 1   No signs or symptoms
Grade 2   Only signs, no symptoms
Grade 3   Proptosis
Grade 4   Extraocular muscle involvement
Grade 5   Corneal involvement (conjunctival oedema, corneal scarring)
Grade 6   Optic nerve involvement leading to loss of sight

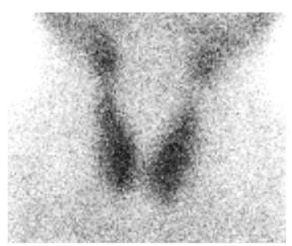

Fig 3.14 Radionuclide thyroid imaging using iodine. There is normal uptake in the thyroid gland.

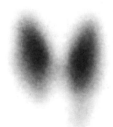

Fig 3.15 Radionuclide thyroid imaging using iodine. There is bilateral increased uptake seen in Graves' disease.

3.10 Thyroid cancer

Thyroid cancer is rare and accounts for 1% of all malignancies. The incidence is 4 per 100 000 per year (UK) with a peak at 30–50 years and a female preponderance (female:male 3:1). Papillary cancers are more common in iodine-rich areas, follicular cancers in iodine-deficient areas.

Aetiology

The aetiology is unknown, but associations include exposure to low-dose environmental radiation or high-dose head and neck radiotherapy. Regions where goitre is endemic have a high incidence.

Pathophysiology

The five histological types of thyroid cancer are papillary, follicular, medullary, anaplastic, and lymphoma.

Papillary carcinoma (70%)

- Most common in children and young adults
- Patients are euthyroid
- Slow-growing well-differentiated tumour, often multifocal
- FNAC demonstrates characteristic nuclear grooves, intranuclear inclusions or 'optically clear nuclei'—Orphan Annie cells and psammoma bodies
- Lymphatic spread to cervical lymph nodes
- Good prognosis

Follicular carcinoma (20%)

- Patients are euthyroid
- Follicular adenoma is a benign tumour that grows in a glandular or follicular pattern. It is well encapsulated and leads to compression of normal thyroid tissue
- There are two histologically distinct groups of carcinoma: (1) minimally invasive follicular cancers are small, encapsulated neoplasms that show invasion only into the tumour capsule. Vascular and lymphatic invasion is normally absent. They are associated with an excellent prognosis; (2) widely invasive follicular cancers exhibit invasion through the capsule into the surrounding thyroid tissue and local structures
- Haematogenous spread to the lungs

Medullary carcinoma (10%)

- Rare cancer—75% are sporadic, and the rest are familial
- Derived from calcitonin-secreting parafollicular C cells
- Sporadic tumours tend to be single and unilateral
- Familial tumours are often multicentric and bilateral and feature as part of the MEN 2 syndrome.

Anaplastic carcinoma

These tumours are very rare and extremely aggressive. They are characteristically seen in older women and present as a hard woody goitre. They are diagnosed on FNAC or core biopsy. Following surgical excision, patients are treated with external beam radiotherapy.

Thyroid lymphoma

Rarely, lymphomas of the mucosa-associated lymphoid tissue (MALToma) can occur. The majority are non-Hodgkin's lymphomas. Longstanding Hashimoto's thyroiditis may predispose to thyroid lymphoma.

Clinical assessment

Most thyroid nodules are asymptomatic and a chance discovery by the patient or during a routine general examination.

History

- Previous neck irradiation
- Family history of thyroid carcinoma
- Symptoms of altered thyroid status (see Topic 3.9)
- Rare symptoms: pain, haemoptysis, vocal cord paralysis, carcinoid symptoms

Examination

- Solitary versus multiple nodules
- Nodule characteristics: firm/hard or fixed nodules are more likely to be a cancer. Rapid increase in size of a previously static longstanding nodule is worrying (particularly in an elderly patient)
- Signs of altered thyroid status
- Cervical lymphadenopathy
- Voice changes: recurrent laryngeal nerve palsy suggests an invasive cancer
- Retrosternal extension should be assessed

Investigations

- Bloods—thyroid function tests are usually normal
- FNAC is the first line diagnostic test for all thyroid nodules but cannot reliably distinguish between follicular adenomas and follicular cancer
- USS of the neck can localize and determine whether a nodule is solitary or part of a multinodular goitre
- Radionuclide thyroid imaging with iodine (^{123}I or ^{131}I) or technetium 99m pertechnetate have been largely superseded by FNAC and USS
- Unenhanced CT or MRI scans are used for staging

Table 3.9	Classification of thyroid FNAC
Thy1	Insufficient material
Thy2	Benign (e.g. colloid nodule)
Thy3	Follicular lesion (i.e. either an adenoma or a carcinoma, the distinction being possible only after excision biopsy and histological analysis
Thy4	Suspicious but not diagnostic of malignancy
Thy5	Definite malignancy

Management

Operative

Surgical resection is the mainstay of treatment. There are a number of options:

- Lobectomy and isthmusectomy is the minimum operation for thyroid tumours. It is curative for colloid nodule (alleviating pressure symptoms), enables full histological diagnosis in suspicious (Thy3) follicular lesions, and it is considered curative for micropapillary cancers (<1 cm) and for minimally invasive follicular cancers
- Completion thyroidectomy after initial lobectomy is necessary for papillary thyroid cancers larger than 1–2 cm in diameter and for widely invasive follicular cancers

- Subtotal thyroidectomy
- Total thyroidectomy is indicated for all palpable thyroid cancers diagnosed on FNA
- Selective neck dissection is performed in patients presenting with palpable cervical lymphadenopathy and in all patients with medullary thyroid cancer

Postoperative medical management

T_3 substitution (liothyronine) is used in the immediate postoperative period in patients due to undergo ^{131}I ablation of the thyroid remnants after total thyroidectomy. The shorter half-life of T_3 means it can be stopped for only 2 weeks to allow a raise in TSH that would favour uptake of ^{131}I in any remaining thyroid cells.

T_4 replacement (thyroxine) is used to maintain a suppressed TSH. This has been shown to decrease the risk of contra-lateral disease in patients undergoing lobectomy and to reduce the risk of local recurrence or metastatic disease in patients following total thyroidectomy.

Iodine-131 is used after total thyroidectomy to destroy any remaining thyroid or metastatic cells.

Recombinant human TSH (rhTSH, Thyrotropin®) has recently become available as a means of inducing ^{131}I uptake without having to stop thyroid hormone replacement therapy (therefore avoiding the distressing symptoms of hypothyroidism in the weeks before and after the ^{131}I scan).

Complications and prognosis

Papillary and follicular carcinomas have excellent long-term survival (up to 90% at 20 years). Patients with anaplastic cancers rarely survive more than a few months.

✛ Total thyroidectomy

Check that patient is euthyroid or that hyperthyroidism is well controlled on medication.

Assess for possible retrosternal extension of a goitre that would have implications for the anaesthetist. Preoperative laryngoscopy documents recurrent laryngeal nerve function.

Procedure

- Position the patient supine with the neck extended
- Skin-crease incision (collar) ~2 cm above sternal notch, extending 3–5 cm from the midline
- Lift subplatysmal flaps, identify midline between strap muscles, lift and retract laterally the sternohyoid and sternothyroid muscles, and expose the thyroid lobe
- Upper pole of the thyroid is dissected and superior thyroid artery ligated above the thyroid (avoiding injury to superior laryngeal nerve)
- Lower pole is mobilized and recurrent laryngeal nerve identified and followed up to entry point in the larynx
- Parathyroid glands are identified. They should be mobilized away from the thyroid capsule, preserving their vascular supply
- Close in layers (strap muscles and platysma separately)
- Drains are not routinely used

Complications

Intraoperative and early	Intermediate and late
- Primary haemorrhage	- Hypocalcaemia
- Acute airway obstruction	- Hypothyroidism
- Recurrent laryngeal and/ or superior laryngeal nerve injury	
- Thyrotoxic crisis	

Haemorrhage

Postoperative haemorrhage can cause acute airway obstruction. The mechanism is usually severe laryngeal oedema caused by venous congestion as a result of an expanding haematoma rather than direct compression of the trachea. Immediate management includes:

- ABC and call for senior anaesthetic and surgical assistance
- evacuation of the haematoma by removing the skin and deep sutures should *not* be delayed by putting in lines or waiting for assistance
- sit the patient up and give 100% O_2
- secure wide bore IV access

Nerve injury

Bilateral incomplete right laryngeal nerve injury leaves the cords adducted and causes airway obstruction and respiratory distress. Patients require re-intubation and tracheostomy. Bilateral complete right laryngeal nerve injury leaves the cords abducted in the cadaveric position. There is limited dyspnoea and the voice is absent.

Superior laryngeal nerve injury is usually to the external branch which is the motor supply to the cricothyroid. This adducts and tenses the cords. Unilateral weakness causes a change in voice.

3.11 Parathyroid conditions

There are usually four parathyroid glands (paired inferior and superior glands) situated posterior to the thyroid gland. They secrete parathyroid hormone (PTH) which is involved in calcium homeostasis (see box).

Primary hyperparathyroidism

Primary hyperparathyroidism (PHP) is overactivity of one or more parathyroid glands, leading to secretion of excessive PTH and subsequent hypercalcaemia. Incidence is 3 per 1000 per year (UK) and is highest in postmenopausal women (female:male 2:1).

Aetiology

- Single adenoma (87%) or multiple adenomas (3%)
- Hyperplasia of multiple glands (9% of sporadic cases but almost all MEN cases)
- Primary parathyroid carcinoma is rare (<1%)

Pathophysiology

High circulating levels of PTH result in excessive resorption of calcium and phosphate from bone. This leads to osteopenia and, rarely, osteitis fibrosa cystica, and brown tumour (osteoclastoma) of long bones. The rest of the pathology is a result of hypercalcaemia.

Clinical assessment

Most patients are said to be asymptomatic but there are often occult symptoms that can be attributed to PHP. The diagnosis is often made following a routine blood test showing hypercalcaemia.

Symptoms are related to the elevated PTH or hypercalcaemia, sometimes remembered as 'stone, bones, abdominal groans, and psychic moans.'

- Raised PTH: urinary tract stones owing to excessive calcium excretion, and bone pains and pathological fractures due to osteopenia
- Hypercalcaemia: fatigue, abdominal pain (peptic ulcers, pancreatitis), vomiting, constipation, polyuria, polydypsia, psychiatric disturbance (depression, confusion)

Investigations

- Bloods—high ionized calcium and PTH with a low phosphate is diagnostic. Patients with bone metastases have a suppressed PTH and a small subset of patients have normocalcaemic hyperparathyroidism. Vitamin D levels are taken as deficiency can lead to elevated PTH
- High 24 h urinary calcium excludes familial hypocalciuric hypercalcaemia
- Tumours are localized by a combination of high resolution ultrasound and technetium-99m sestamibi scanning. CT or MRI is rarely helpful except in cases of mediastinal parathyroid tumour
- Venous sampling and angiography are helpful in locating missing glands in redo parathyroid surgery

Management

Surgical excision of affected glands offers the only cure for PHP. This should be offered to all symptomatic patients and those asymptomatic patients with Ca^{2+} >2.90 mmol/L.

Operative

Complete neck exploration identifies all of the glands. Single adenomas are excised with the other glands left alone. Multiple gland hyperplasia is treated by subtotal parathyroidectomy, leaving only half of one gland behind. This is often grafted into the forearm to avoid further neck surgery if there is recurrence.

Minimally invasive parathyroidectomy (MIP) is feasible when imaging studies reliably identify the position of the adenoma. This is a focused neck exploration though a lateral cervical incision aiming to remove the adenoma visualized on scanning without exploring the other parathyroid glands.

Complications and prognosis

Serum calcium is monitored twice daily as there is a risk of marked hypocalcaemia caused by the 'hungry bone syndrome', hypomagnesaemia, and hypofunction of parathyroid remnants or grafts.

Recurrent hyperparathyroidism occurs in 8% of cases and is a result of incomplete removal of diseased tissue.

Hypocalcaemia may be transient if parathyroid tissue is left but will be permanent if all the glands are removed. This requires lifelong calcium and vitamin D supplements.

Secondary hyperparathyroidism

Secondary hyperparathyroidism (SPH) is caused by excessive secretion of PTH in response to a chronic abnormal stimulus.

Chronic renal failure and vitamin D deficiency are the most common causes. The mechanisms include hyperphosphataemia, a deficit of calcitriol synthesis owing to decreased hydroxylation of vitamin D precursors by the kidney, and reduced expression of vitamin D receptors.

A low calcium intake and calcium-depleted dialysate increase the risk of developing SPH in patients with CRF.

All four glands become hyperplastic in an attempt to normalize serum calcium levels. This may progress from diffuse to nodular hyperplasia and possible adenoma formation.

Clinical assessment

History

Pruritus is a disabling symptom that affects most patients on haemodialysis for CRF. Muscle weakness, proximal myopathy, and easy fatiguability are often present.

Examination

- Osteitis fibrosa cystica or osteomalacia may eventually lead to skeletal deformities or fractures, e.g. funnel chest deformity and sternal bowing owing to rib deformities
- Reduced height—kyphosis and vertebral crush fractures
- Soft tissue calcification may compress adjacent structures, causing pain, organ dysfunction, and cosmetic deformities
- Calciphylaxis is a rare condition in which patients develop severe calf pain and tenderness caused by extensive non-ulcerating, hard and tender subcutaneous calcification. These cutaneous lesions progress to skin and subcutaneous necrosis, deep non-healing ulcers and gangrene

Investigations

- Bloods—high serum PTH and phosphate with low or normal calcium. High serum alkaline phosphatase is associated with bone disease. Vitamin D levels
- Radiographs are not routine. Skull radiograph may show a 'pepper pot' appearance owing to irregular demineralization.

Management

Medical management aims to maintain calcium and phosphate levels close to normal levels, to suppress PTH secretion, and to prevent the bone disease. The definitive treatment in patients with CRF is renal transplantation.

- Oral calcium supplements and calcium added to dialysate
- Oral vitamin D supplements
- Dietary phosphate restriction, phosphate-binding agents
- Pruritus is ameliorated by charcoal haemoperfusion in conjunction with standard haemodialysis
- Calcimimetics (Cinacalcet®) stimulate the parathyroid calcium-sensing receptor, hence inhibit PTH synthesis and secretion, and decrease parathyroid cell volume and potentially prevent development of SPH

Operative

- Total parathyroidectomy: all four glands are located and resected. Transcervical thymectomy should be routine, aiming to remove supranumerary glands or embryonic remnants. This method is currently favoured in most centres
- Subtotal parathyroidectomy: resection of 3½ glands, leaving approximately 50 mg of viable parathyroid tissue *in situ*
- Total parathyroidectomy plus autotransplantation: the parathyroid gland which macroscopically looks most normal and on frozen sections shows predominantly diffuse hyperplasia (i.e. not nodular hyperplasia) is selected for autografting in the forearm flexor mass

Tertiary hyperparathyroidism

Tertiary hyperparathyroidism is the autonomous hypersecretion of PTH without an abnormal stimulus. It classically occurs In patients with longstanding SPH caused by CRF. Following renal transplantation there is resolution of the renal stimuli and normalization of serum calcium, but continued hypersecretion of PTH. Most cases resolve spontaneously. Parathyroidectomy is indicated if there is no resolution by 1 year.

⊙ Hypercalcaemic crisis

Hypercalcaemia is seen in up to 5% of hospital inpatients. In the majority of cases it is mild or moderate and clinically asymptomatic. A hypercalcaemic crisis (serum Ca^{2+} >14 mg/dL) is life-threatening.

Aetiology
- Malignancy—bone metastases, primary tumours secreting PTH-related peptide, multiple myeloma, lymphoma
- Hyperparathyroidism—PHP, familial hypocalciuric hypercalcaemia, MEN, lithium
- Increased bone turnover—prolonged immobilization, hyperthyroidism, thiazide diuretics
- Excess vitamin D—vitamin D intoxication, sarcoidosis
- Renal failure

Clinical assessment
- Acute confusion
- Dehydration and oliguria
- Weakness and malaise
- Abdominal pain with nausea and vomiting

Management
- First aim is fluid resuscitation which increases the renal excretion of calcium. It is guided by severity and until adequate urine output is achieved

- Loop diuretic increases urinary excretion of calcium
- Bisphosphonates are an effective treatment for acute hypercalcaemia in patients with metastatic bone disease, but should be avoided in patients with PHP as they impair the ability to maintain normocalcaemia following parathyroidectomy

⊙ Calcium homeostasis

Calcium is essential for many bodily functions, including bone formation, clotting, muscle contraction, regulation of membrane potentials, and intracellular signalling.

Calcium is absorbed by the intestine and excreted by the kidney. The majority of body calcium is stored in bone (99%). The daily flux between these three sites leads to tight regulation of serum calcium (2.12–2.65 mmol/L).

Parathyroid hormone
PTH is released by the chief cells in the parathyroid gland in response to hypocalcaemia. It plays the most important role in calcium homeostasis.

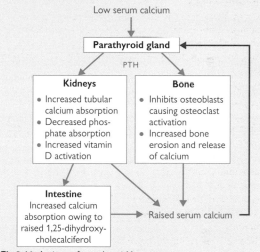

Fig 3.16 Actions of parathyroid hormones.

Vitamin D
The primary source of vitamin D is from the conversion of 7-dehydrocholesterol to cholecalciferol (D_3) by ultraviolet activation in the skin. Cholecalciferol then undergoes further metabolism in the liver and kidney to produce the active product, 1,25-dihydroxycholecalciferol.

Activated vitamin D increases absorption of calcium and phosphate in the kidneys, stimulates osteoblasts to form new bone, and increases calcium and phosphate absorption in the intestine.

Calcitonin
Calcitonin is not essential for calcium homeostasis. It is secreted by parafollicular cells in the thyroid gland in response to hypercalcaemia. It acts by inhibiting the reabsorption of calcium and phosphate by the kidney and osteoclast activity in bone.

The two adrenal glands are retroperitoneal structures that sit on the upper poles of the kidneys. Microscopically they have an outer cortex and an inner medulla.

The cortex is divided into three layers. The zona glomerulosa secretes mineralocorticoids (e.g. aldosterone); the zona fasciculata is the largest zone and secretes glucocorticoids (e.g. cortisol); and the zona reticularis secretes sex hormones. The medulla secretes catecholamines (norepinephrine and epinephrine) and dopamine.

Primary hypoadrenalism

Primary hypoadrenalism is an uncommon condition in which there is adrenal insufficiency following destruction of the entire adrenal cortex.

Ninety per cent of cases are caused by autoimmune adrenalitis (Addison's disease), although historically tuberculosis was the main cause. Rarer causes include bilateral adrenalectomy and metastatic deposits.

Clinical assessment

Symptoms are often vague, with non-specific malaise, weakness, anorexia, and weight loss. It can also present as an emergency (Addisonian crisis), with vomiting, weakness, and profound hypovolaemic shock.

Common signs include postural hypotension from salt and water loss; grey–brown pigmentation of the buccal mucosa, flexor creases, and new scars owing to excess ACTH stimulation of melanocytes. Other signs include loss of body hair and vitiligo.

Acute insufficiency requires urgent treatment before formal investigation. Blood tests may show a low plasma cortisol with high ACTH, hyponatraemia, hyperkalaemia, raised urea, and hypoglycaemia. The short synacthen test is usually diagnostic.

Management

Acute adrenal insufficiency is treated with intravenous steroids (hydrocortisone 100 mg IV), fluid resuscitation, and 50 mL of 50% dextrose if hypoglycaemia is present.

In the long term, patients need lifelong glucocorticoid and mineralocorticoid replacement therapy. Higher doses are needed during periods of stress (e.g. infection and surgery. www.addisons.org.uk). They should also wear a MedicAlert bracelet and carry a 'steroid card' detailing their condition.

Secondary hypoadrenalism

Secondary hypoadrenalism is caused by low ACTH. This is caused by either hypothalamic–pituitary disease or long-term steroid therapy causing suppression of the adrenal axis. The long synacthen test differentiates between primary and secondary hypoadrenalism. Management is with a glucocorticoid in patients not already on steroids.

Cushing's syndrome

Cushing's syndrome is the collection of symptoms and signs associated with excess circulating corticosteroids.

Aetiology

The causes are either ACTH-dependent or independent. The commonest cause is long-term steroid therapy.

ACTH-dependent

- Pituitary adenoma secreting ACTH (Cushing's disease)
- Ectopic secretion of ACTH by small cell lung cancer and carcinoids (25%)

ACTH-independent

- Iatrogenic long-term steroid therapy
- Adrenal cortical adenoma or carcinoma (50%)
- Bilateral adrenal hyperplasia (rare)

Clinical assessment
History

Symptoms are non-specific and include weight gain, lethargy, muscle weakness, menstrual irregularities, and psychological disturbance (depression, psychosis).

Examination

Common signs include facial plethora, truncal obesity, kyphosis, and buffalo hump (Fig 3.18). Proximal muscle wasting and myopathy add to the overall appearance of a 'lemon on sticks'. Other problems include hypertension, osteoporosis, pathological fractures, and impaired glucose tolerance or diabetes.

Investigations

- High midnight cortisol level >50 nmol/L is diagnostic and confirms loss of the cortisol diurnal rhythm which has a morning peak and night-time low
- High 24 h urinary cortisol reflects the elevated plasma cortisol level
- Dexamethasone suppression tests establish cause
- CT or MRI scans are used to localize suspected adrenal, pituitary or ectopic lesions
- Chest radiograph may identify an ACTH-secreting bronchial carcinoma

Management
Operative

Surgery is the preferred option for both adrenal and pituitary disease.

Unilateral laparoscopic adrenalectomy is used to excise adrenocortical adenomas. Carcinomas are often larger tumours and are removed via an open approach.

Pituitary adenomas are excised via a trans-sphenoidal approach. Bilateral adrenalectomy is indicated if the pituitary surgery is unsuccessful (~40% of cases) or if there is an unidentified ectopic source of ACTH.

Medical

Metyrapone and ketoconazole can be used preoperatively to decrease cortisol synthesis.

Steroid replacement therapy is vital after unilateral or bilateral adrenalectomy. Patients with solitary adrenal tumours have an atrophied contralateral adrenal gland which may take a year to return to normal function.

Table 3.10 Tests used in the diagnosis of adrenal conditions

ACTH (synacthen) tests used in the diagnosis of hypoadrenalism	
Test and protocol	**Result and clinical use**
Short • 250 mcg tetracosactrin IM given at time 0 • Plasma cortisol measured at time 0 (baseline) and at +30 min	Normal patients have a 30 min cortisol >600 nmol/L with a rise of >330 nmol/L. An inadequate rise suggests hypoadrenalism
Long • 1 mg tetracosactrin IM given at time 0 • Plasma cortisol measured at time 0 (baseline) and +1, +4, +8, and +24 h	Normal patients have a 4-h cortisol of >1000 nmol/L. Primary hypoadrenalism gives low cortisol levels throughout. Secondary hypoadrenalism gives a delayed but normal response
Dexamethasone suppression tests used in the diagnosis of Cushing's syndrome	
Test and protocol	**Results and clinical use**
Overnight • 1 mg dexamethasone given at bedtime (22.00) • Plasma cortisol measured the next morning (09.00)	Normal patients have a suppressed morning cortisol which is not seen with Cushing's syndrome. This is a useful outpatient screening test
Low dose • 0.5 mg dexamethasone given qds for 48 h • Plasma cortisol measured day 0 (baseline) and day 2	Normal patients have a suppressed day 2 cortisol which is not seen with Cushing's syndrome. This establishes the diagnosis of Cushing's syndrome
High dose • 2 mg dexamethasone given qds for 48 h • Plasma cortisol and urinary steroids measured day 0 (baseline) and day 2	A day 2 cortisol <50% of baseline suggests pituitary rather than adrenal disease as it inhibits ACTH secretion. This helps to establish the cause of Cushing's syndrome

⊙ Glucocorticoid axis

Biochemistry

All steroids are derived from cholesterol and share a basic structure. Glucocorticoids are so named because one of their main actions is to increase gluconeogenesis and glycogen deposition. Other effects include increased protein catabolism and fat deposition.

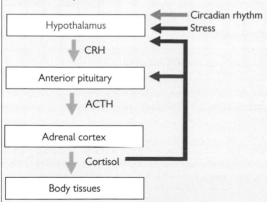

Fig 3.17 Hypothalamic–pituitary–corticotrophic axis

1. Hypothalamus secretes corticotrophin-releasing hormone (CRH) in response to stress and the circadian rhythm. This stimulates the anterior pituitary to secrete ACTH
2. ACTH acts on adrenocortical cells and stimulates cortisol production from cholesterol
3. Cortisol is secreted by the zona fasciculata into the systemic circulation. It acts on the body's tissues and has an inhibitory effect on the hypothalamus and anterior pituitary

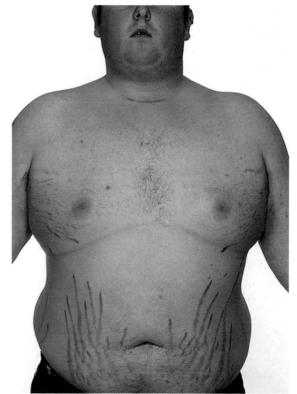

Fig 3.18 A young man with Cushing's syndrome. Note the facial plethora, moon face, truncal obesity, and purple abdominal striae.

Primary hyperaldosteronism

Primary hyperaldosteronism is the excessive secretion of the mineralocorticoid hormone aldosterone independent of the renin–angiotensin system.

Secondary hyperaldosteronism is caused by elevated renin as a result of stimulation of the renin–angiotensin system (e.g. renal artery stenosis, diuretics, left ventricular dysfunction).

Aetiology

Dr Jerome W. Conn [1907–1981, American endocrinologist] first described the condition in 1955.

- Unilateral adrenocortical adenoma secreting aldosterone accounts for over 50% of cases (Conn's syndrome)
- Idiopathic bilateral adrenal hyperplasia (30%)
- Rare causes: glucocorticoid-remediable aldosteronism (GRA), adrenocortical carcinomas, and ovarian tumours.

Clinical assessment

Hypertension is usually asymptomatic. Symptoms of hypokalaemia are rare but patients may experience muscle weakness, cramping, intermittent paralysis, headaches, polydypsia, polyuria, and nocturia.

Investigations

- Bloods—serum K$^+$<3 mmol/L with 24 h urinary K$^+$>40 mmol/L
- Ratio of serum aldosterone to renin activity is the screening test of choice. Aldosterone is elevated and the plasma renin activity is suppressed. False-positive results occur in patients on beta-blockers, clonidine, NSAIDS, the contraceptive pill or those with renal impairment. False-negative results can be obtained in patients on diuretics, ACE inhibitors, renovascular hypertension, calcium blockers, and very low sodium diet
- Abdominal CT or MRI used for tumour localization
- Sampling of aldosterone and cortisol concentrations in each adrenal vein are used to demonstrate unilateral secretion of excessive amounts of aldosterone. Patients in whom localization is not confirmed may have bilateral adrenal hyperplasia and should be treated medically

Management

The aim of treatment is to reduce the morbidity associated with hypertension and hypokalaemia.

Conn's syndrome is treated surgically with laparoscopic adrenalectomy. Hypokalaemia is corrected preoperatively with spironolactone and/or oral potassium supplements. The blood pressure response to spironolactone preoperatively is a predictor of the blood pressure response to unilateral adrenalectomy.

Bilateral adrenal hyperplasia is treated with spironolactone or amiloride diuretics.

Phaeochromocytoma

Phaeochromocytomas are rare neuroendocrine tumours of the adrenal medulla that secrete excessive amounts of catecholamines and related products. They are usually sporadic, benign, and unilateral. However, approximately 10% are malignant, bilateral, or ectopic (extra-adrenal).

They are rarely associated with familial conditions such as MEN, neurofibromatosis, and von Hippel–Lindau syndrome.

Clinical assessment

Paroxysmal secretion of excess catecholamines gives rise to intermittent 'attacks' characterized by headache, sweating, palpitations, paroxysmal hypertension, and a feeling of impending doom. These episodes are often triggered by activities that cause mechanical pressure on the tumour.

Only 50% of patients have persistent hypertension. The rest are normotensive or hypotensive between episodes. The diagnosis should be considered in patients with characteristic paroxysmal episodes, unusually labile or intermittent hypertension, family history of phaeochromocytoma or related conditions (📖 Topic 3.14), and in hypertensive children.

Investigations

- 24 h urinary metanephrines are high (metabolites of catecholamines)
- Plasma metanephrines and free catecholamine levels are also high but difficult to measure
- Abdominal CT or MRI scans demonstrate the side of the adrenal tumour
- Functional imaging with MIBG (iodine-131-meta-iodobenzylguanidine) scintiscan demonstrates characteristic uptake in the adrenal tumour and ectopic sites of chromaffin tissue

Management

Once the diagnosis is made, the patient should be immediately blocked with alpha-adrenergic drugs (phenoxybenzamine or doxazosin). Once these are well established a beta-blocker (propranolol) can be added to control tachycardia.

Laparoscopic adrenalectomy is the treatment of choice for small benign tumours. Open adrenalectomy is reserved for large or malignant tumours.

Adrenal incidentaloma

Adrenal masses are found incidentally in approximately 1% of abdominal CT or MRI scans. There is a long list of differential diagnoses, many of which require no further investigation or treatment.

A careful clinical assessment looks for imbalance in the adrenal axis, such as Cushing's syndrome, hypertension, and diabetes. Simple investigations, including routine bloods and a chest radiograph, may reveal the cause. If this is not endocrine, investigations will be required and potentially further imaging and biopsy.

Non-secreting masses <3–4 cm in diameter can be followed up with annual CT scans. Larger masses should be excised as 30% turn out to be adrenocortical carcinomas.

⊙ Renin–angiotensin–aldosterone axis

The renin–angiotensin system regulates arterial blood pressure. Inactive renin is stored in the juxtaglomerular cells of the kidney. It is released in response to three main stimuli:

1. Reduced renal perfusion due to systemic hypotension or renal artery stenosis
2. Sympathetic stimulation acting via beta$_1$-adrenoceptors

3. Reduced sodium delivery to the distal tubules of the nephron.

Atrial and brain natriuretic peptides (ANP and BNP) oppose the effects of renin by increasing water and salt excretion (natriuresis) by the kidney. They are released in response to raised blood pressure (i.e. increased atrial stretch).

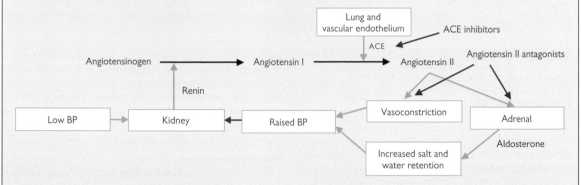

Fig 3.19 Renin–angiotensin–aldosterone axis

1. Low perfusion pressure in the kidney stimulates the juxtaglomerular apparatus to release renin
2. Renin catalyses the cleavage of angiotensin I from angiotensinogen (a circulating alpha2-globulin)
3. A further two amino acids are cleaved from angiotensin I to form angiotensin II. This is catalysed by angiotensin-converting enzyme (ACE) which is mainly found in the lung and vascular endothelium

4. Angiotensin II causes powerful and rapid vasoconstriction. It also stimulates adrenal cells in the zona glomerulosa to produce aldosterone. Angiotensin II is rapidly metabolized
5. Aldosterone causes sodium retention from urine, sweat, saliva, and gastric juice, and increased potassium excretion by increasing the exchange between Na^+ and K^+/H^+ in the renal tubules. This slowly increases the extracellular fluid volume over hours to days
6. Both vasoconstriction and salt and water retention increase renal perfusion, which reduces renin release

61

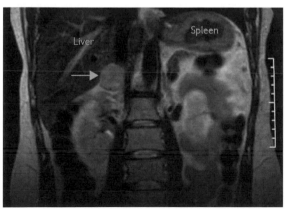

Fig 3.20 Abdominal MRI (coronal section) showing a mass in the right adrenal gland (arrow). This is a large phaeochromocytoma that went on to be resected.

3.14 Multiple endocrine neoplasia

Multiple endocrine neoplasia (MEN) syndromes are characterized by the occurrence of tumours in two or more endocrine glands. They are rare inherited autosomal dominant disorders with two major forms: MEN Type 1 (Wermer's syndrome) and MEN Type 2 (Sipple's syndrome).

MEN 1

MEN 1 is characterized by tumours of the parathyroid (95%), pancreatic islet cells (40%), and anterior pituitary (30%). The gene for MEN 1 is located on chromosome 11q13 and encodes a nuclear protein named MENIN whose role in endocrine cell growth control is yet to be defined.

Clinical assessment

Hyperparathyroidism is the most common manifestation of MEN 1. The majority of pancreatic islet cell tumours are non-functioning and clinically silent, although they may be radiologically and biochemically detectable. Prolactinomas are the most commonly detected pituitary tumours.

Management

Primary hyperparathyroidism can be managed with subtotal or total parathyroidectomy. Transcervical thymectomy is recommended at the same time.

Insulinomas are usually excised, but other pancreatic islet cell tumours respond to medical management (e.g. proton-pump inhibitors to treat gastrinoma). The indications and timing of surgery in these cases are controversial.

Prolactinomas can be treated with dopamine agonists. Hypophysectomy and external beam irradiation are considered for other pituitary tumours.

Screening

Lifelong clinical, biochemical, and radiological screening is required in patients with MEN 1 owing to the multiple and metachronous nature of tumours. Genetic screening can be used for offspring of known index cases. Because 10% of MENIN mutations are *de novo*, siblings of an index case are not necessarily at risk.

- Parathyroid adenoma: serum ionized Ca^{2+}, PTH
- Pancreatic islet cell: serum glucose, insulin, gastrin, glucagon, somatostatin, VIP, pancreatic polypeptide
- Anterior pituitary: prolactin and insulin-growth factor 1
- MRI scan is performed every 3–5 years after age 20

Table 3.11 Tumours associated with MEN 1

Endocrine gland	Tumours
Parathyroid	Adenoma
Pancreatic islet cells	Gastrinoma Insulinoma Glucagonoma VIPoma Pancreatic polypeptide-producing tumour
Anterior pituitary	Prolactinoma (20%) Non-functioning tumour Somatotropinoma Corticotropinoma
Other tumours	Bronchial and intestinal carcinoids Adrenocortical tumours Cutaneous lipomas Facial angiofibromas

MEN 2

MEN 2 can be subdivided into several discrete forms.

- MEN 2A is defined by medullary thyroid carcinoma (MTC) associated with phaeochromocytoma (50%) and primary hyperparathyroidism (15%)
- MEN 2B is defined by MTC and phaeochromocytoma associated with a marfanoid habitus, decreased upper to lower body ratio, mucosal neuromas, and gastrointestinal ganglioneuromatosis
- Familial MTC is described as occurrence of MTC in 10 or more family members without the other characteristic associations of MEN 2 syndrome

The gene for MEN 2 is *RET*, a proto-oncogene located on chromosome 10q11. It encodes a cell-surface glycoprotein member of receptor tyrosine kinases. Point mutations in specific parts of the *RET* gene determine the severity of the clinical syndromes.

Clinical assessment

Although MEN 2 can present with many different signs and symptoms, a thyroid nodule as a result of MTC is the most common. Phaeochromocytomas present in a similar way to sporadic disease and are frequently bilateral. Hyperparathyroidism is usually asymptomatic.

Screening

Genetic screening with demonstration of point mutations of the *RET* gene identifies gene carriers with 100% accuracy. This allows identification of children at risk before the biochemical screening becomes positive.

- MTC: serum calcitonin and carcinoembryonic antigen
- Phaeochromocytoma: 24 h urine metanephrines and normetanephrines
- Primary hyperparathyroidism: serum ionized Ca^{2+}, PTH

Management

Management for MTC is by total thyroidectomy and ipsilateral neck dissection. Prophylactic total thyroidectomy is indicated in patients identified as high risk by genetic screening.

Phaeochromocytoma and primary hyperparathyroidism are managed in the same way as sporadic cases.

Specific gastrointestinal tumours

Insulinoma

Insulinomas arise in pancreatic beta cells and are the most common endocrine tumours of the pancreas. Most are sporadic although some present as part of the MEN 1 syndrome. They are usually solitary and small (<2 cm in diameter).

Clinical assessment

Patients describe intermittent 'attacks' characterized by neuroglycopenia (confusion, change in behaviour, fatigue, seizures, loss of consciousness) and high sympathetic drive (palpitations, tremor, sweating, flushing, and anxiety). Many patients are overweight because they eat excessively in an attempt to prevent the 'attacks'. Diagnosis is based on demonstrating the Whipple's triad. Symptoms of hypoglycaemia:

- Low serum glucose and symptomatic relief with the administration of glucose
- Low glucose levels (<2.5 mmol/dL) in the presence of an inappropriately elevated insulin level

- Serum C-peptide and proinsulin are used to differentiate insulinoma (high levels) from factitious administration of insulin preparations (no C-peptide)
- Serum sulphonylurea: these drugs induce endogenous secretion of insulin and C-peptide identical to those seen in insulinomas
- Endoscopic ultrasound (EUS), MRI or CT scans
- Selective angiography shows a 'blush' on injection of contrast medium in a small arterial branch supplying the tumour

Management

Controlled diet, diazoxide, and somatostatin analogues are used preoperatively. Intraoperative ultrasound confirms the position of tumour within the pancreas. Small superficial tumours can be enucleated; tumours in the tail of the pancreas require distal pancreatectomy.

Gastrinoma

Gastrinomas are rare gastrin-secreting tumours of non-beta pancreatic islet cells. They are most common in middle age and have a male preponderance. Most are sporadic, although 25% are associated with MEN type 1.

Tumours associated with MEN tend to be found in the duodenum and are often multifocal. Sporadic tumours are more commonly located in the pancreas and have a greater malignant potential. Overall, the majority of tumours are located in the 'gastrinoma triangle' bounded by the cystic duct superiorly, second and third parts of the duodenum inferiorly, and the head of the pancreas medially.

Clinical assessment

Zollinger–Ellison syndrome describes the triad of gastrinoma, hypergastrinaemia, and severe peptic ulcer disease. Over 90% of cases present with peptic ulcer disease or its complications (e.g. upper GI haemorrhage). Diarrhoea may result in dehydration, weight loss, and muscle wasting.

Medical management and *Helicobacter pylori* eradication is usually unsuccessful.

Investigations

The biochemical diagnosis is based on three tests.

1. High fasting serum gastrin of >150 pg/mL. A level of >1000 pg/mL is virtually diagnostic of Zollinger–Ellison syndrome
2. High basal acid output >10 mEq/h
3. Secretin and calcium stimulation tests are used to differentiate gastrinomas from other conditions associated with hypergastrinaemia (in patients with Zollinger–Ellison syndrome, gastrin increases by 100% over basal levels in response to calcium IV)

- Gastroscopy shows multiple ulcers in unusual locations (e.g. distal duodenum and jejunum)
- EUS, CT, and MRI scans can be used to localize the tumour and identify regional spread to lymph nodes or the liver
- Somatostatin receptor scintigraphy (Octreoscan) localizes the tumour and metastases

Management

Gastric acid secretion is controlled by multiple daily doses of proton-pump inhibitors.

Surgery is now indicated for local control of the disease; it is curative in 30% of patients. Whipple's procedure is advocated in patients with locally advanced or large tumours and patients with MEN 1 as it removes the whole gastrinoma triangle. An aggressive dissection of local lymph nodes is beneficial in patients with metastatic disease.

Gastrointestinal carcinoid

Gastrointestinal carcinoids are rare neuroendocrine tumours that account for over 95% of all carcinoids. They arise in the enterochromaffin cells found in the gastrointestinal, urogenital, and bronchial tracts. The tumours secrete serotonin (5-hydroxytryptamine, 5-HT) and other histamine-like substances that are metabolized by the liver. The vast majority are sporadic but they can also occur in MEN 1 and MEN 2 syndromes.

Immunohistochemistry differentiates the histological characteristics of carcinoid tumours according to their developmental location (foregut, midgut or hindgut).

Tumours <1 cm are rarely malignant; those >2 cm often exhibit metastatic spread to regional lymph nodes and liver. Carcinoid tumours are the most common small bowel malignant tumours.

Clinical assessment

Most tumours are small and asymptomatic. Symptoms and signs are either related to the tumour (e.g. abdominal pain, intestinal obstruction, palpable mass or, rarely, bowel perforation) or carcinoid syndrome.

Carcinoid syndrome occurs when vasoactive compounds (e.g. bradykinin, serotonin) escape detoxification by the liver and reach the systemic circulation. This usually only occurs in the presence of metastatic liver disease or with tumours that drain directly into the systemic circulation (e.g. ovarian carcinoid). It is characterized by hepatomegaly, diarrhoea, and flushing in 80% of patients; right heart valvular disease in 50%; and bronchospasm in 25%.

Investigations

- High urinary levels of serotonin and 5-hydroxyindole acetic acid (5-HIAA). Because the amount of hormone varies, multiple assessments may be necessary
- Midgut carcinoids are initially too small to be diagnosed on bowel contrast studies. Localization of such tumours remains challenging
- CT scans can demonstrate the presence of metastases
- Somatostatin receptor scintigraphy (Octreoscan) is very sensitive in localizing the tumour

Management

Conservative management with chemotherapy is used for symptom control. Surgical excision offers the only chance of cure. Bowel resection is either limited or segmental, depending on the size, invasive nature, and anatomical location of the tumour.

3.15 Case-based discussions

Case 1

A 21-year-old student has discovered a pea-sized lump in her right breast. She is extremely anxious because her 75-year-old maternal grandmother has recently undergone a mastectomy for breast cancer.

- What effect does having a grandmother with breast cancer have on her own risk of breast cancer?
- What is your differential diagnosis of a breast lump in a woman of her age?
- What are the characteristics of a malignant breast lump?
- Describe your approach to assessment of the breast lump?

Case 2

A 40-year-old woman has noticed a change in the profile of her breasts. Her left breast has a 'dent' on the lateral border which becomes more prominent when raising her arms.

- What other symptoms would you ask about?
- For what other signs would you examine?
- What symptoms and signs are suggestive of a malignant breast lump?

A core biopsy and mammogram confirm the clinical diagnosis of breast cancer.

- What information should the histopathology report give you?

The tumour is 2 cm in diameter and is in the upper outer quadrant.

- What are her options for breast surgery?
- What are the indications and options for an axillary procedure?

The patient has a wide local excision of her tumour, but the histology report shows a high grade tumour with both invasive tumour and DCIS at two opposing margins.

- What further surgery would you recommend?
- If you recommend a mastectomy, what options for reconstruction does she have?

Case 3

A 32-year-old telephonist presents with progressive hoarseness of her voice. She can also feel a lump on the right side of her neck. On examination the lump is in the right anterior triangle of the neck and it moves up when she swallows.

- How would you determine her risk of thyroid malignancy?
- What is the significance of her voice changes?
- What other features of the lump would be relevant?

She has a FNAC of the lump. The cytology shows thyroid cells with nuclear grooving and intranuclear inclusions. It is described as Thy 5.

- What does the report mean?
- What is the significance of finding similar types of cells in a small lump in the posterior triangle that you might have missed during your examination?

The patient undergoes a total thyroidectomy and right modified radical neck dissection. Three days after her discharge from hospital you receive a call from the GP who queries the fact that the patient has not been prescribed thyroid hormones.

- What adjuvant therapy do patients with differentiated thyroid cancer receive after thyroidectomy and why?
- What advice would you give female patients who want to have children but who have received radioactive iodine treatment?

Case 4

A 52-year-old woman presents to her GP with a few months' history of right upper quadrant pain suggestive of biliary colic. An abdominal ultrasound confirms the presence of gallstones and reveals a 4 cm mass in the right loin; further imaging is arranged.

- What other investigations would you organize?

The patient is diagnosed with Cushing's syndrome. Whilst gaining her consent for a right laparoscopic adrenalectomy, she asks whether she will have to take medication after operation.

- What are the causes of Cushing's syndrome?
- What are the signs and symptoms of Cushing's syndrome?
- Can you comment on the pituitary–adrenal axis function after unilateral adrenalectomy for an adrenal adenoma associated with Cushing's syndrome?

Chapter 4

Upper gastrointestinal surgery

➕ Technical skills and procedures

- Oesophagogastroduodenoscopy
- Laparoscopic cholecystectomy

◎ Clinical skills

- Jaundice
- Nutritional support algorithm
- Urgent 2-week wait referral for suspected upper gastrointestinal cancer
- Dysphagia
- Post-splenectomy prophylaxis

4.1 Gastrointestinal physiology I

The gastrointestinal (GI) tract, including its adnexae is involved in a wide range of homeostatic and physiological processes. Control is via complex neural and hormonal systems which are intrinsic to the tract, but both influence and are influenced by systemic nervous and hormonal systems.

The systems act to:

- control peristaltic and 'sphincteric' activity and food movement
- modulate biosynthetic pathways
- modulate GI tract neurohormonal function

Enteric neuroendocrine system

The enteric neuroendocrine system is derived from neural crest tissue. It comprises scattered mucosal cells and paraneurones which interface with the cells of the intrinsic nervous system of the GI tract (□ Topic 5.1).

These cells predominantly release amine-/peptide-derived small chemicals which may act on adjacent cells (paracrine activity) or distant/systemic target tissues (endocrine activity). The molecules released may act as vasoactive substances, neurotransmitters, hormones or regulators of cellular function, depending upon where they are released and on the target tissue affected. Almost all tissues of the GI tract have membrane-bound receptors to some or all of these substances, making them potent effectors of GI tract function.

Table 4.1 Examples of enteric peptides/hormones

Substance	Actions
5-hydroxytryptamine (5-HT)	Vasoconstriction Smooth muscle contraction
Gastrin	Secretion of pepsinogen Secretion of HCl Secretion of somatostatin/histamine Increased gastric motility Pyloric canal relaxation
Secretin	Secretion of pancreatic juice Reduced gastric acid/pepsin secretion
Vasoactive intestinal peptide (VIP)	Reduced gastric and gallbladder motility Reduced gastric secretion Secretion of pancreatic and intestinal juice Vasodilatation
Gastric inhibitory peptide (GIP)	Reduced gastric motility and secretion
Cholecystokinin (CCK)	Release of pancreatic enzymes and juice Contraction of the gallbladder Reduced gastric emptying Reduced small bowel motility
Substance P	Vasodilatation Reduced upper GI tract motility
Somatostatin	Inhibits enteric neuroendocrine cell function Reduced splanchnic blood flow Reduced motility of all GI tract hollow viscera Reduced GI hormone production.

Enteric motility

The contents of the GI tract are propelled along by non-striated smooth muscle under enteric and autonomic control. The only exceptions to this are the mouth, tongue, pharynx, and external anal sphincter which contain striated smooth muscle under voluntary control.

Autonomous smooth muscle activity creates self-induced electrical activity, and pacemaker cells are distributed through the muscular layers which create a low frequency slow-wave potential which determines the inherent rate of GI tract contractile activity.

Tonic contractions are either low pressure sustained contractions (e.g. gallbladder) or high pressure (e.g. sphincters). Phasic contractions occur throughout the tract. They may be shortlived, local, and bidirectional, such as gastric churning and 'mixing', peristalsis or prolonged, propagating, and unidirectional such as propulsive peristalsis and colonic mass movements.

Oesophageal physiology

Motility and swallowing

Swallowing is initiated by a bolus voluntarily forced by the tongue into the pharynx, triggering touch receptors, and initiating a reflex action (the first phase of swallowing.) The impulses are transmitted to the swallowing centre in the medulla and lower pons; efferent impulses are then returned via the cranial nerves to the pharynx and oesophagus.

The pharyngeal phase inhibits respiration and takes less than a second; during this time the position of the tongue, epiglottis, and uvula prevent the food re-entering the mouth or nasal passage. The soft palate is elevated, the vocal cords close, the upper oesophageal sphincter (cricopharyngeus) relaxes, and the superior constrictor muscle contracts.

Finally, the oesophageal phase begins as the upper oesophageal sphincter contracts. The swallowing centre initiates a primary peristaltic wave, at a rate of 5 cm/s that forces the bolus ahead of it for the length of the oesophagus. Secondary, more forceful, peristaltic waves can be initiated by pressure receptors if food is still present, mediated by intrinsic nerve plexuses at the level of the distension. Distension also reflexively increases salivary secretion to aid trapped boluses.

Lower oesophageal sphincter

The lower 1–2 cm of the oesophagus forms a zone of high pressure (HPZ), often referred to as the lower oesophageal sphincter (LOS). The mechanisms which contribute to this HPZ are:

- intrinsic hypertonicity of the lowermost oesophageal wall muscles modulated by intrinsic and extrinsic innervation
- endoluminal gastro-oesophageal mucosal rosettes filling the lumen
- external compressive action of the diaphragmatic crural sling
- acute gastro-oesophageal angle

The LOS responds to oesophageal peristalsis, gastric contractility, and external innervation.

Stomach physiology

The stomach has several functions; to store ingested food and convert a relatively intermittent oral intake to a more controlled progressive flow into the small intestine; to begin the process of digestion, and to modulate other GI tract function via the enteric neuroendocrine system.

Gastric secretion and digestion

- **Cephalic**—excitatory stage (via odours and thoughts, processed in the cerebral cortex, hypothalamus and medulla) is responsible for saliva production, some pancreatic fluid production, and 10% of stimulus to gastric secretion
- **Gastric**—mediated by the short gastric reflex (via local neurohormonal pathways in the stomach wall) and the long vagus reflex (via the vagus and brainstem nuclei). This is responsible for 80% of gastric secretion. It also has an inhibitory element
- **Intestinal**—responsible for 10% of gastric secretion, but is also inhibitory to reduce stomach activity once emptying begins. Acids, fatty acids, peptides, and increased osmolarity in the duodenum, via neural and hormonal feedback, act on the stomach to decrease gastric motility and regulate chyme volume, propelled through the pylorus

Gastric motility

Following relaxation of the LOS (resulting from the relaxation of oesophageal peristaltic waves), the stomach relaxes reflexively. Gastric distension increases gastric secretion and motility. Gastric body contractions mix food and gastric juice; churning action is created by more forceful antrum contractions (retropulsion). Only small volumes pass through the pyloric sphincter (3 mL/min), owing to its closure as waves arrive. Gastric emptying takes 3–4 h (fluid first, fat last), ensuring that the duodenum and jejunum can neutralize gastric acid and process chyme.

The rate of gastric motility and emptying is related to gastric volume, degree of fluidity; presence of fat, acid, hypertonicity, distension of the duodenum, emotion, pain, and decreased glucose utilization in the hypothalamus have a role.

Small intestinal physiology

Duodenum

The duodenum receives contents from the stomach which it mixes with bile and pancreatic secretions. It admits the conjoined common bile duct and main pancreatic duct via the ampulla of Vater on the medial wall of the second part. The alkaline pancreatic juice neutralizes gastric acid and renders the luminal pH suitable for the action of the pancreatic proenzymes which contribute to digestion. Iron and calcium are preferentially absorbed in the duodenum.

Jejunum and ileum
Motility

Segmentation, mixing, and circulation of intestinal contents occur. This is not very powerful and the slow rate ensures the mixing of chyme, facilitating digestion and absorption by mechanical disruption and reduction of food particle size. Ringlike contractions occur along the length of the small intestine; within seconds, the contracted segments relax and the previously relaxed areas contract.

Digestion

The small intestine is the main site of digestion and absorption of nutrients, and several factors are important.

- The mucosa is arranged into numerous villi and circular folds (plicae circulares) which increase the surface area for absorption. In addition, the epithelial cells have microvilli which increases this further
- Solubilization and emulsification allows insoluble particles (e.g. fat) to be broken down and then absorbed
- Digestion is both luminal and membranous. Luminal digestion mainly involves the pancreatic enzymes. Membranous digestion involves enzymes which are in the luminal aspect of the membranes of the epithelial cells, i.e. the brush border. Absorption is accomplished by active transport, co-transport, and passive diffusion; transcellular and paracellular absorption
- Control of pH is important. Saliva is weakly acidic, stomach acid is very acidic (pH<5), and the small bowel has an alkaline environment (pH 8.5). The gastric acid kills microbes and denatures proteins. The alkaline environment of the small bowel facilitates the action of pancreatic enzymes and aids absorption
- Some nutrients need special factors or specialized membrane functions for absorption, e.g. intrinsic factor for vitamin B_{12} absorption in the terminal ileum, folic acid in the jejunum, and bile acids in the terminal ileum

Immune function

The small intestine also has an immune function. Throughout its length, there are lymphoid aggregates (Peyer's patches). Goblet cells also secrete IgA antibodies, helping to protect against intraluminal microbes.

Liver physiology

The liver is an exceptionally complex physiologically active organ involved in many homeostatic processes. The most significant of these are outlined below. It receives approximately 30% of cardiac output and most of this comes via the portal system. Hepatocytes are able to proliferate following injury, giving the liver regenerative potential.

Function

- **Lipid metabolism** releases cholesterol, phospholipids, and triglycerides
- **Carbohydrate metabolism** includes gluconeogenesis (formation of glucose from amino acids, fats or lactic acid), glycogenolysis (breakdown of glycogen to glucose), and glycogenesis (formation of glycogen from glucose)
- **Protein metabolism** releases amino acids with ammonia as a byproduct. Ammonia is converted to urea and excreted
- **Protein synthesis** of non essential amino acids, plasma proteins, enzymes, and blood clotting factors
- **Vitamin D activation** to aid calcium metabolism and absorption; vitamin D is converted to 25-hydroxycalciferol
  - **Breakdown and excretion** of lipid-soluble compounds (drugs, steroids, hormones)
  - **Breakdown of haemoglobin** and release of pigments which are added to the excreted bile salts
  - **Storage** of glycogen, iron, copper, folate, and vitamins (A, D, K, and B_{12}.)
  - **Bile secretion**—bile is composed of cholesterol, bile salts, inorganic salts, water, and phospholipids. It is secreted according to hormonal and neural feedback mechanisms

Pancreas

The pancreas is a mixed endocrine and exocrine gland. Pancreatic secretion is regulated by vagal stimulation, secretin (released in response to acid in the duodenum), cholecystokinin (CCK; released in response to amino acids, peptides, and fatty acids in the duodenum), and gastrin.

Endocrine secretion

- Insulin from beta-cells increases tissue uptake of glucose, amino acids and lipids, stimulates glycogenesis and protein synthesis, and lipid oxidation
- Glucagon from alpha-cells stimulates conversion of glycogen to glucose. Its actions oppose insulin
- Somatostatin from delta-cells (reduces digestion by reducing GI tract motility, GI secretions, nutrient absorption and digestion, insulin, and glucagon secretion)
- Pancreatic polypeptide secreted from F-cells acts to regulate digestion (stimulated by fasting, decreased blood sugar, and protein).

Exocrine secretion

Pancreatic juice has two components, produced by the acinar cells and ductal epithelial cells.

- Acinar tissue produces a digestive secretion containing enzymes (e.g. amylase, trypsinogen, phospholipase) and inactive proenzymes (preventing autodigestion). They are stored in the pancreas within granules, which fuse with the cell membrane and exocytose to be converted (via catalysts) to their active forms in the duodenum
- Ductal epithelium produces an aqueous secretion comprising water, bicarbonate, and sodium. This increases the endoluminal pH to allow pancreatic enzymes to work

Colonic physiology

The main functions of the colon are to reabsorb water and store faecal material. Its bacterial flora also helps to synthesize vitamin K and some B vitamins as well as providing a significant part of the nutritional requirement of the colonic epithelium from metabolism of residual enteric contents.

The colonic mucosa is smooth and consists of closely packed tubular glands containing absorptive and goblet cells. The goblet cells produce mucus which lubricates the faeces, provides a neutral pH layer which protects the brush border from the acidic products of fermentation, and provides a microenvironment in which normal bacterial flora can proliferate.

The largest part of the colonic water reabsorption takes place in the proximal half of the colon, and the distal half functions primarily for storage and expulsion of faeces. Only water and some electrolytes (Na^+) are absorbed by colonic action. The maximum volume of water absorbed is 7 litres/day. Bacteria account for about 30% of the dry weight of faeces.

Motility

Various hormones and neurotransmitters can affect the colonic transport by the intrinsic nervous plexus:

- CCK increases postprandially and increases colonic activity
- electrolyte imbalances such as hypokalaemia can affect smooth muscle function
- sleep decreases colonic activity, stress increases it

Anorectal physiology

The rectum extends from the confluence of the taeniae coli at the rectosigmoid junction to the anorectal junction and is approximately 15 cm long. The anal canal extends from the junction to the anal verge (usually taken as the lower border of the external sphincter complex) and is between 1.5 and 4 cm long. The dentate line is about 2 cm distal to the anal verge and is the point at which columnar epithelium (endoderm) undergoes transition to become squamous epithelium (ectoderm).

Together, the rectum and anus maintain faecal continence by acting as a reservoir and an expulsion unit for faeces.

Continence

Continence is maintained by several mechanisms.

- **Anorectal angle** is partly due to the embryology of the formation of the anorectum and partly maintained by the anterior pull of the puborectalis, but is not of major importance
- **Internal anal sphincter** has a constant low resting tone under autonomic control. Reflex increases in tone in response to straining and coughing prevent leakage of gas, liquid, and small volumes of solids
- **Endoanal cushions** formed from submucosal vascular and connective tissue help physically to plug the anal canal and make it gas- and fluid-'tight'
- **External anal sphincter** is under voluntarily control. The tone can usually be increased to defer defaecation until appropriate

Sampling is a phenomenon by which reflex relaxation of the upper anorectal canal allows small volumes of rectal content into contact with the upper anal canal (which lies within the puborectalis). A combination of impulses from thermoreceptors in the mucosa and proprioceptors in the muscles enable differentiation between liquids, gas, and solids to be made fairly accurately.

Defaecation

1. Solid stool descends into the rectum, causing distension and the urge to defaecate
2. Relaxation of the internal anal sphincter in response to rectal distension (rectoanal inhibitory reflex) and voluntary relaxation of the external anal sphincter allows stools to pass into the anal canal
3. Relaxation of the pelvic floor muscles and contraction of the rectum acts to straighten the anorectal angle
4. Continued rectal contraction empties the lower third of the rectum
5. Tonic contractions of the pelvic floor and anal canal help to empty and cleanse the anal canal and restore the anal canal and anorectal angle

⊙ Jaundice

Jaundice (icterus) is yellow discoloration of the skin, conjunctiva, and mucous membranes. It is a result of abnormalities in bilirubin production, metabolism or excretion, resulting in hyperbilirubinaemia. Serum bilirubin >40 μmol/L is usually clinically apparent. It can be classified as pre-hepatic, hepatic, and post-hepatic.

Pre-hepatic (haemolytic)

Haemolysis of red blood cells results in levels of unconjugated bilirubin that exceed the liver's metabolic capacity. Serum unconjugated bilirubin is elevated but there are normal levels of conjugated bilirubin. Urine is a normal colour as unconjugated bilirubin is insoluble.

Hepatic

Hepatocellular causes such as hepatitis and Gilbert's syndrome involve an inability of hepatocytes to conjugate bilirubin and/or excrete it.

Post-hepatic

Post-hepatic jaundice is a result of bile duct obstruction. This is often due to bile duct calculi or pancreatic cancer. Serum conjugated bilirubin and alkaline phosphatase are elevated; serum transaminases (AST/ALT) are usually normal. The urine may become dark as conjugated bilirubin is freely filtered by the kidney.

4.3 Nutrition in surgical patients

Abnormalities of nutrition are problems seen every day on surgical wards in the UK. At any one time, an estimated 35% of patients are overweight (body mass index >25); 65% of those staying in hospital for more than 1 week lose weight, and 40% of patients admitted demonstrate moderate–severe malnutrition, particularly the elderly and those with malignancy or chronic illness.

Malnutrition is important as it has been implicated in:
- delayed wound healing
- impaired organ function (particularly respiratory muscles but also cardiac, CNS, GI and skin system dysfunction)
- impaired immune function

There is a probable increase in morbidity and mortality rates from major surgery in the nutritionally compromised. Indeed, any patient fasted for more than 3 days should be considered for nutritional support, using the GI tract wherever possible (thereby maintaining gut mucosal integrity and deterring bacterial translocation).

Nutritional assessment

Clinical assessment
Clinical assessments are based on a diet history, medical history, and physical examination. They are easily performed and give a good overall picture of long-term status.
- 10% weight loss=mild malnutrition; 30%=severe malnutrition
- Body mass index (weight in kg/height in m^2) also aids assessment; BMI<18.5=significantly underweight

Anthropometric assessment
- Triceps skinfold measurement (fat measurement)
- Midarm muscle circumference (lean muscle measurement)
- Handgrip strength

These methods are useful in normal healthy individuals, but have limited use in the critically ill since skeletal muscle is preferentially lost early in the stress response to sepsis, surgery or starvation.

Laboratory data
- Proteins—serum albumin is slow to decline and slow to recover during periods of starvation as well as being affected by liver and renal disease. Prealbumin has a shorter half-life and responds more quickly to changes in nutrition. Transferrin is a protein with a very short half-life and is the best monitor of liver protein biosynthesis
- Trace elements, vitamins, and electrolyte deficiencies are the most useful
- Immunological studies such as total lymphocyte count and immune function response can also be analysed but are non-specific

Nutritional support

Enteral nutrition
If the GI tract is functioning and access to it safe, enteral feeding is the preferred method of nutritional support. It is cheaper, safer, and has physiological advantages such as the prevention of gut mucosal atrophy and bacterial translocation, the promotion of biliary flow, and decreasing nosocomial pneumonia.

Indications for typical routes of enteral nutrition
- **Oral**—this should be the first 'port of call' unless there are contra-indications. Supplementation should be considered for all but mild malnutrition
- **Nasogastric/nasojejunal fine bore feeding tube**—poor intake despite attempted supplementation (commonest problem in surgical wards), loss of gag/swallow reflex, intubated/sedated patient, gastric ileus (requires a nasojejunal tube)
- **Tube enterostomy (gastrostomy/jejunostomy)**—oesophagogastric surgery/injury, long-term inability to eat/swallow (e.g. head injury, oesophageal stricture)

Contraindications to enteral feeding: obstructed GI tract (which cannot be bypassed by feeding tube), protracted vomiting, high output (proximal small bowel) fistula, proximal small bowel injury or acute bowel ischaemia.

Forms of enteral nutrition
- Normal diet—sometimes modified according to situation (e.g. high in gelatine for enterostomy patients)
- Supplemented normal diet with fortified nutritional supplements (e.g. Fortisip®, Enlive®)
- Specialized diets (e.g. low residue, elemental, polymeric)
- Specialized tube feeds (e.g. Fresubin®)

Complications of enteral feeding
- Related to feed—feed intolerance, hyperosmolar diarrhoea
- Related to nasoenteric intubation—aspiration of feed, nasal/pharyngeal/oesophageal ulceration
- Related to tube enterostomy—tube displacement/migration/obstruction, visceral injury, fistulation, wound infection, peritonitis

Parenteral nutrition
Parenteral nutrition (PN) delivers elemental feed intravenously.

Indications: any contraindication to enteric feeding, but commonly used in enterocutaneous fistulae, prolonged vomiting, short bowel syndrome, severe inflammatory bowel disease, acute pancreatitis, mechanical bowel obstruction, severe malnutrition, major trauma, and burns.

Forms of parenteral nutrition
- Partial peripheral nutrition (PPN)—may be supplemental (i.e. not full protein-calorie requirements) or complete. Administered via peripheral venous cannula or via proximal venous catheter (e.g. PICC line)
- Total parenteral nutrition (TPN)—always complete initially but may become partial if enteric nutrition is re-introduced later. Administered via central venous cannula (conventional central line or tunnelled line if long term)

Complications of parenteral feeding
- Related to feed—hyperglycaemia, refeeding syndrome (rapid, potentially fatal transcellular shifts in electrolytes), electrolyte imbalances, micronutrient deficiencies (e.g. hyposelenism, vitamin B$_6$ and folate deficiency)
- Related to liver dysfunction—bile stasis and infection, intra-hepatic cholestasis, deranged liver enzymes (related mostly to fatty acid content of TPN)
- Related to cannula—cannula infection, central line infection/bacteraemia, catheter blockage, venous thromboembolism

In view of the above complications, it is important (especially when using TPN) to liaise closely with the nutritional team and dietitians, to maintain meticulous sterility, and to review fluid balance and monitor blood markers of nutrition on a regular basis.

Monitoring nutritional status

Patients on TPN require regular review and monitoring, including:

- urea and electrolytes (initially daily then twice-weekly once established)
- glucose (initially daily then twice-weekly unless signs of abnormal glucose levels
- liver function tests (twice-weekly)
- micronutrients, including Mg, PO_4, Mn, Cu (weekly)

Central venous catheters require specific attention. In particular, they should not be used for non-TPN infusions and *never* used for phlebotomy as this increases the risk of catheter sepsis dramatically. Dressings should be changed regularly and the catheter entry site kept clean.

⊚ **Nutritional support algorithm**

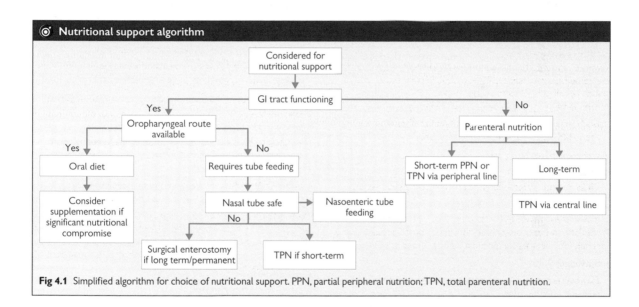

Fig 4.1 Simplified algorithm for choice of nutritional support. PPN, partial peripheral nutrition; TPN, total parenteral nutrition.

Gastro-oesophageal reflux disease

The incidence of gastro-oesophageal reflux disease (GORD) is estimated at 40% of the adult population.

Reflux occurs up to 5% of the time in 'normal' individuals. GORD can be defined as excessive amounts of reflux associated with significant symptoms or complications.

Aetiology

Several factors may be involved.

- Failure of function of the LOS complex is the most common feature and may be caused by destruction of mucosal rosettes, e.g. by ongoing reflux and reduced endogenous tone, perhaps caused by drugs (sedatives, alcohol, anti-cholinergics) or secondary to neurological disease (MS, CVA)
- Defective oesophageal contraction/emptying, e.g. scleroderma, hiatus hernia
- Abnormal gastric emptying, e.g. gastric outlet obstruction
- Duodenogastric reflux worsens symptoms, e.g. after gastric resection, obesity, raised intra-abdominal pressure

Pathology

Reflux exposes the lower oesophageal mucosa to low acid or alkaline (bile) injury, increasing the risk of mucosal injury (oesophagitis). *Helicobacter pylori* gastritis may protect against GORD by reducing gastric acid secretion.

Clinical presentations/assessment

During the assessment establish the onset, frequency, and period of reflux symptoms. A symptom diary is often helpful. Also exclude other diagnoses such as a chest infection.

Heartburn

- Intermittent epigastric/retrosternal pain, may be shortlived or prolonged, may radiate to the jaw/neck (angina-like pain). Painful dysphagia is rare and suggests other oesophageal pathology
- May or may not be associated with any endoscopic features of reflux (oesophagitis or secondary changes such as stricture)

Frank food reflux

- May present with acid entering the throat, especially on lying down/at night
- Pulmonary aspiration (nocturnal coughing, hoarse voice)

Dysphagia

- Secondary to stricture, Barrett's oesophagus or adenocarcinoma

Investigations

- Oesophagogastroduodenoscopy (OGD) ± biopsy to exclude other diagnoses (e.g. carcinoma); assess for presence and extent of oesophagitis, and for the development of complications
- 24 h pH monitoring—a naso-oesophageal probe is placed 5 cm above the LOS for 24 h. A pH <4 for over 1% of the time when supine or >6% when erect is diagnostic
- Dynamic contrast swallow—if there is the possibility of alternative/additional motility disorder

Management

Conservative

Conservative management is successful in 90% of cases and centres around lifestyle changes and gastric acid suppression.

Table 4.1 Savary–Miller classification of GORD

Grade	Features
I	Erosions isolated to one mucosal fold
II	More than one erosion on more than one fold
III	Circumferential erosions
IV	Ulceration, shortening or stricture formation
V	Barrett's epithelium formation

Table 4.2 Los Angeles classification of GORD

Grade	Features
A	Erosions <5 mm on single folds
B	Erosions >5 mm on single folds
C	Erosions across two or more folds <75% of circumference
D	Erosions across >75% of circumference

- Lifestyle modification (weight loss, alcohol avoidance, smoking cessation, raising the bed head)
- Prokinetics (e.g. metoclopramide)
- Proton-pump inhibitors (PPI) such as omeprazole and lansoprazole. H_2 antagonists (e.g. ranitidine) are rarely used.

Surgery

Surgery is indicated for:

- failure of symptoms to respond to medical therapy
- long-term dependence on medical therapy in young adults (recurrent symptomatic relapses)
- development of complications
- possibly bile reflux or documented evidence of LOS deficiency

Open or laparoscopic fundoplication is the procedure of choice, with the gastric fundus being mobilized and wrapped around the oesophagus. Complications include dysphagia (3%), and gastric bloating (11%).

Complications and prognosis

- Oesophageal stricture/shortening (10%)—treated by balloon dilatation, although surgery might be considered in the young; recurrent strictures, undilatable (rare) or shortened oesophagus
- Haemorrhage (rare)
- Barrett's oesophagus (adenocarcinoma)

Barrett's oesophagus

Barrett's oesophagus is defined as the presence of columnar epithelium lining the distal oesophagus (usually taken to be >3 cm above the gastro-oesophageal junction), replacing normal squamous epithelium.

It is a premalignant condition, with the risk of developing high-grade dysplasia and adenocarcinoma of around 0.5% per year (and increasing the risk of cancer by 30%).

Surveillance should be considered, although the best policy and the optimum frequency are yet to be defined.

Evidence suggests that this should be considered for those with Barrett's and chronic symptoms of GORD (greater than 5 years).

The American College of Gastroenterology suggests:
- no dysplasia—OGD every 3–5 years
- low-grade dysplasia—OGD every 6–12 months
- high-grade dysplasia—endoscopic ablative therapies or oesophagectomy, since up to 30% will have an undiagnosed coincident adenocarcinoma

Gastritis

Gastritis is defined as the presence of non-ulcerative inflammation or changes in the gastric mucosa.

Aetiology/classification

Atrophic causes
- Type A—autoimmune
- Type B—associated with *H. pylori* infection

Non-atrophic causes
- Infective (*H. Pylori*-related, tuberculous, HIV-related)
- Inflammatory (biliary reflux gastritis, stress-induced (e.g. burns/ITU), drug-induced, eosinophilic, lymphocytic)

Pathology

May have any or all of the following:
- chronic inflammatory infiltrate
- acute inflammatory infiltrate
- glandular atrophy
- intestinal metaplasia

Clinical presentations/assessment

Bleeding
- Acute, intermittent UGI bleeding (coffee ground vomiting, melaena)
- Chronic intermittent bleeding (iron deficiency anaemia, positive faecal occult bloods)

Dyspepsia
- Progression to ulceration and complications

Investigations
Gastroscopy (OGD) to confirm diagnosis, exclude alternative diagnoses (e.g. carcinoma, peptic ulceration), and to obtain biopsy classification of cause.

Management
- Lifestyle modifications (avoid alcohol and NSAIDs)
- Symptomatic treatment with drugs (see GORD)
- *H. pylori* eradication therapy in proven infections

Complications
- Development of lymphoid follicular hyperplasia and possible MALT lymphoma in *H. Pylori*-related gastritis

⊕ Oesophagogastroduodenoscopy

Pre-procedure
- Symptoms of high oesophageal dysphagia should be excluded since a high oesophageal tumour or stricture can be extremely difficult to identify and may prevent intubation
- Pulse oximetry monitoring is always desirable and is required if IV sedation is used
- A toothguard should be used to protect the teeth from the endoscope and vice versa
- Ensure the patient is comfortable in the left lateral position with the neck slightly flexed

Procedure
- Oropharyngeal local anaesthesia is almost always used with additional sedation (e.g. midazolam) at the patient's request
- The endoscope is inserted straight under direct vision and flexed once the soft palate is passed. Direct visualization of the inlet of the larynx allows passage of the endoscope posterolaterally into one of the piriform fossae and then medially to the level of cricopharyngeus
- Intubation should be coordinated with swallowing
- General principles are: to visualize the oesophagus during slow intubation, evaluate the body and antrum of the stomach, intubate the duodenum, where possible, to the second part, inspect the duodenal cap during withdrawal, and inspect the gastric fundus by scope retroflexion prior to extubation

Complications
- Perforation (most commonly oesophageal) 1/5000
- Bleeding
- Aspiration

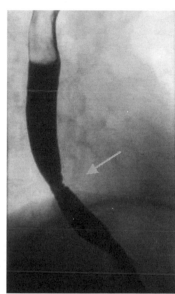

Fig 4.2 Barium swallow showing a benign mid-oesophageal stricture.

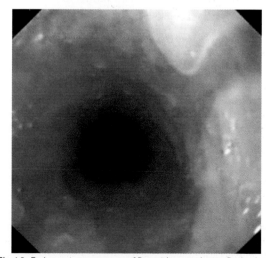

Fig 4.3 Endoscopic appearance of Barrett's oesophagus. Red columnar epithelium is extending proximally above the gastro-oesophageal junction.

4.5 Peptic ulcer disease

Peptic ulcer disease is defined as the presence of complete, established defects in the columnar mucosa of the lower oesophagus, stomach or duodenum.

Aetiology/epidemiology

Proximal gastric (type I) ulcer

The commonest sites are the lesser curvature and the antrum/body junction.

The condition is associated with reduced mucosal protection owing to:

- drugs: NSAIDs, bisphosphonates, K^+
- smoking, alcohol (modest)
- a weak association with *H. pylori* infection
- an association with low or normal acid production
- age (peak incidence 30–55 years)
- male sex (M:F 3:1)

The incidence is 0.2% of the population per annum.

Distal gastric/duodenal (type II) ulcer

Eighty per cent are found in the duodenum, and 80% of these are solitary (half of which are <2 cm in diameter).

Of the duodenal ulcers, 90% are in the first part, on the anterior wall within a few centimetres of the pylorus.

These ulcers are associated with increased mucosal damage:

- strong association with *H. pylori* infection of the antrum
- drugs: NSAIDs, bisphosphonates, K^+
- smoking, alcohol (strong)
- high acid production (including Zollinger–Ellison syndrome)
- age (peak incidence 20–35 years)
- male sex (M:F 4:1)

The incidence is 0.8% of the population per annum.

Helicobacter pylori is a Gram-negative spiral microaerophilic bacillus found in the mucous layer of human gastric mucosa. It produces alkaline urease and is found in 90–100% of duodenal ulcer cases and 70–75% of gastric ulcers.

Macroscopically, peptic ulcers are usually chronic, round or oval punched out lesions of variable depth with a base relatively free of exudate owing to peptic digestion. Vessels may be prominent, predisposing to haemorrhage; scarring may be evident underlying the ulcer (spokes or spicules are visualized), and the surrounding mucosa tends to be oedematous and erythematous. Although suggestive of malignancy, heaped or rolled edges may occur in chronic benign ulcers.

Clinical assessment

Dyspepsia/pain

Type II ulcers (e.g. duodenal) present with epigastric pain, worse when fasting and at night, relieved by food. Relapsing and remitting course (2 weeks of symptoms every few months.) Pain may radiate to the back.

Type I ulcers (e.g. gastric) present with epigastric pain on eating. Weight loss, nausea, and vomiting may occur.

Chronic bleeding

Chronic bleeding usually presents as iron deficiency anaemia (low ferritin), manifest as tiredness, lethargy, dyspnoea (usually exertional but may be at rest), exertional angina.

Acute bleeding

Acute bleeding usually presents with haematemesis (fresh or altered blood), with or without melaena.

Perforation

Perforation usually presents as acute, sudden onset central/upper abdominal pain, upper abdominal peritonism, and features of shock.

Investigations

- Hb, ferritin—anaemia
- U+Es may be abnormal in rare causes such as Zollinger–Ellison syndrome
- Non-invasive *H. pylori* testing—CO_2 breath testing (tests for CO_2 produced by the action of urease on stomach contents), *H. pylori* serology
- Gastroduodenoscopy—diagnostic and enables biopsies and testing for *H. Pylori*, e.g. rapid urease tests such as the Clo test
- Barium meal—this is usually only done where endoscopy is not possible. Good at hiatus hernia identification and some ulcers, although reduced specificity for benign versus malignant ulcers

Management

Medical

- Lifestyle changes: stopping smoking, reduce alcohol intake
- Control of medication: stop NSAIDS where possible
- Reduction of acid production: PPIs are the gold standard with 80–90% healing at 8 weeks (e.g. omeprazole, lausoprazole). H_2 antagonists have a high recurrence rate, especially of gastric ulcer in patients on NSAIDs.
- *H. pylori* eradication therapy, e.g. PPI twice daily plus clarithromycin 500 mg bd and amoxicillin 1 g bd.
- Research shows that treatment with PPIs twice daily is superior to once daily, and that poor compliance and bacterial resistance (depending on geographical location) can lead to treatment failure, and therefore the choice of antibiotics used. First line eradication success varies from 70 to 95% and 10–14-day regimes have been found to be 7–9% more effective than 7-day treatment.

Operative

Elective surgical intervention is now extremely rare for peptic ulcer disease (once Zollinger–Ellison syndrome has been excluded). The main indication is failed medical treatment (non-compliance, non-healing/frequently relapsing ulcer).

Gastric ulcer

- Bilroth I partial gastrectomy (excision of the distal third of the stomach and gastroduodenostomy)
- Bilroth II (Polya) partial gastrectomy (excision of the distal two-thirds of the stomach and gastro-jejunostomy)

Duodenal ulcer

- Highly selective vagotomy
- Bilroth II (Polya) partial gastrectomy (excision of the distal two-thirds of the stomach and gastro-jejunostomy)

Complications and prognosis

Complications of gastric surgery

- Diarrhoea owing to rapid gastric emptying and fast intestinal transit
- Dumping syndrome results from rapid gastric emptying after pyloroplasty or gastrectomy and may be early (owing to a hypertonic load in the small intestine causing large volume fluid shifts) or late (owing to reactive hypoglycaemia), and is characterized by an autonomic response (faintness, palpitations, sweating, tachycardia, and nausea)
- Alkaline reflux gastritis (duodenal contents)— treatment consists of cholestyramine and occasionally roux-en-Y jejunostomy
- Malabsorption of folate, vitamin B_{12}, iron, and vitamin D
- Gastric remnant carcinoma—benign disease gastrectomy increases the risk of adenocarcinoma 3-fold over 20 years due to metaplasia

Complications of ulceration

Haemorrhage
📖 Topic 8.15 and 8.16. This presents with haematemesis or melaena.

Perforation
📖 Topic 8.18. Perforation usually presents with acute onset severe upper abdominal pain but may be delayed in presentation with secondary sepsis.

Gastric outlet obstruction ('pyloric' stenosis)
This condition is most commonly secondary to chronic peri-pyloric antral or proximal duodenal ulceration. There is usually a history of projectile vomiting of undigested food only, weight loss, epigastric pain, dehydration, and a hypochloraemic, hypokalaemic, metabolic alkalosis. On examination, the abdomen may be distended, with visible peristalsis and a succussion splash. Endoscopy is diagnostic and may allow balloon dilatation of the stricture. Surgery is usually either gastrojejunostomy or proximal gastric vagotomy with duodenoplasty.

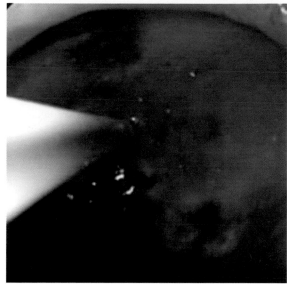

Fig 4.4 Endoscopic view of an ulcer on the posterior wall of the first part of the duodenum. A Gold Probe is being used to cauterize bleeding points within the ulcer. Ulceration of this area has the potential to cause significant haemorrhage as the gastroduodenal artery lies deep to the posterior wall.

4.6 Gallstone disease

Aetiology and pathology

Twelve per cent of men and 24% of women will develop gallstones, although only 10–20% of all stones become symptomatic.

Cholesterol stones (15%)

- Cholesterol stones form when bile becomes supersaturated with cholesterol, the exact reason being unclear
- Risk factors include raised cholesterol (obesity, female, increasing age) and decreased bile salts (oestrogen-related or increased gut loss, e.g. cystic fibrosis, Crohn's disease)
- Stones are generally solitary, large (0.5–3 cm), round, faceted, and yellow in colour

Bilirubin pigment (5%)

- Pigmented stones are caused by bilirubin forming insoluble calcium precipitates; there is a predisposition to formation with increased hepatic secretion of bilirubin
- Risk factors include genetic background, e.g. Asians and ethnic North American groups, chronic haemolysis, cirrhosis, chronic biliary infection, and ileal resection
- Stones generally have an irregular outline, measure up to 1 cm, and are brown, black or occasionally dark green in colour

Mixed stones (80%)

- These are a mixture of cholesterol and bilirubin

Clinical presentations

Gallbladder-related non-septic presentations

Biliary colic

Typical features are recurrent, intermittent periods characterized by right upper quadrant and epigastric pain radiating to the right flank, scapula, and shoulder. Pain is often induced by food, especially food that is high in fat content. It may be continuous for 24–48 h or have a periodicity of 20 min. Nausea and vomiting are common.

Mucocoele of the gallbladder

Obstruction to the cystic duct (usually by stones) results in bile resorption with epithelial secreted mucin filling the gallbladder. The wall itself is thinned and the mucosal surface smooth. It is characterized by features similar to biliary colic with a persistent, unresolving pain, and a palpable right upper quadrant mass which is mildly tender.

Chronic cholecystitis

Chronic cholecystitis is a histological diagnosis, and may be associated with a history of recurrent biliary colic or acute cholecystitis episodes. Longstanding fatty intolerance and 'flatulent dyspepsia' is only weakly associated with gallstone carriage.

Histologically there is wall hypertrophy, submucosal fibrosis, and chronic inflammation (out-pouches of mucosa into the wall, forming small cystic spaces called 'Aschoff–Rokitansky sinuses'). Secondary changes include calcification of the gallbladder—'porcelain gallbladder'.

Gallbladder-related septic presentations

Acute cholecystitis

This is typified by gradual onset, constant right upper quadrant pain lasting several days, associated with fever, tachycardia, nausea, and anorexia. There is usually right upper quadrant tenderness, accentuated during inspiration ('Murphy's sign'). Severe right upper quadrant peritonism suggests either severe pericholecystic inflammation or gallbladder necrosis.

Empyema of the gallbladder

Empyema usually results from obstruction to the cystic duct in the presence of acute cholecystitis rather than infection of a pre-existing mucocoele. The development of constant severe right upper quadrant pain with a mass and a high, swinging fever on the background of acute cholecystitis suggests the diagnosis.

Treatment is by percutaneous cholecystostomy and/or cholecystectomy in addition to IV antibiotics.

Presentations involving jaundice

Obstructive jaundice due to choledocholithiasis

This typically involves dark urine (high in bilirubin), pale stools (low in sterco/urobilinogen) with moderate jaundice (high serum conjugated bilirubin). It is often described as 'painful', to differentiate it from 'painless' causes which suggest malignancy, although at the time of presentation the patient does not necessarily complain of pain. Often the pain is a background history of biliary colic.

The underlying gallstones are typically multiple small stones which can migrate via the cystic duct.

The gallbladder is very rarely palpable since it is usually fibrotic secondary to recurrent episodes of inflammation due to cholecystolithiasis ('Courvoisier's law').

Acute (ascending) cholangitis

This is usually secondary to the presence of chronic common bile duct stones. It is characterized by clinical and biochemical features of obstructive jaundice with right upper quadrant pain and fevers ('Charcot's triad').

Mirrizzi's syndrome

Mirrizzi's syndrome is the presence of features of obstructive jaundice with cholecystitis caused by the presence of inflammation or stone impaction in the neck of the gallbladder causing compression of the common hepatic duct at or above the level of the entry of the cystic duct. A long, parallel cystic duct ± a low insertion into the common bile duct predisposes to this condition.

Other presentations

Acute pancreatitis (📖 Topic 8.19)

Acute pancreatitis is caused either by the passage of stones through or impaction at the ampulla of Vater or occasionally just by the presence of common bile duct stones.

Gallstone ileus

This is obstruction of the ileum secondary to intraluminal gallstone(s). The site of impaction is commonly the distal but not the true terminal ileum where the ileum is at its narrowest. There is usually a pre-existing cholecystoenteric (duodenal) fistula via which a single large stone enters the small bowel.

Clinical assessment

Investigations

- Bloods—raised WCC and CRP suggest septic complications. Raised bilirubin and ALP suggest bile duct obstruction or cholangitis
- Abdominal USS should be arranged for all acute presentations, ideally within 24 h. It detects 95% of gallstones, features of acute cholecystitis (thickened, oedematous gallbladder wall with pericholecystic fluid), is the first line investigation for probable obstructive jaundice (to evaluate intrahepatic and extrahepatic duct size and possibly identify distal bile duct obstruction)

- CT scan—for the evaluation of a right upper quadrant mass, investigation of possible gallbladder infarction/necrosis/perforation, investigation of possible malignancy
- Magnetic resonance cholangiopancreatography (MRCP) for the diagnosis of obstructive jaundice (bile duct stones, cholangiocarcinoma, pancreatic head lesions)
- Endoscopic retrograde cholangiopancreatography (ERCP) for the diagnosis and treatment of obstructive jaundice
- HIDA (hydroximinodiacetic) scan (radioactive isotope) scan is only rarely used, occasionally to demonstrate functional gallbladder disease

Management

- 95%+ of acute biliary colic settles with dietary restriction (low fat) and analgesia alone
- 80%+ of acute cholecystitis will settle with analgesia, dietary restriction, and antibiotics
- 70%+ of patients suffering episodes of symptoms of biliary colic will improve/resolve with dietary manipulation (low fat)

Elective (laparoscopic) cholecystectomy

Asymptomatic gallstones need no intervention. Elective laparoscopic cholecystectomy is considered in:

- symptomatic gallstones failing conservative management (dietary manipulation) or by patient choice
- episodes of septic gallbladder complications to prevent recurrence (in patients fit for surgery)
- episodes of complications (e.g. pancreatitis) to prevent recurrence of complications

Management of complications

Identification

- Consider a CT scan for pain, inflammatory features or septic features which fail to resolve with treatment—these may indicate the development of an empyema, gallbladder necrosis or intrahepatic abscess
- Consider an urgent ERCP for proven common bile duct obstruction (dilated extrahepatic bile ducts on USS) with features of ascending cholangitis

Treatment

- **Percutaneous cholecystostomy**—indicated for acute empyema of the gallbladder or unresolving acute cholecystitis with a distended gallbladder in patients unfit or unwilling to undergo acute cholecystectomy
- **ERCP**—indicated for obstructive jaundice (urgently if associated with cholangitis or pancreatitis). Stone extraction or insertion of endoluminal stent to relieve obstruction and ensure adequate bile drainage
- **Acute laparoscopic cholecystectomy**—indicated for uncomplicated biliary presentations (colic or cholecystitis) provided the patient would require/elect to have an elective procedure *and* the presentation is early in the course of the disease. 'Same admission' surgery is advocated to reduce the risk of recurrent symptoms and improve efficiency of the use of medical resources. The risk of conversion to open surgery and complications depends on the patient and the timing, but may be slightly higher if there have been previous inflammatory episodes or the disease process is established
- **Acute open cholecystectomy**—indicated for unresolving severe cholecystitis (particularly with an associated mass), septic complications associated with cholecystolithiasis which cannot be treated by ERCP—requires common bile duct exploration (CBDE)

- **Laparotomy**—indicated for proven 'gallstone ileus' diagnosed on AXR or CT scan or gallbladder necrosis (diagnosed as diffuse peritonitis or on CT scan)

✚ Laparoscopic cholecystectomy

Ninety per cent of cholecystectomies are performed laparoscopically in the UK. The only absolute contraindication to this approach is a bleeding diathesis.

- Consent should include conversion to open procedure (~5%), infection, bleeding, bile leak, bile duct injury (<1%)
- 'Paperwork' to check—what are the recent LFTs? If there were common bile duct stones, is there documented evidence that they have been treated?

Procedure—principles

- CO_2 pneumoperitoneum is induced using open (Hasson) technique (preferred method) or Verress needle (blunt sprung hollow needle) in the subumbilical region to form a 10 mm port
- Intra-abdominal pressure is usually kept between 12 and 15 mmHg (lower pressures can be used if the anaesthetist notes problems with excessive pulmonary inflation pressures or decreased venous return leading to low cardiac output)
- Three further ports: 10 mm midline below the xiphisternum, 5 mm subcostal, 5 mm right lateral/flank
- The patient is positioned head up and tilted to the left
- Perform a general laparoscopic abdominal survey
- Dissection proceeds as follows: 1) exposure of Calot's triangle, 2) exposure of cystic duct and artery, 3) cystic duct identified by seeing direct continuity with gallbladder neck, 4) division of cystic duct followed by cystic artery between clips, 5) retrograde dissection of gallbladder from liver bed by diathermy dissection

Calot's triangle is formed by the cystic duct inferiorly, the common hepatic duct medially, and the liver edge superiorly; it contains the cystic artery, often with a lymph node adjacent to it.

- Cholangiography may be performed via the cystic duct prior to clipping to confirm biliary anatomy or if CBD stones are suspected
- Subhepatic drains may be placed
- During exsufflation, port sites should be inspected for bleeding into the abdomen

Complications

- Bleeding—suggested by persistent hypotension or excessive abdominal pain
- Bile leak—suggested by excessive abdominal pain

4.7 Oesophageal neoplasia

- Oesophageal carcinoma is the sixth leading cause of cancer deaths worldwide
- Fifty per cent of patients have unresectable disease at presentation
- The UK incidence is 7000, with 6700 deaths per annum
- Squamous and adenoma carcinoma are essentially different diseases
- Benign tumours are rare—leiomyomas (GISTs) derived from the smooth muscle of the muscularis propria, neural tumours such as schwannomas, and neurofibromas

Aetiology

Squamous carcinoma

- Squamous carcinoma has an incidence of 2–3 per 100,000 in the UK, which is decreasing. It is twice as common in men and is seen in older patients (>65 years).
- Strong relationship to dietary and inhaled carcinogens: smoking, smoked food (China/Iran), raw fish/nitrosamines (Japan, Russia, Scandinavia), alcohol
- Low intake of vitamins A/C/B_6
- Pre-existing abnormalities of squamous epithelium; tylosis, caustic strictures

Adenocarcinoma

Adenocarcinoma is more common in developed countries (incidence >5 per 100,000 in the UK) and the incidence is rising rapidly. It is seen in younger patients (>40 years).

There is a strong relationship to:

- gastro-oesophageal reflux disease (📖 Topic 4.3)—acid or biliary
- columnar epithelium in the lower oesophagus—Barrett's oesophagus (📖 Topic 4.3). The relative risk doubles, increasing with symptom duration, especially in male Caucasians

Pathology

Squamous carcinoma

Squamous carcinoma is most commonly found in the middle third (upper 10%, middle 60%, distal 30%).

Adenocarcinoma

This is most common in the lower third owing to the relationship with GORD (upper rare, middle 15%, lower 85%).

Morphologically, the tumours may be an intraluminal mass, polypoid, ulcerating, stenosing predominantly extraluminal mass, or a focus of carcinoma arising in Barrett's oesophagus.

Spread can be direct local spread, lymphatic or haematogenous. Metastases are established in 30% of patients at diagnosis.

Clinical assessment

Primary disease

- Dysphagia is typically progressive, initially worst for solids, with worsening symptoms for liquids as the intraluminal tumour increases. It is accompanied by weight loss
- Dyspepsia/retrosternal pain is persistent, typically resistant to acid suppression
- Haematemesis is rare and may indicate invasion and erosion of local vascular structures. Anaemia is more common

Features of locoregional spread

- Hoarseness/bovine cough—recurrent laryngeal invasion
- Recurrent cough—oesophagotracheal fistula or aspiration
- Supraclavicular mass
- Jaundice, upper abdominal mass—liver/para-aortic node involvement

> ⊘ **Urgent 2-week wait referral for suspected upper gastrointestinal cancer**
>
> - New onset dysphagia
> - Dyspepsia with weight loss, anaemia or vomiting
> - Dyspepsia with family history, Barrett's or previous peptic ulcer surgery
> - New dyspepsia in a patient over 55 years of age
> - Jaundice
> - Upper abdominal mass

Investigations

- Bloods—FBC (anaemia)
- OGD + biopsy/brush cytology to achieve a (tissue) diagnosis and may be required for tumour dilatation and stent insertion
- Thoracoabdominal CT scan used for locoregional staging and preoperative assessment of tumour
- Barium swallow may be required for diagnosis of lesions presenting with very high dysphagia where flexible endoscopy is either impossible or contra-indicated due to risk
- Endoscopic ultrasound (EUS) assesses local mural invasion and operability in the absence of metastases
- Liver ultrasound, liver MRI, and CT PET scan may help to assess possible metastatic disease
- Laparoscopy is often used to exclude small volume peritoneal disease in patients considered for resection

Staging

TNM classification

Primary tumour

TX	Cannot be assessed
T0	No evidence of primary tumour
Tis	Carcinoma *in situ*
T1	Invades submucosa
T2	Invades muscularis propria
T3	Invades up to serosa
T4	Invades adjacent structures

Regional lymph nodes

NX	Cannot be assessed
N0	No regional lymph node metastasis
N1	Regional lymph node metastasis

Distant metastasis

MX	Cannot be assessed
M0	No distant metastasis
M1	Distant metastasis

Management

Palliative

The majority of tumours are incurable or unresectable at presentation. They will require some form of palliative care during their clinical course. General symptoms requiring palliation including dysphagia pain, nausea, and cough.

Treatments for dysphagia

- Radiotherapy—most effective for squamous carcinoma; may result in tracheo-oesophageal fistula
- Dilatation—may result in tumour perforation
- Stent insertion—self-expanding metal (SEM). May be used in conjunction with radiotherapy and endoluminal treatments. Cannot be used for tumours in the upper third owing to resulting continuous sensation of stent presence
- Endoscopic tumour ablation—alcohol injection, laser ablation (may result in tumour necrosis-related perforation)

Treatments for oesophagotracheal fistula

- Covered metal stent
- Chemotherapy has a limited role in younger patients

Operative

Surgery is offered only for potentially curative treatment (i.e. where there is no determinable metastatic disease and no nodal disease other than possible peritumoral nodes. All other nodal disease carries an increasingly poor prognosis.

Neoadjuvant chemoradiotherapy may be used to downsize tumours and improve both resectability and chance of cure.

Surgical principles

The aim is radical excision of tumour and locoregional lymph nodes followed by restoration of gut tube continuity. The tumour location guides the surgical approach, extent of resection, and the conduit used for reconstruction.

Abdominal surgery and some thoracic surgery may be laparoscopically and/or thoracoscopically assisted.

- Distal oesophageal/oesophagogastric junction: transabdominal approach, proximal oesophago-gastrectomy, and oesophagogastric anastomosis
- Mid-oesophageal—combined abdominothoracic approach (Ivor–Lewis/Lewis–Tanner), oesophagectomy, intrathoracic gastro-oesophageal anastomosis
- Proximal oesophagus—abdominothoracocervical approach, proximal oesophagectomy, colonic or jejunal interposition

Complications and prognosis

Complications of surgery

- Chest infection/pneumonia/pleural effusion
- Anastomotic leak (should be less than 5%)
- Chylothorax
- Recurrent laryngeal nerve damage
- Benign anastomotic stricture

Prognosis

Fewer than 50% of cases are suitable for potentially curative treatment. Of those undergoing surgery, 1-year survival is approximately 75% but 5-year survival is only 25–30%.

⊙ Dsyphagia

Dysphagia is defined as difficulty in swallowing. Aphagia is the inability to swallow. Odynophagia is painful swallowing.

Dysphagia can be caused by oropharyngeal or oesophageal conditions. The causes can be divided into mechanical and neuromuscular conditions.

Extrinsic mechanical

- Bronchial carcinoma
- Retrosternal goitre
- Thoracic aortic aneurysm

Intrinsic mechanical

- Oesophageal carcinoma
- Foreign body (luminal)
- Benign stricture (peptic/caustic/postsurgical)
- Plummer–Vinson syndrome (oesophageal web)
- Pharyngeal pouch
- Systemic sclerosis

Primary neuromuscular

- Achalasia
- Diffuse oesophageal spasm
- Nutcracker oesophagus

Secondary neuromuscular

- Myasthenia gravis
- Bulbar palsy or poliomyelitis
- Multiple sclerosis

Investigations

- Barium swallow (dynamic video)
- OGD
- Others possible: CT, MRI, EUS, and oesophageal manometry

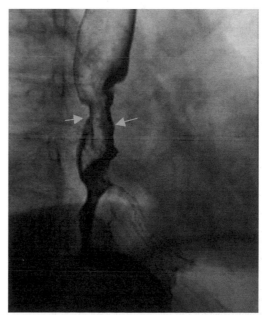

Fig 4.5 Barium swallow showing an adenocarcinoma of the distal oesophagus with an irregular outline of both the anterior and posterior walls. Above this the oesophagus is dilated and there is some 'shouldering'.

4.8 Gastric neoplasia

Primary gastric neoplasias include:

- adenocarcinoma—95% of tumours
- gastrointestinal stromal tumours (GISTs)—include tumours previously called leiomyomas, leiomyosarcomas (1–3% of tumours)
- Gastric carcinoid—1%
- Gastric lymphoma—2%
- Tumours of mucosal-associated lymphoid tissues (MALTomas)

Gastric carcinoma

- 10% of all new cancer diagnoses and 12% of all cancer-related deaths in the Europe

Aetiology

Gastric adenocarcinoma is the fourth most common cause of cancer deaths in Europe. It is more common in men and has a peak incidence around 55 years of age. The highest incidence is in Japan.

- Environmental factors:
  - diet high in nitrosamines (smoked fish)
  - carcinogen exposure (smoking, high alcohol intake
  - *H. pylori* exposure
- Mucosal factors:
  - gastritis (atrophic, autoimmune with pernicious anaemia—excess cell proliferation within gastric epithelium)
  - Family history (e.g. E-cadherin mutation)

Pathology

The incidence of tumours in the cardia is rising but falling for the antrum and corpus. Macroscopically, appearance of tumours varies.

- Malignant ulcers typically have raised everted edges with a necrotic base
- 'Polyp' carcinomas grow out into the stomach lumen and are rare
- Colloid tumour—a massive gelatinous growth
- Leather-bottle stomach (linitis plastica) is a diffuse infiltration within the mucosa and submucosa with marked fibrosis leading to a shrunken, inelastic, thickened stomach

Microscopically, adenocarcinomas have varying differentiation; intestinal gland-like spaces confer a better prognosis whilst diffuse sheets of anaplastic (signet ring cells) give a poor prognosis (Lauren classification).

Tumour spread may be local, lymphatic (the main route, to lesser and greater curvature, left gastric, and supraclavicular nodes) or via the portal system (commonly to the liver, lungs, and brain). Spread to the ovaries leads to the development of a Krukenberg tumour.

Clinical presentations

Dyspepsia

New onset of dyspepsia over age 50 years is suspicious as is constant dyspepsia, worsening dyspepsia or resistance to treatment. Weight loss, early satiety, and epigastric mass are worrying signs

Upper GI bleeding

Upper GI bleeding is often low volume/occult, leading to iron-deficiency anaemia, and possibly haematemesis or melaena.

Gastric obstruction

Regurgitation, early postprandial vomiting, and dysphagia suggest a proximal gastric obstructing tumour.

Late postprandial vomiting, often copious, projectile/effortless, old altered food without bile suggests obstruction to the gastric outlet/pyloric canal.

Perforated malignant ulcer

See Topic 8.18.

Distant metastases/diffuse disease

- Ascites suggests peritoneal metastases
- Jaundice suggests liver metastases
- Left supraclavicular node: Virchow's node, Troisier's sign
- Umbilical nodule: Sister Mary Joseph nodule is a hard, red, painless mass at the umbilicus associated with advanced malignancy. It is the result of local tumour spread along the falciform ligament. Over 90% are adenocarcinomas from the stomach or ovary

Clinical assessment

Investigations

- Bloods—FBC (anaemia), LFTs (liver metastasis)
- Gastroscopy + biopsy are usually diagnostic. Barium meal is occasionally useful when OGD is contraindicated
- Abdominothoracic CT scan to assess regional and distant spread
- Endoluminal ultrasound is superior to CT for local staging
- Laparoscopy for staging to identify peritoneal metastases if resection is considered possible
- CT PET scan occasionally used to assess possible resectable disease

Staging

TNM classification

Primary tumour

TX	Cannot be assessed
T0	No evidence of primary tumour
Tis	Adenocarcinoma confined to the mucosa
T1	Invading submucosa
T2	Invading muscularis propria
T3	Invading subserosal tissues
T4	Invading serosal or into adjacent organs

Regional lymph nodes

NX	Cannot be assessed
N0	No nodal metastases
N1	1–6 nodes involved
N2	7–15 nodes involved
N3	>15 nodes involved

Distant metastasis

MX	Cannot be assessed
M0	No distant metastasis
M1	Metastases (Hep—liver, Per—peritoneal, Pul—lung)

Management

The majority of tumours are incurable at presentation. Surgery offers the only hope of cure in those suitable.

Potentially curative

Surgery

Extent of stomach resection:

- tumours of cardia/gastro-oesophageal junction—proximal/total gastrectomy and distal oesophagectomy
- middle third—total gastrectomy
- distal (antral) tumours—subtotal gastrectomy

The extent of lymph node resection depends on location but is usually described as D2, meaning radical locoregional nodes according to tumour location. For proximal cancers this may include splenectomy.

Chemotherapy

- Neoadjuvant—may have a role in some patients
- Adjuvant—no clear evidence of survival benefit
- Locoregional relapse may still occur following gastric cancer complete resection (with curative intent) in the form of distal metastases and/or peritoneal carcinomatosis, i.e. in many ways it is a systemic disease

Palliative

Surgery

Limited gastrectomy may be used to palliate bleeding tumours, perforated tumours, or, very rarely, symptomatic tumours or bypass-obstructing distal tumours.

Interventional procedures

Endoscopic laser ablation, endoluminal stenting for obstructing tumours of the oesophagogastric junction or pylorus.

Chemotherapy

Has a limited role in palliation where there may be some quality of life and survival benefit.

Radiotherapy

For palliation, radiotherapy can be particularly helpful in reducing bleeding.

Complications and prognosis

- Early gastric cancer (Tis or pT1 with pN0, pM0)— 80% 5-year survival if resected with clear margins
- Localized gastric cancer (pT2/pT3 with pN1 pM0)— 20–60% 5-year survival if resected with clear margins
- Advanced gastric cancer—3% 5-year survival
- Mortality 12.4 per 100 000 population/year

Gastrointestinal stromal tumours

Gastrointestinal stromal tumours (GIST) is the correct term for all tumours arising from non-epithelial and non-lymphoid tissues of the GI tract.

They include tumours of benign, malignant, and indeterminate malignant potential, including those previously known as:

- leiomyoma/leiomyosarcoma
- lipoma/liposarcoma
- fibrosarcoma
- gastrointestinal autonomic nerve cell tumours (GANTs)

Malignant potential is related to and assessed from mitotic rate (number of divisions per high power microscopic field), cellular atypia, and evidence of non-neoplastic tissue 'invasion'.

The commonest sites are:

- stomach—typically benign 'leiomyomas' and submucosal 'lipomas'
- small intestine—submucosal 'lipomas'
- rectum—various

Common presentations are:

- acute upper GI bleeding (gastric or small bowel 'leiomyoma')
- palpable abdominal mass (intramesenteric fibro(sarco)ma)

Management

Principles of treatment are:

- small lesions should be excised (locally or radically if necessary); clear margins are required to prevent recurrence
- large lesions, lesions involving vital structures or metastatic GISTs may be treated by anti-CD-117 antibody ('Glivec') prior to surgery

Gastric lymphoma

- Commonest site for GI primary lymphoma
- Almost always non-Hodgkin's type; commonly B cell
- Low grade MALT lymphomas may be related to *H. pylori* infection
- Presentations are similar to adenocarcinoma

Management

Principles of treatment are:

- resection of isolated primary disease ± chemotherapy
- chemo(radio)therapy for more extensive disease

4.9 Pancreaticobiliary neoplasia

This is the fourth commonest site of GI tract neoplasia.

- Adenocarcinoma (pancreas commonest but also ampullary and gallbladder)
- Cholangiocarcinoma
- Neuroendocrine pancreatic tumours

Adenocarcinoma of the pancreas

Adenocarcinoma of the pancreas is increasing in incidence. There are over 6000 cases per year in the UK. There is a male preponderance and the majority of cases occur over the age of 60 years.

Aetiology

Risk factors:

- cigarette smoking
- chronic pancreatitis
- adult onset diabetes <2 years' duration
- hereditary pancreatitis (50–70-fold risk)
- familial pancreatic cancers
- familial cancer syndromes (such as *BRCA2* mutations, familial adenomatous polyposis, and hereditary non-polyposis colorectal cancer)

Pathology

Ninety per cent of adenocarcinomas of the exocrine pancreas arise from the ductal epithelium, while 10% originate from glandular tissue of lobules.

The main routes of spread are: local (into distal common bile duct, duodenal wall, portal vein, IVC, and peri-aortic nerve sheaths), lymphatic (peripancreatic, para-aortic, hepatic), and haematogenous (liver, lung, adrenals).

Clinical assessment

Carcinoma of the head of the pancreas (70%)

- Early obstructive jaundice is painless and progressive, and may be associated with a palpable distended gallbladder
- Courvoisier's law: 'If, in the presence of jaundice, the gallbladder is palpable then it (*the jaundice*) is unlikely to be due to stone,' i.e. stones lead to gallbladder fibrosis which resists distension when the CBD is obstructed.
- Exceptions are a distended but impalpable (intrahepatic) gallbladder or a gallbladder mucocoele due to stone leading to a palpable gallbladder coincidental with CBD stones.
- Features of obstruction of the main pancreatic duct include anorexia, a mild degree of steatorrhoea, and postprandial epigastric pain radiating to the back (a poor prognostic sign)
- Acute pancreatitis (rare)
- Other periampullary tumours (i.e. ampulla and lower common bile duct) may have similar presentation
- Precipitating an episode of acute pancreatitis (rare)

Carcinoma of the neck (5%)/body (20%)/tail (5%) of pancreas

- Typically present late with features of advanced disease: constant back pain, anorexia and weight loss, hepatomegaly, palpable (left) supraclavicular lymph node ('Virchow's node,' 'Troisier's sign'), and ascites
- Features of systemic effects of malignancy—anaemia, migratory superficial thrombophlebitis ('Trousseau's syndrome')
- Rarely, features of endocrine pancreatic failure—acute onset diabetes mellitus

Investigations

- Bloods—FBC (anaemia), deranged LFTs (liver metastases, jaundice)
- Ca 19-9 can be used as a tumour marker to assess prognosis and recurrence
- Abdominal ultrasound is the first line investigation and may identify a mass
- Thoracoabdominal CT scan defines resectability and assesses local and distant disease
- ERCP + biopsy/cytology excludes stones and ampullary disease

For possible resectable disease:

- CT angiography may be used to assess local vascular invasion
- Endoluminal ultrasound (ELUS) is possibly the most sensitive investigation to assess local invasion if resection is considered
- MRCP is used to evaluate local bile duct involvement
- Laparoscopy is used for staging to identify peritoneal metastases if resection is considered possible
- CT PET scan is occasionally used to assess possible resectable disease

Management

The majority of tumours are incurable at presentation, usually because of local invasion of vital structures (portal/mesenteric vessels).

Surgery offers the only hope of cure in those suitable and the majority of these are carcinoma of the head of the pancreas, involving the distal CBD early in its course, or periampullary carcinomas.

Potentially curative

Surgery

Surgery is considered for tumours <4 cm in diameter, confined to the pancreas, with no local invasion or metastases (distant or peritoneal).

Whipple's procedure (proximal pancreaticoduodenectomy + distal gastrectomy) is performed for head tumours. This can be modified to be pylorus-preserving.

Left-sided resection (with splenectomy) is very rarely possible for localized pancreatic body and tail carcinomas.

Preoperative biliary drainage remains controversial (and should only involve plastic stents). It is not a routine procedure, but may be justified in jaundiced patients, the reduced complications from resolved jaundice post-stenting being offset by greater biliary sepsis and inflammatory tissue response. However, trials indicate that surgical outcome is not improved and, indeed, may increase the risk of infective outcomes.

Chemotherapy

Adjuvant/neoadjuvant (gemcitabine/fluorouracil) demonstrates no clear evidence of survival benefit, and may be the subject of clinical trials.

Palliative

Endoscopic procedures: endobiliary stenting (metal/plastic) is preferable to transhepatic stenting, although it still carries the risk of cholangitis and perforation.

Surgery

Choledochojejunostomy and gastrojejunostomy (open or laparoscopic) may be used for patients with a prognosis >6 months or those with an uncertain diagnosis.

Complications and prognosis

Pancreatic ductal adenocarcinoma has a 0.4–4% 5-year survival (6–10-month median survival); i.e. since survival is so poor, incidence and mortality figures are almost identical. Following Whipple's procedure, the median survival time is extended to 18 months, with a 5-year survival rate of around 10% (failure occurring owing to local recurrence ± hepatic metastases).

Cystic tumours

These constitute less than 1% of tumours and, although most are benign, half are mucinous types, which are considered premalignant. They tend to present in women of a young age group, and care must be taken to differentiate these tumours from pseudocysts, especially as they have a good prognosis. On CT, tumours have septa within the cyst and a calcified rim of the cyst wall without other pancreatic calcification.

Endocrine tumours

Endocrine tumours have an incidence of approximately 1.2 per million of the population. They are either sporadic in nature or part of the multiple endocrine (MEN) syndrome. Tumours either produce high levels of pancreatic hormones, such as insulin and glucagon, or non-pancreatic hormones like gastrin or vasoactive peptide. Presentation therefore tends to be with clinical syndromes of hormonal excess. Except for insulinomas, most endocrine tumours are malignant, but survival following surgical resection is generally good (10-year survival for malignant lesions is around 50%).

Adenocarcinoma of the gallbladder

Most tumours arise in the fundus and histologically are moderately differentiated adenocarcinomas.

They are usually associated with gallstones and are discovered incidentally at cholecystectomy or at advanced stages.

The incidence rises over the age of 50 years, and they are more common in women over the age of 70.

Curative treatment involves radical cholecystectomy (with resection of segment IV of the liver) if diagnosed preoperatively. Salvage surgery or surgery for advanced disease is rarely possible due to liver involvement.

Chemotherapy has little impact.

Cholangiocarcinoma

This is carcinoma arising from the bile duct epithelium (most commonly the extrahepatic biliary tree, but it may be intrahepatic). Cholangiocarcinoma may be multifocal or spread within the biliary tree.

Cholangiocarcinoma is usually primary but it is associated with cystic dilatation of the bile duct and chronic inflammation, chronic cholecystolithiasis, and sclerosing cholangitis.

It usually presents with obstructive jaundice or cholangitis.

Surgical resection is the only chance of cure but is rarely possible owing to local invasion of vital liver hilar structures (median 5-year survival following resection is 14%; median survival of unresected cases is 6 months).

Palliative treatment is biliary decompression via ERCP or percutaneous transhepatic stenting.

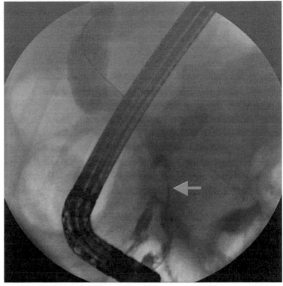

Fig 4.6 ERCP showing irregular malignant-looking stricture of the distal common bile duct (arrow) and pancreatic duct (not shown). The biliary tree is markedly dilated. These findings are consistent with a neoplasm of the pancreatic head. A stent was placed and achieved good drainage. The patient went on to have a CT scan for further assessment (see below).

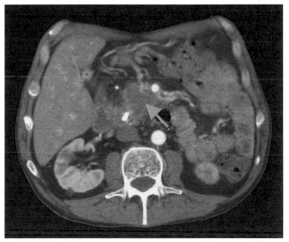

Fig 4.7 Abdominal CT scan showing an irregular hypodense mass in the region of the head of the pancreas (green arrow). The common bile duct stent inserted at ERCP is seen to run along the right side of the mass. There is no intrahepatic bile duct dilatation, and no focal liver lesions.

Liver

Liver neoplasia

Liver tumours can be benign or malignant and primary or metastatic. Metastatic tumours are common, probably because of a high blood flow and immunological factors.

Primary hepatocellular carcinoma is uncommon in the UK, but has a higher incidence in areas where hepatitis and chronic alcoholic cirrhosis is prevalent. Benign tumours, including haemangiomas and adenomas, are rare.

Metastatic liver disease

Common primary tumours that metastasize to the liver include lung, breast, colorectal, pancreas, and stomach. Early disease is usually asymptomatic.

Assessment

- Weight loss, anorexia, jaundice, and ascites suggest advanced disease
- Blood tests depend on the stage of disease and whether there is biliary obstruction, but may show raised bilirubin, ALP, and AST
- CT scan is the diagnostic and assessment modality of choice. CT or ultrasound-guided biopsy is used in inoperable cases to gain a tissue diagnosis but only once operability has definitely been excluded. Operable cases may be assessed with laparoscopy to avoid seeding

Treatment

- Even multiple or multilobar metastases may be considered for resection with a view to cure or significantly increased life expectancy if all deposits can be resected with clear margins (35% 5-year survival)
- Ablation (thermal, ultrasonic or radiofrequency) may be used for palliation or may be combined with resection for residual lesions not resectable
- Palliative chemotherapy offers a good prospect for increased life expectancy: it is usually delivered systemically rather than by intra-arterial chemoembolization.

Extrahepatic abscesses

Intra-abdominal abscesses are a common problem. There is often a delay in making the diagnosis, difficulty in localizing the abscesses, and they are associated with significant morbidity and mortality rates.

They may complicate pancreatitis, cholecystitis, or perforation in diverticular disease, acute appendicitis, and peptic ulcer disease. Other causes include trauma and posteroperative anastomotic leak.

Abscesses can form in six spaces around the liver: superiorly in the left and right subphrenic spaces (anterior and posterior), inferiorly below the left lobe and around the lesser sac. Other positions in the abdomen include pelvis, right and left paracolic gutters, and in the interloop spaces of the small intestine.

Clinical presentations are variable. Abscesses may cause persistent abdominal pain, localized tenderness, spiking fevers, and prolonged GI dysfunction. CT scan or ultrasound is usually diagnostic. Patients need high dose parenteral antibiotics and percutaneous or open drainage of the abscess.

Spleen

The spleen is situated in the left upper quadrant beneath the left hemidiaphragm. It has a number of functions, including:

- removal of old blood cells
- modification of circulating red blood cells—removal of inclusion bodies and remodelling of their surface membrane
- production of antibodies and complement activation
- production and maturation of B cells, T cells, and plasma cells
- filtering of circulating pathogens and particulate matter. It is the largest collection of lymphoid tissue in the body
- storage of bloods, particularly platelets and leucocytes

Hyposplenism and hypersplenism

Hyposplenism

Hyposplenism is confirmed by abnormalities of red blood cells on the peripheral blood film. These include Howell–Jolly bodies, Pappenheimer bodies, target cells, and irregular contracted cells. Causes include:

- splenectomy
- acquired hyposplenism: coeliac disease, inflammatory bowel disease, SLE, sickle cell disease
- congenital splenic agenesis

Hypersplenism

Hypersplenism is defined as excessive splenic function as indicated by anaemia, thrombocytopenia, leucopenia or pancytopenia (caused by sequestration and destruction of cells in the spleen's reticuloendothelial system) in the presence of splenomegaly. It may present with anaemia, infection or bleeding.

Primary hypersplenism is due to disorders of the reticuloendothelial system.

Secondary hypersplenism is due to overactivity induced by splenomegaly owing to other causes (mostly liver disease and portal hypertension).

Splenomegaly

There are numerous causes of splenomegaly. Their incidence varies with geographical location. In the UK, hepatic cirrhosis and haematological conditions are most common. The spleen is usually palpable when at least twice its normal size.

- **Congestion**: cirrhosis, portal vein thrombosis, splenic vein thrombosis, congestive cardiac failure, Budd–Chiari syndrome
- **Haematological**: sickle cell disease, thalassaemia, iron-deficiency anaemia
- **Infection**: hepatitis, mononucleosis, cytomegalovirus, AIDs
- **Neoplastic**: acute and chronic leukaemia, lymphoma
- **Storage disorders**: Gaucher's disease, Wilson's disease
- **Miscellaneous**: congenital, cysts, trauma

Splenectomy

Splenectomy has a number of indications (see below). Laparoscopic splenectomy is the preferred approach as it has a low complication rate and shorter hospital stay. Patients need careful perioperative management as they will have an increased risk of sepsis (see box).

Indications for splenectomy

- Unsalvageable splenic injury (📖 Topic 8.10) (occasionally iatrogenic injury)
- Spontaneous rupture occurring with massive splenomegaly
- Hypersplenism: hereditary spherocytosis, idiopathic thrombocytopenic purpura
- Neoplasia of the spleen or *en bloc* resection of other local GI tumours
- Parasitic splenic cysts, splenic abscess

⊙ Post-splenectomy prophylaxis

Patients are at risk of severe systemic infection following splenectomy sepsis. Overwhelming post-splenectomy infection (OPSI) is rare but has a high mortality rate (>50%). The risk is higher for children than adults and is also related to the underlying condition (low risk following trauma, highest in patients with thalassaemia).

Complications of splenectomy

- Thrombocytosis: platelet count peaks at 7–10 days. Aspirin may be indicated for very high counts (>1000 g/dL)
- Overwhelming post-splenectomy infection is usually due to encapsulated bacteria such as *Streptococcus pneumoniae*, *Haemophilus influenzae*, and *Neisseria meningitides*.

Prophylaxis

Follow British Committee for Standards in Haematology guidelines.

- Vaccination should be given 2 weeks before elective splenectomy or as soon as possible following emergency splenectomy
- *H. influenza* type B (HIB) vaccine in unimmunized patients and annual influenza vaccination
- Pneumococcal vaccine
- Meningococcal serogroup C conjugated vaccine for unimmunized patients
- Lifelong prophylactic antibiotics (penicillin V) are recommended, although the first 2 years are most important as this is when most infections occur
- Patients should be educated in the risks of OPSI and to identify early symptoms and signs so that they can seek treatment
- Patients should be registered and carry a Medic-alert bracelet and card

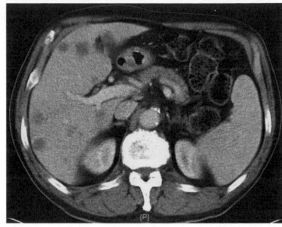

Fig 4.8 Abdominal CT scan showing multiple liver metastases.

4.11 Case-based discussions

Case 1

A 57-year-old year old man presents to the outpatient department with a 7-week history of intermittent dysphagia, worse particularly in the last 2 weeks. He is an ex-smoker, drinks moderate alcohol, and has mild angina on exertion.

- What features of the dysphagia might help you to a differential diagnosis?

There are no obvious abnormalities on examination. The dysphagia is mostly felt at the lower end of the sternum.

- What initial investigations would you request?

He has a borderline anaemia (Hb 11.2 g/dL), normal U+Es, and LFTs. Chest radiograph is normal. An OGD the following week reveals an ulcerated, bleeding stricture at the lower end of the oesophagus which is passable by the endoscope. Biopsies confirm an adenocarcinoma.

- What are the possible risk factors for this development?
- What investigations would you arrange?

A thoracoabdominal CT scan reveals a locally confined thickening of the distal oesophagus with no evidence of lymphadenopathy or metastases. A CT PET scan is normal. ELUS suggests the tumour is at the outer limit of the oesophageal muscle.

- What are principles of treatment for this lesion?

Case 2

A 44-year-old woman is seen in the outpatient department complaining of upper abdominal pain, nausea, and mild anorexia.

- Describe what features of the pain you would elicit to clarify a differential diagnosis

The pain is worse after meals, particularly those high in saturated fats. The lady is mildly overweight and there is a family history of gallstones (mother and grandmother).

- What investigations would you request?

Her blood investigations are normal, including LFTs. Upper abdominal ultrasound reveals multiple small gallstones and a common bile duct of 10 mm (larger than expected in a lady of her age).

- What further investigations might be requested?

An MRCP shows no evidence of common bile duct stones.

- What advice would you give to the patient
- When would you recommend surgery?
- How would you consent the patient for the surgery?

Case 3

A 44-year-old woman is admitted into the surgical assessment unit where you are on duty. She is pale and sweaty, complaining of severe epigastric pain.

- What is the initial differential diagnosis?

After analgesia, she is able to tell you that she has had the pain for 6 h; it radiates to the back, is worse on movement and she's never had it before. She has vomited several times (bilious) and has no urinary symptoms or change of bowel habit. Her observations reveal a temperature of 36.1°C, BP 110/70, pulse 100, SaO$_2$ 96% on air and respiratory rate 24.

On examination of the abdomen there is guarding in the epigastric region and a mildly distended abdomen; there is no organomegaly and bowel sounds are present but quiet.

- What diagnostic investigations would you request?

An ECG is performed and shows a sinus tachycardia; the erect chest radiograph shows no free air below the diaphragm. The bloods come back, revealing an amylase of 2600 iu, with mildly deranged LFTs.

- What other tests are needed to score the severity of the patient's pancreatitis?

The patient is transferred to a high dependency unit and managed conservatively for 24 h before transfer back to the main ward.

- What complications were most likely to have occurred whilst on HDU and how would they present?

An ultrasound is performed whilst she is on HDU and multiple gallstones are demonstrated with biliary tree dilatation.

- When is a suitable time to perform a cholecystectomy?
- How would you consent the patient and what are the basic principles of the procedure?

Chapter 5

Colorectal surgery

◎ Clinical skills

- Extraintestinal manifestations of IBD
- Colorectal screening
- Urgent 2-week wait referral for suspected colorectal cancer
- Rigid sigmoidoscopy
- Classification of fistula-in-ano
- Goodsell's Law

⊕ Technical skills and procedures

- Ileostomy and colostomy formation
- Ileostomy closure
- Inguinal hernia repair
- Femoral hernia repair
- Banding of haemorrhoids
- Injection of haemorrhoids
- Drainage of perianal abscess
- Setons
- Drainage of infected pilonidal sinus
- Excision and primary closure of pilonidal sinus
- Excision of anal warts/tags

5.1 Gastrointestinal embryology and overview

Embryology of abdominal contents

The primitive gut tube forms from the fourth week. The gut tube components are derived from:

- endodermal epithelium: mucosa and glands of the GI tract, biliary tract, and parenchyma of the liver and pancreas
- splanchnopleuric mesenchyme: submucosa, muscularis propria, and mesenteric connective tissue
- splanchnopleuric coelomic epithelium: serosa
- angiogenic mesenchyme: blood vessels and lymphatics
- neural crest: autonomic nerves and enteroendocrine cells
- mesoderm: intestinal mesentery

Embryological division of GI tract

1. **Foregut** gives rise to the hypopharynx, oesophagus, stomach, first half of duodenum (to ampulla of Vater in the mid second part of the duodenum), liver, dorsal pancreas, and biliary tract
2. **Midgut** gives rise to the duodenum distal to the ampulla of Vater, ventral pancreas, jejunum, ileum, caecum, vermiform appendix, ascending colon, and proximal two-thirds of the transverse colon
3. **Hindgut** gives rise to the distal third of the transverse colon, descending colon, sigmoid, and rectum to the anorectal junction

Key points in the embryological development

1. Initial development (stages 7–15)—within the intraembryonic coelom; the gut tube is axial
2. Mid development (stages 15–23)—rotation occurs initially of the stomach and subsequently the midgut loop owing to growth in size and length not being matched by the increase in coelomic cavity size. The intestinal loop continues its development outside the peritoneal cavity as a physiological hernia. Rotation of the gut occurs to the right of the yolk stalk and the anticlockwise rotation is continued, forming the pattern of intestinal loop position within the peritoneum
3. Late development (stage 23 on)—midgut loop returns to the coelomic (peritoneal) cavity owing to an increase in size of the cavity

GI tract general structure

From the oesophagus to the rectum, the wall of the gut tube has a general structure outlined below (inside to outside). There is some specialization in certain areas.

1. Mucosa—the innermost layer. It is divided into the epithelium, lamina propria, and muscularis mucosae. Its structure at various sites in the GI tract reflects their specialist needs
2. Submucosa—a dense connective tissue layer containing blood vessels, nerves, and lymphatics
3. Muscularis externa (propria)—a circular inner muscular layer and a longitudinal outer muscular layer
4. Adventitia or serosal layer—formed from mesothelium and submesothelial connective tissue

GI tract vascular supply

The coeliac axis arises from the anterior aspect of the aorta at the level of the L1 vertebral body and supplies the foregut. The three main branches are splenic, common hepatic, and left gastric arteries. Multiple common variants occur, including absence of branches and accessory or replaced arteries arising from the superior mesenteric artery.

Superior mesenteric artery and vein—the artery arises from the anterior aspect of the aorta at the level of the lower border of the L1 vertebral body, and supplies the midgut. Normal branches are: middle colic artery, right colic artery, jejunal arteries, ileal arteries, and ileocolic artery. Multiple common variants occur, including absence of the right colic artery, common middle/right colic origin, accessory arteries from the coeliac trunk.

Each branch of the artery is accompanied by one or more veins. These join to form the superior mesenteric vein, which in turn joins the splenic vein to form the portal vein behind the neck of the pancreas.

Inferior mesenteric artery and vein—the artery arises from the aorta at the level of L3 vertebral body and supplies the hindgut. Normal branches are: left colic artery, three or four sigmoid arteries, and the superior rectal artery (although the sigmoid arteries are effectively branches of the superior rectal).

The inferior mesenteric vein receives tributaries similar to the branches of the artery. It lies to the left of the artery in the left colonic mesentery and ascends laterally to drain into the splenic vein behind the tail of the pancreas.

Middle and inferior rectal arteries and veins—the rectum is also supplied by two middle rectal arteries (variably sized branches of the internal iliac artery or its superior vesical or vaginal branches); two inferior rectal arteries (branches of the pudendal branch of the internal iliac artery) and a rectal branch of the median sacral artery—a branch of the aorta.

The rectal veins correspond to the arterial supply and anastomose freely in both the submucosal internal rectal plexus and the perimuscular external rectal plexus outside the rectal wall and with veins of the anal canal.

The portal vein arises from the confluence of the splenic and superior mesenteric veins behind the neck of the pancreas. It drains the GI tract from the lower oesophagus to the anorectal junction.

Venous channels exist between the portal system and veins draining to the vena cavae at:

- the lower oesophagus and gastro-oesophageal junction
- umbilicus and ligamentum teres
- retroperitoneum around the pancreas and colon
- anorectal junction

GI tract lymphatics

All lymph from the stomach, small intestine, and colon drains via the submucosal lymphoid channels into lymph nodes lying in the peritoneal attachments at the margin of the gut (perigastric, peri-ileal, pericolic, perirectal nodes).

These nodes drain back to nodes along the feeding mesenteric arteries (with the same names as those vessels) to the pre-aortic nodes at the origin of the coeliac, superior, and inferior mesenteric arteries ('highest' nodes of the relevant part). All pre-aortic nodes drain via the cisterna chyli to the thoracic duct.

Lymph from the rectum drains into pararectal, superior rectal, and pre-aortic nodes. Significant drainage to internal iliac nodes via the middle rectal pedicles is rare and then is probably only important in pathological conditions. Drainage to the inguinal nodes via the inferior rectal pedicle is only seen in tumours involving the lower anal canal tissues.

GI tract innervation

The GI tract tube has both an intrinsic enteric nervous system and extrinsic innervation from the autonomic nervous system. The peritoneum surrounding the gut has somatic and autonomic innervations.

Intrinsic (enteric) nervous system

Plexuses of neurons lie at several levels within the GI tract wall. They can function autonomously with local reflex arcs and intrinsic activity although there is much communication with the central nervous system (mostly the autonomic system). Plexuses also contain sensory neurons and interneurons that create intrinsic reflex arcs in response to pain, luminal pressure, and intestinal pH.

There are ganglionated intramural plexuses, submucosal (Meissner's) and intermuscular myenteric (Auerbach's), and non-ganglionated plexuses at multiple levels.

Extrinsic nervous system

The extrinsic nervous system modulates the enteric nervous system's control of secretomotor activity and blood supply.

Sympathetic

Sympathetic nerves innervate the entire GI tract and carry afferent pain impulses and efferent vasomotor impulses. They also modulate enteric nervous system function (mostly inhibitory).

- Greater splanchnic nerve—fibres originate in the T5–9 segments (possibly also T1–4) and travel via the thoracic sympathetic chain to the nerves which receive their distribution mainly via the coeliac, superior, and inferior mesenteric, intermesenteric, and pre-aortic plexuses
- Lumbar sympathetics—fibres arise in the lowest thoracic and lumbar segments, travel via the lumbar sympathetic chain into the pre-aortic, intermesenteric, and inferior mesenteric plexuses
- Pelvic sympathetics—fibres arise in the lower lumbar and sacral segments, travel up via the lumbar cord into the lumbar sympathetic chain, down into the sacral chain, and via the sacral nerves to the inferior hypogastric plexus

Parasympathetic

Parasympathetic nerves innervate the GI tract carrying afferent sensory impulses, form extrinsic reflex arcs, and modulate enteric nervous system function, mostly to enhance motor and secretomotor activity.

- Vagus—supplies as far as the distal third of the transverse colon via the anterior vagus (supplies mainly the stomach, liver, and biliary tree) and the posterior vagus (supplies the pancreas, small bowel, and proximal colon)
- Pelvic parasympathetics—originate in segments S2, 3, and 4, supply the distal colon, rectum, and upper anal canal via the inferior and superior hypogastric plexuses

Peritoneal innervation

Visceral peritoneum

Visceral peritoneum is innervated by autonomic nerves, which are sensitive to tension (of a hollow viscus wall or mesentery), visceral muscle spasm, and ischaemia. It receives no somatic innervation and so is insensitive to mechanical, thermal, and chemical stimulation.

Visceral pain is interpreted centrally as poorly localized, vague abdominal discomfort, e.g. initial central, colicky abdominal pain in appendicitis.

Visceral pain is experienced at the dermatome innervated by somatic nerves sharing common afferent pathways with autonomic nerves at that spinal level. This in turn relates to the anatomical relationship of the embryonic foregut, midgut, and hindgut to the developing anterior abdominal wall ($\square$ Topic 8.12).

Parietal peritoneum

Parietal peritoneum is segmentally innervated by somatic nerves, which also supply the abdominal wall musculature and skin in a segmental distribution.

Mechanical, thermal or chemical stimulation of these somatic pain fibres causes reflex (involuntary) contraction of abdominal wall muscles by the corresponding spinal nerve segments ('guarding') and hyperaesthesia of the skin sharing their segmental sensory innervation.

Somatic pain is interpreted centrally as high localized, sharp abdominal pain, e.g. right iliac fossa pain in acute appendicitis.

Oesophagogastric anatomy

The oesophagus commences at the lower border of the cricopharyngeus and ends at the gastro-oesophageal junction. The majority is intrathoracic but approximately 5 cm lies intra-abdominally. The mucosa is stratified non-keratinizing squamous epithelium for all but the lower few centimetres of the intra-abdominal portion, which is a columnar epithelium, and extension of this into the anatomical thoracic oesophagus is pathological. The submucosa is particularly thin and the muscular wall is striated muscle in its upper third but becomes progressively interspersed with and is then replaced with smooth muscle in the lower two-thirds.

The stomach is divided into four portions.

- Fundus—that portion of the stomach above the level of the gastro-oesophageal junction. Mucosa contains little secretory or glandular elements and it functions mostly to store food
- Body—that portion above the line of the incisura angularis and below the gastro-oesophageal junction. Mucosa contains the bulk of acid-producing parietal (oxyntic) cells and a large number of chief (peptic) enzyme-producing cells
- Antrum—that portion below the incisura angularis and above the pyloric canal. Mucosa contains mostly mucus-secreting glands and scattered neuroendocrine (G) cells
- Pyloric canal—mucosa often contains mucus glands and neuroendocrine cells

The greater curvature gives attachment to the greater omentum and the lesser curvature to the lesser omentum.

The gastric mucosa has coarse folds (ruggae) and is protected from the acidic stomach contents by a mucus layer. Specialized cells in the gastric glands secrete various substances: hydrochloric acid (parietal and oxyntic cells), mucus (goblet cells), and pepsin (chief cells).

Small bowel anatomy

The small bowel comprises the duodenum, jejunum, and ileum. The duodenum is divided into four parts and occupies an approximately 'C'-shaped position in the epigastrium between the level of the L1 and L3 vertebral bodies. It admits the conjoined common bile duct and pancreatic duct in the form of the ampulla of Vater on the medial wall of the second part.

The remaining small bowel is arbitrarily divided into the jejunum (proximal one-third) and ileum (distal two-thirds). There are no defining features but the characteristics of the two parts are:

	Jejunum	Ileum
Calibre	Thick-walled, large calibre	Thin-walled
Colour	Red-pink	Purple
Arterial supply	Single or double arcades with long vasa recta	Multiple arcades with short vasa recta
Lymphoid tissue	Sparse	Numerous

Colonic anatomy

The colon starts at the point just distal to the ileocaecal valve and terminates at the rectosigmoid junction. It is about 1.5 m long, and consists of the caecum, and ascending, transverse, descending, and sigmoid colon.

The colonic mucosa is smooth and consists of closely packed tubular glands containing absorptive and goblet cells. The goblet cells produce mucus which has several functions; these include

lubricating the faeces in its passage through the colon and providing a neutral pH layer which protects the brush border from the acidic products of fermentation and provides a microenvironment for digestion and absorption.

The rectum starts at the level of S2 (although a length of 15 cm above the anorectal junction is often used in surgical practice). It characteristically has three semilunar mucosal folds ('valves') within the lumen.

Anal canal anatomy

The anal canal comprises several layers which are, in order (inside to out):

- mucosa—lined by columnar epithelium in the upper third and non-keratinized squamous epithelium in the lower third with a variable zone of columnar, squamous, and transitional cells in the middle third
- submucosa—loosely bound to the mucosa in the upper two-thirds with a profuse arterial and venous plexus derived mostly from terminal branches of the superior rectal vessels. In the lower third the submucosa is replaced by subdermis
- internal anal sphincter—derived from a continuation of the circular smooth muscle of the rectal wall; present to the lower third of the canal and innervated by the autonomic nerves supplying the lower rectum
- conjoint longitudinal coat—derived from fibromuscular fibres which form the continuation of the longitudinal rectal muscle; help to tether and support the lower anal canal mucosa
- external anal sphincter—striated skeletal muscle surrounding the entire length of the canal; innervated by branches of the pudendal nerve

Liver anatomy

The liver occupies the right upper quadrant of the abdomen; the biliary epithelium (the ductal system of the liver) is derived from the endodermal bud arising from the distal foregut, and the parenchyma (the hepatocytes) is derived from the mesenchyme of the septum transversum.

It is supplied by the portal vein (PV) and the hepatic artery (HA) and their left and right branches, and is drained by the hepatic bile ducts (HD) and the hepatic veins (HV) into the inferior vena cava.

The liver is divided according to macroscopic external appearance into the large right lobe (lying to the right of the falciform ligament superiorly and the groove for the ligamentum venosum inferiorly) and the left lobe, which is smaller. The quadrate and caudate lobes visible on the inferior surface are said to be part of the right lobe macroscopically.

Internally and functionally, the liver is divided into two lobes, each containing four segments.

- The right lobe (lies to the right of an approximate line joining the inferior vena cava and gallbladder fossa) is supplied by the right branch of the HA, PV, right HD, and right and middle HVs. It contains segments VIII (right of the middle HV and above the right PV), V (right of the middle HV and below the right PV), VII (right of the right HV and above the right PV), and VI (right of the right HV and below the right PV)
- The left lobe (lies to the left of the above line) is supplied by the left branch of the HA, PV, left HD and left, middle and central HVs. It contains segments I (caudate), II (left of the left HV and above the right PV), III (left of the left HV and below the left PV), and IV (between middle and left HVs)

Pancreatic anatomy

The pancreas lies in the retroperitoneum of the upper abdomen running from slightly to the right of the midline within the 'C' of the duodenal curvature across the midline to the base of the lienorenal ligament.

It is formed from a larger dorsal part derived from the foregut and a smaller ventral part derived from the midgut which forms the uncinate process.

It is divided into head (to the right of the portal vein), neck (overlying the portal vein), body to the left of the portal vein), tail (in the lienorenal ligament), and uncinate process (lying anterior to the superior mesenteric vessels).

It is supplied by pancreatic branches of the coeliac axis (anterior and posterior superior pancreaticoduodenal vessels, pancreatic branches of the splenic artery) and smaller inferior pancreaticoduodenal and jejunal branches from the superior mesenteric vessels.

Secretions usually drain via the main pancreatic duct and a smaller, superiorly placed accessory duct, but multiple variants of the ductal drainage occur.

Splenic anatomy

The spleen occupies part of the left upper quadrant of the abdomen and is derived from coelomic epithelium (epithelial cells) and dorsal angiogenic mesenchyme of the foregut (the vascular structures).

It is supplied by the splenic artery (the largest branch of the coeliac axis) and drains via the splenic vein into the portal vein.

The spleen has two main suspensory ligaments: the lienorenal and gastrolienal. The capsule is often attached to important surrounding structures by congenital peritoneal adhesions (lienocolic from the inferior pole, lieno-omental from the anterior border, and lienophrenic from the posterior surface).

5.3 Intestinal stomas

Any hollow GI viscus brought out or connected directly to the skin surface is an enteric stoma.

Common stomas are:

- ileostomy (usually distal ileum)
- colostomy (commonly left colonic but occasionally from the caecum—'caecostomy')
- urostomy (disconnected loop of ileum used as a conduit for urine)
- gastrostomy (usually indirect involving a tube)

Any stoma may be:

- end (i.e. single lumen), double-barrelled (i.e. two adjacent but disconnected lumens) or loop (i.e. one loop opened to form twin lumens)
- permanent or temporary
- spouted or flush. Spouts are *much* commoner in ileostomy and urostomy

Ileostomy

Ileostomy output is chyme; semi-liquid, heavily bile-stained and between 400 and 1000 mL/24 h on a 'normal' diet. Above this, fluid and electrolyte imbalance may occur. Treatment is by replacement of losses, either orally or intravenously, and reduction of loss by dietary manipulation and slowing the transit of contents through the bowel with codeine phosphate or loperamide.

The high bile content is caustic, and prolonged contact with skin will cause excoriation. Hence the fashioning of a spout so that the contents empty directly into the bag.

Common indications—loop ileostomy

- Temporary diversion of ileal contents (chyme) away from more distal bowel (e.g. to 'protect' a high-risk anastomosis such as low anterior resection after radiotherapy to the pelvis)
- To rest distal bowel affected by disease to induce remission or relief of symptoms (e.g. colonic Crohn's disease)
- To divert chyme away from a pathological process (e.g. a distal ileal fistula or traumatic injury)

Common indications—end ileostomy

- After resection of the colon, rectum, and anus (panproctocolectomy)
- A permanent alternative to any of the loop ileostomy indications

Colostomy

Colostomy output is faeces; (semi) solid and usually less than 500 mL/24 h on a 'normal' diet.

Common indications—loop colostomy

- Temporary diversion of colonic contents (faeces) away from more distal bowel (e.g. to protect a rectovaginal fistula repair or during pelvic radiotherapy for rectal cancer)
- To rest distal bowel affected by disease to induce remission or relief of symptoms (e.g. colonic Crohn's disease)
- To divert faeces away from a pathological process (e.g. unresectable perforated diverticular disease with a mass)

Common indications—end colostomy

- After resection of the rectum and anus (e.g. abdominoperineal resection), or sigmoid and rectum where re-anastomosis is not performed (e.g. 'Hartmann's' type resection)
- As permanent treatment for faecal incontinence

Stoma complications

Early

- Mucocutaneous separation—rarely requires refashioning of the stoma)
- Ischaemia/infarction—usually a technical error by interruption of the blood supply. It may require reoperation if the ischaemia extends beyond just the spouted portion in an ileostomy
- Pre-stomal obstruction—most common at the level of the rectus sheath owing to too small an opening or angulation

Late

- Parastomal hernia—associated with problems of appliance adherence. It is often difficult to repair, may require mesh placement in the area around the stoma by open or laparoscopic surgery or re-siting of the stoma completely
- Stricturing of the stoma—may be due to ischaemia or fibrosis of the adjacent skin, may need regular dilatation or refashioning
- Ulcers and overgranulation over the stoma—may be caused by repeated trauma of the appliance. Granulation tissue may be cauterized by application of silver nitrate
- Prolapse of the stoma may require local mobilization, excision, and refashioning if troublesome

⊕ Ileostomy and colostomy formation

A stoma specialist nurse should see all elective patients preoperatively. Ideally, they should also see emergency cases if stoma formation is likely; however, this is not always practicable. The stoma site should be marked before surgery.

Procedure

- Points to consider when positioning a stoma if not already preoperatively marked
- Avoid skin creases, bony prominences, depressed scars, and any obvious belt line
- Avoid the lower abdomen in obese or pendulous abdomens; the stoma may lie beyond view and make management difficult
- Choose the rectus abdominis through which to bring the stoma and use the smallest orifice that will comfortably accommodate the bowel to be used to give the lowest risk of herniation
- May be formed as part of laparotomy or in a smaller procedure of trephine of the abdominal wall and exteriorizing the underlying bowel. The procedure may also be aided by laparoscopic mobilization
- Use fine absorbable sutures (e.g. 3/0 PDS or maxon) for the mucocutaneous stitches
- Ensure the sutures are placed from submucosa to subdermis to avoid burying skin or mucosa
- Ensure any ileostomy spout is an adequate length (3–4 cm once formed). Colostomies are very occasionally formed with a small spout, especially in obese patients to help appliance adherence
- Use a bridge to support a loop stoma with care and only if it looks necessary. Always check first that there is enough length in the bowel loop being used

⊕ Ileostomy closure

Always check for yourself that the integrity of the distal bowel has been confirmed before closing the stoma (e.g. contrast studies of an anastomosis).

Closure within 8 weeks of formation is usually hampered by adhesions, but these soften and decrease after this time.

Procedure

- Usually done as a trephine mobilization but occasionally requires a mini-laparotomy
- Usually done with a circumstomal incision, bringing the dissection down into the peritoneal cavity
- Ensure the intraperitoneal portion is free enough to allow easy return to the peritoneal cavity
- If in doubt, check the integrity of the two limbs with saline wash before forming the join
- Anastomosis is either end-to-end or side-to-side, and is closed with sutures or staples

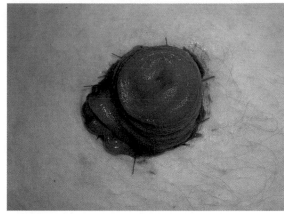

Fig 5.1 Loop ileostomy.

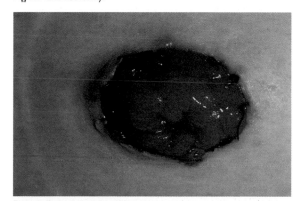

Fig 5.2 End ileostomy.

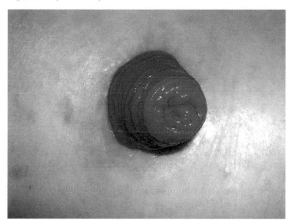

Fig 5.3 End colostomy.

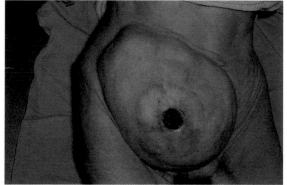

Fig 5.4 Parastomal hernia in an elderly woman.

5.4 Abdominal wall hernias

A hernia is defined as an abnormal protrusion of a viscus through its normal coverings or into an abnormal position.

Inguinal hernia

Relevant anatomy

The inguinal canal runs obliquely from the internal to the external inguinal ring. In men it contains the spermatic cord and ilioinguinal nerve; in women it contains the round ligament and ilioinguinal nerve.

'Walls' of the inguinal canal

- Anterior wall—formed by the external oblique aponeurosis reinforced by muscle fibres of the internal oblique in the lateral third, superficial fascia, and skin
- Posterior wall—formed by peritoneum and transversalis fascia reinforced by the conjoint tendon and reflected portion of the inguinal ligament in the medial half
- Inferior wall—formed by the in-rolled inguinal ligament and lacunar ligament in the medial quarter
- Superior wall—formed by the arched conjoint tendon fibres (from internal oblique and transversus abdominis)

Inguinal rings

- Deep inguinal ring—formed by medial border of the edge of transversus abdominis and the lateral edge of the inferior epigastric vessels
- Superficial inguinal ring—formed by the medial and lateral edges of the opening in the external oblique aponeurosis, and the inguinal ligament and pubic periosteum inferomedially

Types of hernia

- Direct—sac originates medial to the inferior epigastric vessels. Usually formed from a defect in the posterior wall transversalis fascia
- Indirect—sac emerges lateral to the inferior epigastric vessels. May be closely applied to or contained with the coverings of the spermatic cord or separate from it. May extend through the superficial ring or into the upper scrotum
- Infantile hernia—always a congenital indirect sac within the spermatic cord. May be associated with a hydrocele.

Natural history

- Direct hernia—often wide-necked, tend to increase in size over time, low risk (e.g. <0.5% per annum) of acute complications (incarceration or strangulation)
- Indirect hernia—may be narrow-necked, may be medium to high risk (e.g. 2–5% per annum) of acute complications, especially if symptomatic in young men

Presentations

- Painless, intermittent or variable groin lump
- Groin or upper scrotal pain, discomfort or ache with or without a lump
- Acute painful irreducible groin lump
- Incarcerated—content held within the hernial sac often but not always with intestinal obstruction, with or without compromise of the vascular supply
- Strangulated—incarcerated hernia with compromise of the vascular supply

Diagnosis

- Inguinal herniae tend to be palpable medial and superior to the pubic tubercle
- Direct—tends to emerge directly anteriorly. Often difficult to maintain reduction ('control') by specific direct digital pressure
- Indirect—sac emerges lateral to the inferior epigastric vessels. Reduction ('control') may be maintained by digital pressure over the deep ring

Diagnosis may be helped by groin ultrasound, abdominal wall CT scan, peritoneography or laparoscopy if uncertain.

Management

Non-surgical

- No treatment—used for low risk hernias where there are few or no symptoms or the patient does not wish to have surgery
- A truss—used to reduce symptoms by stopping the hernia from protruding by direct pressure. For this to work effectively, it needs to be fitted well by the surgical appliance officer. It may be used for patients unsuitable for any form of surgery, even under local anaesthesia

Operative

Inguinal hernia repair can be performed via open or laparoscopic approaches (see box). The majority of elective repairs are done as a day case procedure.

⊕ Inguinal hernia repair

Principles

- Define anatomy, isolate sac, and reduce or excise it
- Repair the defect in the canal
- Reinforce the canal with synthetic material (mesh or suture)
- Mesh may be simple sheets, shaped sheets, plugs, combined sheet/plugs; may be simple permanent (e.g. polypropylene) or composite permanent/dissolvable (e.g. polypropylene/collagen)
- Mesh should be secured medially to the level of the pubic symphysis, along the inguinal ligament, and superiorly to the internal oblique
- The ilioinguinal nerve should be identified and protected. If it is necessary to sacrifice it, it should be cut as laterally as possible so that the nerve does not grow back into the scar tissue and cause pain

Elective repair options

- Open, 'in-lay' mesh repair (Lichtenstein)
- Open nylon-sutured (darn) repair ('Shouldice', 'Oxford')— very rarely used
- Laparoscopic totally extraperitoneal mesh repair (TEP) is best suited to recurrent or bilateral hernias
- Laparoscopic transabdominal preperitoneal mesh repair (TAP) is best suited to recurrent hernias with previous lower abdominal scars/incisions

In laparoscopic approaches, if the mesh is not bonded to a biological membrane it is usually placed in the preperitoneal position to avoid contact with the intra-abdominal viscera and reduce the risk of adhesions or fistulation.

Emergency repair

Same approach as for elective repair. Mesh may be omitted if a bowel resection has been performed or secondary infection is present.

Complications

- Recurrence ~2% in 10 years for most mesh repairs
- Wound infection (5%) is usually transient and self-limiting
- Mesh infection (<1%) can be chronic and persistent, and often needs a mesh excision
- Chronic groin pain (2%) may be due to incorporation of nerve endings into the scar
- Testicular atrophy (<1%) is usually due to ischaemia, and is more common in redo repairs

Femoral hernia

Relevant anatomy

Femoral canal

- Located below and lateral to the pubic tubercle
- Borders are: medial—lacunar ligament, lateral—medial wall of the femoral vein, anterior—inguinal ligament, posterior—pectineal ligament
- Femoral canal contents = lymph gland(s) and fat

Natural history

- Half present primarily as complications (incarceration or strangulation)
- Half of acute presentations will require a bowel resection
- Risk of acute presentation is >10% per annum

Presentations

- Painless, intermittent or variable groin lump
- Groin or upper scrotal pain, discomfort or ache with or without a lump
- Acute painful irreducible groin lump
- Incarcerated—content held within the hernial sac often but not always with intestinal obstruction, with or without compromise of the vascular supply
- Strangulated—incarcerated hernia with compromise of the vascular supply

Diagnosis

- Femoral herniae tend to be palpable lateral and inferior to the pubic tubercle
- A common, subtle feature is loss of the groin skin crease whereas inguinal herniae tend to accentuate the groin skin crease

Diagnosis may be helped by groin ultrasound, abdominal CT scan or laparoscopy if uncertain.

Management

Femoral hernia have a high risk of complications and so the majority undergo elective repair under local anaesthetic. Conservative management is rarely indicated.

⊕ Femoral hernia repair

- Skin incision may be low (Lockwood) below the inguinal ligament which is more direct but gives limited exposure, or high (McEvedy) above the ligament which allows a transinguinal dissection to approach the peritoneal cavity/involved bowel or internal aspect of the femoral canal
- Define anatomy, isolate sac, and reduce it
- Ensure contents have been evaluated if emergency presentation to exclude necrotic bowel
- Close the femoral canal without narrowing of femoral vein. This is usually done by two or three interrupted permanent sutures apposing the inguinal and pectineal ligaments

Complications

- Wound infection
- Recurrence
- Femoral vein injury or narrowing

Other hernias

Incisional hernia

- Acquired defect in surgical scar tissue, often larger than clinically anticipated
- Repair for small defects is occasionally by open sutured closure but larger defects require mesh (open or laparoscopic)

Para-umbilical hernia

- Acquired defect in the linea alba close to the umbilicus
- Often symptomatic, usually contains preperitoneal fat, may strangulate
- Repair may be open with sutures or mesh or laparoscopic with composite mesh

Umbilical hernia

- Congenital defect in the umbilical cicatrix, may present in childhood or early adulthood. Requires repair if present over the age of 6 years
- Repair is usually by open sutured closure (combined with mesh for larger established defects)

Epigastric/ventral hernia

- Acquired defect in the linea alba usually above the umbilicus
- Repair is by mesh—open or laparoscopic

Spigelian hernia

- Acquired defect in the posterior rectus sheath at the level of the arcuate line, at the lateral edge of the rectus muscle
- Repair can be via an open approach, using mesh in the extraperitoneal layer followed by apposition of the overlying muscles. This can also be repaired via the transabdominal laparoscopic approach

Stomal/parastomal hernia

- Acquired defects at or about the abdominal wall defect used for a stoma

5.5 Crohn's disease

Crohn's disease is an idiopathic, chronic, transmural inflammatory bowel disease that can affect any part of the GI tract from the mouth to the anus.

- Incidence: 50 per 100 000 of the population
- Age: 25–40 years and second peak >70 years
- Sex: F>M
- Geography: temperate climates

Aetiology

- Genetic factors—several are implicated and there is a definite familial tendency, but the precise genetic factors are unknown
- Microbiological—there is some evidence for an association with GI infection but little direct evidence for mycobacterial or bacterial causation
- Faecal content—definite evidence for 'activating' factors present in chyme which aggravate pre-existing inflammation
- Vascular—underlying pathology is related to vascular damage in submucosal arterioles; smoking induces vascular damage and definitely worsens disease and makes recurrence more likely

Pathology

Microscopic

- Initial lesion starts as a focal inflammatory infiltrate around the crypts, followed by ulceration of superficial mucosa
- Later, inflammatory cells invade deep layers and, in that process, begin to organize into non-caseating granulomas. The granulomas extend through all layers of the intestinal wall and into the mesentery and the regional lymph nodes. Although granuloma formation is typical of Crohn's disease, the diagnosis is not dependent on their presence

Macroscopic

- The initial abnormality is hyperaemia and oedema of the involved mucosa
- Later, discrete superficial ulcers form, which become deep serpiginous ulcers located transversely and longitudinally over an inflamed mucosa, giving the mucosa a cobblestone appearance. The lesions are often segmental, being separated by healthy areas ('skip lesions')
- Transmural inflammation results in thickening of the bowel wall and narrowing of the lumen. As the disease progresses, it is complicated by obstruction, fistulation, abscess formation, adhesions, and malabsorption

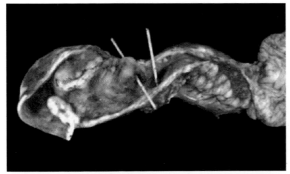

Fig 5.5 Gross features of small intestinal Crohn's disease showing fistula formation, fat wrapping, and ulceration.

Distribution

- May affect any area of the GI tract and extraintestinal organs/tissues
- The most common site of disease is the ileocaecal region (80% of patients have one focus of disease within 2 feet of the ileocaecal valve)
- Colon—may be focal or pancolonic, similar to ulcerative colitis
- Small intestine—often multifocal and prone to multiple recurrences
- Stomach and the mouth—the oesophagus is involved very rarely
- Perianal Crohn's disease occurs in nearly 30% of patients. This may precede the development of intestinal symptoms. Manifestations include atypical anal fissure, perianal fistula or abscess, and atypical skin tags

In addition to local complications, a variety of extraintestinal manifestations may be associated with Crohn's disease. The usual sites are skin, joints, mouth, eyes, liver, and bile ducts.

> ### ⊙ Extra intestinal manifestations of IBD
>
> Both Crohn's disease and ulcerative colitis may be associated with extraintestinal conditions affecting many different systems.
>
> #### Local
>
> - **Perianal** disease is most common with Crohn's disease, and includes anal fissure, fistulae, abscess, and rectal prolapse
>
> #### Systemic
>
> - **Skin** manifestations include erythema nodosum, aphthous ulcers of the oral mucosa, and pyoderma gangrenosum (predominantly with UC)
> - **Eye** manifestations include conjunctivitis, iritis, uveitis, episcleritis (📖 Topic 11.17), and are much more common in Crohn's
> - **Arthritis** involving peripheral joints (migratory, non-deforming, seronegative) is common in Crohn's; ankylosing spondylitis and sacroiliitis are common in UC
> - **Hepatic** disease includes pericholangitis, primary sclerosing cholangitis (UC), and gallstones (Crohn's)
> - **Haematological**: megaloblastic or iron-deficiency anaemia and hypercoagulable state

Clinical presentations

'Fibrostenosing/stricturing' presentations

- Acute intestinal obstruction—colicky pain, distension, vomiting
- Chronic incomplete intestinal obstruction—abdominal pain after meals, bloating, 'food fear', weight loss

'Perforating' presentations

- Acute peritonitis—fever, constant pain, rigid abdomen
- Enteroenteric fistula—fever, diarrhoea, malabsorption
- Enterocutaneous fistula—recurrent abdominal wall abscesses, enteric discharge, fever

'Inflammatory' presentations

- Chronic inflammation—abdominal pain, diarrhoea (may be bloody with colitis), tender abdominal mass, weight loss, anaemia
- Malnutrition—weight loss, delayed puberty, short stature (in children)
- Haemorrhagic colitis

Investigations

- Bloods—FBC, WCC, CRP, albumin—markers of inflammation and chronic disease activity; positive ASCA, negative perinuclear-ANCA
- Flexible sigmoidoscopy or colonoscopy—assessment of colonic or terminal ileal disease
- Barium follow through/small bowel enema, contrast-enhanced abdominal CT—assessment of ileal disease
- MRI—assessment of pelvic and perianal disease

Management
Medical

- Acute inflammatory exacerbations—systemic (oral, IV) steroids, infliximab (anti-TNF-alpha monoclonal antibody)
- Chronic inflammatory disease—anti-inflammatories (5-ASA compounds), immunosuppression (azathioprine, infliximab, cyclosporin A), specialized diet (elemental, semi-elemental)
- Perforating complications—antibiotics, infliximab, parenteral nutrition
- Stricturing complications—endoscopic balloon dilatation

Surgical
Absolute indications

- Acute obstruction
- Peritonitis
- Haemorrhage

Relative indications

All indicated by a balance of: response to medical therapy, side effects of therapy, severity of symptoms, risk of surgery.

- Recurrent obstruction
- Chronic inflammatory features
- Chronic fistulizing complications
- Unacceptable side effects of medical treatment
- Side effects on growth/development

Principles

- Only deal with bowel causing the symptoms indicated
- Conserve bowel length where possible (e.g. strictureplasty for stenoses)
- Defunctioning may be used for refractory colonic and peri-anal disease
- Consider side-to-side (possibly stapled) anastomosis over end-to-end anastomosis—possibly less prone to restricting
- Perianal disease and sepsis may require drainage, often involving seton insertion for underlying fistula. Enterocutaneous fistulae may require input of specialist units that can manage intestinal failure

Prognosis

There is spectrum of disease, some who relapse repeatedly may have complications of long-term immunosuppression and/or short bowel.

The risk of high-grade dysplasia and malignant change in long-standing disease is similar to that in ulcerative colitis.

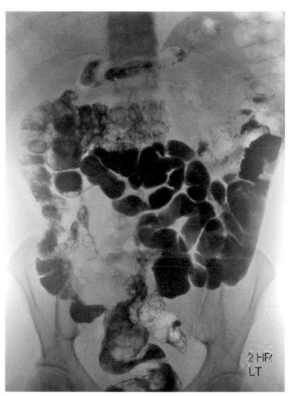

Fig 5.6 Barium meal and follow through showing distal small bowel Crohn's disease in a patient who presented with recent onset of diarrhoea, rectal bleeding, weight loss, and abdominal pain.

There is marked cobblestoning, ulceration, and separation of loops of the terminal ileum. The rectum and distal sigmoid colon are also opacified by contrast prior to filling of the descending colon owing to passage through a fistula from the distal ileum into the sigmoid colon.

5.6 Ulcerative colitis

Ulcerative colitis is an idiopathic acute and chronic inflammatory bowel disease originating in the mucosa and submucosa of the large intestine.

- Incidence >6000 new cases per year in the UK
- Age: 20–40-years-old
- Sex: M = F
- Geographic: more common in western countries which are in the temperate climate zone

Aetiology

- Genetic factors—several implicated, definite familial tendency but precise genetic factors unknown. Similar candidate genes to Crohn's disease. Association with HLA B27
- Microbiological—no evidence for causation but may precipitate attacks and infections may coexist with UC

Pathology

Macroscopic

- Ulceration of mucosa, usually starting at the rectum with varying degree of ulceration and inflammation proximal to the rectum; rarely presents as rectal sparing disease
- Pseudopolyps are areas of regenerated mucosa on a background of severe ulceration
- May find areas associated with complications of bleeding, perforation, stricture formation, toxic megacolon in fulminant colitis, dysplasia leading to invasive malignancy. May affect terminal ileum (so called backwash ileitis)

Microscopic

Mucosocentric disease but may involve changes in other layers with increasing severity. There is goblet cell depletion, no granuloma formation, increased inflammatory cell infiltration in the lamina propria, and crypt abscesses

Neoplasia associated with UC

Dysplasia may be low or high grade, may arise in flat mucosa or be associated with visible mucosal abnormalities (dysplasia-associated lesion or mass, DALM). Proven high-grade dysplasia or the presence of DALMs is usually an indication for surgery.

Adenocarcinoma is often preceded by high-grade dysplasia, and is commonest in chronic disease.

Clinical assessment

- Clinical examination looking for fever, abdominal distension or tenderness, peritonism
- Ensure the stool chart records frequency, consistency, and blood content of stools

Acute severe colitis

- Bloody diarrhoea, abdominal pain, fever, systemic septic features
- May progress to fulminant colitis (previously known as 'toxic megacolon'). Characterized by colonic dilatation, severe systemic upset, risk of perforation, and severe haemorrhage. Suggested by sudden reduction in stool frequency and worsening of vital signs
- May be the first presentation of UC

Relapsing intermittent proctocolitis

- Typically episodes, 'attacks' of increased frequency and urgency of bloody, loose stools interspersed with normal function
- May be confined to rectum (proctitis), distal colon (proctosigmoiditis, left-sided colitis) or pancolitis
- Any relapse may progress to acute severe colitis

Chronic proctocolitis

- Variable degree of chronic loose stools, urgency, frequency. May be accompanied by weight loss

Investigations

- Bloods—Hb, WCC, platelet count, CRP, albumin—markers of inflammation and disease activity
- Electrolytes (Na^+, K^+)—deranged in acute exacerbations
- Stool microscopy and culture for infections, cysts, parasites, and ova
- Plain abdominal radiograph is the initial assessment in acute presentation but is not reliable for extent or severity
- CT scan assesses the extent of disease and complications in acute presentations
- Flexible sigmoidoscopy confirms initial diagnosis or limited assessment of acute exacerbations
- Colonoscopy gives a definitive assessment of disease and is also used for surveillance

Management

Medical

- Acute exacerbations: systemic IV steroids +/- 5-aminosalicyclic acid (5-ASA) to induce remission in pancolitis, topical steroid, and 5-ASA suppositiories/enemas in proctitis. Pancolitis may require additional IV ciclosporin or infliximab
- Antibiotics may be required to treat any coincident infection
- Maintenance therapy: anti-inflammatories (5-ASA) and immunosuppression (azathioprine, mercaptopurine)
- Fulminant or complicated disease may need supplementary nutrition either enterally or parenterally

Surgery

Emergency surgery

Urgent or emergency surgery may be needed in acute exacerbation failing to respond to maximal medical therapy, bowel perforation, and for life-threatening bleeding. Options for acute surgery include:

- subtotal colectomy with ileostomy formation. The rectal stump is usually closed and left in the pelvis but may be left as a longer rectosigmoid stump which is closed and secured in the laparotomy wound or left open as a mucus fistula incorporated into the wound or as a separate stoma
- subsequent surgery—excise the rectum and either leave a permanent ileostomy or undertake ileal pouch formation

Elective surgery

Elective surgery should be considered for patients with chronic disease which is poorly controlled by medical therapy, with complications of medical therapy or those who develop malignancy or premalignant high-grade dysplasia.

Options for elective surgery include:

- proctocolectomy ('panproctocolecotmy') with end ileostomy
- restorative proctocolectomy with ileoanal pouch with or without defunctioning loop ileostomy

Complications and prognosis

Once the colon is excised there is no further risk of colitis but it is associated with extraintestinal manifestations, e.g. iritis, erythema nodosum, pyoderma gangrenosum, sclerosing cholangitis (📖 Topic 5.5).

The risk of high-grade dysplasia developing and progressing to adenocarcinoma is approximately 10% after 10 years of active disease (highest in acute severe colitis at presentation, recurrent exacerbations, family history of colonic carcinoma). Colonoscopic surveillance (chromoendoscopy and biopsies) is recommended regularly after 10 years of disease.

Complications of surgery

Early—stump blow out, continued uncontrolled inflammation, poor wound healing, and infection owing to pre-existing malnutrition and immunosuppression, anastomotic leak, and pelvic sepsis.

Late—pelvic sepsis and deep pelvic dissection may affect sexual function and fertility, stoma problems (📖 Topic 5.3).

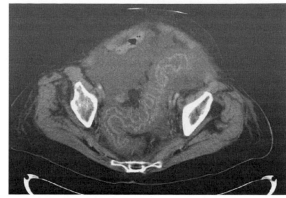

Fig 5.7 CT scan of a patient with acute severe colitis. The colon has a grossly thickened wall with pericolic fat stranding and mucosal hyperenhancement. There is also free intraperitoneal fluid.

5.7 Diverticular disease

A diverticulum is a pouching from the wall of a hollow viscus and may occur at any point in the GI tract. A congenital diverticulum contains all of the layers of the wall (e.g. Meckel's diverticulum).

Acquired diverticula are formed of mucosa, submucosal connective tissue, and serosa, and occur most commonly in the colon but may also occur in the jejunum or ileum.

The exact prevalence is unknown. Up to 50% of people over the age of 75 years have one or more colonic diverticula. Incidence increases with age but may occur in young adults and there is a female preponderance with advancing age. It is predominantly seen in western populations.

Aetiology

- Diet—may be related to low intake of dietary fibre
- Colonic hypersegmentation—increase in intracolonic pressure owing to complete segmentation caused by hypercontractility
- Inherent weakness of the bowel wall—occurs at the site of colonic vascular entry; may have a familial tendency
- Rarely congenital

Pathology

- Diverticula are out-pouches containing only mucosa, submucosa, and serosal covering
- They tend to occur at sites of vascular entry in the colon wall
- Acquired diverticula are commonest in the sigmoid and descending colon. They almost never occur in the rectum (with a complete external longitudinal muscle coat)
- Congenital diverticula are more likely to be pancolonic or right-sided
- In oriental populations, right-sided diverticula are more common

Clinical presentations

'Painful' diverticular disease

A presentation with intermittent left iliac fossa pain may be due to diverticular disease with colonization by bacteria; this may respond to courses of antibiotics.

PR bleeding

Acute, usually large-volume bright and dark red clotted blood pr, often no prodrome, not usually associated with features of inflammation, very rarely a cause of anaemia or small volume bleeding (suspicious for coincidental carcinoma).

Acute diverticulitis

Gradual onset left iliac fossa pain, fever, anorexia. Usually tender of left iliac fossa, may be associated with loose stools.

Complicated acute diverticulitis

Pericolic/paracolic abscess

Persisting symptoms of acute diverticulitis, swinging fever, possible left iliac fossa fullness/mass.

Abscess may be pericolic (associated with bowel wall) or paracolic (into retroperitoneal or pelvic tissues).

Peritonitis

May be caused by direct perforation of an area of diverticular disease (usually acutely inflamed)—leads to faecal peritonitis.

May be due to perforation of a pericolic or paracolic abscess—leads to purulent peritonitis.

Acute onset severe generalized pain and tenderness/peritonitis.

Table 5.1 Hinchey classification of complicated diverticulitis	
Stage	**Features**
1	Pericolic/mesenteric abscess
2	Pelvic/retroperitoneal abscess
3	Purulent peritonitis
4	Faecal peritonitis

Large bowel obstruction

This is usually caused by acute inflammatory mass occurring on the background of chronic scarring.

Chronic diverticulitis

Persistent, recurrent abdominal pain, weight loss, left iliac fossa mass.

Occasionally gives rise to stricturing and obstruction.

Diverticular fistulae

Usually occur with the rupture of a chronic paracolic abscess into adjacent organs:

- vagina (especially if patient had previous hysterectomy)—'wind' and faecal discharge pv
- bladder—recurrent enteric organism-related urinary infections, pelvic pain
- small bowel—diarrhoea, 'short gut' syndrome
- abdominal wall—faecal fistula

Clinical assessment

Clinical examination looking for tenderness, localized or generalized peritonism or a mass.

Investigations

- Bloods—WCC, CRP, raised in acute inflammation; low Hb and ferritin suggests iron-deficient anaemia associated with neoplasia
- Plain abdominal and erect chest radiograph shows free gas or features of obstruction
- Abdominopelvic CT scan assesses the extent of local inflammation, the presence of abscesses, perforation or obstruction
- Barium enema assesses possible stricture
- Colonoscopy to exclude neoplasia

Management

Initial management of acute presentation

- Patients may need resuscitation. Acute complications, e.g. perforation, should be identified and managed appropriately
- Acute diverticulitis can initially be treated with broad spectrum oral or IV antibiotics
- Pericolic/paracolic abscess can be treated by radiologically-guided drainage if there are no signs of peritonitis

Emergency surgery

Indications:

- generalized peritonitis
- localized peritonitis not resolving with medical treatment
- bowel obstruction
- unresolving haemorrhage

The principles are:

- where possible, resect the inflammatory segment responsible for the presentation; only use defunctioning alone where resection is impossible/hazardous
- ensure all collections are dealt with and drained if necessary
- primary anastomosis depends on the extent and type of peritoneal contamination, patient age, and co-morbidity and surgical experience

Outpatient management

Patients should be advised to try a high-fibre, high-fluid diet. Those with chronic diverticulitis may benefit from a trial of low-dose antibiotics.

Elective surgery

Indications:

- recurrent acute inflammatory episodes (rarely indicated after first episode)
- recurrent chronic symptoms proven to be due to diverticular disease
- symptomatic stricture
- symptomatic fistula

The principles are:

- resect all colon involved by diverticular disease (usually all of the sigmoid and part of the descending colon)
- primary anastomosis unless complicated surgery
- organs affected by fistula can usually be simply repaired
- consider a defunctioning stoma for symptomatic fistula in the very elderly or those unfit for resection

Complications of surgery and prognosis

- Anastomotic leak (where present)
- Intra-abdominal abscess formation (after surgery for acute complications)
- 'Recurrence' of diverticular disease most likely where initial resection is limited (may fail to excise all disease)

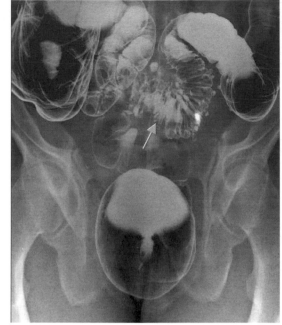

Fig 5.9 Barium enema showing diverticular disease of the sigmoid colon (arrow). There are no mucosal lesions or strictures demonstrated.

101

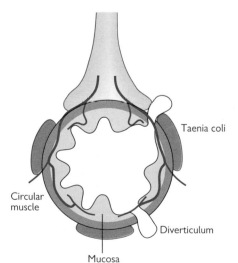

Fig 5.8 Sites of diverticula formation.

5.8 Colorectal polyps

Classification

Pathological

- Adenomatous—true neoplasia (i.e. structurally abnormal tissue with growth not controlled by the tissue of origin). May show low- or high-grade dysplasia (premalignant cellular and structural abnormality)
  - Villous—10% of polyps
  - Tubulovillous—15% of polyps
  - Tubular—75% of polyps
- Metaplastic—not true neoplasia (possibly reversible) change from colonic to other type intestinal epithelium, very common in the colon
- Hamartomatous—not true neoplasia, contain tissues of several types
- Pseudopolyps—include inflammatory

Macroscopic appearance

- Polypoid—possess a stalk attachment to the normal bowel wall
- Sessile—no discernible stalk, large may be referred to as 'carpet'
  - Elevated—more than twice the height of the surrounding mucosa
  - Flat—similar to height of surrounding mucosa
  - Depressed—part or all lower than the level of the surrounding mucosa

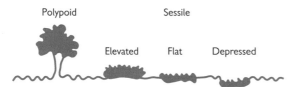

Polypoid   **Sessile**

Elevated   **Flat**   **Depressed**

Fig 5.10 Macroscopic forms of colorectal neoplasia.

Aetiology

Single gene germline abnormalities
~5% of polyp sufferers.

- **Familial adenomatous polyposis** (FAP)—*APC* gene abnormality, chromosome 17, increases production of adenomas which have the same risk of malignant progression as sporadic ones, associated with adenoma formation in the upper GI tract and small bowel, associated with bone cysts, skin cysts, desmoid tumour development
- **Hereditary non-polyposis colon cancer** (HNPCC)—abnormality in one of several DNA mismatch repair (*MMR*) genes (e.g. *hMLH1*), increased rate of progression to malignancy, associated with other GI tract, gynaecological, endocrine, and soft tissue tumours
- **Peutz—Jeghers syndrome**—multiple hamartomatous tumours, mostly in the small bowel, associated with small bowel carcinoma development
- **Juvenile polyposis**—tyrosine kinase gene abnormality, multiple hamartomatous polyps, occur throughout the GI tract

Multiple (unknown) genetic germline abnormalities
~15% of polyp sufferers.

- **Familial polyps**—multiple adenomatous polyps, tend to occur in several members of a family, suggesting multifactorial genetic influences

Sporadic (somatic abnormalities)
~80% of polyp sufferers.

- Single or few polyps not associated with family history, owing to acquired somatic gene abnormalities
- Most associated with environmental factors

Factors increasing polyp formation and growth

- Smoking
- Age
- Obesity
- Diet rich in red meat

Factors decreasing polyp formation and growth

- Diet rich in fruit and vegetables
- Diet rich in antioxidants (selenium, vitamin C)
- NSAIDS—?influence growth within polyps via prostaglandin/prostacyclin inhibition
- Oral contraceptive/hormone replacement therapy

Malignant transformation

Adenoma–carcinoma sequence

- All but a small minority of carcinomas arise in an adenoma
- Direct malignant proliferation may occur in high-grade mucosal dysplasia (e.g. ulcerative colitis)
- Adenoma–carcinoma sequence reflects sequential 'acquisition' of genetic abnormalities until invasive capability occurs

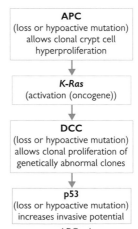

Adenoma carcinoma sequence. APC-adenomatous polyposis coli gene; DCC-deleted in colon cancer gene

Factors influencing risk of transformation

- Adenoma risk features
  - Size (>1 cm)
  - Villous architecture
  - High-grade dysplasia
  - Flat/depressed morphology
- Metaplastic polyps—low risk of transformation unless multiple

Colorectal screening

Principles

- Identification of carcinoma at an earlier, more favourable stage, i.e. more treatable and potentially curable
- Identification of premalignant polyps suitable for endoscopic treatment to prevent carcinoma development
- Targeted screening for high-risk groups
  - Previous personal history of colorectal cancer or multiple polyps
  - Proven familial cancer syndromes (e.g. FAP)
  - High-risk family history of multiple colorectal tumours
  - Chronic colitis (ulcerative or Crohn's)
- Consider screening for medium risk groups
  - Moderate-risk family history of colorectal neoplasia
- Population screening is based on age only and is targeted at peak age of polyp prevalence (50–65 years)

Methods of screening

- Faecal occult blood testing (guiac test) is currently the preferred method for population screening
- It has moderate sensitivity and specificity. A high false-positive rate, most sensitive for carcinomas and less so for adenomas
- Colonoscopy is indicated in response to positive result
- Flexible sigmoidoscopy has been proven in randomized trial as an effective population screening tool, used mostly for symptomatic patients
- Colonoscopy is not used for population screening, but is used for targeted screening in medium/high risk groups

National bowel cancer screening program

- Central handling of 'call-up' of individuals
- Invitations sent to all individuals in age bands between 50 and 65 years
- Positive test results invited for full colonoscopy in designated regional screening centres ('hub and spoke')

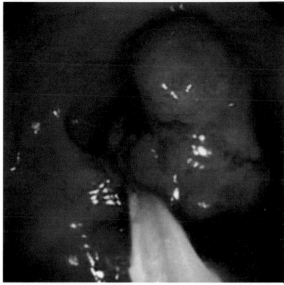

Fig 5.11 Polypoid adenoma in the sigmiod colon seen on colonoscopy. It has been snared and is about to be excised.

5.9 Colorectal cancer

Colorectal cancer is the second most common cancer to affect women and the third most common to affect men. There are 35 000 new cases per year in UK, and the peak age of incidence is over 60 years.

Aetiology

- Pre-existing adenoma (📖 Topic 5.6)
  - FAP
  - HNPCC
  - Family history of colorectal neoplasia
  - Personal history of colorectal neoplasia
- Colorectal disease
  - Ulcerative or Crohn's colitis
  - Ureterosigmoidostomy
- Environmental factors

Pathology

- 98% adenocarcinomas, 2% adenosquamous carcinoma or adenocarcinoid carcinoma
- Adverse features include mucinous differentiation (including 'signet ring cell type'), poor differentiation
- Spread may be direct into adjacent organs (e.g. duodenum, bladder, uterus), blood (liver and lungs preferential sites), lymph (pericolic and mesenteric nodes) or transcoelomic
- Distribution: caecum/ascending (20%), transverse colon (10%), descending/sigmoid colon (30%), rectum (40%)

Clinical presentations

Right-sided colonic carcinoma

This includes the caecum, ascending, and transverse colon.

- Anaemia (iron-deficient)
- Right-sided abdominal mass
- Abdominal pain

Left-sided colonic carcinoma

This includes the descending and sigmoid colon.

- Change in bowel habit (more often to looser more frequent than to more solid less frequent)
- Large bowel obstructive symptoms
- Colicky left-sided, lower abdominal pain
- Intermittent distension and bloating
- Dark blood mixed with stool

Rectal carcinoma

This includes the rectum and the rectosigmoid junction.

- Change in rectal habit
  - Urgency and frequency of stools
  - Sensation of incomplete evacuation
  - Sensation of inability to pass stool (tenesmus)
- Dark or bright red blood and mucus
  - Mixed with stools, on surface, clots, mixed with mucus

> ⊙ **Urgent 2-week wait referral criteria for suspected colorectal cancer**
>
> *For all ages*
> 1. Rectal bleeding with change in bowel habit to looser stools and/or increased frequency of defaecation persistent for 6 weeks
>
> 2. Palpable right-sided abdominal or rectal mass
> 3. Unexplained iron-deficiency anaemia Hb <11 in men and <10 in women
>
> *Over 60 years old*
> 4. Change in bowel habit to looser stools and/or increased frequency of defaecation persistent for 6 weeks without rectal bleeding
> 5. Rectal bleeding persistently without anal symptoms, e.g. soreness, discomfort, itching, lumps, prolapse, and pain

Investigations

- Bloods—Hb (anaemia), LFTs (metastases); CEA is only useful if elevated in primary disease to monitor postoperative recurrence
- Flexible sigmoidoscopy or colonoscopy and biopsy chosen according to symptoms have the highest diagnostic sensitivity and specificity
- Double contrast barium enema
- CT colography (with pneumocolon) is useful for frail/elderly patients (lower sensitivity and specificity for small polyps)
- CT chest/abdomen/pelvis is used for staging
- MRI pelvis—local extension of rectal cancer
- Transrectal ultrasound is used to assess depth of invasion of particularly early rectal cancer

Follow-up

Reasons for active follow-up

- Identification of local or systemic recurrence when treatment may be possible (rarely to attempt cure or extend life expectancy)
- Identification of metachronous disease (either adenomas or carcinomas)
- Psychological support for the patient
- Clinical audit and monitoring of quality/outcome of treatment/care given

Methods of follow-up

- Clinical examination (including rectal examination and rigid sigmoidoscopy)
- CEA levels—useful when raised prior to treatment of the primary and falls to normal after potentially curative surgery. Subsequent increase is highly predictive of recurrent disease
- Cross-sectional imaging
- CT thorax/abdomen/pelvis—to detect systemic recurrence (metastases) and intra-abdominal local recurrence
- MRI pelvis—to detect local recurrence of rectal cancer
- Colonoscopy—usually offered to all patients (unless of advanced age) since removal of metachronous adenomas confers protection against future primary carcinomas

There is intense debate regarding the form of follow-up which is optimal—from 'no follow-up' to 'intensive follow-up.' As the survival of patients after surgery for liver and lung metastases continues to improve, more intensive follow-up may be justified.

Staging

Staging is usually by the TNM classification although the Dukes' classification is still quoted for its simplicity. Pathological reporting should include tumour differentiation, staging, margins, and extramural vascular invasion.

Dukes' classification of colorectal cancer

A   *Confined to bowel wall with no positive lymph nodes*
B   *Extends beyond the muscularis propria with no positive lymph nodes*
C   *Positive lymph nodes (with any extent of primary)*

Modified classification includes stage D for disease that has metastasized.

TNM classification
Primary tumor

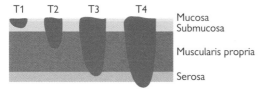

Mucosa
Submucosa
Muscularis propria
Serosa

Regional lymph nodes

N0   No positive nodes
N1   1–3 positive nodes
N2   >4 positive nodes

Distant metastases

M0   No metastases
M1   Metastases

Principles of management

All colorectal cancer patients should be discussed in the local multidisciplinary meeting where the case is presented to the surgeons, gastroenterologists, oncologists, radiologists, pathologists, and the colorectal nurse specialist.

Neoadjuvant therapy

- Radiotherapy for rectal cancer
- Given as 'short course' five fractions over 5 days, or 'long course' 25 fractions over 5 weeks with low-dose chemotherapy
- Indicated for rectal cancers which are invading local structures, close to or at the mesorectal fascial limit or large and technically difficult to excise
- Acts to downsize the tumour and reduce the chance of viable microdeposits remaining after surgery

Surgical resection

- The primary objective is to resect the primary tumour *en bloc* with all potentially directly involved tissue (including adjacent organs if necessary) to obtain clear resection margins (both bowel, distal and proximal, and circumferential)
- Resection should include the vascular supply and lymphatic drainage related to or potentially draining the primary tumour. The objective is to clear all potential micrometastatic-bearing tissue as well as to provide maximal tissue for histological assessment and staging, and guide the decision regarding adjuvant therapy
- Resection may be open (via midline or tranverse incisions) or laparoscopically-assisted (still requires a mini-laparotomy to deliver the specimen)
- Primary anastomosis is usual unless there is acute obstruction, significant peritonitis, a severely ill patient or a grossly malnourished patient
- Low rectal anastomoses are usually protected by a temporary loop ileostomy

Choice of procedure

The extent of resection of uninvolved normal bowel is determined by the vascular territories resected.

- Right hemicolectomy: ileocolic (and right colic) artery
- Extended right hemicolectomy: ileocolic, right colic, and middle colic arteries

- Left hemicolectomy: left colic and sigmoid arteries
- Total colectomy: ileocolic, right, middle and left colic and sigmoid arteries
- Anterior resection (high and low): superior rectal or inferior mesenteric artery
- Abdominoperineal excision of the rectum (APER): inferior mesenteric and pudendal arteries

Adjuvant therapy
Chemotherapy for colonic or rectal cancer

- Usually given as 5FU-based infusions
- Multiple other agents can be used (e.g. irinotecan, oxaliplatin)
- Proven survival benefit (up to 5 percentage points) for:
- lymph node-positive
- positive extratumoral vascular invasion
- Also offered for poorly differentiated, mucinous differentiation, serosal involvement (T4)

Radiotherapy for rectal cancer

- Usually only given for unexpected positive surgical margins where neoadjuvant treatment has not been given.

Liver and lung metastases

- 50% of patients develop liver metastases
- Resection of isolated liver or lung metastases can offer significant survival advantage
- Criteria for resection are (broadly):
- 20% of the liver spared
- no inferior vena cava involvement
- fewer than three lesions

Palliative procedures

- Transanal resection—for inoperable rectal cancer
- Endoluminal stenting—for obstructing left-sided colon cancer

Prognosis

The commonest 5-year survival figures are quoted for Dukes' classification:
Dukes' A—up to 90%
Dukes' B—60–85%
Dukes' C—35–65%
'Dukes' D'—5–15%

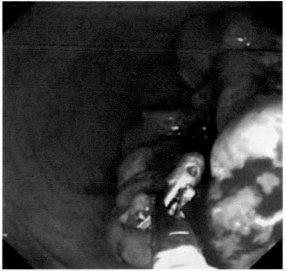

Fig 5.13 Colonoscopic appearance of a suspected carcinoma being biopsied.

5.10 Haemorrhoids

Aetiology

Normal anatomy/physiology

- Anorectal vascular cushions are normally present in the anal canal
- They commonly form three prominent cushions but there may be more
- Their normal function may be to help to maintain continence for liquid and gas, and to allow the sampling of the lower rectal contents to distinguish between gas, liquid, and solid.
- They are formed from mucosa, submucosal connective tissue, and (extensive) associated blood vessels
- Arterial supply to the cushions comes mainly from the lower rectal submucosal vascular network (from the superior rectal artery) reinforced by perforating branches from the inferior rectal artery (from the pudendal artery)
- Venous drainage occurs mostly upwards to the rectal submucosal plexus but to a lesser extent downwards to the subcutaneous perianal venous plexus

Pathological anatomy

- Expansion of the endoanal cushions (vascular and supporting connective tissue) results in haemorrhoids
- Precipitating factors include: constipation, prolonged straining at stool, obesity, family history, previous rectal surgery
- Portal hypertension may result in rectal varices *not* haemorrhoids

Classification

Anatomical

- Internal—formed only from the upper anorectal cushions, lined by columnar and transitional epithelium, minimal nociceptor innervation
- External—formed predominantly from the lower anorectal cushions and perianal skin, lined by transitional and squamous epithelium, dense supply of cutaneous nerves (including nociceptors)
- Interoexternal—extensive, involves all levels of cushions

Clinical

- First degree—non-prolapsing with local symptoms
- Second degree—intermittent prolapse during/after defaecation but reduce spontaneously
- Third degree—prolapse frequently and require manual reduction

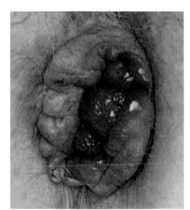

Fig 5.14 Fourth degree haemorrhoids.

- Fourth degree—continuously prolapsed

Clinical assessment

Local symptoms

- Bright red bleeding *per rectum*—typically on the paper, on the surface of the stools, and in the water of the bowl
- Seepage of fluid or mucus from the anal canal which can cause itching, irritation, and excoriation of the perianal skin
- Palpable, uncomfortable prolapsing tissue

Secondary complications

- Thrombosed external 'piles'—painful, constantly prolapsed tissue with intramucosal bleeding and thrombosis

Investigations

- Digital rectal examination—to exclude other anorectal pathology prior to sigmoidoscopy
- Rigid sigmoidoscopy and proctoscopy—diagnose the presence, number, extent, and size of haemorrhoids
- Flexible sigmoidoscopy should be performed for any 'new' haemorrhoidal symptoms or where the extent of haemorrhoidal tissue does not 'match' with the clinical history

> ### ⏱ Rigid sigmoidoscopy
>
> This is actually a misnomer—it is more correctly called 'rigid proctoscopy' since only the rectal mucosa is truly visualized.
>
> #### Pre-procedure
>
> - Ensure the patient is comfortable in the left lateral position. Maximal flexion of the hips, only partial flexion of the knees, and the anal canal close to the edge of the couch 'pointing' out into the examination room will all help a thorough examination
> - Always have a nurse to assist/chaperone
> - Always perform a rectal examination to check for anal stenosis/spasm or low rectal pathology
>
> #### Procedure
>
> - Insert the sigmoidoscope initially along the axis of the anal canal and then angle posteriorly by 45° to allow for the anorectal angle
> - Insufflate gently, never 'push' to advance the scope and always keep the lumen in full view
> - A slight pressure anteriorly onto the prostate in men and the cervix in women may help open out the upper rectal curve/rectosigmoid junction
> - Do not attempt to intubate the distal sigmoid specifically—if it is necessary to view the sigmoid colon, arrange a flexible sigmoidoscopy

Management

Outpatient therapy

- Topical creams—with or without corticosteroids, best directed at local irritative symptoms or associated perianal dermatitis
- Reduction of haemorrhoidal tissue—usually rubber band ligation, best suited to symptoms or prolapse of large internal haemorrhoids without an external component. Should be avoided in patients who have previously had a haemorrhoidectomy or significant reduction of endoanal tissue and those on anticoagulation

- Ablation and fixation of haemorrhoidal tissue—sclerosant injection (e.g. 5% phenol in almond oil), laser ablation or cryotherapy, usually best suited to symptoms of bleeding and discharge. Should be avoided in patients with nut allergy (for injection) and used with care in those on anticoagulation
- Devascularization of haemorrhoid—Doppler-guided suture ligation of feeding artery

Surgical treatment
Haemorrhoidectomy
- Usually reserved for failure of repeated outpatient therapy or symptomatic haemorrhoids with an extensive external component
- Variety of techniques—excision without closure of the wounds (Milligan Morgan), submucosal excision (Parks operation)
- Excision ensures the internal sphincter is preserved with ligation of the supplying vessels at the anorectal junction
- It is important to leave sufficient mucosal bridges in place to prevent anal stenosis
- Complications include urinary retention, bleeding, postoperative anal fissure

Stapled haemorrhoidectomy
- Stapled haemorrhoidectomy uses a modified circular stapler and excises a cuff of mucosa from above the haemorrhoids, which pulls any prolapsed tissue back into the anal canal and disrupts the supplying vessels. It is usually reserved for circumferential prolapsing haemorrhoids not suitable for excision

Complications
Post-haemorrhoidectomy
- Bleeding
- Pain
- Infection of wound or surrounding tissues
- Anal stenosis (usually only with extensive surgery)
- Recurrence of symptoms.

Thrombosed external piles are usually treated by continued conservative management (topical treatment, analgesia, and rest), but are very occasionally operated on to excise the affected portion with a very mild anal dilatation to relieve the anospasm associated.

Banding of Haemorrhoids

Pre-procedure
- Check that the patient has transport or company to leave the clinic—topical treatment may cause a vasovagal reaction
- Ensure the assisting nurse has the suction bander and additional bands available before starting
- Always perform the rigid sigmoidoscopy before giving topical therapy

Procedure
- Insert the proctoscope to the limit of the upper anal canal and withdraw slowly until the upper third of the haemorrhoids begin to 'bulge' into the lumen. A gentle 'in–out' movement may help to accentuate them. Ensure that the lowest limit of the area to be banded is no lower than the dentate line
- Place the end of the banding device over the cushion and apply suction for 1 or 2 seconds
- Deploy the band before releasing the suction

Complications
- Pain: immediate pain may indicate inclusion of the lower anal canal epithelium and may require band removal if severe
- Bleeding may occur after sloughing of the banded pedicle. This usually settles spontaneously

Injection of Haemorrhoids

Pre-procedure preparation as for banding.

Procedure
- Insert the proctoscope as for banding
- Insert the needle obliquely into the submucosa in the upper third of the haemorrhoid. Inject up to 3 mL per location. The submucosal 'bleb' should be easily visible. If it is not, consider whether the needle tip is too deeply placed (into the rectal wall or pararetal tissues)
- Inject in up to three locations—more may give troublesome swelling after the procedure

Complications
Immediate pain may indicate injection too low in the anal canal. Delayed pain may indicate sterile or infected abscess formation in the rectal wall or pararectal tissues. Patients re-presenting with significant pain should under go EUA or urgent MRI scanning.

5.11 Fissure in ano

A fissure in ano is a longitudinal split in the anal mucosa running from the anal verge to a point below the dentate line. They occur in all ages but are most common between the ages of 30 and 50 years.

Aetiology

Normal anatomy/physiology

- Tone in the anal canal at rest is maintained, in part, by contraction in the internal anal sphincter generated by autonomic innervation and local neurohormonal mechanisms
- Recruitment of contraction by the external anal sphincter occurs in response to voluntary contraction
- Acute transient fissuring of the anal canal lining is common and is usually self-limiting without symptoms

Pathological anatomy/physiology

- Pathological, excessive contraction of the internal anal sphincter occurs in response to fissuring of the anal canal which is painful or prolonged
- Recruitment of additional pathological, spontaneous, contraction of the external anal sphincter and posterior pelvic floor muscles may occur in response to pain

Proposed mechanism of chronic 'high pressure' fissure formation

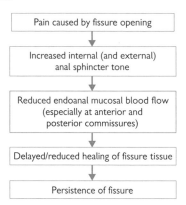

Pain caused by fissure opening

↓

Increased internal (and external) anal sphincter tone

↓

Reduced endoanal mucosal blood flow (especially at anterior and posterior commissures)

↓

Delayed/reduced healing of fissure tissue

↓

Persistence of fissure

Classification

- Idiopathic 'high pressure' fissure—persistence and aggravation of simple acute fissure by the above mechanism
- Postpartum 'low pressure' fissure—fissure induced by vaginal delivery, persistence related to delayed healing not anospasm
- Secondary fissures—related to underlying anal mucosal disease, e.g. Crohn's disease, endoanal sepsis, chronic anal infections

Clinical assessment

Patients usually present with severe anal pain on defaecation. This may last from minutes to hours afterwards. Over 80% are associated with a small amount of bright red bleeding.

On examination there may be a sentinel tag (Fig 5.15).

- Digital rectal examination should be attempted to exclude other anorectal pathology prior to sigmoidoscopy. Acute pain on eversion of the anal margin or attempted digital rectal examination is often diagnostic

Management

Reduction in endoanal 'trauma'/pain

Act to reduce trauma and induced pain. This results in spontaneous fissure healing in approximately 50% of patients after 6 weeks of compliant treatment.

- Stool softeners, e.g. sodium docusate
- Defaecatory habit; avoidance of straining
- Topical analgesics/anaesthetics, e.g. emollient cream, local anaesthetic gel
- Oral simple analgesia

None of these treatments is associated with significant side effects.

Pharmacological reduction in anal (sphincteric) tone

Act to reduce anospasm by inducing anal sphincter relaxation by inhibition of smooth muscle contraction. This results in spontaneous fissure healing in between 60 and 80% of patients after 6 weeks of compliant treatment.

- Nitrate ointments, e.g. glyceryl trinitrate (GTN)
- Calcium channel blocker ointments, e.g. diltiazem
- Both are associated with headaches, facial flashing, and palpitations in up to 15% of patients. Transient reduction in anal tone may result in minor perianal soiling in 5% of patients
- Botulinum A toxin, e.g. Botox®, blocks motor end-plate acetylcholine release. It is given as a single injection in the intersphincteric groove. Maximal effect starts 48 h after injection and lasts until motor end-plate proteins regenerate (6–8 weeks minimum)

This is associated with transient reduction in anal tone (for the duration of effect) and associated perianal soiling in 5% of patients.

Surgical reduction in anal (sphincteric) tone

Act to reduce anospasm by permanently weakening the internal anal sphincter. This results in spontaneous fissure healing in more than 80% of patients by 6 weeks.

- Lateral internal sphincterotomy—division of the lower one-third of the internal anal sphincter
- Manual anal dilatation—forced anal dilatation under anaesthetic. This should never be performed in the elective treatment of anal fissure owing to the risk of uncontrolled anal injury (often diffuse and not amenable to simple repair)
- Both techniques are associated with a 5% risk of permanent noticeable reduction in anal tone and associated perianal soiling/incontinence

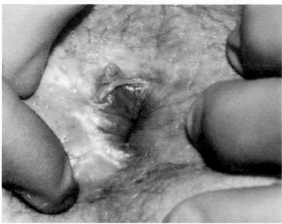

Fig 5.15 Chronic anterior fissure in ano with associated 'sentinel' skin tag .

Typical strategy for treatment of fissure

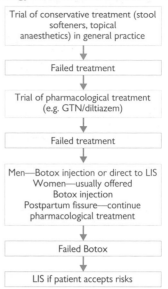

5.12 Perianal infection and fistula-in-ano

A fistula-in-ano is a granulation tissue-lined track connecting a primary opening inside the anal canal to a secondary opening in the perianal skin. Secondary tracts may be multiple and from the same primary opening and tracks may become epithelialized.

Aetiology

'Parkes' cryptoglandular theory

- The anal canal possesses between eight and twelve glands opening into the midzone of the canal, with the bulk of the gland lying deep to the submucosa and part deep to the internal anal sphincter fibres
- Infection of the gland results in pus tracking into the submucosal and intersphincteric plane
- Normal anal pressure at rest prevents discharge into the anal canal and the pus tracks to present in the perianal tissues (usually first presents as an acute perianal abscess)
- Tracking may occur in the submucosal or intersphincteric planes or may pass along the spreading fibres of the conjoint longitudinal coat of the rectum into the extra or suprasphincteric tissues
- Persistence of the underlying anal gland with its internal opening results in a persistent source of infection and the resulting granulation tissue-lined track forms a fistula

Other causes of fistula

- Chronic inflammatory or infectious conditions (e.g. Crohn's disease, actinomycosis, syphilis)
- Radiation-induced tissue damage (e.g. post-prostatic brachytherapy)
- Traumatic (e.g. surgical instrumentation, postrectal anastomosis, after excision of anorectal lesions, penetrating trauma)
- Obstetric-related (e.g. after third-degree tear or episiotomy)—usually rectovaginal or anovaginal
- Tumour (very rarely primary, may result after treatment)

Clinical assessment

Presentations

Perianal abscess

- Acute pain and swelling in the perianal tissues, usually associated with systemic features of fever, sweating, and tachycardia
- May not be obvious on external inspection (all symptoms of perianal sepsis deserve an EUA even if an abscess is not obvious)

Chronic discharge/recurrent perianal 'infections'

- May be simple seropurulent fluid, recurrent minor episodes of 'flare-up' or recurrent perianal abscesses

Air/fluid per vagina

- Usually a feature of post-obstetric fistulae

Necrotizing perineal infection

- Very rare in non-diabetics. Presents with rapidly worsening pain, spreading sepsis with local signs of skin discoloration, crepitus, and offensive odour (of anaerobic sepsis). Patients may be systemically relatively well.

Examination

- Inspection—describe sites, sizes, and appearances of external openings, scars of previous interventions, anal contour, and signs of previous surgery/trauma

> ### ⊙ Classification of fistula-in-ano
>
> #### Anatomical (Parks' classification)
> Anatomical classification depends upon the precise track a given fistula takes:
> - submucosal (5%)—superficial to all sphincteric structures (1)
> - intersphincteric (60%)—passes deep to part or all of the internal anal sphincter (2)
> - trans-sphincteric (25%)—passes through the external sphincter to lie deep to part or all of it. Divided into low (<½) and high (>½) according to the amount of sphincter encircled (3a, 3b)
> - suprasphincteric (5%)—passes above the external anal sphincter below the levator ani (4)
> - extrasphincteric (5%)—passes above the levator ani. May originate in the rectum rather than the anal canal (5)
>
>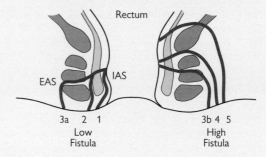
>
> **Fig 5.16** Types of fistula-in-ano. EAS, External anal sphincter; IAS, internal anal sphincter.
>
> #### Clinical classification
> - Low—effectively defined as those fistulae for which fistulotomy will divide less than 50% of the external anal sphincter (submucosal, intersphincteric, and low trans-sphincteric)
> - High—effectively defined as those for which fistulotomy would divide more than 50% of the external anal sphincter (high trans-sphincteric, suprasphincteric, and extrasphincteric)
> - Complex—involve multiple tracks, multiple openings (internal or external) or a combination of both

> ### ⊙ Goodsell's Law
>
> Goodsell's Law states that for external openings behind the line drawn from 3 to 9 o' clock across the anus as viewed in the lithotomy position, the fistula track will curve and open into the midline. For those with external openings in front of this line, the internal opening will be in a straight line at the same 'clockface' position in the anus.
>
> Exceptions are:
> - non-cryptoglandular sepsis
> - long anterior fistula may curve to the posterior midline
> - previously operated fistulae

- Digital rectal examination—to exclude other anorectal pathology, may locate internal opening(s), feel for tenderness or mass of deep abcess/inflammation
- Rigid sigmoidoscopy and proctoscopy—seek underlying rectal pathology and locate internal opening(s)

Investigations

Flexible sigmoidoscopy—if a diagnosis of non-cryptoglandular cause is suspected

- EUA may be required to identify the track. Techniques used during EUA include: probing with a blunt silver probe, injection of H_2O_2 or dye
- Endoanal ultrasound scan (EAUS) with or without H_2O_2 injected into it to highlight the track
- MRI scan provides the best delineation of pararectal tissues and complex/obscure fistulae

Management

Acute perianal abscess

- Drain all pockets of infection, clean the cavity, and keep external opening open to allow continued drainage
- Identify any underlying anorectal pathology
- Identify any obvious underlying fistula without creating artificial tracks

Non-operative therapy

- Not all fistulae require treatment. Some patients may settle for a chronic discharge in preference to surgery

Elective operative treatment

Low fistulae

Low fistulae can be laid open, cleaned, and left to heal by secondary intention (without packs) ('fistulotomy'). Fistulotomy may be performed as a primary procedure unless there is acute active sepsis.

High fistulae

High fistulae must be treated without complete fistulotomy to avoid the risk of incontinence. A non-cutting seton suture will prevent acute sepsis/abscess formation. Options for definitive treatment include:

- cutting setons—large calibre permanent suture material tied tightly and sequentially tightened over many weeks to slowly 'cut' thought the tissues
- fistula track obliteration—filling of the track with fibrin glue or collagen plug
- endorectal advancement flap—formation of a full thickness rectal wall flap, cleaning of fistula track, destruction of residual gland tissue, closure of the internal opening by the flap, and obliteration of the existing track with surgery, fibrin glue or collagen plug. May require a stoma.

Non-cryptoglandular fistulae

- This should always be treated as high fistulae and may not be suitable for surgery

> ### ⊕ Drainage of perianal abscess
>
> Consider preoperative imaging (MRI scan) if the patient has recurrent infections or previous surgery has failed to find an abscess/fistula.
>
> #### Procedure
>
> - Inspection and palpation will identify 90% or all pathology—take your time, feel all quadrants of the anus and anorectal junction, including palpation against the levator sling
> - Incise over any external collections—make the cut circumferentially not radially; this reduces the risk of accidental sphincter injury
> - Lavage the cavity and track—the internal opening of a fistula may become obvious
> - Gently probe with a blunt silver probe, with a finger in the anal canal. Do not press too hard. Insert a non-cutting seton if a fistula is found
> - Place a light, loose pack of soft material to keep the cavity open
>
> #### Post-procedure
>
> - Give a course of oral antibiotics
> - Request a change/removal of pack before discharge and regular district nurse review
> - Outpatient review is only necessary for a non-healing wound (i.e. a probable underlying fistula)
>
> #### Complications
>
> - Pain, if continuous, may indicate failure of drainage of all sepsis
> - Bleeding
> - Incontinence is usually due to an underlying fistula rather than sphincteric injury, and is usually transient

> ### ⊕ Setons
>
> There are three main types of seton.
> 1. **Loose setons** are usually Silastic slings tied into a loop. They are used to control/prevent recurrent infections, prevent secondary tracks developing, and encourage fibrosis in the track. They may be temporary (e.g. in high or complex fistulae) or semi-permanent (e.g. fistula in Crohns', malignancy, radiotherapy, immunosuppressed patients, and patients unsuitable for fistulotomy owing to previous surgery or incontinence risk)
> 2. **Cutting setons** are usually hard suture material such as nylon. They are used to divide high or complex fistulae progressively.
> 3. **Chemical setons** are organic thread impregnated with chemicals

5.13 Other anorectal conditions

Pilonidal sinus disease

Aetiology

Implantation theory

Shed hairs from the skin of the midline natal cleft become trapped within the follicle by pressure and local irritation. This accounts for the increased incidence in lorry drivers, hairy individuals, and men.

Chronic build up of follicular secretions enlarges the follicle into a sinus. Secondary infection further scars and enlarges the sinus with resulting acute or intermittent infections. Secondary tracks may arise from the original sinus which discharge out onto previously normal lateral natal cleft or buttock skin.

Congenital theory

Pre-exisiting sinus 'pits' exist in the natal cleft midline, resulting from the fusion of the body wall mesoderm. Shed hairs become entrapped in these sinuses with a similar course as above.

Clinical presentations

- **Acute pilonidal abscess**—pain, swelling, and 'lump' in the natal cleft. This is distinct to perianal infection but often the terms are confused. Always assess both the perianal area/perineum and the natal cleft.
- **Chronic discharging pilonidal sinus**—intermittent haemopurulent discharge with discomfort, skin irritation, and occasional swelling
- **Extensive sinus and fistula formation**—lateral tracking of sinus leads to fistula openings onto lateral buttocks

⊕ Excision and primary closure of pilonidal sinus

Principles

- Excise the midline pits and deal with the underlying sinuses either by excision or by surgical toilet
- Excise lateral tracks and fistulae
- Attempt primary closure in all but the largest sinus complexes
- Closure should flatten the natal cleft, produce an asymmetrical scar lying *off* the midline, and result in primary healing in most cases

Procedures

- Karydakis flap involves deep excision of affected tissue with 'stepped' excision of natal cleft tissue, mobilization of both medial buttock skin flaps, and sutured closure
- Bascom II procedure involves elliptical excision of natal cleft pits, cleaning, and/or excision of underlying tissue without deep excision, unilateral skin flap mobilization, and sutured closure
- Rhomboid flap involves a diamond-shaped excision of natal cleft pits and underlying tissue, mobilization of a wide unilateral buttock skin/fascial flap in the form of a rhomboid flap, and suture of flap into the natal cleft defect

Complications

- Wound infection and dehiscence in 10%
- Haematoma

⊕ Drainage of infected pilonidal sinus

Ensure the diagnosis is correct. Perianal and pilonidal abscesses are often confused or misrecorded.

Procedure

- The patient is usually best in the lateral position
- Aim to open the abscess as close to the midline as possible—this will help with any subsequent surgery
- Ensure the abscess is washed out and a light temporary pack placed
- Do not attempt to open up lateral tracks or fistulae unless they are frankly involved by the abscess
- Discharge home can be the same day but district nurse dressings are usually required initially

Pruritus ani

Aetiology

Primary

Pruritus ani is idiopathic in 50%. It is possibly due to a combination of incomplete perianal skin cleaning, susceptible perianal skin, and local irritation by hygiene products, clothes, and prolonged sitting/close fitting underwear. It is associated with obesity and sedentary jobs.

Secondary

- Dermatological (10%)—secondary to underlying skin condition (e.g. psoriasis, lichen planus, lichen sclerosis et atrophicus (LSA), contact dermatitis)
- Infection (15%)—secondary to anorectal infections (e.g. *Candida*, pinworms, syphilis)
- Anorectal (25%)—secondary to anorectal disorders (e.g. haemorrhoids, fissure in ano, fistula-in-ano, anal tumours)

Management

- Always perform a rigid sigmoidoscopy to exclude rectal pathology
- Recommend loose natural fibre underwear, avoidance of scented soaps/deodorants/talcum powder, washing regularly, use of petroleum jelly-based ointments on clean skin to improve waterproofing and prevent friction chafing
- Treat associated infections (e.g. mebendazole for pinworms)
- Deal with underlying anorectal conditions (e.g. topical treatment of haemorrhoids)

Anal stenosis

Aetiology

- Post-surgical—this is the commonest cause, usually due to anal surgery (e.g. extensive haemorrhoidectomy, multiple fistula surgeries, local excision of anal lesions)
- Postradiotherapy—usually following radical (chemo) radiotherapy for anal or vulval squamous carcinoma
- Postinfective—rare, e.g. after tuberculosis
- Postinflammatory—rare, e.g. after chronic anal Crohn's disease, after severe fissure in ano healing

Management

- Anal dilatation—may be under anaesthetic if severe or can be home dilatation by the patient using anal dilators. Great care must be taken, especially under general anaesthesia, to avoid overdilatation since 'a fixed closed anus is better than a fixed open anus'

- Advancement flaps—over reduction of endoanal tissue may be augmented by rectal mucosa (advanced flap) or perianal/buttock skin (cutaneous V–Y advancement flap)

Condylomata acuminata (warts)

- Caused by HPV virus infection (commonly types 6 and 11)
- May occur in isolation or as part of generalized wart infection and not all (peri)anal condylomata are sexually transmitted
- May be associated with cervical infection (including CIN) and vulval infection (including VIN) especially with HPV types 16 and 18
- Anal infection may be associated with the development of anal intraepithelial neoplasia (AIN)
- Treatment for small lesions is topical chemical therapy (e.g. podophyllin resin)
- Excision should be reserved for large or recurrent lesions
- Giant condylomata—'Buschke–Löwenstein tumours'— may develop in immunosuppressed or susceptible patients

---

⊕ Excision of anal warts/tags

Procedure

- Dilute adrenaline may be used as subcutaneous infiltration if sharp excision is used
- Excision is performed to include unaffected surrounding skin, by sharp dissection or cutting diathermy (with smoke plume evacuation)

Hidradenitis suppurativa (perianal)

Aetiology

- Chronic, recurrent infection of apocrine glands of the perianal and groin skin
- Secondary infection leads to multiple lateral tracks and skin fistula formation
- Presents as recurrent infection in the groin, perineal, and perianal skin

Management

- Acute abscesses are drained by simple incision
- Excision of all affected skin is required for prevention of recurrent sepsis. This may involve primary sutured closure or skin flaps. Local debridement and cleaning rarely produces long-term 'cure'

5.14 Case-based discussions

Case 1

A 35-year-old asymptomatic man is referred to your clinic for consideration of screening colonoscopy.

- What family history criteria would you use to determine his risk status?
- What is the underlying process of colorectal cancer development from an adenomatous polyp to frankly invasive tumour?

He has a 47-year-old brother, a 68-year-old father, and two paternal cousins all affected by colorectal cancer or adenomatous polyps.

- What screening investigation would you recommend for him?
- How would you consent him for a colonoscopy and what are the principles of the procedure?

Case 2

The following history is presented at the weekly multidisciplinary team meeting.

A 60-year-old man who complains of new onset rectal bleeding is found to have an ulcerated tumour 10 cm from the anal verge. He is otherwise fit and well.

- What investigations would you request and why?

Biopsies taken in clinic confirm an adenocarcinoma of probable bowel origin.

A colonoscopy confirms that this is an isolated lesion with no other tumours found in the colon.

A thoracoabdominopelvic CT scan shows no evidence of metastases.

A pelvic MRI scan suggests that the tumour is invading into the mesorectal fat close to the seminal vesicles anteriorly.

- What neoadjuvant treatments are possible for rectal cancer and would this patient be suitable?

Following long-course chemoradiotherapy the patient comes to theatre for surgery.

- What is the lymph node drainage and blood supply of the rectum and what operations would be considered for the patient?

He undergoes a radical low anterior resection with resection of the inferior mesenteric artery at its origin and the mesorectal tissue and associated lymph nodes. He has a temporary loop ileostomy formed.

- What factors would determine whether he is offered adjuvant chemotherapy?

Case 3

A 20-year-old woman presents to the emergency department with lower abdominal pain, bloody diarrhoea 12 times per day, temperature 38°C, HR 100, weight loss and dehydration.

- What is the differential diagnosis and how would you differentiate the possible alternatives?
- What is your initial management of this patient?

Fresh stool samples are negative for infectious causes and a diagnosis of probable ulcerative colitis has been made on the basis of the appearances at flexible sigmoidoscopy. Biopsies are awaited.

- How would you treat this patient at this stage? What features would you be concerned about if she did not improve?

She continues to have marked bloody diarrhoea with increasing abdominal tenderness, falling albumin, rising white cell count, and an abdominal radiograph showing severe colonic oedema.

- What non-surgical options are available?

She fails to respond to high-dose steroids and is too ill to consider immunomodulation.

- What urgent surgical procedures might be considered?
- How would you optimize her for surgery?

She undergoes acute total abdominal colectomy and ileostomy formation and recovers well.

Case 4

A 55-year-old woman is seen in outpatients complaining of painful troublesome 'haemorrhoids'.

- What is the differential diagnosis and what features are typical of each?
- What procedures would you perform and how?

On examination she has an external skin tag with three large internal haemorrhoids on rigid proctoscopy and nothing of note in the rectum on rigid sigmoidoscopy.

- What procedures could she be offered and what are the principles of their execution?

Chapter 6

Urology

Basic principles

Knowledge

Covered elsewhere

Clinical skills

- Incontinence in the elderly
- Urodynamics
- Interpreting urinalysis
- Interpreting PSA levels
- Digital rectal examination

Technical skills and procedures

- Male urethral catheterization
- Suprapubic catheterization
- TURP and bladder neck incision
- Percutaneous nephrostomy
- Intravenous urography
- Extracorporeal shock wave lithotripsy
- Percutaneous nephrolithotomy
- Retrograde ureteroscopy and ureteric stent insertion
- Hydrocele excision (Lord's procedure)
- Male sterilization
- Urinary diversion (urostomy formation)
- Flexible cystoscopy
- Transurethral resection of the bladder (TURBT)
- Radical orchidectomy

Renal blood flow

The kidneys receive ~20% of the cardiac output (~1000 mL/min). The renal arteries arise at slightly different levels at approximately the level of the L2 vertebral body. They subdivide into segmental, lobar, interlobar, and arcuate arteries which supply the afferent arterioles to the glomeruli (as end arteries).

Renal blood flow (RBF) is maintained over a wide range of perfusion pressures (80–180 mmHg) by autoregulation. This involves:

- sympathetic nerves (arising from the lumbar spinal segments travelling via the least splanchnic and first lumbar sympathetic nerve and the para-aortic and renal plexuses) mediating principally arteriolar vasoconstriction
- smooth muscle contraction (intrinsic myogenic tone) in afferent arterioles
- endocrine mechanisms (angiotensin II and antidiuretic hormone (ADH) act via arteriolar vasoconstriction and atrial natriuretic peptide (ANP) increases RBF by afferent arteriole vasodilatation
- paracrine mechanisms (local release of endothelins and nitric oxide act to cause arterial and venodilatation)

Glomerular filtration

The afferent arteriole supplies the glomerulus, which is effectively a unique interarteriolar capillary bundle draining into the efferent arteriole. The glomerulus sits within Bowman's capsule and is supported by mesangial tissue.

Glomerular filtration produces ultrafiltrate which is a rich solution of anions, cations, micronutrients and small proteins and unbound molecules (below 69 kDa). It is affected by several mechanisms:

- hydrostatic pressure gradient across the capillary wall (owing to arterial pressure, glomerular blood flow, and afferent/efferent arteriolar tone)
- oncotic pressure across the glomerular wall (caused by tissue and intravascular oncotic pressure)
- capillary permeability—affected by local and systemic mediators and capillary wall charge. This is usually negative and so resists protein, lipid, and polysaccharide filtration
- mesangial cell tone controlling glomerular capillary dimensions

Common measures of urinary function

Glomerular filtration rate

- The glomerular filtration rate (GFR) is measured by the principle that GFR=clearance for any substance completely filtered, not metabolized or reabsorbed, and passed unaltered in the urine
- Inulin is an ideal substrate but has to be administered and requires specific testing
- Creatinine clearance is used clinically to estimate GFR. It is freely filtered by the glomerulus but is secreted in small amounts by the tubules. Its plasma levels are also affected by age, sex, weight, starvation, nutrition, and disease
- GFR is approximated from serum measurements by the Cockroft-Gault formula (typically approximately 120 mL/min in healthy adults)

Renal clearance

- Renal clearance is the volume of plasma completely cleared of solute by the kidneys in 1 min
- It is measured by the principle that GFR=clearance for any substance completely filtered, not metabolized or reabsorbed, and passed unaltered in the urine

$$\text{Clearance (mL/min)} = \frac{UV}{P}$$

U=urinary concentration of substance, V=urine flow rate per minute, and P=plasma concentration of substance

Tubular/ductal function

Tubular and ductal functions are divided into four zones.

Proximal convoluted tubule

- Performs the reabsorption of the vast majority of ultrafiltrate contents—water, cations, anions, micronutrients (glucose, amino acids, etc.) via mostly passive and some active transport processes
- Actively secretes urea
- Mostly affected by blood flow in the efferent arteriole

Loop of Henlé

- Provides the mechanism for the generation of hypertonic medullary osmotic pressure required to effect collecting duct function of water reabsorption via the countercurrent multiplication effect generated by Na^+/K^+ pumps
- Highly dependent on blood flow and the provision of adequate quantities of energy (ATP) to power the membrane pumps

Distal convoluted tubule

- Performs the reabsorption ('fine control') of the balance of the cations (Na^+, K^+, Mg^{2+}, and Ca^{2+}) via active transport across a semi-permeable membrane
- Actively secretes H^+ via active transport
- Mostly affected by ADH altering membrane permeability and aldosterone affecting $Na^+/K^+/H^+$ membrane pumps

Proximal collecting duct

- Performs the reabsorption ('fine control') of the balance of the water required to determine final urine osmolarity
- Affected by ADH altering membrane permeability
- Dependent on medullary osmotic gradient

Micturition physiology

Innervation of the lower urinary tract

Sympathetic innervation

- **Upper ureter**: originate in T12–L5 spinal segments, distributed via the renal and pre-aortic plexuses
- **Lower ureter and bladder**: originate in L3–S2 spinal segments, distributed via superior and inferior hypogastric plexuses
- **Base of bladder, prostate, and upper urethra** (including sphincter): distributed via inferior hypogastric plexus via periprostatic plexus

Parasympathetic innervation

- **Ureter, bladder, urethra, and periurethral pelvic floor smooth muscle**: originate in the S2, 3, and 4 spinal segments via the pelvic parasympathetic nerves to the inferior and superior hypogastric plexuses.

Somatic innervation

- **Lower urethra, external urethral sphincter (EUS) and pelvic floor**: enables voluntary control of inhibition and initiation of micturition

Process of micturition

- As the bladder fills, the capacity expands without increase in intravesical pressure. The elastic properties of the detrusor muscle allows considerable compliance
- Gradually, local myogenic activity of the bladder wall tends to increase but stretch sensation, mediated mainly by parasympathetic fibres, initiates a spinal reflex with inhibition of the parasympathetic fibres acting to reduce bladder wall contractility and increase sphincter tone
- With further filling, the conscious sensation of bladder distension develops by stretch receptors sending afferent fibres to the frontal cortex via the dorsal columns and a further involuntary reflex contraction of the EUS and pelvic floor occurs. In men, conscious contraction of the muscles of the root of the penis may also help to increase tone in the proximal urethra and inhibit micturition
- Initiation of micturition is usually voluntary and results from stimulatory signals sent to the rostral pontine micturition centre. When stimulated, this centre sends signals to Onuf's nucleus at the level of S2/3. This nucleus contains motor neurons of the parasympathetic system which innervate the detrusor muscle profusely and, when activated, lead to detrusor contraction
- Simultaneous inhibition of sympathetic and somatic input causes coordinated relaxation of the bladder neck and EVS, and possibly also contraction of periurethral pelvic floor smooth muscles. This is further enhanced by local reflexes and nitric oxide release from specific nitrergic neurons of the parasympathetic system which innervate just the 'internal' sphincter and bladder neck muscle fibres (Fig 6.2).

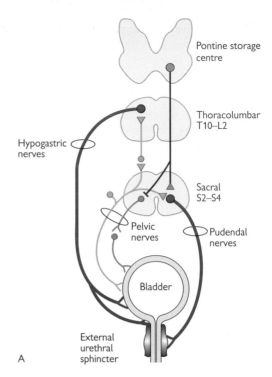

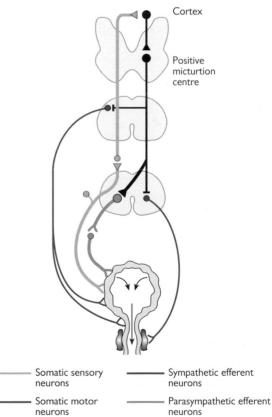

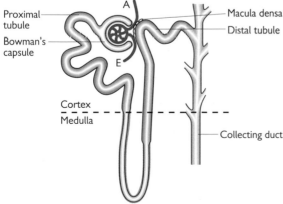

Fig 6.1 The basic anatomical components of a nephron. A – afferent arteriole; E – efferent arteriole.

Somatic sensory neurons — Sympathetic efferent neurons

Somatic motor neurons — Parasympathetic efferent neurons

Fig 6.2 Neural pathways involved in controlling urinary continence and micturition (A) Gradual bladder distension causes low level sensory firing. This in turn causes sympathetic stimulation which inhibits detrusor contraction and maintains internal sphincter tone. Also, it stimulates motor outflow to the EUS. (B) Significant distension of the bladder causes intense afferent firing. This stimulates parasympathetic firing, via the PMC, which inhibits the sympathetic and pudendal outflow. This results in detrusor contraction and relaxation of the EUS.

117

Embryology

Key points of embryology related to the development of congenital abnormalities:

- The kidneys are formed from the metanephros (of the intermediate mesoderm) which forms in the region of the pelvis and migrates cranially as it buds and divides. Failure to migrate or division of the metanephros into multiple segments produces ectopic or multiple kidneys. Fusion of the two metanephric tissue masses produces a horseshoe kidney (Fig 6.3)
- The lower ureter, ureteric orifices, and trigone of the bladder are derived from the mesonephric duct(s). Duplication of the ducts gives rise to duplex ureters, and obliteration of the mesonephric duct leads to congenital stenosis/obstruction
- The bladder forms from the urogenital sinus which connects to the peritoneal cavity via the allantois. Failure of closure of the external part of the urogenital sinus/cloacal membrane leads to extrophy, and persistence of the allantois leads to urachal abnormalities
- The urethra forms (in its upper part in males or entirely in females) from a combination of the distal part of the mesonephric ducts and the urogenital sinus, and (in its distal part in males) the fusion of the genital folds forming the shaft of the penis. Abnormal or incomplete closure of the folds gives rise to distal urethral abnormalities, e.g. hypospadias, and abnormalities of the junction of the two portions give rise to urethral valves in males

Kidney

Renal cysts

- Incidence: increases markedly with age (up to 60% at 80 years)
- Non-malignant, do not connect with any part of the nephron and are of no clinical consequence (unless massive)
- Difficulty exists when cysts are not simple (thick walls, calcification, and septae). These may represent cystic renal cancers

Polycystic kidney disease

- Autosomal dominant polycystic kidney disease presents in the fourth decade as large abdominal masses (95% bilateral), haematuria, and renal failure
- Treatment—symptomatic and preserving renal function. Eventual dialysis or transplant is inevitable

Ureter

Ectopic ureter

- Usually associated with a duplex system (upper and lower renal poles with its own renal pelvis and ureter)
- If the two ureters do not join before the bladder, they implant as two ureteric orifices (UO), the upper pole ureter inserting distally (Weigert–Meyer principle)
- Usually asymptomatic, occasionally associated with UTIs, rarely incontinence in women (UO below external sphincter)
- Treatment—heminephrectomy for poorly functioning symptomatic hemi-kidney

Pelviureteric junction (PUJ) obstruction

- This is caused by congenital failure of mesonephric duct formation
- Typically presents on antenatal USS as an aperistaltic segment
- Adult presentation is usually in adolescents with loin pain, especially after drinking alcohol. It is due to PUJ stenosis or crossing vessel
- Diagnosis by isotope (MAG-3) renogram and plain axial X-ray. Retrograde ureterogram may be useful intraoperatively
- Treatment—balloon dilatation, endopyelotomy or pyeloplasty (open or laparoscopic)

Bladder

Urachal abnormalities

- Failure of the urachus to close can lead to a fistula from bladder to umbilicus presenting as urinary discharge
- Partial closure can lead to a sinus or urachal cyst which may become infected
- Treatment—excision of cysts with closure of fistula if present
- Urachal adenocarcinoma occurs rarely

Extrophy of the bladder

- The urogenital membrane involutes and the posterior wall of the bladder and ureteric orifices are exposed on the anterior abdominal wall
- Incidence: 1 in 30 000 live births
- Usually occurs with the presence of epispadias
- Associated with pelvic (pubis and ilium) bony, genital, and anorectal defects
- Treatment—at birth cover the bladder with clingfilm and seek expert advice. The principles of surgery are correct bony pelvis, close bladder and abdominal wall, correct genitals, and later bladder neck reconstruction.

Urethral valves

- Incidence: 1 in 5000 live births
- Mucosal folds obstruct the prostatic urethra causing bladder outflow obstruction
- In-uterine diagnosis of severe obstruction is by eventual bladder wall hypertrophy, hydronephrosis, reduced amniotic fluid, and hence pulmonary hypoplasia.
- Presentation *in utero* is by oligohydramnios or postnatally with oliguria and in children by recurrent UTIs and bladder outflow obstruction. Diagnosis is by micturating cystourethrogram
- Treatment is by valve ablation. Impaired renal function may already exist at diagnosis and is always an indication for intervention

Penis

Hypospadias

- Hypospadias is the failure of preputial folds to fuse ventrally during penis development
- Depending on its severity, it can cause an excessive ('hooded') foreskin which is deficient ventrally, an ectopic urethral meatus, and chordee

- Incidence is 1 in 300 live male births, and there is an increased risk if siblings or parents are affected
- The ectopic urethral meatus is proximal and ventral compared with normal
  - Anterior (meatus between glans and subcoronal groove; 50%)
  - Midshaft (meatus along penile shaft; 30%)
  - Proximal (meatus between perineum and penoscrotal junction)
- It is commonly associated with developmental anomalies affecting other organs. When occurring together with undescended testes, intersex must be excluded
- Treatment—a wide range of plastic reconstruction aiming for a straight penis capable of voiding, erection, and pain-free sexual intercourse

Epispadias

- Incidence: 1 in 100 000 live male births
- It is related to bladder extrophy, the urethra opens on the dorsal penile shaft, often proximally with splaying of corpora cavernosae

Maldescent of the testis (Topic 13.12); vesicoureteric reflux and congenital scrotal swellings (Topic 13.11).

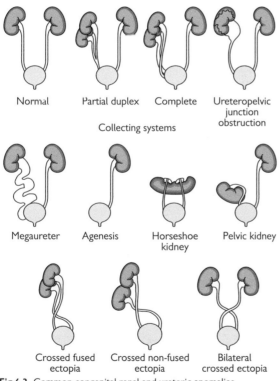

Fig 6.3 Common congenital renal and ureteric anomalies.

6.3 Urinary retention

Acute retention of urine may be defined as the rapid onset of a painful inability to pass urine. This is a common urological emergency with a lifetime risk of 1–2% in men.

Chronic retention of urine may be defined as a gradual onset of painless inability to pass urine normally.

Pathophysiology

Bladder emptying depends on appropriate relaxation of the bladder neck/sphincter muscles, correct elevation of the anterior bladder neck, and coordinated detrusor contraction.

Acute retention

Acute retention may cause disordered bladder function and prevents emptying, although the volume in the bladder may be little more than normal voiding volume.

1. 'Precipitated'—normal underlying anatomy/physiology + acute precipitating event, e.g. constipation, post-surgery, long car journey triggers retention
2. 'End of the road'—long history of deteriorating function with 'acute on chronic' retention

Chronic retention

In chronic retention owing to outflow obstruction, the bladder responds along a 'Starling curve' by initially compensating (bladder thickening, hyperactivity, and hypersensitivity); chronic overdistension eventually results in decompensation (bladder thinning, painless hypocontractility) with increased residual volumes and ultimately retention.

Aetiology

The causes of urinary retention are the same for acute (*) and chronic (+) although the spread of causes is different and either may be multifactorial.

- Bladder outflow tract obstruction
  - BPH (+) (📖 Topic 6.4)
  - Tumours (prostatic, bladder neck)(*)
  - Prostatitis (*)
  - Urethral strictures/trauma/tumours/valves (+)
- Pelvic pathology
  - Masses (fibroids, tumours, faeces, fetus)
  - Inflammation (diverticulitis, PID) (*)
- Neurological disorders
  - Cord compression/disc prolapse (*)
  - Peripheral neuropathies (including diabetes mellitus) (+)
  - Central nervous disease (MS), amyotrophic lateral sclerosis (AMLS)
- Pharmacological (disorders of autonomic function)
  - Post-anaesthesia (GA, spinal, epidural)
  - Drugs (anticholinergics)

Beware of the unwell patient referred as having retention because they have not passed urine for hours and have low abdominal pain. This may reflect reduced urine output secondary to some intra-abdominal pathology. If catheterization of a patient with 'acute retention' yields little urine then think again.

Clinical/assessment

Acute retention

- Painful inability to pass urine
- Precipitating factors/underlying disease (preceding lower urinary tract symptoms)
- Tense bladder distension (painful on palpation)

Chronic retention

- New nocturnal incontinence (may be caused by overflow)
- Deteriorating background function
- Often still able to pass urine in small volumes (painless)
- Patients often smell of urine (overflow incontinence)
- Bladder often lax, difficult to palpate, dull to percussion (often up to the umbilicus)
- Signs of chronic renal failure

Check for rare external causes (phimosis, penile cancer), common prostatic causes by DRE (benign prostatic hypertrophy (BPH), carcinoma), and features of neurological disease

Investigations

- Bladder ultrasound scan in cases of doubt
- Catheterization is diagnostic
- Full blood count, U&Es
- Catheter specimen of urine on catheterization
- Do not perform prostatic-specific antigen (PSA) acutely (retention raises PSA)
- Urodynamics in chronic retention
- Flexible cystoscopy to assess for cause
- USS in chronic retention may show hydronephrosis

Management

Acute retention

- Initial therapy is emergency catheterization to relieve symptoms. This is usually urethral but a suprapubic catheter (SPC) can be used if this is not possible
- Subsequent management depends on presentation.
  - In 'end of the road' patients or higher residual volumes (greater than 900 mL) owing to prostatic disease, TURP (or equivalent) performed 2–4 weeks after the retention (less blood loss than immediate TURP)
  - In patients with 'precipitated' retention or lower residual volumes, consider a trial without catheter (TWOC) performed 1 week after retention, with preceding alpha blockers

Chronic retention

- Initial therapy is catheterization. This is usually urethral, but a suprapubic catheter can be used if this is not possible
- Rapid decompression of a grossly distended bladder may result in haemorrhage from the bladder wall; this can be managed by clamping the catheter to allow gradual progressive decompression
- If a post-obstructive diuresis occurs after catheterization (diuresis >200 mL/h for 12 h), monitor by daily weights, U&Es, standing/lying BP, and give IV normal saline replacement
- BPH/Ca prostate treatment. Common treatments include: TURP, intermittent self-catheterization (ISC) or long-term catheter if unfit
- If renal function is normal, book for urgent TURP but catheterization can be avoided (less risk of pre-operative urinary infection)
- If renal function is abnormal, catheterize and consider TURP in 2–4 weeks

Urethral stricture

Periurethral scarring causing reduced urethral calibre sufficient to render symptoms

Clinical assessment

Patients may present with a slow, prolonged stream, urinary retention or UTI.

On examination there are usually no external findings. It may be impossible to pass a urethral catheter.

Investigations

- Urodynamics show a prolonged duration and low flow rate with raised residual volume
- Flexible cystoscopy demonstrates stricture

Management

- SPC for acute retention
- Urethral dilatation
- Optical urethrotomy
- Excision and reanastomosis or grafting

➕ Male urethral catheterization

Urinary catheters are measured in Charriere (CH), which relates to the outer circumference of the catheter. The smallest diameter should be used (12 Ch or 14 Ch) apart from when blood clots or debris are present. For clot retention, a three-way irrigation catheter should be used (20 Ch or 22 Ch).

Indications

- Acute urinary retention
- Close monitoring of urine output
- Pass urethral obstruction
- Incontinence
- Bladder irrigation
- Instil drugs into bladder

Procedure

1. Place a sterile field centred on the penis
2. One hand is 'dirty' and holds the penis. Retract the fore-skin and clean the glans with normal saline 0.9%
3. Inject some anaesthetic gel into the urethra. Leave for 5 min to take effect
4. Elevate and angle the penis towards the umbilicus
5. Use minimal force to advance the catheter down the urethra. It should be held with sterile forceps or the 'clean' hand. Resistance suggests stricture or false passage
6. There may be increased resistance at the external sphincter. Ask the patient to try and pass water and this should relax the sphincter
7. When urine begins to flow, advance the catheter up to the hilt and inject the balloon with the required volume of water (usually 10 mL). If inflating the balloon causes pain, the catheter is in the wrong place and the balloon should be deflated immediately. Connect the catheter bag
8. Clean any excess gel and reposition the foreskin
9. Note the residual volume

Complications

Procedural and early	Intermediate and late
• Trauma to urethra/prostate/ bladder	• Encrustation and blockage
• Clot retention	• Urethral erosion/stricture
• Acute UTI	

➕ Suprapubic catheterization

A percutaneous stab or open cystotomy.

Indications

- Urethral trauma
- Urinary retention when urethral catheter not possible
- Long-term catheterization

Procedure

1. Confirm bladder by percussion +/- ultrasound
2. After skin preparation, locate the bladder by aspiration using long hollow bore needle usually just to the side of the midline
3. Pass guide wire ('floppy' end first) into the bladder
4. Withdraw the needle and make a small stab incision alongside the wire
5. Ensure the trochar and disposable sheath are assembled and locked together
6. Feed the trochar over the wire and advance into the bladder using a rotating action
7. Use other hand on SPC at entry site to prevent sudden plunge
8. Unlock the trochar from the sheath and withdraw to check correct insertion as far as the bladder (copious urine should flow out of the sheath)
9. Occlude the sheath with thumb so bladder does not empty and immediately insert catheter down sheath, inflate balloon, and remove sheath by tearing apart into two halves

Complications

Procedural and early	Intermediate and late
• Injury to bowel/bladder	• Encrustation and blockage
• Clot retention	• Urethral stricture
• Acute UTI	• Bypassing

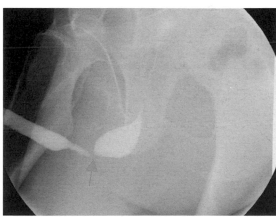

Fig 6.4 Urethrogram showing a urethral stricture.

121

Lower urinary tract symptoms (LUTS) is an umbrella term for symptoms of different aetiology.

The major cause of LUTS is bladder outflow obstruction (BOO). This is usually caused either by 'static' or 'dynamic' effects of the prostate.

Static effects cause mechanical obstruction owing to benign prostatic enlargement (BPE), and occur most commonly because of BPH.

Dynamic prostate obstruction occurs when the bladder neck/prostate junction fails to relax at voiding. Hence small prostates can cause obstruction.

Classification of lower urinary tract symptoms

Filling (irritative—'storage') symptoms

- Nocturia
- Frequency
- Urgency
- Urge incontinence

Voiding (obstructive) symptoms

- Weak stream
- Incomplete emptying
- Hesitancy
- Straining

Nocturnal enuresis

- Classic symptom of chronic retention

For differential diagnosis of LUTS, see Topic 6.3.

Investigations

- Bloods—FBC, U+Es (raised creatinine)
- Urinalysis
- International prostate symptom score (IPSS) quantifies severity of symptoms
- PSA
- Flow rate
- Residual volume (urodynamics)

Benign prostatic hyperplasia

BPH arises in the transition zone of the prostate (periurethral glands and stroma). It is common and incidence increases with age. It is histologically present in 60% of 60-year-olds, and half will be symptomatic.

Pathophysiology

5-α-reductase converts testosterone to dihydrotestosterone (DHT). DHT stimulates growth factors, especially epidermal growth factor (EGF), inducing cell proliferation and inhibition of TGF-beta leading to reduced apoptosis. These growth factor changes result in smooth muscle (with α-adrenoreceptors), connective tissue, and epithelial hyperplasia, and an increase in prostate size. Prostate volumes increase by approximately 1 cm^3 per year, and flow rate reduces by 0.2 mL/s/year.

Clinical assessment

History

As the prostate enlarges, the patient usually develops LUTS.

- 15% of patients' symptoms improve with time
- 30% of patients' symptoms are unchanged
- 55% of patients' symptoms deteriorate with time

Examination

- Large palpable (precussable) bladder of chronic retention
- DRE for size and consistency of prostate
- External genitalia examination to exclude associated phimosis
- Neurological examination to exclude associated causes

Management

Medical

This is suitable for patients with a short history, minimal inconvenience, and normal investigations.

Medical management produces moderate improvements in flow rate and symptom scores:

- α-blockers relax bladder neck/prostate smooth muscle. They have a rapid onset of action but 5% of patients suffer postural hypotension
- 5-α-reductase inhibitors reduce prostate volume, but have a slow onset (3–6 months). Side effects include reduced libido and erectile dysfunction in 10% and a reduction in PSA, making monitoring difficult. They can reduce the risk of acute retention.

Surgical

Surgical management leads to a large improvement in flow rates and symptom scores.

Indications for intervention

- Acute retention (relative indication)
- Chronic retention (relative indication)
- Renal insufficiency
- Recurrent UTI/haematuria
- Bladder stones
- Large diverticula
- Patient choice/severe symptoms

Options for intervention

- Intermittent self-catheterization
- Transurethral resection of prostate (TURP)
  - 80% achieve reduction in symptoms
- Laser 'prostatectomy'
- Open prostatectomy
  - Superior to TURP at symptom relief
  - Greater morbidity/mortality rates than TURP
  - Usually reserved for very large prostates (greater than 100 cm^3)
- Prostatic stents
  - Usually reserved for unfit patients with limited life expectancy
- Microwave ablation of the prostate

> **→ Extra**
>
> *Laser TURP*
>
> Newer generation lasers, e.g. Greenlight/KTP lasers appear to maintain the benefits of lasers (decreased blood loss/day case surgery) without losing effectiveness as seen with older lasers.

⊕ TURP and bladder neck incision

Bladder neck incision divides bladder neck sphincter and prostate tissue.

Open TURP is the removal of prostatic tissue.

Pre-procedure

Consent should include the risks of bleeding, infection, altered continence (2%), perforation, erectile dysfunction (10%), and retrograde ejaculation.

Procedure

1. DRE on table (re-evaluate size)
2. Preliminary cystoscopy
3. Smaller prostate and high bladder neck—perform bladder neck incision (BNI). Incise with Collin's knife from just distal to ureteric orifice to veru at 5 or 7 o'clock position
4. Larger prostates require TURP
5. Many different techniques; for example
6. Trench at 6 o'clock from bladder neck to veru
7. Then trench at 2 o'clock (or 10) from bladder neck to level of veru
8. Resection of 'dislocated' intervening prostate has reduced blood supply
9. Repeat from 10 o'clock to 2 o'clock
10. Evacuate resected chips of tissue
11. Never transgress distal to the veru owing to the risk of external striated sphincter injury
12. Care at 6 o'clock position (easy to undermine bladder neck)
13. For a larger perforation/venous sinus, insert catheter and inflate balloon plus or minus traction
14. Better to do one lobe well than two badly

Complications

Intra-procedural and early	Intermediate and late
• Bleeding (requiring trans-fusion 5%)	• Incontinence (1%)
• Clot retention	• Impotence (10%)
• Acute UTI	• Retrograde ejaculation (80%)

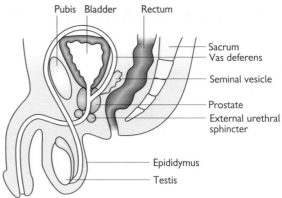

Fig 6.5 Sagittal cross-section showing the anatomical relations of the prostate gland.

Urinary incontinence is the involuntary loss of urine.

- Incidence: 20–30% of women >65 years
- Age: increases with age
- Sex: F>M

Neuropathic bladder is the broad term for dysfunction of the bladder secondary either to upper motor neuron, lower motor neuron or intrinsic bladder neuromuscular disease.

Aetiology

Bladder abnormalities

- An 'overactive' bladder with normal compliance which is 'unstable' and contracts spontaneously. Causes:
  - idiopathic
  - secondary to BOO/pelvic surgery/damage during pregnancy and delivery
  - secondary to bladder pathology (stones, tumours)
  - secondary to an upper motor neuron neurological cause, e.g. MS, spinal cord injury
- A flaccid bladder with normal compliance which overfills and leaks due to 'overflow,' e.g.
  - secondary to a lower motor neuron neurological cause, e.g. pelvic nerve damage, peripheral neuropathies
- A bladder with low compliance which results in failure to relax and fill, e.g.
  - after pelvic radiotherapy
  - chronic bladder infection (TB, schistosomiasis)
  - after bladder surgery
- Hypermobility of bladder base/urethra resulting in descent through weakened pelvic floor, disrupting normal sphincter mechanism
  - childbirth
  - after pelvic surgery

Sphincter abnormalities

- Disruption of sphincter complex (intrinsic sphincter deficiency; ISD) in which the bladder neck and sphincter are open at rest
  - After surgery (TURP/BNI)
  - After trauma

Risk factors

- Obesity
- Pregnancy and childbirth
- Age—reduced oestrogens and atrophic vaginitis/bladder instability
- Chronic cough—raised intra-abdominal pressure

Special cases

- **Overflow incontinence**: new nocturnal incontinence is the classic sign of chronic retention
- **Post TURP/radical prostatectomy** causes severe incontinence in up to 5%. Wait 1 year for spontaneous improvement and consider pelvic floor exercises, anti-cholinergic for instability, urethral bulkers, artificial sphincter
- **Vesicovaginal fistula** may develop following prolonged childbirth (developing countries), postoperative radiotherapy, and malignancy (developed countries). Cystogram demonstrates fistula (associated ureterovaginal fistula in 10%). Small fistulas may settle with catheterization,

but most require surgery which can be vaginal or transabdominal.

Clinical assessment

History

- Severity of symptoms (quality of life, pads)
- Urgency and urge incontinence (typically overactive bladder)
- Stress incontinence is characterized by incontinence on coughing, sneezing, etc.
- About one-third of women with symptoms have mixed overactive bladder and sphincter abnormalities

Examination

- Abdominal examination (palpable bladder in chronic retention or abdominal masses)
- DRE to assess prostate
- Vagina—leak, vaginal wall prolapse on coughing
- Neurological examination—anal sensation and tone, lower limb neurology

Investigations

- Patient diary—frequency, volume, incontinent episodes, use and the number of pads
- Urinalysis to exclude UTI
- Flexible cystoscopy for cases with severe symptoms, sudden onset, and where bladder irritability is the predominant feature to exclude intrinsic bladder pathology, e.g. stone, tumour
- Bladder USS—chronic retention, other urological symptoms
- Urodynamics—differentiate between detrusor instability and sphincter abnormalities
- CT—associated chronic retention and hydronephrosis
- MRI lumbar spine—lower cord/spinal nerve lesions

Management of bladder instability

Conservative

- Weight loss
- Stop smoking
- Avoid caffeine, alcohol
- Bladder retraining (consciously delay micturition)
- Treat obvious cause (bladder stone, tumour, TURP)

Medical

Fifty per cent will improve with medical management.

- Anticholinergics inhibit contractions. They are contraindicated with closed angle glaucoma, and side effects include dry mouth and constipation
- Tricyclic antidepressants can be beneficial
- Desmopressin is an antidiuretic which is good for nocturnal polyuria

Surgical

Interventions

- Neuromodulation—sacral nerve root stimulators. This is available at specialist centres only
- Intravesical treatment for those failing medical therapy
- Botulinum toxin A injected cystoscopically into detrusor muscle

Operative

Increase bladder capacity and decrease detrusor contraction pressure by interrupting detrusor muscle continuity.

- Detrusor myomectomy removes muscle, leaving intact urothelium
- Clam ileocystoplasty interposes a segment of small bowel to bisected bladder
- Ileal conduit is used in extreme cases

Management of bladder hypermobility/sphincter abnormality

Conservative

- Weight loss
- Stop smoking
- Pelvic floor exercises
- Electrical stimulation (sacral neuromodulators)

Surgery

- Injections—periurethral and bladder neck bulkers. Ideal for intrinsic sphincter deficiency. This can be performed under LA. It lasts for a shorter time than other treatments but is easily repeated. Risks include retention
- Slings support bladder neck and sphincter, e.g. tension-free vaginal tape (TVT). This can be performed as day case surgery and provides 80% long-term cure rates. Risks include erosion
- Retropubic suspension—elevate and fix the bladder neck/sphincter within pelvis. This can be done by:
  - Needle suspension, e.g. Stamey
  - Open suspension, e.g. Burch colposuspension. Good initial success but significant operation risks—retention, development of overactive bladder
- Artificial urinary sphincter—post-prostatectomy incontinence and when other methods for sphincter abnormalities fail
- Self-operated cuff and reservoir system. Risks include infection/erosion

---

⊙ Incontinence in the elderly

The aetiology is the same as previously described but, in addition, the mnemonic DIAPPERS can be used.

- **D**ementia
- **I**nfection
- **A**trophic vaginitis
- **P**sychological depression
- **P**harmacological—constipating drugs
- **E**xcess fluid—diuretics/CCF
- **R**estricted mobility
- **S**tool impaction

⊙ Urodynamics

Simple

- Flow rates
- Post-voiding residual volume

Advanced

- Cystometry is the combination of bladder and rectal transducers. Measurements derived include:
  - bladder pressure and stability during filling
  - minimum pressure on leakage (abdominal leak point pressure). A pressure <60 cmH$_2$O suggests intrinsic sphincter deficiency (ISD) and >90 cmH$_2$O urethral hypermobility

When combined with flow rate studies, information can be obtained on the degree of obstruction.

- Fluoroscopy (video urodynamics) to assess the movement of the urethra/bladder neck during micturition

Urinary tract infection (UTI) is significant bacteriuria associated with symptoms. It is an inflammatory response of the urothelium to bacterial infection. It covers a wide range of conditions.

A **simple UTI** occurs in an anatomically and functionally normal urinary tract.

A **complicated UTI** is one that occurs in an anatomically or functionally abnormal urinary tract or in a compromised host, e.g. diabetic or immunosuppressed patient.

UTI is the second commonest infection to present to GPs (after URTI), and accounts for 30% of hospital-acquired infections.

Incidence: women 20%+ lifetime risk
Age: increases with age (except in neonates)
Sex: M<F (reversed in neonates)

Aetiology
- Most UTIs arise from ascending infection from perineal organisms
- Common organisms are *E. coli*, faecal streptococci, *Proteus* spp., *Klebsiella* spp., and staphylococci

Pathophysiology
Susceptibility to infection is a balance between host defences and bacterial virulence factors.

Host defences
- Urethral length (increased UTI in women)
- Maintained commensal flora ('good' bacteria, e.g. lactobacilli compete for nutrients, cell surface receptors) affected by menopause in women, and intercourse in susceptible women
- Maintained urine flow, complete bladder emptying, and normal urine composition (e.g. absence of glucose)
- Intact bladder surface mucins/IgE/mucosal white cells

Bacterial virulence
- Adhesion ability—*E. coli* has fimbriae (pili) that aid adhesion to urothelium
- Specific virulence factors, e.g. haemolysins, capsular antigens
- Drug resistance—intrinsic or acquired through mutation/plasmid acquisition

Clinical assessment
History
- Increased urinary frequency
- Urgency of micturition
- Dysuria (pain on micturition)
- Pungent smelling urine
- Lower abdominal pain (cystitis) or loin pain (pyelonephritis)
- Haematuria

Examination
- Fever (typically >39°C in pyelonephritis)
- Abdominal examination (suprapubic discomfort)

Investigations
- Urinalysis (clean mid-stream collection) may look turbid and show leucocytes and be positive for nitrites—80% sensitive
- Urine sent for microscopy, sensitivity, and culture. Urinary infection is suggested if there are >10 WBC per mL on microscopy and $>10^5$ CFU per mL of urine on culture
- Bloods are not indicated in a simple UTI. FBC, U+Es, and CRP may show elevated inflammatory markers

- Renal USS is indicated in men, children, and recurrent/complicated infections. It is not required in simple infections in women
- CT or CT urogram (CTU) if stones are suspected
- Flexible cystoscopy is performed following resolution in men and older women with recurrent infections

Management
Medical
Lifestyle advice
- Increase fluid intake
- Eat probiotic yoghurt
- Drink cranberry juice (decreases bacterial adhesion)
- Void following sexual intercourse (reduces colonization of the urethra with perineal bacteria)

Drug therapies
- Empirical antibiotics (follow local guidelines for hospital- or community-acquired infection). A 3 day course is adequate for a simple UTI. Male patients, patients with symptoms of more than 1 week's duration, and complicated UTIs should be treated for longer

Operative
- Treat complicating factors (stones, bladder outflow obstruction, etc.)

Complications and prognosis
Simple UTIs in healthy patients rarely have complications. The main issues are with resistant organisms or re-infection.

The prognosis is worst in elderly patients or those with chronic disease or abnormal urinary tracts.

In patients with non-resolving UTI, consider:
- antibiotic sensitivity/compliance
- vesicoenteric fistula (pneumaturia plus debris in urine)
- radiolucent calculi—CTU

Recurrent UTIs
Consider other diagnoses, especially if MSU is negative, e.g. pelvic inflammatory disease, STI or interstitial cystitis. In those with genuine recurrent UTIs practising lifestyle advice, consider:
- long-term low dose antibiotics taken at night (rotate monthly between two or three types)
- rapid self-start treatments from home supply
- postcoital single dose antibiotics

UTI in special groups
- Indwelling urethral catheters induce bacterial colonization of urine (bacteriuria) within days. Only symptomatic bacteriuria needs to be treated (about two to three episodes per year)
- Pregnancy—treat asymptomatic bacteriuria as 30% will progress to acute pyelonephritis with risk of premature labour. Avoid tetracyclines (discolour teeth) and trimethoprim (neural tube defects)
- Elderly patients often have a bacteriuria. Treat those who are symptomatic
- Children—there is a risk of renal damage if young and vesicoureteric reflux is present. Treat with a 7 day course of antibiotics and refer for a paediatric opinion/investigation

Acute pyelonephritis

This is acute infection of the renal parenchyma. It is almost always an ascending infection from a bladder UTI (very occasionally haematogenous).

Clinical assessment

History and examination

- Dysuria, loin pain, pyrexia, rigors, flu-like symptoms
- Loin tenderness, temperature
- Positive urine dipstick for leucocytes and nitrites (reconsider if negative)

Investigations

- MSU (Dipstix, Gram stain, MC+S)
- FBC (↑WBC)
- Blood cultures if pyrexial
- IVU excludes obstruction and infection (not if creatinine raised/GFR impaired)

Management

- IV antibiotics (e.g. Gentamicin and Augmentin initially)
- IV fluids if cardiovascular signs
- Switch to oral antibiotics for 14 days when temperature settles
- Consider abscess and re-image if temperature fails to settle in few days

 Extra

A rare but severe form of acute pyelonephritis called emphysematous pylonephritis typically occurs in diabetics. Patients are more unwell. Imaging shows gas within/around kidney. This condition may require urgent nephrectomy.

Chronic pyelonephritis

This is the end result of repeated episodes of UTIs/acute pyelonephritis, usually in abnormal renal tract.

Chronic pyelonephritis is often asymptomatic and is diagnosed following a deterioration in renal function.

Imaging shows deformed calyces with cortical scars and shrunken kidney.

Management

- Treat UTI and prevent others if possible
- Estimate overall (GFR) and split renal function (DMSA)
- Consider nephrectomy if split renal function less than 20%

Interstitial cystitis

Interstitial cystitis is characterized by suprapubic pain, frequency, urgency, and nocturia in the absence of other explanations. Often patients believe they are having recurrent UTIs but MSU tests are negative.

The aetiology is unknown, but an abnormal glycosaminoglycan (GAG) layer in the bladder or increased inflammatory mast cells are seen.

The diagnosis is made by seeing 'glomerulations' (or rarely Hunner's ulcer) on cystodistension of the bladder.

Management

Cystodistension helps many patients; intravesicle GAG analogues are second line. Rarely symptoms are so intractable that cystectomy is needed.

⊚ Interpreting urinalysis

Look for nitrite- and leucocyte-positive. Many bacteria convert nitrates to nitrites which are detectable on dipstick. Specificity is high (greater than 90%), but sensitivity is low (35–85%). A positive nitrite strongly suggests a UTI and negative nitrites do not exclude one.

Leucocyte esterase from neutrophils in urine causes a dipstick colour change. Twenty per cent of patients with UTI have minimal pyuria, giving false-negative results. False-positives (pyuria but no infection) occur with TB, calculi, and interstitial cystitis.

6.7 Inflammation and infection of the urinary tract II

Renal and perirenal abscess

Abscess is usually secondary to ascending UTI and acute pyelonephritis.

It is more common in patients with diabetes mellitus, IV drug users, and those who are immunocompromised (possible haematogenous spread).

Clinical assessment

These conditions can present acutely but often there is a more insidious onset, with a history of 'chills', loin pain, weight loss, malaise, and night sweats.

On examination there may be a palpable loin mass.

Investigations

- Urinalysis: leucocytes but no organisms is typical
- Bloods—FBC (raised WBC), U+Es, raised CRP
- Blood cultures
- USS—to look for features of renal parenchymal abnormality

Management

- Small abscesses can be managed conservatively with intravenous antibiotics
- Larger abscesses need percutaneous or open surgical drainage. Emergency nephrectomy or delayed nephrectomy (loss of function)
- Once resolved, a delayed DMSA should be performed to estimate renal function
- Mortality rates are 5–10% in untreated sepsis

Pyonephrosis

Pyonephrosis is expansion of an upper urinary tract abscess, usually associated with obstruction resulting in destruction and degeneration of the renal parenchyma. This condition is potentially life-threatening.

Clinical assessment

- Presentation is similar to 'simple' abscess formation but with increasing signs of sepsis and deterioration of renal function
- IVU shows poor function/obstruction
- USS confirms hydronephrosis

Treatment

- Urgent nephrostomy with IV antibiotic and IV fluid cover (may precipitate septic crisis if patients are inadequately fluid-resuscitated)
- Once resolved, any underlying obstruction must be corrected
- Nephrectomy may be indicated for failure to extirpate sepsis, non-functioning kidney or secondary hypertension

Genitourinary tuberculosis

This is usually secondary to previous pulmonary infection, with haematogenous spread to the upper renal tract (especially kidney with seeding down the urothelial tract).

Clinical assessment

- Previous history of TB or chronic 'cystitis'
- Examination is usually normal but may see draining sinus

Investigations

- In patients with sterile pyuria, obtain three early morning urines for TB culture
- IVU—calyceal abnormalities, ureteric strictures
- Cystoscopy—inflamed contracted bladder, 'golf hole' ureteric orifices

Management

- There is minimal infection risk (without pulmonary TB) to contacts
- One year combination anti-TB therapy
- Surgery for local complications (e.g. chronic renal abscess, secondary hypertension, ureteric strictures)

Schistosomiasis (bilharzia)

- Schistosomiasis is a parasitic disease caused by trematode flatworms (schistosomes). It is particularly prevalent in tropical regions of Africa and Asia
- Life cycle involves freshwater snail and man
- It is usually a chronic condition affecting many body systems, but causing few symptoms
- Microscopy of urine or stool shows schistosome eggs
- A number of drugs are used, including praziquantel
- Schistosomiasis is a major risk factor for subsequent bladder squamous cell carcinoma (SCC). In Egypt, this is more common than bladder transitional cell carcinoma (TCC), although the latter is catching up because of increased smoking

Prostatitis

Acute bacterial prostatitis

- An acute bacterial infection of the prostate is uncommon
- Clinical features of an abscess are severe perineal pain, malaise, frequency, urgency, and intense dysuria
- Treatment is with antibiotics or de-roofing the abscess endoscopically into the urethra

Chronic bacterial prostatitis

- Common in 40–60-year-olds
- Possibly related to infection (associated with recurrent UTIs) or more likely to chronic prostatic inflammation, although pelvic floor muscle dysfunction may cause some symptoms (better termed chronic pelvic pain syndrome)
- Clinical features are of fluctuating perineal, groin, thigh, and scrotal pain which typically waxes and wanes
- Treatment—reassurance, 6–12 weeks Ciproxin, α-blockers, prostatic massage

Sexually transmitted diseases

Gonococcal urethritis

- Gonococcal urethritis is caused by *Neisseria gonorrhoea*. It is a significant public health problem and is a notifiable disease. It has an incubation period of 3–10 days
- History should include sexual history, use of contraception, and details of previous STD
- Men present with urethral discharge and women with urethral and vaginal discharge, dysuria (often without frequency

or urgency), and lower abdominal pain. Disseminated gonococcal infection occurs in 1%

- Gram staining of either urine or urethral discharge is usually
diagnostic. Ultrasound should be considered if pelvic inflammatory disease (PID) is suspected
- Treatment for uncomplicated infections is ciprofloxacin for
1 week or single dose cefotaxime. Contact tracing is
recommended
- Complications in women include PID, leading to infertility
(15% after one episode), and an increase in ectopic
pregnancies

Non-gonococcal urethritis

- *Chlamydia trachomatis* is the commonest cause of non-
gonococcal urethritis. It has an incubation period of
1–5 weeks. Others include *Ureaplasma urealyticum* and
Mycoplasma hominis
- Clinical presentation is with dysuria, urethral discharge +/−
epididymitis, but is often asymptomatic in women or
presents with chronic pelvic pain
- Nucleic acid amplification tests are more sensitive than culture for diagnosing *C. trachomatis*
- Treatment is with doxycycline for 1 week or single dose of
azithromycin

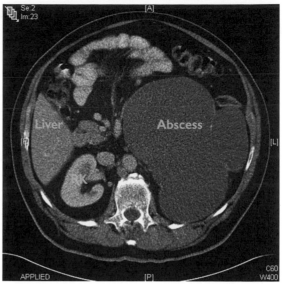

Fig 6.6 Abdominal CT scan showing a left perinephric abscess.
(RK = right kidney.)

⊕ Percutaneous nephrostomy

Percutaneous nephrostomy is used for the emergency drainage of an obstructed or infected upper tract and those not fit
for surgery.

Procedure

- Ensure clotting normal
- Under ultrasound or fluoroscopic control
- Local anaesthetic
- Needle puncture through calyx—not pelvis
- Guidewire to pelvis/ureter, then nephrostomy tube over
guidewire

Complications

Haemorrhage requiring embolization or nephrectomy occurs
in 1 per 200 cases. Acute infection is also a risk.

6.8 Urinary tract calculi—basics

Urinary tract calculi (nephrolithiasis) are common. The incidence peaks between 25 and 50 years of age, and they are more common in men (M:F 3:1).

Aetiology

Urinary stone formation is increasing as countries become more affluent and diets change accordingly (increased animal protein).

The UK lifetime prevalence for stones is about 7%, rising to 20% in some Middle Eastern countries.

Risk factors

- Hot climate
- Low fluid intake (concentrated urine)
- Diet with excess purines (meat) and oxalates
- Genetic disorders are implicated for certain rarer stones

Pathophysiology

- Epithelial cells or cell debris provide a nucleus around which crystals form if the urine is supersaturated or contains high concentrations of salts
- Foreign bodies in the urinary tract may act as the initial nucleus, e.g. non-absorbable sutures/clips, worm infestation debris
- Aggregation of crystals forms a stone 'particle' which tends to become lodged in the urinary tract—this process is exacerbated by low urine flow
- Particles grow with further aggregation and crystallization of salts—this is modulated by the presence of salts which act to reduce crystal formation (e.g. citrate and magnesium)

Upper urinary tract stones

- Commonest site for stone formation
- Origin is usually within the collecting system
- Natural sites of obstruction occur at narrowings in the pelvi-ureteric junction and ureter

Primary bladder stones

Primary bladder stones are more common in developing countries owing to infestation, chronic untreated infection or recurrent UTIs.

Calcium oxalate stones

- 75% of stones in UK patients
- Typically small, extremely hard, irregular ('spiky'), and radiodense
- 10% of patients have elevated serum calcium levels (primary hyperparathyroidism should be excluded—increased PTH, decreased phosphate)
- ~30% of patients have normal serum calcium levels but raised urinary calcium; this is caused by high intake (e.g. very high dairy product intake, calcium-containing medications) and excessive renal calcium excretion
- The remainder have a combination of small changes in urinary composition, including: ↑urinary oxalate, ↑urinary uric acid/urate, ↓urinary citrate/magnesium
- Prophylactic treatment is by increasing fluid intake and a low oxalate diet (spinach, strawberries, and bananas are high in oxalate). Consider a thiazide diuretic, magnesium or citrate supplements

Calcium phosphate stones

- 20% of stones in UK patients
- Typically soft, chalky, large, radiodense
- Associated with renal tubular acidosis (RTA), causing excessive calcium and phosphate excretion
- Prophylactic treatment is by alkalinizing urine (to counter systemic acidosis) with potassium bicarbonate orally and general measures

Infection stones

- 10% of stones in UK patients
- Also known as staghorn, struvite or triple (calcium, magnesium, ammonium) phosphate stones
- Occur secondary to UTI with urea-splitting organisms, especially *Proteus* spp.
- Infection stones are the most common stone seen in women
- Most are partly radiolucent
- Prophylactic treatment is by antibiotics
- High morbidity of staghorn calculi if left untreated and can lead to loss of kidney function

Uric acid and urate stones

- 5% of stones in UK patients
- Typically small, pale, yellow
- Associated with ↑excretion of uric acid in urine (gout, glycogen storage disease) and very acid urine (pH less than 5.5)
- Prophylactic treatment is with high fluid intake and alkalinization of the urine and allopurinol for gout-related stones

Cystine stones

- Extremely rare—autosomal recessive renal amino acid transport defect
- Typically very small, extremely dense, and hard
- Affects younger patients and stones very hard so lithotripsy has only variable success
- Prophylactic treatment is with very high fluid intake, alkalinization of the urine, D-penicillamine for congenital causes

Clinical assessment

Symptoms and signs depend on the site of the stone. Renal colic is a misnomer as it is usually ureteric colic.

Kidney

Intraparenchymal renal stones are usually asymptomatic but may cause a dull ache.

Ureter

- Severe colicky loin to groin pain (sometimes to testis/labia). Patients often move around as they are unable to get comfortable
- Assess for features of super-added infection, including fever, rigors, and tachycardia
- A typical feature is the patient indicating the site of pain by putting the fingers of one hand posteriorly on the lower ribs with the thumb anteriorly pointing to the umbilicus
- Bladder stones cause suprapubic and perineal discomfort, and bladder irritability
- Abdominal examination is usually normal with minimal guarding

Differential diagnoses

- Acute appendicitis
- Acute cholecystitis
- Acute pancreatitis
- Acute pyelonephritis
- Leaking abdominal aortic aneurysm
- Acute diverticulitis

Investigations

Acute presentation

- Urinalysis (microscopic haematuria seen in 85%)
- Bloods—FBC, U+Es, LFTs, amylase, CRP (inflammation, infection, pancreatitis, renal dysfunction)
- Plain abdominal radiograph ('KUB'—kidneys, ureters, bladder)
- CT urography has now superseded IVU as the investigation of choice. It can identify radiolucent stones, other intra-abdominal pathology, and avoids the need for contrast
- Renal ultrasound is not so good at identifying small stones (<5 mm), but can quickly identify hydronephrosis

Further investigations

All patients should be evaluated shortly after acute presentation.

- Bloods—U+Es, calcium, phosphate, uric acid
- Stone analysis
- Two 24 h urine collections for volume, pH, calcium, oxalate, uric acid, and citrate are usually reserved for recurrent stone formation

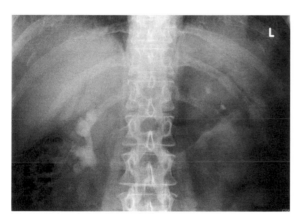

Fig 6.7 Right-sided staghorn calculus on a plain radiograph (not a KUB).

⊕ Intravenous urography (IVU)

Indications

- Haematuria
- Renal colic/suspected stones
- Structural abnormalities/trauma

Pre-procedure

- Ask about general atopy (asthma) and specific allergy to contrast and iodine
- Consider steroids as pre-med (needs to be longer than 12 h) or non-contrast CTU
- Avoid using contrast in patients with significant renal failure as this can be exacerbated

Procedure

- Plain abdominal radiograph ('control film') used to look for calcification (Fig 6.8)
- Inject non-ionic contrast rapidly
- 2–3 min film shows nephrogram phase
- 15 min film shows pyelogram phase
- Compression, tomograms, and delayed films all add further information if required
- Ureteric calculi causing obstruction are diagnosed on the 3Ds: dense, delayed nephrogram and dilated ureter

Complications

There is a 1% risk of a minor contrast reaction (urticaria, minor respiratory symptoms). Major or anaphylactic reactions are rare. Death from contrast reaction is 1 in 100 000 procedures.

Initial management of suspected anaphylaxis:

- ABC
- call for help
- give high flow oxygen
- **intramuscular** epinephrine 0.5 mL 1/1000 solution (1 mg/mL) is the most important drug to administer
- Give rapid bolus of crystalloid fluid IV
- IM/slow IV chlorpheniramine 10 mg
- IM/slow IV hydrocortisone 200 mg

6.9 Urinary tract calculi—management

Acute renal colic

Acute renal colic is very painful and causes significant distress. Most stones will pass spontaneously (90% are <4 mm, 50% are 4–6 mm, and 30% are >6 mm) and symptoms will subside within 24 h.

Initial

- Intravenous access for administration of analgesia, antiemetics, and fluids
- Analgesia: NSAIDs (e.g. pr diclofenac is as effective as opiate analgesia)
- Intravenous fluids if dehydrated
- Antiemetics as required or with opiate analgesia
- Once obstruction and infection have been excluded the patient can go home if comfortable
- Hospital admission is indicated for pain control, ureteral obstruction in a solitary or transplanted kidney, and obstruction associated with infection (pyonephrosis; 📖 Topic 6.7)

Long-term care

Renal calculi

- Small stones (<1.5 cm maximum diameter) are managed with extracorporeal shock wave lithotripsy (ESWL; see box). Flexible ureteroscopy is used if this fails or there are retained fragments
- Larger stones (>3 cm) are managed by percutaneous nephrolithotomy (PCNL; see box)
- Open surgery is less frequently used owing to the success of ESWL and PCNL. It is still indicated for:
  - large staghorns
  - anatomical abnormalities
  - multiple failed ESWL/PCNL
- Surgical techniques include radial nephrotomy, anatrophic nephrolithotomy, partial nephrectomy, and nephrectomy for poor function (open or laparoscopic)

Ureteric stones

- Indications for operative intervention:
  - continued symptoms after conservative management
  - large stones
  - a solitary kidney
- Large upper ureteric calculi or those associated with acute renal failure need ureteric stenting with delayed ureteroscopic extraction
- Small, lower ureteric calculi are managed with ureteroscopic extraction (directly with graspers if small, with fragmentation by ultrasound, lithoclast or laser if large)
- Associated upper tract UTI requires urgent nephrostomy

Ureteric injury occurs in around 5%. It is usually minor and settles with stenting. Strictures occur in 1–2% (related to stone +/– ureteroscopy).

Other options

ESWL has a 50–90% success rate depending on the position in the ureter.

Open or laparoscopic ureterolithotomy may be used for large ureteric calculi.

Bladder calculi

- Small stones can undergo fragmentation with cystoscopic ultrasound or lithoclast
- Large stones need open vesicolithotomy
- Bladder calculi usually occur in the setting of bladder outflow obstruction, which should be dealt with at the same time (TURP, open prostatectomy)

Complications and prognosis

The recurrence rate for upper tract calculi is greatest in the first few years after presentation (3 years—25%), and the majority of patients will develop more than one stone in their lifetime.

⊕ Retrograde ureteroscopy and ureteric stent insertion

Retrograde ureteroscopy and stent insertion under GA is indicated in ureteric calculi where conservative management has failed or is inappropriate.

Procedure

1. Single shot gentamicin or oral ciprofloxacin
2. Ureteric catheter introduced into bladder
3. Flush ureteric catheter to remove air bubbles
4. Insert catheter into ureteric orifice
5. Inject contrast media while screening to detect level of calculus
6. Insert safety guidewire through ureteric catheter to renal calyces
7. Insert ureteroscope adjacent to guidewire
8. Use irrigation under pressure to negotiate intramural ureter
9. A second guidewire through the ureteroscope can help
10. Look on the way up and back. The ureter is easily traumatized so be gentle. Fragment or extract stone if possible
11. Railroad stent over guidewire
12. Once the stent is in the renal pelvis, withdraw the guide wire 15 cm to allow for stent to curl.
13. When last 4 cm visible in bladder withdraw guidewire completely

Complications

Intraoperative and early	*Intermediate and late*
• Ureteric injury	• Ureteric injury
• Haemorrhage	
• Acute UTI	

⊕ Extracorporeal shock wave lithotripsy

ESWL is focused ultrafrequency sonic shockwaves directed at the stone under fluoroscopy or ultrasound guidance.

- Induced vibrational energy causes the incompressible structure of the stone to shatter
- Performed on outpatient basis
- Increased success with smaller stones (<1 cm 90%), locations in upper pole versus lower pole, hardest stones (calcium oxalate versus cystine)
- Repeated treatments may be required

Contraindications

- Pregnant women
- Uncorrected bleeding disorders
- Unresolved obstruction below stone

Complications

- Transient haematuria
- Pain
- Septic complications
- Steinstrasse (stone fragments blocking lower ureter)

⊕ Percutaneous nephrolithotomy

- PCNL is used for larger renal calculi, especially staghorns/failure of ESWL
- Stone-free rate 80%
- ESWL used for residual fragments
- Performed under GA by serially dilating a percutaneous tract to the kidney
- Calculi fragmented (ultrasound, lithoclast) and extracted through tract

Complications

- Injury to colon, pneumothorax, bleeding, sepsis

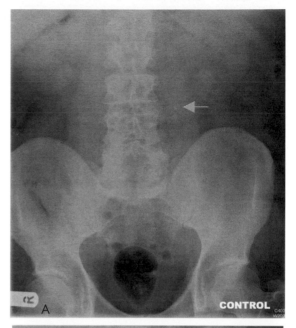

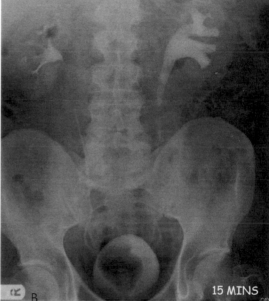

Fig 6.8 Intravenous urography. (A) Control KUB showing a left-sided calcified mass opposite L4 (arrow). (B) 15 min film showing a dilated left ureter and renal pelvis owing to obstruction by the calculus.

Hydrocele

A hydrocele is a collection of fluid between the testis and tunica vaginalis. They can be divided into three types: congenital (communicating), acquired (non-communicating), and hydroceles of the cord. Congenital hydroceles and the relevant embryology are discussed in Topic 13.11.

Adult hydroceles are almost all non-communicating, and 10% are bilateral. Many are idiopathic: causes include trauma, infection, and cancer.

Clinical assessment

- Gradual onset hemi-scrotal swelling
- Occasional discomfort/heaviness
- Hydroceles lie anterior to the testis
- Fluctuant, transilluminates, often difficult to feel underlying testis
- Abdominal examination is usually normal
- An acute scrotum must be excluded. Have a high index of suspicion for testicular torsion in younger patients

Investigations

- Urinalysis (exclude UTI)
- Inguinoscrotal ultrasound may be indicated if underlying testis pathology is suspected

Treatment

Conservative

- Small hydroceles with minimal symptoms and no underlying testicular pathology do not need treatment
- Needle aspiration only if patient unfit for surgery but symptomatic as this risks infection

Operative

- Aspirated hydroceles often reaccumulate and so surgical excision (Jaboulay) or plication (Lord's) is indicated. Scrotal haematoma requiring drainage occurs in 1%

Fournier's gangrene

Fournier's gangrene is necrotizing fasciitis of the scrotum and perineum. It may be associated with local trauma or urethral instrumentation and is usually an aerobic and anaerobic synergistic infection. It is more common in those with diabetes, and may follow urethral or perineal trauma.

Clinical assessment

- Rapid clinical course with severe pain out of proportion to the apparent examination findings is highly indicative of subcutaneous infection
- On examination the patient may be very unwell with signs of systemic sepsis
- There may be scrotal skin necrosis, discoloration, and crepitus
- The diagnosis may only be made at surgery and so whenever the diagnosis is suspected exploratory surgery should be considered

Management

- ABC
- Resuscitation with intravenous fluids
- Analgesia

- Broad spectrum antibiotics (typically include benzylpenicillin, metronidazole, flucloxacillin, and gentamicin)
- Aggressive surgical debridement of skin and subcutaneous tissue is always required
- Second look surgery is often needed followed by delayed plastic surgical reconstruction
- Mortality rate is up to 50%

Epididymal cyst and spermatocele

These cysts usually arise in the head of the epididymis superior to the testis. They are common and are usually asymptomatic. However, there may be associated anxiety about testicular cancer when first discovered.

Clinical assessment

- Noticed incidentally or on ultrasound for another reason
- Occasional discomfort
- A smooth, well defined swelling arising distinct from body of testis which is fluctuant and transilluminates is usually a cyst
- Can be multiple and bilateral
- Epididymal cysts and spermatoceles cannot be clinically differentiated

Investigations

- Ultrasound may be indicated but is often unnecessary to make a diagnosis
- Needle aspiration should be avoided

Management

- Conservative unless symptoms direct or there is concern over diagnosis
- Surgery for large (>3 cm) or symptomatic conditions. Avoid surgery in young men as postoperative scarring may interfere with sperm transport. There is also a risk of scrotal haematoma and infection
- Aspiration and sclerotherapy may be considered in older men

Varicocele

A varicocele is 'varicose veins' of the scrotum caused by dilatation of the paminiform venous plexus and internal spermatic vein. It initially presents in the 15–30-year age group. Left varicoceles are much more common than right ones as the left testicular vein enters the left renal vein (high pressure) rather than IVC and there are no antireflux valves.

Clinical assessment

- Ill-defined peritesticular swelling with dull testis ache.
- Examination performed with the patient standing up
- 'Bag of worms' above and behind testis (Fig 6.9)
- Enhanced by Valsalva manoeuvre

Investigations

- Scrotal and renal ultrasound. A left renal cancer may block drainage of left testicular vein

Management

- Conservative management is used if symptoms are mild
- Radiological embolization is probably the treatment of choice
- Surgery to ligate the dilated veins can be perfomed open or laparoscopically

⊕ Hydrocele excision (Lord's procedure)

Procedure

- Midline incision just big enough to 'deliver' testis
- Stab incision through tunica vaginalis into hydrocele sack
- Babcock or Allis forceps on edges
- Deliver testis
- Plicate tunica vaginalis with 6–10 absorbable sutures
- Meticulous haemostasis
- Scrotal support for 36 h
- Insert drain if very large hydrocele for 24 h
- For very large hydroceles, the hydrocele sac can be excised (Jaboulay), but this has a higher rate of postoperative haematoma

Complications

- Scrotal haematoma
- Infection
- Recurrence

⊕ Male sterilization

The procedure is intended to be permanent and the majority are carried out under local anaesthetic.

The usual indication is for the prevention of pregnancy in a stable relationship with children in which no further children are desired.

Informed consent is very important; the risks and complications of the procedure should be outlined, and the postoperative procedure before unprotected intercourse can be started.

Procedure

- Midline or bilateral incisions
- Identify and strip vas deferens of coverings
- Ligate and divide. Cauterize ends or ligate folded back on itself (+/– excise segment)
- Fertility requires two clear semen samples prior to unprotected intercourse

Complications

- Scrotal haematoma <5%
- Infection <5%
- Early failure 3 per 1000 (active sperm fail to disappear)
- Late failure (recanalization with risk of pregnancy) 1 in 3000
- Chronic scrotal pain 5–10%

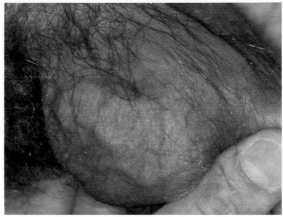

Fig 6.9 Varicocele is visible beneath the scrotal skin more evident on palpation.

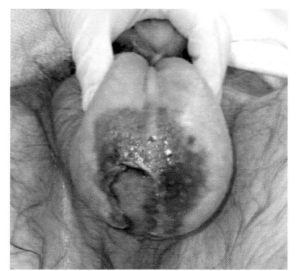

Fig 6.10 Fournier's gangrene before emergency surgical debridement. Reproduced with kind permission of the Nature Publishing Group.

6.11 Penile conditions

Priapism

Prolonged (>4 h) painful erection of the penis. Most cases are idiopathic (80%).

Other causes include intracorporal injection during the treatment of erectile dysfunction, sickle cell disease, leukaemia, and malignant infiltration.

Prolonged erection leads to venous and arterial thrombosis. Following this there is fibrosis of the penile corporal and subsequent erectile dysfunction. Rarely, penile trauma leads to an AV fistula and high flow painless priapism.

Management

- Priapism is a urological emergency
- Blood should be aspirated from the corpora cavernosa
- If this is not sufficient, inject intracavernosal phenylephrine. Failing that, a shunt can be created (commonly between corpora cavernosa and the glans penis)
- Blood should be taken to exclude sickle cell disease and leukaemia

Peyronie's disease

This condition presents with fibrosis within the tunica albuginea, causing penile curvature. The clinical course runs for 18 months.

History and examination

- Occasionally painful erections
- Progressive deformity of erections

Treatment

- For pain—vitamin E and colchicine occasionally help
- Surgery should not be performed before 18 months after onset. It is indicated for difficulty with intercourse
- Nesbit's procedure will straighten erections (but result in penile shortening by ~2 cm)

Condyloma accuminata

Condyloma (penile warts) are caused by cutaneous infection with human papilloma virus (commonly types 6 and 11; types 16 and 18 are associated with intraepithelial neoplasia development). They occur on the foreskin, urethral meatus, corona, and perianal areas.

Managment

- Weekly podophyllin for 6 weeks
- Cryotherapy, laser, surgical excision/diathermy ablation if larger areas

Erectile dysfunction

This condition increases with age.

Aetiology

- Psychogenic (often multifactorial)
- Underlying vascular disease (decreased arterial inflow)
  - Atherosclerosis of distal aortoiliac segments (Leriche's syndrome)
  - Smoking-related arteriolosclerosis
  - Pelvic radiotherapy with fibrosis
- Underlying neurological disease (loss of autonomic parasympathetic inflow)
  - MS
  - Diabetes mellitus
  - Pelvic surgery/radiotherapy
- Underlying hormonal/chemical imbalances
  - Anticholinergic drugs
  - Antihypertensives
  - Hyperprolactinaemia
  - Hypotestosteroneaemia

Clinical assessment

Psychogenic erectile dysfunction is suggested by sudden onset, maintenance of early morning/nocturnal erections, and loss of libido.

Organic erectile dysfunction is suggested by gradual onset, progressive loss of erection, synchronous loss of nocturnal erections, and associated features of vascular or neurological disease.

Investigations

- Serum glucose and urinalysis (diabetes mellitus)
- If libido is low, test FSH/LH, testosterone, prolactin
- Measurement of nocturnal penile tumescence

Management

- Reduce weight
- Stop smoking
- Stop anticholinergic/antihypertensive drugs if possible

Medical

Oral medication is first line (PDE5 inhibitors).

Surgical

- Intra-urethral pellets
- Intracavernosal injections
- Vacuum devices
- Penile prosthesis

Penile cancer

Almost all penile cancers are squamous cell carcinomas. It is rare in the UK but more common in Africa and the Indian subcontinent. The incidence increases with age.

It is rare in men who undergo early circumcision and is associated with poor hygiene and phimosis.

Pathophysiology

- Associated with pre-existing high-grade anal intraepithelial neoplasia (AIN III) caused by HPV infection (types 16 and 18)
- Majority of lesions affect glans +/- foreskin
- Erythroplasia of Queyrat is penile carcinoma *in situ*. It is a red velvety painless lesion. Treatment is biopsy and topical 5FU

Clinical assessment

- There are often long delays in presentation of penile cancer, so lesions can be advanced
- Penile lesions are usually on the foreskin or glans and are ulcerative or nodular

- Fifty per cent of patients have groin lymph nodes at presentation, occasionally with ulceration. Half are infected and half show regional spread

Investigation

- Unless circumcision would remove the entire lesion, perform incision biopsy
- FNA of palpable lymph nodes

Management

Management is considered separately for the penis, regional lymph nodes, and any distant metastases.

Penis

- Surgical approaches include circumcision, glansectomy, and split skin graft, partial penectomy or radical penectomy
- Radiotherapy is an option, but local recurrence is 30% and penectomy for radiotherapy has a complication rate of 10%

Lymph nodes

- If lymph node FNA is negative, treat the penis and give antibiotics for 6 weeks
- If lymph node FNA is positive or if they are still present after the antibiotics, bilateral lymphadenectomy is indicated. Risks include wound breakdown and lymphoedema
- Prophylactic lymphadenectomy is an option for clinically node-negative patients who have higher stage and grade tumours
- Chemotherapy is of limited benefit

Prognosis

- Node-negative 5-year survival is 65–90%.
- Inguinal lymph node-positive 5-year survival 30%.

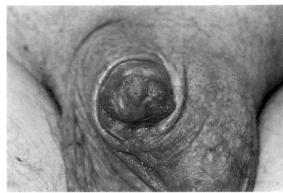

Fig 6.11 Squamous cell carcinoma of the penis.

Renal cell carcinoma

Increasing numbers of renal tumours are being diagnosed as patients have abdominal imaging for other reasons. Incidence is 10 per 100 000 population and peaks >60 years of age. It is more common in men (M:F 2:1).

Aetiology

- The majority of renal cell carcinomas (RCC) are sporadic
- Associated with von Hippel–Lindau (VHL) syndrome (retinal and cerebellar haemangiomas and phaeochromocytomas); have high incidence of RCC (70% by 60 years). Often multifocal and bilateral. Screen VHL patients with USS from 15 years old
- Familial RCC without VHL occurs but is uncommon

Risk factors

Smoking is a weak risk factor except for transitional cell carcinoma (TCC).

Haemodialysis patients develop acquired cystic disease of the kidney. Of these, 15% develop renal tumours.

Pathophysiology

Around 90% of renal malignancies are RCC. The remainder are TCC of the renal pelvis, rarely lymphomas and occasionally secondary tumours, usually in the setting of other widespread metastatic disease. RCC spreads by local invasion through the kidney and renal vein, and is metastatic to bone, liver, and lung.

Clinical assessment

History

- The majority of tumours are now diagnosed incidentally on imaging for another condition or after presentation to a haematuria clinic
- Local symptoms—haematuria, abdominal pain
- Metastatic symptoms—bone pain, shortness of breath, jaundice
- Paraneoplastic symptoms—weight loss, pyrexia of unknown origin, hypocalcaemia, polycythaemia, and raised ESR

Examination

Examination is often normal. Occasionally there is abdominal mass, hepatomegaly, effusion, and cachexia.

Investigations

- Renal ultrasound is better than IVU and can distinguish between cystic or solid masses. A solid mass seen on ultrasound should have a pre- and post-contrast CT scan of chest and abdomen. Look for contrast enhancement, renal vein/IVC involvement
- It is often difficult to determine malignant potential in complex renal cysts
- Biopsy is rarely done because of the high rate of false-negatives (heterogeneous nature of tumour)
- Angiography occasionally before partial nephrectomy
- Bloods—U&Es, creatinine clearance, split renal function if contralateral kidney abnormal on imaging

Staging

TNM classification of renal cancer

Primary tumour
CIS Carcinoma *in situ*
Ta   Superficial tumour
T1   Tumour <7 cm confined to kidney
T2   Tumour >7 cm confined to kidney
T3   Perinephric fat, renal vein or IVC invasion
T4   Tumour outside pararenal fascia

Regional lymph nodes
N0   No regional lymph node metastases
N1   Metastasis in single node
N2   Metastases in two or more nodes

Distant metastasis
M0   No distant metastases
M1   Distant metastases

Management

Operative resection of the tumour is preferable. Conservative treatment is an option for elderly/unfit patients. Some renal tumours grow very slowly and cause minimal symptoms.

Embolization—a palliative procedure for unfit patients with haematuria, pain, and paraneoplastic symptoms.

Surgery

Radical nephrectomy

Radical nephrectomy includes perinephric fat (+/- adrenal gland) and can be open or laparoscopic.

The main risks are bleeding (sometimes massive) and injury to adjacent organs, especially the spleen.

Mortality rate is 1%. Around 5–10% have renal vein/IVC invasion which is amenable to surgery.

Partial nephrectomy

Partial nephrectomy is considered for smaller tumours <4 cm, patients with chronic renal failure, solitary kidneys, bilateral tumours, and VHL.

There are higher perioperative complications than for non-conservative surgery.

Surgery for metastases

Very occasionally patients will have a truly solitary metastasis which can be resected. This leads to some long-term survival.

Palliative nephrectomy

Palliative nephrectomy is performed in the presence of metastatic disease for pain, excessive haematuria or paraneoplastic symptoms.

Medical

- Radiotherapy is of limited use except in painful metastases
- Chemotherapy is not very effective
- Immunotherapy, a combination of interferon, IL-2, and 5FU, may have marginal survival advantages in metastatic disease. Tyrosine kinase inhibitors are effective for metastatic disease

Complications and prognosis

Prognosis of RCC is determined by the stage of the tumour.

Stage	5-year survival
I	80–100%
II	60–80%
III	40–60%
IV	<20%

Other renal tumours

Transitional cell carcinoma (of renal pelvis)

Between 3 and 5% of patients with bladder TCC will develop upper tract TCC. They present with macroscopic haematuria, renal pelvis filling defect on IVU, and positive urine cytology. Treatment is nephroureterectomy.

Lymphoma

Lymphoma is rare as a primary lesion but not uncommon with multifocal lymphoma.

Oncocytoma

Oncocytoma presents as homogeneous masses on CT. This is usually diagnosed only after nephrectomy for renal mass.

Angiomyolipomas

An angiomyolipoma is a renal mass containing fat. There is a strong association with tuberous sclerosis. They have a tendency to bleed in pregnancy or if large.

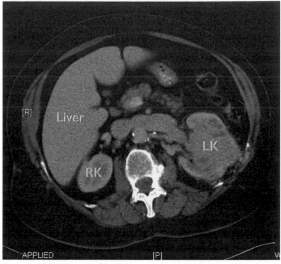

Fig 6.13 CT abdomen showing a mass in the left kidney (LK) which was histologically an adenocarcinoma. RK, right kidney.

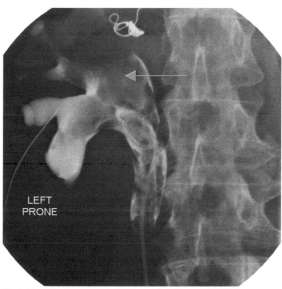

Fig 6.12 Filling defect in the kidney pelvis due to a TCC.

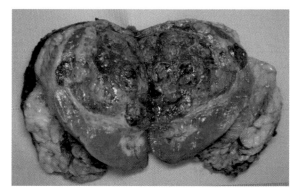

Fig 6.14 Resected kidney divided in half showing a large renal cell carcinoma.

Bladder cancer is the second most common urological malignancy, with an incidence of 30 per 100 000 population. Peak incidence is 60–70 years of age and it is more common in men (M:F 3:1).

Aetiology

- Chromosome 9 abnormalities are common in superficial bladder cancer
- Chromosome 17 abnormalities are common in muscle invasive bladder cancer
- Alterations in the tumour suppressor gene *p53*

Risk factors

- Smoking is the number one risk factor in the western world, increasing risk threefold
- Smokers have higher recurrence rates and higher stage and grade tumours
- Industrial exposure, e.g. aniline dye, rubber manufacture, and printing. Better health and safety is now reducing this
- Cyclophosphamide and previous pelvic radiotherapy
- Chronic infection/inflammation increases the risk of SCC of bladder. Schistosomiasis (bilharzia) in Egypt and long-term catheters in spinal injury patients in the UK also increase risk

Pathophysiology

- Ninety per cent of bladder cancers are transitional cell carcinomas (TCC). Between 5 and 10% are squamous cell carcinomas (SCC) (70% in areas with endemic urinary schistosomiasis). Adenocarcinoma causes 1%
- Three-quarters of new bladder tumours present as 'superficial' bladder tumours (see staging Ta, T1). One-quarter present with invasion into bladder muscle (see staging T2)
- A third entity is carcinoma *in situ* (CIS). This is flat, poorly differentiated intraepithelial change now thought to be the forerunner of muscle-invasive bladder cancer
- Bladder tumours are classified by grade (grades 1–3, increasing degrees of cellular abnormality) and stage (depth of invasion into/through bladder). A proportion of patients with previous superficial bladder tumours progress to muscle-invasive bladder cancer

Clinical assessment

History

- Painless macroscopic haematuria—around 20% will have urinary tract malignancy
- Microscopic haematuria—around 5% will have urinary tract malignancy
- Irritative symptoms, especially without UTI
- UTI—a first UTI should always be investigated in men
- Symptoms of advanced disease—pelvic or loin pain, bone pain, and shortness of breath

Examination

Suprapubic mass is only rarely present (if so, may represent urinary retention owing to bladder neck obstruction by tumour).

Investigations

- MSU—bladder cancer and UTI can present together
- Cytology—poor sensitivity for grade 1 (well differentiated tumours), but 90% sensitive for higher risk grade 3 tumours and CIS

- USS—good for renal tumours and bladder tumours
- IVU (macroscopic haematuria only). Good for renal pelvis and bladder tumours
- Flexible cystoscopy—outpatient procedure using intra-urethral local anaesthetic

Staging

TNM classification of bladder cancer

Primary tumour

CIS	Carcinoma in situ
Ta	Superficial tumour
T1	Superficial tumour but invading subepithelial connective tissue
T2	Invades into bladder wall muscle
T3	Through muscle to perivesical fat (T3a microscopically, T3b macroscopically)
T4	Invades adjacent structures, e.g. prostate, uterus, vagina or abdominal wall

Regional lymph nodes

N0	No regional lymph node metastases
N1	Metastasis in single node <2 cm
N2	Metastases in single lymph node 2–5 cm or multiple lymph node <5 cm
N3	Metastases in single or multiple lymph node >5 cm

Distant metastasis

M0	No distant metastases
M1	Distant metastases

Grading

G1	Well differentiated
G2	Moderately differentiated
G3	Poorly differentiated

Management

Patients with investigations suspicious for bladder tumour should undergo a TURBT (transurethral resection of bladder tumour) under general/spinal anaesthesia. All other abnormal areas should be biopsied. This will make the diagnosis, and give a stage and grade which are the strongest predictors for recurrence and progression.

Subsequent management of TCC

- After first resection of superficial-looking tumour, patients should receive intravesical mitomycin C (see below)
- The risk of recurrence is 30% for low stage and grade tumours (TaG1/G2), rising to 80% for T1G3 tumours
- The risk of progression to muscle-invasive disease is extremely low for TaG1 tumours, rising to 40% for T1G3 tumours
- Follow-up protocols therefore vary with histology, but typically the first check cystoscopy is at 3 months and then 6 monthly before becoming annually
- T1G3 tumours should undergo early (2–4 weeks) re-resection of tumour site to ensure no muscle-invasive elements have been missed
- CIS and T1G3 are regarded as high-risk superficial tumours and should be treated with intravesical (BCG) Bacille Calmette-Guerin (radical cystectomy is an option for widespread disease)

Intravesical therapy

- Mitomycin C—single instillation after first TURBT (of superficial tumour) reduces recurrence rate by 40%. For recurrent multifocal superficial TCC, weekly instillation for 6 weeks. Side effects include irritable bladder in 20%, and, rarely, rash
- BCG for T1G3 and CIS (weekly instillation for 6 weeks) Maintenance treatment every 6 months (weekly instillations x3 weeks) for 3 years for responders. This may delay progression to muscle-invasive cancer. Side effects include irritable bladder in 80%, flu-like symptoms in 25%. BCGosis occurs in <1%; treat with anti-TB drugs for 6 months

Muscle-invasive bladder cancer

Operative

- Ileal conduit or orthotopic neobladder as urinary diversion is the treatment of choice in fit patients, but has a significant perioperative morbidity of 20% and a mortality rate of 3%
- Neoadjuvant chemotherapy has a slight survival advantage. Adjuvant chemotherapy is used for ≥T3 tumour if the patient is fit
- 5-year survival is proportional to local stage and lymph node status: T2 70%, T3 50%, lymph node-positive 30%

Radical radiotherapy

For unfit patients or those who decline cystectomy.

- Survival less than surgery
- Bladder preserved but function may be impaired
- Recurrent tumour or radiation cystitis necessitates cystectomy in 30%
- Palliative radiotherapy is an option for haematuria and bone metastases

Metastatic bladder cancer

MVAC (methotrexate, vinblastine, adriamycin, cisplatin) or gemcitobine/cisplatin achieves response rates in 20%.

⊃ Extra

There is much debate as to whether neoadjuvant or adjuvant chemotherapy should be given with a cystectomy. The advantage of neoadjuvant treatment is the earlier treatment of micrometastatic disease, but the disadvantage is that for patients with non-chemotherapy-responsive tumours, definitive cystectomy is delayed. For adjuvant chemotherapy, the advantage is that treatment can be reserved for higher stage disease once formal pathology is known, but a disadvantage is that any micrometastatic disease at presentation has longer before chemotherapy is started.

⊕ Urinary diversion (urostomy formation)

The commonest diversion is an ileal conduit where a short segment of ileum is isolated. The ureters are joined to the proximal end and the distal end is brought out to the skin as a nipple. It is relatively simple operation but the disadvantages are the permanent stoma, body image, pyelonephritis, and stoma problems (stenosis, retraction, hernia).

Continent diversions are possible by creating a catheterizable pouch or more commonly an orthotopic neobladder. Here 50–60 cm of ileum is detubularized, folded, and reanastomosed to form a neobladder joined to the patient's urethra. An advantage is a 'normal' body image. A disadvantage is increased perioperative complications. Nocturnal incontinence is 20%, with a small risk of bladder rupture.

Intestinal mucosa in contact with urine can develop adenocarcinoma after many years. Surveillance is recommended after 10 years.

⊕ Flexible cystoscopy

Indications

- Investigation for haematuria/UTI
- Surveillance of patients with previous bladder cancer

Procedure

- Aseptic technique with lubricant jelly
- Visualize entire bladder, entering diverticulae
- 'J' manoeuvre to visualize bladder neck

⊕ Transurethral resection of bladder tumour (TURBT)

- Preliminary cystoscopy
- Insert resectoscope
- Resect entire segments vertically from top to bottom of tumour before moving on to the adjacent bit of the tumour
- Resecting horizontally (i.e. all the top of the tumour before moving on to deeper tumour) causes more bleeding
- Consider sending separate biopsy from tumour base and random bladder biopsies
- Increased risk of perforation in female bladders (thinner wall) and near bladder diverticulae (minimal or absent muscle layer). Also take care with tumours at the dome as perforation is likely to be intraperitoneal and require a laparotomy
- TWOC at 24–48 h (5 days if extraperitoneal perforation suspected).

Complications

- Haemorrhage
- UTI
- Bladder perforation
- Urethral strictures

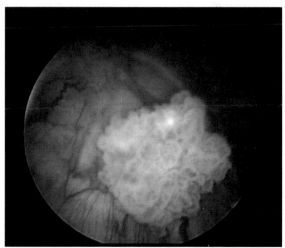

Fig 6.15 Cystoscopic view of a superficial exophytic TCC.

6.14 Prostate cancer

Prostate cancer (CAP) is the second commonest cause of male cancer deaths in the UK. Incidence is 100 per 100 000 population and increases with age. American black population has highest incidence.

Aetiology

Prostate cancer growth is dependent on testosterone and dihydrotestosterone. Eunuchs do not get prostate cancer.

Risk factors

- Age
- Family history
- Race (Black>Caucasian)

Pathophysiology

- Previously undiagnosed incidental histological evidence of prostate cancer is seen very commonly at autopsy (>60% of 80-year-olds)
- Lifetime risk of a clinically diagnosed CAP 10%
- Lifetime risk of death from CAP 3%
- The dilemma is identifying which of the tumours diagnosed incidentally need treatment.

Clinical assessment

History

- Patient requesting PSA test
- LUTS (usually unrelated to any underlying CAP)
- Haematuria
- Occasionally symptoms of metastatic disease

Examination

- Abdominal examination usually normal
- DRE reveals firm irregular prostate with loss of central sulcus and poorly defined lateral margins. The extent of the tumour on DRE is used to give it a clinical stage

Investigation

PSA (prostate-specific antigen) is produced exclusively by the prostate. In patients with prostate cancer, PSA is usually elevated. However, PSA can also be elevated in patients with benign prostate, after urinary tract infection, prostatitis, and after sexual intercourse. To improve the specificity, age-adjusted 'cut offs' are used. Other methods are rate of rise of PSA and free to total PSA subfractions. In patients with either abnormal DRE or elevated PSA, a transrectal ultrasound biopsy of the prostate (TRUS biopsy) should be performed.

Grading

CAP is graded according to architectural changes to give a Gleason grade (1–5). The two commonest Gleason grades are added together to give a Gleason sum out of 10 (e.g. 3+4=7). Gleason 2–4, well differentiated, Gleason 5–7, moderately differentiated, Gleason 8–10, poorly differentiated.

A combination of DRE staging, PSA, and Gleason sum can be used in various algorithms to give an indication of disease extent, e.g. Partin's tables.

Staging

- Clinically by DRE
- Bone scan to exclude bone metastases
- MRI for margins of prostate, lymph nodes
- Laparoscopic lymph node biopsy (when lymph node status unclear but important for management decision)

TNM classification of prostate cancer

Primary tumour

T1	Diagnosed following biopsy for raised PSA or incidentally in TURP chips
T2	Palpable disease or radiological disease confined within prostate
T3	Tumour extends through prostatic capsule (including seminal vesical)
T4	Tumour fixed to adjacent structures, e.g. pelvic side wall

Regional lymph nodes

N0	No lymph nodes
N1	Pelvic lymph nodes

Distant metastases

M0	No distant metastases
M1	Distant metastases (a non-regional lymph nodes, b bone, c other)

Management of non-metastatic disease

Treatment options depend on patient life expectancy, quality of life, and personal philosophy. Options include the following.

Watch and pounce

Continued PSA surveillance and only pounce (to other treatments) if rapid rate of rise:

- Advantages—avoids side effects
- Disadvantages—risks progression, psychological aspects of 'non-treatment'
- Ideal candidate—low PSA and Gleason sum, unfit patients

Radical prostatectomy

- Laparoscopic or open
- Advantages—cancer is 'cut out,' certainty of pathological stage. Secondary radiotherapy for positive margins or salvage radiotherapy for pelvic recurrence is straightforward
- Disadvantages—death rate 1 in 500, incontinence 1% severe, 3% mild/moderate, impotence variable but common
- Ideal candidate—fit, less than 70 years, T1 and T2 disease, erections not important

Radical radiotherapy

Traditional external beam (EBRT) or radioactive seed implants (brachytherapy). This is often used in combination with neoadjuvant +/− adjuvant hormone therapy.

ERBT

- Advantages—avoids surgery, includes 'margin' around prostate. Risk of impotence less than with surgery
- Disadvantages—daily for 6–7 weeks, irritative bowel symptoms 3%, salvage treatments for recurrence difficult
- Ideal candidate—some co-morbidity, greater than 70 years, T1–T3 disease

Brachytherapy

- Implantation under ultrasound guidance under GA
- Advantages—overnight stay, rapid return to normality
- Disadvantages—not suitable for patients with significant LUTS. Long-term data suggest equivalent results to other treatments for low PSA and Gleason sum. Limited data available for higher PSA, stage and grade tumours.
- Ideal candidate—younger sexually active patient, low PSA and Gleason sum. T1 and T2 disease

Newer treatments

Cryotherapy and HIFU (high intensity focused ultrasound) are not routinely used.

Follow-up

- Follow-up is by clinical evaluation and PSA. Initially frequently, progressing to annually
- After radical prostatectomy, PSA should fall to undetectable levels. After radiotherapy the PSA nadir is often higher
- Recurrence is suggested by a rising PSA
- Early recurrence (<6 months from treatment, fast PSA doubling time) suggests metastatic disease
- Late recurrence (>2 years from treatment, slower PSA doubling time) suggests pelvic recurrence
- Metastatic disease should be treated with hormones (see below)
- Pelvic recurrence may be amenable to salvage radiotherapy, cryotherapy, surgery depending on initial treatment and patient status

Management of metastatic disease

Metastatic disease is incurable but the median survival is 3 years with treatment.

Pelvic, spinal, and long bones are the commonest site for bony metastases. Pelvic lymph nodes are the other common metastatic site.

Most CAP is androgen-dependent, and treatment is by hormone deprivation. Options include:

- bilateral subcapsular orchidectomy
- LHRH agonists, e.g. Zoladex, Prostap
- Direct anti-androgens, e.g. Flutamide

Side effects include impotence, lethargy, and occasionally hot flushes and gynaecomastia

Hormone-escaped CAP

Ultimately a subset of CAP cells proliferates without the need for androgens, and standard androgen deprivation treatment fails. Alternative anti-androgens, oestrogens, and steroids may buy temporary remission, but life expectancy is less than 1 year. Chemotherapy is of modest value. Newer growth factor inhibitors show promise.

Bone pain (common)—treatment is local radiotherapy to painful areas or weightbearing bones (decrease fracture risk).

Strontium infusion is performed for widespread painful metasteses.

Spinal cord compression is a medical emergency requiring immediate steroids, radiotherapy or neurosurgery.

Complications and prognosis

Anaemia, ureteric obstruction, and pelvic venous obstruction all occur.

⊙ Interpreting PSA level

PSA rises with age and size of prostate, and so no such thing as a 'normal' PSA exists. However, certain age-adjusted cut offs exist. These are: in the 40s PSA <2.5; 50s PSA <3.5; 60s PSA <4.0; 70s PSA <6.5; 80s PSA<20. If the patient has a recent history of UTI or instrumentation, the PSA should be repeated after 4–6 weeks.

Some tumours are so poorly differentiated that they do not secrete PSA. It is possible, therefore, to have a below 'normal' PSA and still have cancer.

Equally, many patients with an above 'normal' PSA will not have cancer. Therefore the decision whether to advise a TRUS biopsy is a combination of the DRE findings and the PSA. This combination also gives the likelihood of diagnosing cancer.

	Likelihood of diagnosing CAP		
PSA	0–4	4–10	>10
DRE normal	10%	20%	30%
DRE abnormal	25%	50%	75%

⊙ Digital rectal examination (DRE)

Procedure

- Consent patient verbally
- Lay the patient in a left lateral position with knees in close to chest; elevate the couch to a comfortable height
- With a gloved finger first test anal and perianal sensation
- Use a small amount of lubricant jelly to help gently insert index finger through the anus into the rectum
- Insert the finger into the anus pulp first, not tip first, by a flexion motion and not by pushing
- Assess anal tone and feel for rectal masses
- Turn the finger anteriorly to assess prostate size, consistency, medium sulcus, and lateral margins
- Finally, withdraw finger and wipe away excess jelly

143

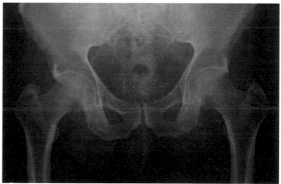

Fig 6.16 Plain pelvic radiograph showing the radio-opaque beads used in brachytherapy.

6.15 Testicular cancer

A man's lifetime risk of developing testicular cancer is approximately 1 in 500 in the UK. Peak incidence is between 20 and 45 years of age. It has a very high cure rate which is in excess of 90%.

Aetiology
Risk factors
- Undescended testes
- Family history (brother-increased x10, father-increased x5)
- Testicular atrophy

Pathophysiology
In patients with undescended testes (crypt orchidism), the risk of developing testicular tumour is 5%. If the testis is surgically positioned in the scrotum, the risk is not significantly decreased, but testicular self-examination (and therefore earlier diagnosis) is easier. Ninety five per cent of testicular tumours arise from the germ cells of the testes. Classification is complex, but relevant for adjuvant treatment. Broadly, testis tumours are either seminomas or non-seminomatous germ cell tumours (NSGCT), including teratomas, yolk sac tumours, and choriocarcinomas. Occasionally tumours arise from supporting sex cord stroma, e.g. leydig cell or sertoli cell tumours.

Clinical assessment
History
- Testis enlargement—global enlargement
- Testis irregularity—hard/irregular
- 'Heaviness'
- Rarely, shrinking testes, gynaecomastia, abdominal mass, haemoptysis

Examination
- Global enlargement or firm mass in body of testis
- Central abdominal mass suggests para-aortic lymphadenopathy

Investigations
- USS—highly sensitive in conjunction with examination
- CXR—preoperatively if any chest signs
- Tumour markers
  - Beta-human chorionic gonadotrophin (βHCG), half-life 1 day, is produced by some seminomas and some NSGCT
  - Alpha-fetoprotein (AFP), half-life 5 days, produced by some NSGCT. Between 50 and 70% of testis tumours have elevation of one marker or another, but normal tumour markers do not exclude testis tumour. LDH is less specific but is a marker of disease burden

Staging
Staging investigations are often performed after initial surgical resection.
- Serial tumour markers—initially weekly, should fall to normal according to half-lives. Failure to do so indicates metastatic disease
- CT scan chest, abdomen, and pelvis

Royal Marsden staging:

Stage 1	Tumour limited to testis
Stage 2	Retroperitoneal lymph nodes
Stage 3	Tumour in lymph nodes above the diaphragm
Stage 4	Extralymphatic

Management
Operative
Unless there is a high level of uncertainty, in which case serial USS and tumour markers should be performed, treatment is by inguinal exploration and radical orchidectomy.

Medical (oncological)
Stage 1 seminoma
- Prophylactic para-aortic radiotherapy, or
- Surveillance (better histological features, compliant patient), or
- Prophylactic single course carboplatin chemotherapy

Stage 1 NSCGT
- Surveillance (better histological features), or
- Two courses of BEP (bleomycin etoposide cisplatin) for poor histological features

Metastatic tumours (stages 2–4)
- Patients can be divided into good, intermediate or poor prognosis groups depending on sites of metastatic disease and levels of tumour markers
- Radiotherapy is an option for low stage 2 seminomas
- All others will require chemotherapy, usually initially BEP
- Residual or recurrent disease may be amenable to other chemotherapy or surgical resection

Follow-up
Exact schedules vary depending on histology, stage, and adjuvant treatment. But regular follow-up, including physical exam, tumour markers, CXR, USS and CT scanning, is vital for several years.

Aims are to detect relapse early whilst avoiding excessive radiation from CT scans.

> ### ➲ Extra
> Premalignant carcinoma *in situ* (CIS) of the testis is seen in 0.5% of the general population, but 5% in the contralateral testis of men with testis cancer. It is estimated to progress to invasive cancer in 50% of these cases within 5 years. The risk is increased if the testis is small or the patient has a previous history of cryptorchidism. In these groups, routine contralateral biopsy is recommended. If CIS is found, progression can be prevented by radiotherapy but this has significant implications for fertility.

✚ Radical orchidectomy

Procedure

1. Confirm correct patient, correct side, and mark
2. Ensure preoperative tumour markers sent
3. Standard prep and drape
4. Inguinal incision, open inguinal canal
5. Clamp cord at deep ring. Some ligate and divide cord now
6. Some deliver testis for final examination prior to ligation and division of cord
7. A prosthesis can be inserted, but complications may delay adjuvant treatment so many surgeons delay this
8. Scrotal support for 24 h

Complications

- Wound infection
- Scrotal haematoma
- Hernia

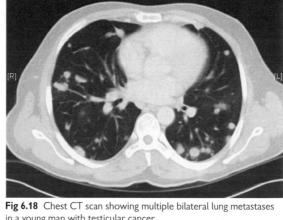

Fig 6.18 Chest CT scan showing multiple bilateral lung metastases in a young man with testicular cancer.

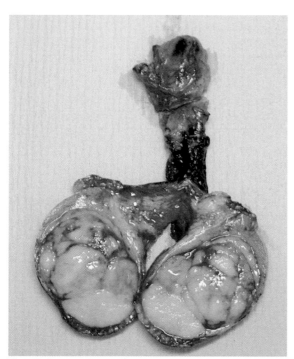

Fig 6.17 Specimen from radical orchidectomy showing a testicular tumour.

6.16 Case-based discussions

Case 1

You are asked to review a 17-year-old schoolboy who has been brought to the emergency department by his parents complaining of acute scrotal pain following a game of rugby at school that afternoon.

- As you walk down to the emergency department, what differential diagnosis is in your mind and what are your priorities?

History reveals the patient to have a unilateral scrotal/testicular pain of rapid onset without an obvious precipitating event. The pain has been present for nearly 4 h.

- What features in the examination would you seek to differentiate a possible testicular torsion from acute traumatic haematocele? What investigations would you request?

The scrotum is exquisitely painful to examination. The testicle is not easily palpable but may be in a high position and swollen. Quite correctly, you elect to forego any investigation and recommend immediate exploration.

- What would you include in your consent for the operation?

At surgery, the testicle is indeed torted but appears to be just viable after de-torsion and prolonged warming. It is fixed in position and a contralateral orchidopexy also performed.

- What, if any, are the long-term risks for this individual having had a torsion?

Case 2

The following history is presented at the weekly multidisciplinary team meeting. A 60-year-old male smoker has been referred under the 2WW system complaining of painless haematuria.

- What are the possible causes and what investigations would you request initially?

There is macroscopic haematuria present on MSU. Blood tests are normal, as is a PSA. Renal tract ultrasound is normal with no renal abnormalities seen.

A flexible cystoscopy performed under LA reveals a papillary growth of the dome of the bladder.

- What further investigations would you now request and what is the initial management?

An abdominopelvic CT urogram scan reveals no evidence of tumour outside of the bladder or tumours of the upper urinary tract, and a transurethral resection of the bladder tumour is performed under general anaesthetic. It reveals a well-differentiated transitional cell malignancy, apparently confined to the subepithelial connective tissue.

- How should this patient be managed now and what strategies are there for prevention of recurrence/progression of the tumour?

A repeat cystoscopy in 8 weeks reveals no evidence of regrowth and apparent complete resection of the lesion. Intravesical chemotherapy is used and repeated follow-up cystoscopies are planned.

Case 3

A 20-year-old woman presents to the emergency department with lower abdominal and left loin pain, dysuria, and frequency. She has been having repeated urinary tract infections, treated at home with cranberry juice and lately on at least two occasions by the GP with antibiotics. She is mildly pyrexial (37.9°C), slightly tachycardic (HR 92 bpm), and feels anorexic. MSU dipstick is positive to blood, white cells, and nitrites.

- What is the differential diagnosis? What is your initial treatment and investigation?

She appears to have an ascending UTI with possible developing pyelonephritis. After IV fluids, taking blood cultures and starting IV antibiotics you request a CT urogram.

- What possible underlying abnormalities might be present to explain the recurrent nature of her infections?
- What possible complications might occur if the ascending infection fails to respond to first line antibiotics and how might they be managed?

Chapter 7

Vascular surgery

◎ Clinical skills

- Vascular imaging
- Non-invasive assessment of PAOD
- The 6Ps
- Ultrasound assessment of deep venous reflux
- Swollen lower limb

✚ Technical skills and procedures

- Lower limb bypass procedures
- Carotid endarterectomy
- Elective open AAA repair
- Saphenofemoral junction ligation and strip and stab avulsions
- Lower limb amputation

7.1 Haemostasis and coagulation

Haemostasis is the normal physiological response to bleeding from an injured blood vessel. It relies on vascular factors, platelet function, the coagulation system, and fibrinolysis. Disorders of these components can lead to excessive bleeding or thrombosis.

Vascular factors

- Blood vessel injury causes release of myogenic factors, resulting in vasoconstriction and reduced blood loss
- Vascular endothelium usually secretes antithrombotic substances, but injury disrupts their production and also exposes the underlying prothrombotic subendothelium. This leads to activation of the tissue factor ('extrinsic') pathway

Platelet function

- Platelets adhere to the exposed subendothelium using a collagen-specific glycoprotein IIb/IIIa receptor enhanced by circulating von Willebrand factor
- Adherence causes activation, release of vasoactive substances, and recruitment of more platelets. Platelet aggregation occurs by binding of fibrin between their surface glycoprotein IIb/IIIa receptors
- The activated platelets also provide a surface on which the coagulation cascade proceeds

Coagulation (clotting)

The coagulation cascade is a series of catalytic reactions involving the activation of clotting factors circulating in the blood. It results in the production of thrombin, which converts fibrinogen to fibrin. This stabilizes the primary platelet plug to form a clot (secondary haemostasis).

Control of coagulation

Haemostasis is regulated so that under normal conditions it delivers a localized and proportionate response to vessel injury.

Inactivation of coagulation factors

Coagulation factors are inactivated by various serum protease inhibitors, including antithrombin, tissue factor pathway inhibitor (TFPI), and heparin.

Protein C and protein S are activated by thrombin bound to thrombomodulin on endothelial cells. Together they inactivate factors VIIIa and Va by proteolysis.

Fibrinolysis

Fibrinolysis counterbalances the tendency to thrombosis and contributes to remodelling and eventual removal of the blood clot during the repair process.

Coagulation disorders

Vessel wall and platelet abnormalities leading to bleeding are discussed in Topic 15.21.

Inherited

Von Willebrand's disease

Von Willebrand's disease is an autosomal dominant disorder that causes a deficiency of von Willebrand's factor (vWF). This results in reduced platelet adherence to exposed subendothelium and instability of factor VIII:C.

It is the most common inherited bleeding disorder, with some degree of deficiency detectable in 1% of the population.

Clinical features are usually mild. Bleeding may follow minor trauma or surgery; haematomas and haemarthrosis are uncommon. Desmopressin (DDAVP®) is given preoperatively and a short course of antifibrinolytic therapy (e.g. tranexamic acid) postoperatively.

Haemophilia

Haemophilia A is a deficiency of factor VIII. Haemophilia B (Christmas disease) is a deficiency of factor IX and is clinically indistinguishable from haemophilia A but is very rare. Both are X-linked recessive disorders.

Clinical features depend on the factor levels. Severe disease results in spontaneous bleeding from an early age. Milder forms may not present until adulthood.

The deficient factors are replaced with plasma-derived concentrates or recombinant factors. The leading cause of death in patients with haemophilia was intracerebral haemorrhage, but it is now AIDS due to HIV transmitted in the blood products.

Acquired

Vitamin K deficiency

Vitamin K is required in the production of factors II, VII, IX, and X, protein C, and protein S. It is fat-soluble and requires bile for absorption. Deficiency is caused by depleted stores, malabsorption or vitamin K antagonists such as warfarin.

Liver disease

The liver is involved in the manufacture of many of the clotting factors. Liver disease reduces their synthesis and can also lead to complications such as thrombocytopenia and DIC.

Disseminated intravascular coagulation

DIC is uncontrolled generalized activation of the coagulation cascade. There is widespread platelet aggregation and consumption of clotting factors, resulting in paradoxical bleeding. There is also marked fibrinolysis and release of fibrin degradation products.

Causes include malignancy, sepsis, trauma, haemolytic transfusion reactions, and severe liver disease.

It often presents as widespread bleeding in a critically ill patient; oozing from line insertion sites is characteristic. Microthrombosis can lead to irreversible organ damage.

Correction of the underlying cause is the most important therapeutic measure, followed by correction of the clotting factor deficiency. Fresh frozen plasma (FFP) in doses of 12–15 mL/kg (raises clotting factor levels by 12–15%) should be given, and cryoprecipitate will be needed to correct low fibrinogen levels. Prognosis is poor.

Coagulation investigations

Routine coagulation tests

- Activated partial thromboplastin time (APTT) is a marker of the contact activation pathway and common pathway. It is also used to monitor heparin therapy
- Prothrombin time (PT) is a marker of the tissue factor pathway and common pathway. It is expressed as the international normalized ratio (INR) when used to monitor warfarin dosing

Other coagulation tests

- Thrombin time (TT) is prolonged if there are low fibrinogen levels or if the patient is heparinized
- Bleeding time is the time taken for a puncture site to stop bleeding. It is a measure of platelet function
- D-dimers are fibrin degradation products (FDP) unique to blood clot breakdown. They can be used in the diagnosis of venous thromboembolism and DIC

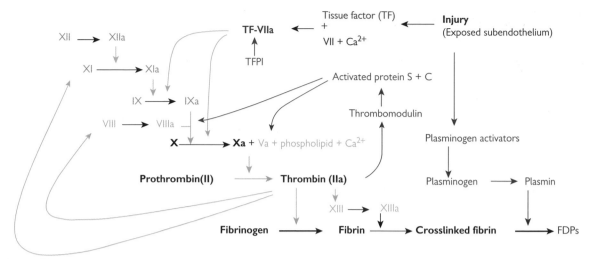

Fig 7.1 Diagram showing the coagulation cascade and its regulation (red). The coagulation cascade is now described in terms of the tissue factor pathway (blue), contact pathway (orange), and common pathway (black). The tissue factor pathway is the primary initiator of coagulation cascade and results in a thrombin 'burst' that is important in activating other factors, including those in the contact pathway. Tissue factor is a lipoprotein expressed on cells not normally in contact with plasma.

Table 7.1 **Laboratory results for common bleeding disorders and anticoagulants**						
	Platelet count	**INR**	**APTT**	**TT**	**Fibrinogen**	**Other**
Haemophilia A	Normal	Normal	Prolonged	Normal	Normal	Low VIII
vWD	Normal	Normal	Prolonged	Normal	Normal	Low VIII, low vWF, and prolonged bleeding time
Liver disease	Normal or low	Raised	Prolonged	Normal	Normal or low	Low V
Vitamin K deficiency	Normal	Raised	Prolonged	Normal	Normal or low	Low II, VII, IX, X
DIC	Normal or low	Raised	Prolonged	Prolonged	Normal or low	Raised FDP, D-dimers, low II, V, VII
Unfractionated heparin	Normal*	Normal or raised	Prolonged	Prolonged	Normal	Raised anti-Xa
LMWH	Normal*	Normal	Normal	Normal	Normal	Raised anti-Xa
Warfarin	Normal	Raised	Normal or prolonged	Normal	Normal	Low II, VII, IX, X
*Heparin-induced thrombocytopenia is rare.						

7.2 Atherosclerosis

Atherosclerosis is a prevalent disease characterized by focal accumulation of lipids and cellular debris in plaques within the intimal layer of medium and large sized arteries.

Through various mechanisms it causes narrowing or occlusion of vessels, leading to tissue ischaemia. The clinical manifestations of atherosclerosis (e.g. myocardial infarction, stroke, peripheral arterial occlusive disease—PAOD) are the leading cause of death in the developed world.

Aetiology

Non-modifiable risk factors

- Advanced age has the strongest association
- Sex: men do not have the protection of female sex hormones and so develop the disease at an earlier age. Following the menopause, women accumulate the same risk
- Race: risk is influenced by geographical location. However, immigrants appear to acquire a similar risk to their host population
- Family history—first degree relative with cardiovascular disease at an early age (men <55 years; women <60 years) in the absence of other major risk factors

Modifiable risk factors

- Tobacco smoking is a strong independent high risk factor
- Hyperlipidaemia: a high level of oxidized low density lipoprotein (LDL) and a low level of high density lipoprotein (HDL) are associated with atherogenesis. Patients with familial hypercholesterolaemia present with symptomatic cardiovascular disease at a young age
- Diabetes mellitus induces endothelial dysfunction and is a risk factor for hyperlipidaemia
- Hypertension induces intimal changes which contribute to accelerated atherosclerosis

Pathophysiology

A mature atherosclerotic plaque develops over many years and goes through three main stages.

1. **Fatty streaks**: focal deposition of serum lipoprotein in the arterial intima and subsequent migration of monocytes and T cells into the subendothelial space leads to macroscopic fatty streaks. The monocytes differentiate into macrophages which ingest the lipid to become foam cells. This process is found in most 20-year-olds but does not always progress to plaque formation
2. **Intermediate plaques**: smooth muscle cells migrate from the tunica media into the affected intima and secrete the connective tissue components to form a fibrous cap on the luminal side of the lipid core
3. **Mature fibrolipid plaques:** the plaque breaks down at the base to form a core of extracellular lipid and necrotic debris which becomes calcified. It is covered by a collagen-rich fibrous cap

Ischaemia

Mature atherosclerotic plaques are the most important cause of chronic ischaemia. Flow reduction may be caused by increasing plaque stenosis or more commonly by rupture or bleeding into the plaque, causing thrombosis and acute on chronic ischaemia.

Arterial thrombosis

Thrombosis is pathological clot formation. When related to atherosclerosis it is usually preceded by plaque injury. This may be superficial erosion of the vascular endothelium or deep fissuring extending into the lipid core. Both stimulate formation of a thrombus which can propagate along the vessel wall (mural thrombus) or occlude the vessel lumen.

Arterial embolism

An embolus is a mass that passes from one site in the vascular tree to another. It is most commonly a piece of thrombus (i.e. thromboembolus). The embolus travels until it lodges in and occludes a distal vessel.

Clinical assessment

Atherosclerosis usually remains clinically silent until late in life. Symptoms and signs are related to the organ affected and the underlying disease process.

In most cases there is a progression of the clinical condition as the stenosis gradually restricts blood flow. The resulting ischaemia manifests as chronic pain.

Acute onset of symptoms is usually related to a sudden complication of the plaque such as rupture or embolism.

Where possible, all adults over 40 years old with no history of cardiovascular disease (CVD) or diabetes should have their cardiovascular risk assessed in primary care using the Joint British Societies' CVD risk prediction charts. They estimate the 10-year risk of CVD (CAD and stroke) over the following 10 years.

Investigations

Investigations are condition-specific but may include:

- Bloods—FBC (anaemia), U+Es, lipid profile, serum glucose, HbA_{1c}
- ECG—screen for ischaemic heart disease and arrhythmias
- Duplex ultrasound or digital subtraction angiography are routinely used to image atherosclerotic vessels
- Novel predictors of cardiovascular disease include serum CRP, homocysteine, fibrinogen, and lipoprotein

Management

The two main aims are modification of a patient's risk factors and symptomatic treatment of the atherosclerosis.

Primary prevention is the prophylactic treatment of high-risk individuals whilst secondary prevention treats individuals with symptomatic disease.

Lifestyle modification

- Smoking cessation
- Regular exercise
- Weight reduction
- Improve diet (reduce saturated fat)
- Improve glycaemic control in diabetics

Drug therapy

- Tight blood pressure control with antihypertensives
- Reduce serum cholesterol levels with HMG-CoA reductase inhibitors (statins)
- Antiplatelet therapy

Operative

Atherosclerosis causes a number of conditions that need percutaneous intervention or open surgery. These are discussed in the relevant topics.

⊙ Vascular imaging

Vascular laboratory

The vascular laboratory plays an important role in diagnosing and guiding treatment in patients with vascular disease. Services include:

- detection and assessment of arterial disease such as PAOD, aortic and peripheral aneurysms, and extracranial arterial disease
- detection and assessment of venous disease such as DVT, mapping of varicose veins, and investigation of suspected chronic venous insufficiency
- Renal and hepatic transplant follow-up

Ultrasound

Ultrasound involves the analysis of sound waves reflected off soft tissues, tissue interfaces or moving blood. A probe sends high frequency sound energy into the tissues and receives reflected energy back. This can be displayed as grey scale cross-sectional images (brightness mode, B mode), sound or colour (using Doppler shift signal from moving blood), although in practice a combination of all these are used in most vascular assessments (duplex ultrasound).

Angiography

Angiography involves the injection of contrast into vessels either via a catheter placed directly in the vessel or by using CT or MRI to follow intravenously injected contrast during its early phase in the arterial circulation.

Catheter angiography is now most commonly performed as a prelude to endovascular treatment (e.g. angioplasty) as non-invasive imaging using ultrasound is sufficient to guide conservative management. Digitally acquired catheter angiograms are commonly displayed, with bones and soft tissues digitally subtracted leaving images of the vessels only.

Complications

Conventional angiography is now a safe procedure. However, before the procedure patients need to have their renal function checked (creatinine should be <300 μmol). The intravascular contrast is potentially nephrotoxic (peaking at 48 h post-procedure). Risks of the procedure are listed below.

Contrast	**Technique**
• Allergic reaction	• Haematoma 3%
• Toxicity (kidney, heart)	• Vessel occlusion 2%
	• Embolism 0.5%
	• Subintimal dissection
	• Vasospasm
	• Infection

Angiography and diabetes mellitus

Before the procedure, diabetics should be kept well hydrated. Metformin is cleared by the kidney and in patients with pre-existing renal dysfunction the contrast can lead to an acute deterioration in renal function and the accumulation of metformin with a resultant lactic acidosis. In patients with abnormal renal function, metformin should be stopped for 48 h before and after the procedure.

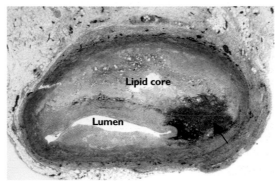

Fig 7.2 Histological section showing a large atheromatous plaque in a coronary artery (low power view). There has been a recent haemorrhage into the plaque (arrow). The properties of a plaque are related to the proportion of fibrous cap and underlying lipid core. Plaques with a core of >40% of total volume are 'unstable' and are much more likely to fissure. Plaques also vary in how much of the vessel circumference they cover. Concentric plaques involve the entire circumference whereas eccentric plaques just involve part of it. Courtesy of Dr Ann Sandison

Peripheral arterial occlusive disease (PAOD) is the chronic obstruction of blood flow to the lower limbs and is almost exclusively caused by atherosclerosis. Incidence of critical ischaemia is 1 per 2500 men (M:F 3:1) and rises with age (peak >60 years).

Aetiology
The principal cause of PAOD is atherosclerosis. Other causes include diabetes mellitus, trauma, vasculitis, and pro-thrombotic disorders.

Pathophysiology
The atherosclerosis causing PAOD is mainly found in the external iliac and superficial femoral vessels. As the narrowing increases, chronic ischaemia promotes the development of collateral vessels. However, severe disease results in cell death, causing ulceration and gangrene.

Basic fluid dynamics and Poiseuille Law
Blood flow in a vessel is determined by vessel diameter (or radius), vessel length, and blood viscosity. Diameter is the most important parameter as it is easily varied and has the greatest influence on vessel resistance.

For instance, doubling either the vessel length or blood viscosity increases resistance 2-fold, but halving the vessel radius increases resistance 16-fold as it is inversely related to the fourth power of the radius.

Resistance equation	$R = (8\eta L)/\pi r^4$
'Ohm's Law' applied to fluids	$Q = P/R$
Poiseuille Law	$Q = (\pi P r^4)/(8\eta L)$

where

R = resistance, η = fluid viscosity, r = vessel radius, L = vessel length, P = pressure gradient, and Q = volumetric flow rate.

Poiseuille's Law combines the first two equations and describes the relationship of flow to pressure, viscosity, vessel radius, and vessel length.

It assumes a straight vessel with uniform diameter and a steady non-pulsatile laminar flow of a Newtonian fluid. These conditions are not met in the body but none the less it demonstrates the detrimental affect of atherosclerotic narrowing.

Clinical assessment
Assessment includes a review of symptoms of PAOD (walking impairment, intermittent claudication, ischaemic rest pain, non-healing wounds), cardiovascular risk, and coexisting vascular disease (e.g. CAD, AAA).

Fontaine classification of PAOD
Stage I   Asymptomatic
Stage II   Intermittent claudication
Stage III   Ischaemic rest pain
Stage IV   Ulceration or gangrene

Intermittent claudication
Intermittent claudication [L. claudicare, to limp] is described as muscular cramplike pain felt in the calf, thigh or buttock that comes on with exercise but is rapidly relieved by rest (2–3 min). Over 50% of patients with claudication pain remain undiagnosed in the community. It is important to find out the:

- site of the pain (predicts level of arterial disease)
- maximum walking distance
- length of pain after stopping exercise

Chronic critical ischaemia
If the disease worsens, pain may develop at rest. It is often described as a severe burning pain, worse at night, but relieved by hanging the leg over the side of the bed.

Chronic critical ischaemia is defined as persistently recurring rest pain, requiring regular analgesia for more than 2 weeks, or ulceration or gangrene affecting the foot, plus an ankle systolic pressure of <50 mmHg. At this point the limb viability becomes threatened.

Examination
A lower limb vascular, neurological, and musculoskeletal examination should be performed along with a general cardiovascular examination. The vascular findings do not always correlate with the severity of PAOD.

Mild to moderate disease
- Pale, cool peripheries
- Atrophic skin changes (thin and shiny, thickened nails)
- Palpate the femoral, popliteal, posterior tibial, and dorsalis pedis pulses. Peripheral pulses are almost always absent. Foot pulses do not necessarily indicate a good blood supply as they may disappear on exercise

Severe disease
- The leg is stone cold but paradoxically appears red owing to the accumulation of vasodilators
- Buerger's test: elevation turns the leg white (note the angle). When returned to a dependent position it turns bluish-red as reactive hyperaemia develops
- Venous guttering may also be evident on elevation of the limb. This is slow to fill when returned to a dependent position
- Ulceration and wet (infected) or dry gangrene indicates advanced disease

General investigations
- Urinalysis (screen for diabetes mellitus)
- Bloods—FBC (polycythaemia, anaemia), U+Es, lipid profile, and serum glucose
- ECG—screen for ischaemic heart disease and arrhythmias

Special investigations
Non-invasive assessment is normally all that is required. Patients requiring surgery will need formal localization and characterization of the lesion.

- Doppler ultrasound (8–10 MHz) to assess pulses and ankle: brachial pressure index (ABPI) should be completed for all patients with suspected PAOD (see box)
- A fixed or graded treadmill walk test estimates an absolute claudication distance. It is useful if the history of intermittent claudication is in doubt
- Identification of the site and significance of the stenosis is achieved by colour duplex ultrasound, conventional angiography, CT angiography or MR angiography
- Clinical evidence of atheroembolism in the lower limb is an indication for aneurysm screening

⊙ Non-invasive assessment of PAOD

Ankle:brachial pressure index

The ABPI gives a quantitative assessment of PAOD. ABPI is initially performed at rest. If this is normal but the symptoms are consistent with intermittent claudication, it should be done following a walk test.

Diabetics may have falsely high readings as medial calcification (Mönckeberg's sclerosis) of their arteries makes them stiff and incompressible. Toe pressures and the pole test are more reliable in diabetics as they are unaffected by vessel calcification.

Procedure

- Lie the patient supine
- Place a blood pressure cuff around the leg. The cuff length should be at least twice the diameter of the limb and is placed just above the malleoli
- Identify the posterior tibial (PT) and dorsalis pedis (DP) pulses using a Doppler probe
- Inflate the cuff above the systolic blood pressure so that the pulses are obliterated
- Slowly deflate the cuff, noting the pressure when the pulses return
- Divide the highest ankle pressure by the average brachial pressure

Value	Suggested clinical interpretation
>1	Normal arterial flow
0.8–0.9	Mild (PAOD present)
0.5–0.8	Moderate (intermittent claudication)
<0.5	Severe (critical ischaemia)

Toe pressures and pole test

In patients with calcified vessels, toe pressures or the pole test can be used instead of ABPI.

Toe pressure is measured in the great toe and is normally 80–90% of brachial systolic pressure. Critical ischaemia is suggested by a toe pressure <30 mmHg.

The pole test involves laying the patient supine and raising the leg whilst holding a Doppler probe over the dorsalis pedis artery. The leg is raised against a pole calibrated in mmHg. The distance up the pole at which there is loss of Doppler signal gives the ankle pressure.

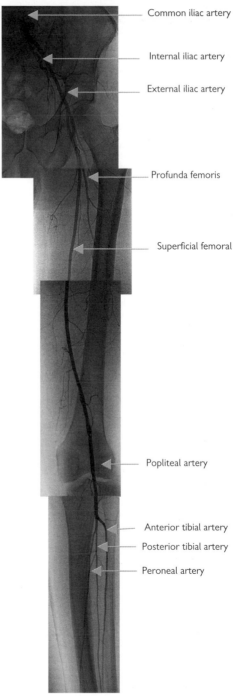

- Common iliac artery
- Internal iliac artery
- External iliac artery
- Profunda femoris
- Superficial femoral
- Popliteal artery
- Anterior tibial artery
- Posterior tibial artery
- Peroneal artery

Fig 7.3 A composite arteriogram of the left lower limb showing a normal arterial tree without digital subtraction of the skeleton.

Patients with symptomatic PAOD can be divided roughly in to three groups.

1. Symptoms improve on their own and do not require further management
2. Stable symptoms tolerated by patient
3. Gradual deterioration in symptoms requiring intervention (<30%)

All patients should undergo risk factor modification. Those with disabling intermittent claudication and critical ischaemia need assessment for percutaneous or surgical intervention.

Conservative

Cardiovascular risk factor modification

- Smoking cessation is most important. Patients go on to have less rest pain and fewer amputations
- Antihypertensives are indicated in hypertensive patients with PAOD. Target blood pressure is <140/90 mmHg. Beta-blockers are generally safe to use
- Antiplatelet drugs such as aspirin reduce associated cardiovascular events but do not improve claudication distance
- Lipid-lowering drugs are indicated in most patients
- Tight glycaemic control in patients with diabetes.

Exercise programme

Regular exercise helps to develop a collateral circulation and encourages better oxygen utilization.

A 6 month period of supervised exercise doubles the claudication and maximum walking distances in over 75% of patients.

Drug therapy for claudication

Cilostazol has been shown in some trials to improve claudication distance and may be valuable in patients unable to exercise or those looking for an early benefit to improve lifestyle limitation.

Percutaneous intervention

Endovascular procedures can offer equivalent or superior long-term outcomes compared to open reconstructive surgery. They also have very low associated morbidity and mortality rates, and are cheaper.

The effectiveness of percutaneous transluminal balloon angioplasty (PTA) in patients with intermittent claudication is dependent on:

1. level of the stenosis/occlusion
2. quality of the distal vessels
3. clinical indication—in certain cases stent placement in addition to angioplasty improves long-term outcomes

Aortoiliac disease treated with PTA is the most successful intervention, with low complication rates and high long-term patency rates. Isolated iliac and superficial femoral disease is also treated successfully with PTA and stent placement.

The evidence for femoropopliteal disease is equivocal and supervised exercise programmes may be more successful.

Operative

Open reconstructive surgery is increasingly being superseded by endovascular intervention. However, it remains an option if endovascular intervention fails or is unsuitable.

Aortoiliac disease

Aortobifemoral bypass is indicated in patients with significant aortoiliac disease which is unresponsive to conservative and percutaneous interventions.

For bilateral iliac occlusive disease, some surgeons will attempt initial iliac stent with a femorofemoral crossover graft, as open aortoiliac surgery has a 10% operative mortality rate.

Indications for extra-anatomical axillofemorofemoral bypass are limited to patients with infrarenal aortic occlusive disease and severe claudication or critical limb ischaemia with significant co-morbidity precluding aortobifemoral bypass.

Femoropopliteal disease

The type of bypass depends on the site and length of disease. It may be femoropopliteal (above or below knee) or femorodistal (tibial, peroneal or pedal). An autologous long saphenous vein is the conduit of choice. It can be left *in situ* or reversed, in which case the valves are destroyed using a valvulotome. Dacron or polytetrafluoroethylene (PTFE) grafts are less successful.

Revision surgery

There are three main complications of arterial reconstruction that can require revision surgery. These are infection, occlusion, and aneurysm formation.

Amputation

Patients with critical limb ischaemia in which arterial reconstruction fails or is inappropriate will need an amputation. It confers a poor prognosis, with a 2-year mortality rate of 40%.

Complications and prognosis

Complications include acute lower limb ischaemia, infection, and, ultimately, amputation. The 5-year mortality rate is 15% in men with intermittent claudication and 50% in those with critical ischaemia.

➕ Lower limb bypass procedures

Femorofemoral crossover

- Bilateral longitudinal groin incisions
- Dissect and control the common femoral artery (CFA), profunda femoris artery (PFA), and superficial femoral artery (SFA) as well as their local branches
- Infuse and circulate up to 5000 IU heparin
- Clamp all three vessels and perform longitudinal arteriotomies
- Flush with heparinized saline and prepare bypass conduit (vein, Dacron or PTFE)
- End-to-side anastomosis of graft to CFA with 5/0 Prolene
- Flush both arteries and graft prior to restoration of circulation
- Reperfuse on completion of anastomosis
- Tunnel graft and undertake contralateral anastomosis
- Check flow and close in three layers

Femorodistal bypass

The femoral component of this is the same as for a fem–fem crossover.

- The popliteal or crural (calf) dissection is undertaken over the vessel and the vessel controlled by rubber slings, with care taken not to damage the accompanying veins in the neurovascular bundle
- Following heparinization, clamps are applied and then the two anastomoses undertaken either simultaneously or sequentially depending on how many surgeons are available
- Care has to be taken to ensure that the length of the graft is correct by straightening the leg on measurement
- The long saphenous vein is the conduit of choice, having the best patency rates and lower infection rates
- Closure is in two layers, after checking patency using on-table angiography, intraoperative Doppler or by palpating the distal pulses

Complications

Intraoperative and early	Intermediate and late
- Haemorrhage	- Graft stenosis
- Graft thrombosis	- Graft infection
- Graft infection	- False aneurysm
- Compartment syndrome and reperfusion syndrome following acute ischaemia	- Progression of disease
	- Amputation
- Wound infection	
- Medical problems	

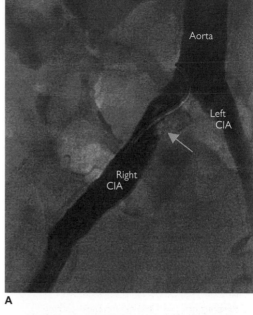

A

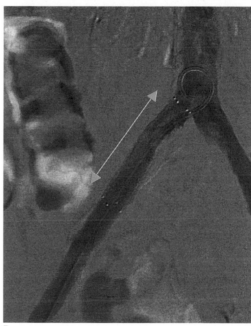

B

Fig 7.4 (A) Digital subtraction angiogram of distal aorta and common iliac arteries (CIA) showing an irregular calcified eccentric tight stenosis of the first 2 cm of the right CIA (arrow). The 4-French pigtail catheter can be seen in the lumen from the right common femoral artery retrograde puncture used to gain access. (B) Right common iliac stenosis was initially angioplastied to 8 mm but, owing to the eccentric calcification and vessel recoil, the stenosis persisted and hence an 8 mm x 4 cm Zilver® stent (arrow) was deployed across the stenosis with good post-stenting appearance.

Acute lower limb ischaemia can be defined as rest pain and/or features of severe ischaemia developing in under 14 days. It can be acute (e.g. cardiac thromboembolus) or acute on chronic (e.g. thrombus formation on a background of PAOD).

Aetiology

Thrombosis (60%) and embolus (30%) are the main causes of acute lower limb ischaemia. Peripheral thrombosis occurs in areas of pre-existing atherosclerosis.

The most common source of emboli is cardiac thrombus caused by atrial fibrillation (80%) or myocardial infarction. Rare causes include atrial myxomas, valve vegetations and paradoxical emboli caused by intracardiac communication of the venous and arterial circulations. Other causes of emboli include atherosclerotic plaques in proximal vessels (e.g. aorta).

Rarer causes of acute limb ischaemia include trauma, iatrogenic (intimal dissection or embolization during interventional procedures), external compression (e.g. supracondylar elbow fractures), compartment syndrome, and vasculitis.

Pathophysiology

Arterial obstruction causes ischaemia which is defined as a level of arterial perfusion that fails to meet the metabolic needs of a tissue or organ. Prolonged ischaemia leads to cellular dysfunction and eventually cell death.

A number of factors influence the effect of ischaemia on the underperfused tissues. These include its metabolic demands, the local blood supply, presence of collateral vessels, and the speed, site, and extent of the blockage.

Clinical assessment

History

- Thrombosis—history of PAOD or pro-thrombotic disorders (e.g. polycythaemia rubra vera)
- Embolism— AF, recent MI, no history of PAOD

Examination

Complete arterial occlusion, without pre-existing collateral circulation, results in the classical presentation of the 6 Ps. This is usually unilateral, but a saddle embolus at the aortic bifurcation may cause bilateral limb ischaemia.

0–6 hours

The limb appears 'marble'-white following acute arterial occlusion owing to intense vasospasm of the distal arterial tree and emptying of the veins.

6–12 hours

Vasodilatation occurs in response to smooth muscle hypoxia. The skin becomes mottled as it fills with deoxygenated blood. This fine light blue/purple reticular pattern usually blanches on pressure.

>12 hours

The stagnant blood coagulates and the thrombus propagates. Capillary rupture causes non blanching coarse dark mottling. Eventually the large areas of fixed staining become blistered and begin to liquefy. Thrombosis in an atherosclerotic vessel does not cause complete limb ischaemia, as borderline perfusion will be achieved by a sufficient number of collateral vessels. Examining the contralateral foot will indicate the presence of pre-existing PAOD and so aid the diagnosis of *in situ* thrombosis rather than embolus.

Investigations

- Bloods—FBC, U+Es, clotting, serum glucose, cross-match
- ECG—screen for arrhythmias and ischaemic disease
- Chest radiograph—cardiomegaly and heart failure
- Echocardiography—identify cardiac thrombus
- Angiography—if the history and examination strongly suggests an embolus, then the patient should proceed to embolectomy and on-table DSA

In patients with likely thrombus and a non-threatened limb there is time to assess the arterial tree formally with DSA (Fig 7.5).

Management

Patients are often elderly and unwell, and may require fluid resuscitation. Patients in a moribund state or with irreversible ischaemia, not suitable for an amputation, require palliation.

Immediate

- ABC
- Supplemental oxygen
- Intravenous fluids
- Analgesia
- Intravenous unfractionated heparin is used to reduce propagation of a thrombus. Heparin acts by potentiating the antithrombotic effect of antithrombin III. A bolus dose is followed by a continuous infusion, keeping the APTT in the therapeutic range

Thrombolysis

Systemic infusion of thrombolytic agents gives poor results, and increases morbidity and mortality rates. Instead, a percutaneous catheter is placed in the thrombus under radiological guidance and infiltrated with streptokinase or tissue plasminogen activator (t-PA).

Embolectomy

Embolectomy is often carried out under local anaesthesia. The artery is mobilized and clamps applied to its branches. A transverse or horizontal incision is made, allowing access for the Fogarty catheter.

The catheter is passed distally along the artery and then inflated and withdrawn. A number of passes are made until the artery is clear of thrombus and this is confirmed by an arteriogram. The artery is closed with either a continuous suture or vein patch.

Reconstructive surgery

Many patients will need urgent bypass surgery, some with on-table thrombolysis and angiography.

Amputation

Amputation can be life-saving and is indicated if the limb has irreversible ischaemia or the patient has significant cardiac or respiratory co-morbidities.

Complications and prognosis

Reperfusion injury is a serious risk following revascularization. Overall acute limb ischaemia has an amputation rate of 40% and a mortality rate of 20%.

The 6 Ps

1. **P**ain is severe, continuous, and resistant to analgesia
2. **P**allor, with the limb initially pale then goes through further colour changes as the ischaemia progresses
3. **P**erishingly cold owing to no arterial flow
4. **P**ulselessness with loss of previously documented pulses is important
5. **P**araesthesia and then paralysis develop later as a result of nerve and muscle ischaemia. Needs emergency surgical intervention
6. **P**aralysis of the muscles

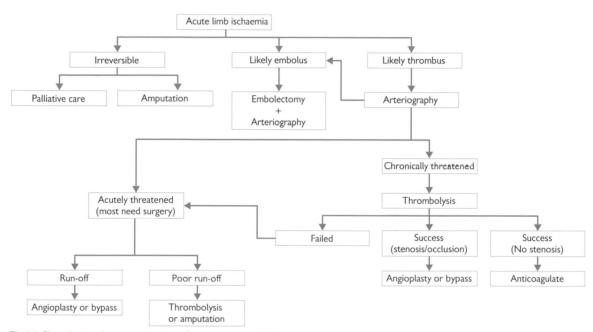

Fig 7.5 Flow chart outlining management of acute lower limb ischaemia.

7.6 Extracranial arterial disease

Atherosclerotic disease of the carotid artery forms the majority of extracranial arterial disease. It is less common for the vertebral arteries or great vessels to be involved. Carotid artery stenosis is responsible for ~30% of all strokes. Incidence is 52 per 1000 male population, with a peak >65 years and male preponderance.

Aetiology

Over 90% of extracranial carotid artery disease is caused by atherosclerosis at the carotid bifurcation. Other rare conditions include fibromuscular dysplasia and carotid body tumours.

Pathophysiology

Atherosclerosis causes narrowing of the carotid lumen. However, emboli rather than flow restriction are the main cause of neurological symptoms.

Blood turbulence results in damage to the vulnerable plaque surface, which can lead to ulceration and rupture. Platelet aggregates develop and can embolize along with the plaque debris. This causes cerebral ischaemia, usually in the anterior circulation.

Very high grade or even complete occlusions may remain asymptomatic if the collateral circulation is good.

Clinical assessment

The main symptoms are related to cerebral infarction (stroke), transient ischaemic attacks (TIA) or retinal infarction.

History

- TIA—neurological symptoms last <24 h
- Stroke—neurological symptoms last >24 h
- Amaurosis fugax—transient loss of vision in one eye
- Contralateral sensory or motor dysfunction
- Higher cortical dysfunction (speech and language deficit)

Examination

- Carotid bruit is not an indicator of disease severity
- Motor, sensory or high cortical dysfunction
- Signs of systemic vascular disease
- Elevated blood pressure

Investigations

- Bloods—FBC, U+Es, serum glucose, lipid profile
- ECG—screen for ischaemia and atrial fibrillation
- Colour duplex ultrasound is the criterion standard for evaluating carotid stenosis
- MRA is more expensive and is used when a brain scan is also indicated
- DSA is usually performed prior to surgery. It gives a very accurate assessment of stenosis but has a 1% risk of CVA. Some surgeons now rely solely on non-invasive investigations (duplex or Doppler + MRA)
- All symptomatic patients must have either a CT or MRI brain to confirm the presence of a cerebral infarct and exclude other intracranial lesions

Management

All patients should be given lifestyle advice as previously discussed to reduce their cardiovascular risk.

In addition, all patients should be started on antiplatelet therapy. Anticoagulation should be considered if they have had an ischaemic stroke or have atrial fibrillation.

Carotid endarterectomy
Asymptomatic patients

The risk of 'stroke prevented' versus 'stroke complication' has to be weighed up. The Asymptomatic Carotid Atherosclerosis Study (ACAS) and Asymptomatic Carotid Surgical Trial (ACAS) showed that asymptomatic patients with a stenosis of 60% or greater benefited from surgery as long as the complication rate was low.

Significant bilateral stenoses pre-CABG is controversial and so only a relative indication.

Symptomatic patients

Carotid endarterectomy is effective in treating patients who have recently had a TIA or stroke with stenosis >70%.

Contraindications

- 100% occlusion of carotid artery
- Severe neurological deficit or acute stroke
- Limited life expectancy (e.g. co-existing metastatic malignancy)

Endovascular procedure

Carotid angioplasty with or without stenting has been shown to be safe and successful in the short term. Ongoing trials are assessing its long-term performance. Its role may be in treating recurrent disease or high risk patients.

Access is gained via the femoral artery under local anaesthetic. A cerebral protection device is used to catch any emboli caused by the procedure.

Complications and prognosis

Asymptomatic disease with a stenosis <75% has an annual cerebral event risk of around 1.5%, but this climbs to 10.5% if it is >75%. Untreated symptomatic disease carries a 20% annual risk of CVA.

⊕ Carotid endarterectomy

Carotid endarterectomy is the most frequently performed procedure to prevent stroke. Preoperatively, the correct side and level of carotid bifurcation must be marked. Transcranial ultrasound is used to confirm patency. It is performed under general or local anaesthetic.

Procedure

- Patient positioned supine with neck extended and turned away
- Skin incision along anterior border of sternomastoid
- Dissect down to, and open, carotid sheath
- Ligate anterior facial vein and divide
- Dissect and control common carotid artery (CCA), internal carotid artery (ICA) and external carotid artery (ECA)
- Heparinize patient (5000 units) and wait 3 min
- Gently occlude carotids and start timing
- A shunt from the CCA to the ICA may be required
- Perform an arteriotomy over the stenosis and then the endarterectomy
- Close the arteriotomy with 6/0 Prolene, wait for haemostasis
- Remove clamps: first from the ECA, then from the CCA, and finally from the ICA. Note the occlusion time
- Place suction drain and close in layers
- Postopertive course: neurological observations and oxygen for 24 h. Repeat carotid duplex at 6 weeks

Complications

Accepted risk for stroke is 3% in asymptomatic patients, 5% for patients with TIA, 7% with CVA, and 10% with recurrent disease.

Intraoperative and early	Intermediate and late
• Intraoperative or postoperative stroke	• Re-stenosis (<20%)
• Bleeding and haematoma	
• Hypoglossal or recurrent laryngeal nerve injury (5%)	
• Hyperperfusion syndrome	
• Postoperative hypertension	
• Death (1%)	

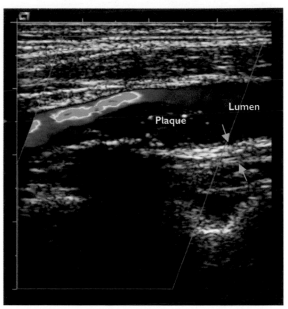

Fig 7.6 Colour duplex ultrasound of a left internal carotid artery (LICA). There is thickening of the intima–media layer (arrows). In the proximal LICA, there is extensive mixed echoplaque measuring 6 mm, which extends along the wall of the LICA for 2 cm. The presence of this plaque significantly narrows the lumen of the vessel. Although the peak systolic velocities in the LICA are elevated (1.8 m/s, IC:CC ratio 3.4 m/s), which would indicate a stenosis of 50–69%, subjectively the degree of stenosis appears much greater, most likely a greater than 70% stenosis.

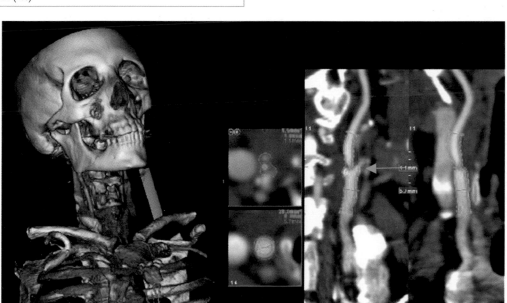

Fig 7.7 Carotid CTA reconstructions showing 90% stenosis at the bifurcation of the right common carotid artery (arrow). The images on the right have been reconstructed to show the vessels in continuity in a single plane.

7.7 Abdominal aortic aneurysm

An aneurysm [Gr. *Aneurysma*, a widening] is a permanent localized dilatation of an artery (≥50% than the expected normal diameter). The infrarenal aorta is the most common site (95%). Other sites include the iliac, femoral, and popliteal arteries; thoracic aorta and cerebral artery aneurysms are rare.

The incidence is 40 per 1000 male population, with a peak >60 years (M:F 5:1).

Aetiology

The aetiology is unknown. Genetic factors predispose to aneurysmal disease, as demonstrated by Marfan's syndrome and Ehlers–Danlos Type IV, which are rare connective tissue disorders associated with arterial aneurysms. Mycotic aneurysms are caused by infection and usually occur in immunosuppressed patients with pre-existing vessel disease.

Risk factors

- Family history
- Tobacco smoking
- Hypertension
- Increasing age
- Male sex

Pathophysiology

Originally, atherosclerosis was thought to have a role in the pathogenesis of aneurysms. Recent research suggests that the overproduction of matrix metalloproteinases (MMP) causes the loss of medial elastin and smooth muscle cells and the excess deposition of adventitial collagen. These extracellular matrix abnormalities lead to a loss in tensile strength of the arterial wall, causing it to dilate. Abdominal aneurysms grow at a rate of 0.1–0.3 cm/year, which increases with size; larger aneurysms are more likely to rupture.

Law of Laplace

Aneurysmal expansion is governed by the Law of Laplace. This states that wall tension is proportional to the pressure multiplied by the radius. With increasing diameter, there is a further increase in wall tension and diameter, leading to an increased risk of rupture.

$$T = PR$$

T = wall tension, P = pressure, R = radius.

Clinical assessment

History

The majority of aneurysms (75%) are asymptomatic at diagnosis. Symptomatic aneurysm can present with:

- back pain (local pressure on vertebral column)
- urinary symptoms (ureteric obstruction)
- acute ischaemia of legs or bowel caused by thromboemboli
- rarely, melaena/haematemesis from aortoenteric fistula

Rupture/leak

- Sudden death (50% die before reaching hospital)
- Severe abdominal pain radiating through to back
- Collapse/shock

Examination

Patients with a contained retroperitoneal leak:

- pale and clammy
- expansile central abdominal mass
- hypovolaemic shock

Differential diagnosis

- Acute pancreatitis
- Perforated viscus
- Renal colic
- Inferior MI

Investigations

Emergency imaging should only be performed in a patient with a suspected rupture if they are stable and the diagnosis is in doubt. A calcified AAA may be an incidental finding on a plain abdominal radiograph.

Routine

- B-mode ultrasound is used as a reliable screening tool
- CT or MRA are used to define the size and relationship of the aneurysm to visceral arteries and other structures
- Angiography or duplex ultrasound is used in patients with evidence of lower limb ischaemia to assess distal vessels

Management

The main aim is to slow the expansion and rupture rates. Conservative measures include smoking cessation (smoking accelerates aneurysmal dilatation), tight control of hypertension, and cardiovascular risk reduction.

Elective repair is either transperitoneal (open) or endovascular. Open repair is usually with a Dacron graft.

Indications for open surgery

- Symptomatic, i.e. back pain
- ≥5.5 cm AP diameter (mortality rate of surgery the same as the annual risk of rupture)
- Rapid increase in size ≥0.5 cm in 1 year
- Peripheral embolization of thrombus in the aneurysm

Endovascular aneurysm repair

Endovascular aneurysm repair (EVAR) was first introduced in 1991 as a technically effective and safe alternative to open aneurysm repair. It has lower short-term morbidity and mortality rates than open surgery, but its long-term efficacy is unknown.

Emergency AAA repair

- Only if the patient is fit; otherwise palliation
- Maintain blood pressure ~100/60 mmHg to reduce the risk of increasing the leak

Complications and prognosis

Rupture is the main consequence of AAA. Other complications are related to thrombosis and embolism. The mortality rate of elective open repair is approximately 5%, and is around 2% for EVAR. Emergency operative mortality rate is 50%.

> ### ➔ Extra
>
> *National screening programme for aortic aneurysm*
> The multicentre aneurysm screening study (MASS) presented strong evidence for both the clinical benefit and the cost-effectiveness of a screening programme for AAAs in men. The Gloucestershire trial successfully reduced AAA rupture rates by screening 65-year-old men using B-mode ultrasound. A screening programme for the UK is currently being developed.

⊕ Elective open AAA repair

Patients require a detailed preoperative assessment, including repeat bloods, cross-match, ECG, and chest radiograph. Echocardiography and lung function tests may also be indicated.

Procedure

- Long midline laparotomy incision
- Retract small bowel and incise peritoneum to expose aorta from left renal vein down to bifurcation
- Give 5000 units IV heparin, wait 3 min, then clamp the aorta above and common iliac arteries below the aneurysm
- Open the aorta and extract mural thrombus
- Cut the Dacron graft to size and suture in place with continuous 3/0 Prolene. Release clamps to evacuate clot
- Check anastomoses
- Aneurysmal sac is closed over the graft to reduce the risk of aortoenteric fistula formation
- Close the sac and then the abdomen in layers
- ITU or HDU until stable

Complications

Intraoperative and early	**Intermediate and late**
<ul><li>Haemorrhage and retroperitoneal haematoma</li><li>Femoral or popliteal embolism; 'trash' foot is rare</li><li>Graft occlusion is rare</li><li>Medical—MI, pneumonia</li><li>Death 5–10%</li></ul>	<ul><li>False aneurysm <5%</li><li>Graft infection <1%</li><li>Male impotence >30%</li><li>Aortoenteric fistula is rare</li></ul>

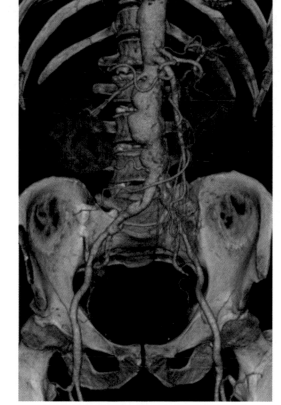

Fig. 7.8 CT reconstruction showing an infrarenal aortic aneurysm (arrow). The vasculature of both kidneys is visible as well as the branches of the aorta going to the bowel. The reconstruction only shows the luminal blood and not the vessel wall.

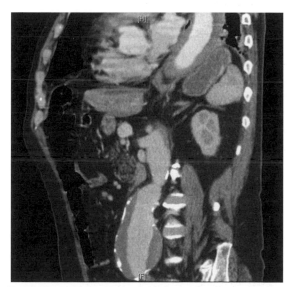

Fig 7.9 CT scan (sagittal section) showing an infrarenal aortic aneurysm with calcification in the wall. There is also a thoracic aortic aneurysm. (See Fig 2.12).

7.8 Chronic venous insufficiency

Chronic venous insufficiency (CVI) refers to the changes that take place in the lower limbs following longstanding venous hypertension. It is a common condition and accounts for up to 1% of healthcare spending.

The incidence is 20 per 1000 population, with a peak >60 years and male preponderance.

Aetiology

Venous return from the lower limb depends on:

1 perfusion pressure across the capillary bed
2 a competent valve system
3 a functioning calf pump

Disruption of these leads to impaired venous return and venous hypertension. Causes include:

- congenital absence of valves
- reflux of superficial, deep or communicating veins
- deep venous occlusion (e.g. DVT)
- abnormality or failure of calf pump (neuromuscular or orthopaedic conditions)

Pathophysiology

There are two main theories as to how sustained venous hypertension causes the clinical manifestations of CVI. The white cell theory is based on the best evidence.

The white cell trapping theory suggests that the reduction in perfusion pressure across the capillary bed leads to white cells plugging the capillaries. This has two consequences: (1) the blocked capillaries cause local tissue ischaemia; and (2) the trapped cells become activated and release oxygen free radicals and proteolytic enzymes which damage the surrounding tissues, causing increased capillary permeability.

The fibrin cuff theory suggests that venous hypertension causes stretching of the capillaries. This leads to the extravasation of larger molecules such as fibrinogen. The fibrin accumulates in the tissues and reduces oxygen diffusion, resulting in localized tissue ischaemia.

Clinical assessment

The condition is usually progressive. Symptoms are best in the morning as the legs have been elevated overnight.

History

- Burning, dull ache or heaviness in the legs after prolonged dependency
- Previous DVT, resulting in acquired deep venous reflux
- Previous varicose vein surgery suggests presence of acquired superficial venous reflux

Examination

- Skin changes (varicose eczema and pigmentation)
- Lipodermatosclerosis
- Inverted 'champagne bottle' legs
- Oedema
- Venous ulceration

Clinical classification of CVI

Class 0 No signs of venous disease
Class 1 Telangiectasia, malleolar flare
Class 2 Varicose veins
Class 3 Oedema but no skin changes
Class 4 Skin changes (lipodermatosclerosis)
Class 5 Skin changes with healed venous ulceration
Class 6 Skin changes with active venous ulceration

Differential diagnosis

- Primary varicose veins
- Post-thrombotic syndrome
- Lymphoedema
- Congestive cardiac failure (CCF)
- Dependency

Investigations

- Doppler ultrasound is used to screen for reflux but is not as sensitive as colour duplex
- Colour duplex ultrasound assesses both the direction and volume of blood flow. It is the gold standard for non-invasive detection of superficial and deep venous reflux

Management

Conservative

- Elevate limbs above the level of the heart
- Graduated elastic compression stockings reduce venous hypertension. They are graded I–IV depending on pressure exerted at the ankle. In CVI use grade II (25–35 mmHg) or above
- Four-layer graduated compression bandages are used to treat venous ulceration

Operative

Approximately 8% of patients will need surgery. Indications include chronic or recurrent ulceration and severe symptoms related to the venous changes.

Superficial venous surgery

Flush ligation of the saphenofemoral junction, long saphenous strip, and saphenopopliteal junction ligation are used in patients with superficial venous reflux.

Surgical treatment of perforating vein reflux is controversial, although subfascial endoscopic perforating vein surgery (SEPS) may have a role.

Deep venous surgery

The surgical correction of deep venous incompetence is controversial. Procedures include valve repair or measures to support the vein walls.

In patients with deep vein occlusion (i.e. failed recanalization following DVT), venous bypass procedures can be considered.

Complications and prognosis

Venous ulceration is the main complication of CVI. Surgical complications include haematoma, nerve damage, and infection. Almost all deaths associated with CVI are caused by venous thromboembolism.

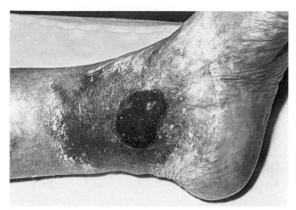

Fig 7.10 Venous ulcer. Reproduced from Mackie (2003) *Clinical Dermatology: An Oxford Core Text*, 5e, with permission from Oxford University Press.

7.9 Varicose veins

Varicose veins are prominent dilated tortuous superficial veins of the lower limb. They are very common (F:M 4:1).

Aetiology

Primary varicose veins develop because of an inherent weakness in the vein walls, making them prone to distension at normal venous pressures.

Secondary varicose veins are caused by a sustained increase in superficial venous pressure. High pressures pass from the deep to the superficial system, causing valvular incompetence. Venous thrombosis, pregnancy or pelvic tumours are causes of raised venous pressure.

Risk factors

Risk factors include family history, age, obesity, and parity. There is no evidence that smoking or social class increase prevalence.

Pathophysiology

The most common scenario is that a single venous valve fails and creates a high-pressure leak between the deep and superficial systems. High pressure within the superficial system causes local dilatation, which leads to sequential failure of other nearby valves in the superficial veins. After a series of valves have failed, the involved veins are no longer capable of directing blood upward and inward.

Without functioning valves, venous blood flows in the direction of the pressure gradient, i.e. outward and downward into an already congested leg. This in turn causes separation of the valve cusps and thus incompetence. In most patients the saphenofemoral valve fails first, leading to failure of the valves below.

Clinical assessment

History

The majority of varicose veins are asymptomatic. Just over 10% have symptoms which may include:

- poor cosmetic appearance
- ache in leg after prolonged standing
- ankle swelling
- pruritus
- concern about future condition (e.g. ulceration)

Examination

- Size, shape, and course of prominent superficial dilated veins
- Oedema
- Ulceration
- Superficial thrombophlebitis
- Varicose eczema
- Perthes' manoeuvre (check deep venous return)
- Trendelenburg test (identify level of incompetent perforator)

Investigations

- Duplex ultrasound scan checks that the deep venous system is intact, especially in post-thrombotic legs. It also maps the source and course of the varicosities. Colour duplex ultrasound is preferred in patients with recurrent varicose veins, a history of DVT or any complications (e.g. superficial thrombophlebitis)
- Venography is invasive and has been superseded by duplex ultrasound

Management

Conservative

- Avoid long periods of standing
- Elevate limbs when resting
- Wear compression stockings (grade II)
- Weight loss advice
- Reassure that varicose ulceration is uncommon

Operative

Common indications are listed below.

- Aching legs
- Haemorrhage from a vein
- Venous skin changes (eczema or lipodermatosclerosis)
- Superficial thrombophlebitis

Surgical options include:

- saphenofemoral ligation, long saphenous strip and stab avulsions (see box)
- saphenopopliteal junction ligation: short saphenous vein is ligated and divided at the saphenopopliteal junction. It is rarely stripped out owing to the potential damage to the sural nerve
- Subfascial ligation (Linton procedure, if open surgery): an endoscope is passed through a small skin incision between the deep fascia and the calf muscle. It is then used to clip perforators. It is useful in patients with ulcerated skin as it causes minimal disturbance

Other options

The following options should be offered to patients as alternatives to traditional open surgical techniques.

- Injection sclerotherapy for small below-knee varicosities. Between 1 and 2 ml 1% sodium tetradecyl sulphate is injected into each vein. This irritant makes the walls stick together and collapse
- Foam sclerotherapy can be performed as an outpatient procedure under Doppler ultrasound guidance. Early results show that up to 30% of patients need two courses of treatment to obtain closure of the saphenofemoral junction, and up to 20% have a recurrence at 2 years
- Radiofrequency ablation is also used with increasing frequency as an alternative to open surgery. The short saphenous vein (SSV) or long saphenous vein (LSV) is cannulated and, under ultrasound guidance, a catheter is advanced to the saphenofemoral or saphenopopliteal junction. Radiofrequency heating then causes collapse and occlusion. This technique has similar results to foam sclerotherapy and avoids the morbidity of open surgery
- Endovenous laser treatment is similar to radiofrequency ablation but uses laser to cause thermal damage to the endothelium

Complications and prognosis

Complications of varicose veins include thrombophlebitis, haemorrhage, ulceration and the other skin changes already described. Thrombophlebitis is an indication for vascular referral. It does not need antibiotics.

⊙ Ultrasound assessment of deep venous reflux

This can be performed in clinic using a Doppler ultrasound, although colour duplex is more sensitive.
- Patient standing
- Probe placed over area to be tested (e.g. sapheno-femoral or saphenopopliteal junction)
- Calf muscles manually compressed, creating an upward flow
- Calf pressure released and a reversal of flow or 'whoosh' is heard if there is reflux

⊕ Saphenofemoral junction ligation and strip and stab avulsions

Incompetent perforating veins should be carefully marked preoperatively.

Procedure
- Patient supine
- Dissect down to the saphenofemoral junction
- Ligate and divide the long saphenous vein along with its tributaries as it enters the femoral vein (i.e. flush ligation of the junction)
- Wire then placed down the long saphenous vein which is stripped out of the leg, disconnecting any branches, including the mid-thigh perforator. Strip to just below the knee, as stripping any lower risks damage to the saphenous nerve. Not stripping risks recurrence from reflux at the mid-thigh perforator level
- Stab skin incisions over varicosities. Pick up vein with Oesch hooks or mosquito forceps and apply traction to avulse it. Direct pressure controls bleeding
- Postoperative care includes compression stockings for 1–3 weeks and early mobilization

Complications and prognosis

Intraoperative and early	Intermediate and late
• Bleeding and haematoma	• Recurrence (5%)
• DVT	
• Wound infection	
• Nerve injury	

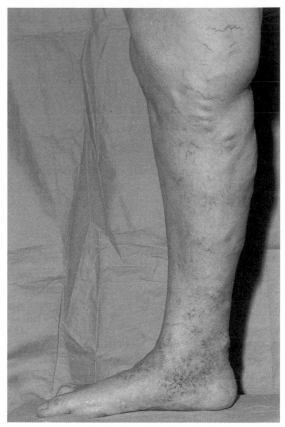

Fig 7.11 Varicose veins in long saphenous vein distribution and spider veins over the medial malleolus. There are no skin changes suggestive of chronic venous insufficiency.

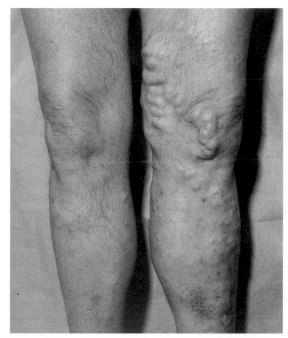

Fig 7.12 Varicose veins of the anterior shin and medial thigh in the long saphenous distribution. The long saphenous vein starts from the venous plexus then travels anterior to the medial malleolus, one hand breadth posterior to knee, and continues up the medial aspect of the thigh to the saphenofemoral junction 2 cm lateral and inferior to the pubic tubercle.

7.10 Lymphatic conditions

The lymphatic system returns interstitial fluid to the intravascular circulation; impairment of flow leads to lymphoedema. The system is at low pressure, with lymph being milked slowly along the vessels by rhythmic contractions. Larger, more proximal, lymphatic vessels have valves which stop reflux.

Lymph nodes are secondary lymphoid organs that support circulating lymphocytes and other immune cells. They filter the circulating lymph for foreign material.

Lymphoedema

Aetiology

Primary

Congenital lymphoedema is very rare and presents at birth or shortly afterwards (<1 year). It has a female preponderance and is either familial (Milroy's disease) or non-familial (often associated with congenital arteriovenous malformations).

The majority of primary lymphoedema is postpubertal and can be divided into lymphoedema praecox (<35 years) and lymphoedema tarda (>35 years). Meige's disease is familial lymphoedema praecox.

Secondary

Worldwide, the commonest cause is filarial infection (*Wuchereria bancrofti*) of lymph nodes. In the UK it is cancer therapy (radiotherapy or lymph node dissection). Only rarely does a tumour itself cause obstructive lymphoedema.

Pathophysiology

The accumulation of interstitial plasma proteins causes an increased oncotic pressure which draws fluid into the tissues. Chronic disease leads to progressive subcutaneous fibrosis and loss of elasticity.

Congenital postpubertal lymphoedema is characterized by three processes.

1. Distal hypoplasia of lymphatic vessels (80%) causes bilateral swelling below the knees
2. Proximal aplasia (10%) causes unilateral swelling
3. Hyperplasia secondary to valve incompetence and subsequent lymphatic dilatation causes bilateral swelling

Secondary lymphoedema is usually due to obstruction which causes valve incompetence and subsequent lymphatic dilatation. It presents with unilateral leg swelling.

Clinical assessment

History

- Painless limb swelling which is worse following periods of limb dependency
- Risk factors: age of onset, family history, previous cancer therapy

General examination

- Site of swelling (starts distally)
- Unilateral or bilateral
- Pitting oedema becomes non-pitting as subcutaneous tissue fibrosis progresses
- Evidence of previous surgery or radiotherapy

Skin

- Pronounced skin creases ('buffalo hump' of dorsum of foot)
- Thickened skin with warty texture (hyperkeratosis)
- Papillomatosis
- Weeping of lymph from vesicles
- Ulceration is very rare

Investigations

- Lymphoscintigraphy—technetium-labelled colloid is injected into the second web space of both feet, followed by imaging with a gamma camera. It is the gold standard, with a negative result excluding the disease
- CT + MRI—both demonstrate the honeycomb appearance of the subcutaneous tissues seen in lymphoedema and are used in combination with lymphoscintigraphy
- Contrast lymphangiography has been superseded by lymphoscintigraphy
- Colour duplex ultrasonography excludes CVI

Management

The aim of treatment is to improve the patient's quality of life, reduce the swelling, and prevent infection. Conservative therapy is usually successful.

Conservative

- Limb elevation
- Exercise improves both passive and active return
- Manual lymphatic drainage (massage by physiotherapist) and compression bandaging
- Careful skin care to prevent infection
- Drug therapy to treat the swelling is ineffective. Swelling that improves with diuretics is unlikely to be lymphatic in origin. Antibiotics or antifungals are used to treat infection

Operative

Surgery is indicated in patients with massive limbs and failure of conservative treatment.

- Debulking procedures: Homan's operation removes ellipses of tissue with primary closure. Charles' operation removes all of the skin and subcutaneous tissue below the knee and requires skin grafting
- Lymphatic bypass is used to treat isolated blockages

Complications and prognosis

Primary lymphoedema is a lifelong but not life-threatening disease. Poor cosmesis and lymphangitis are the main complications. The outcome of secondary lymphoedema depends on the underlying condition.

Lymphatic neoplasia

Lymphatic tumours are rare. Lymphangiomas are benign tumours that are often present from birth (e.g. cystic hygroma). Lymphangiosarcomas are associated with chronic lymphoedema and are aggressively malignant. Mean survival is less than 2 years.

⊚ Swollen lower limb

Unilateral

- Infection (bacterial or fungal)
- Venous disease (CVI, DVT, post-thrombotic syndrome)
- Lymphatic (secondary lymphoedema)
- Arterial (arteriovenous malformation)

Bilateral

- Metabolic (hypoalbuminaemia, pretibial myxoedema)
- Cardiac (CCF, fluid overload)
- Lymphatic (primary or secondary lymphoedema)
- Venous (pelvic or IVC obstruction)
- Chronic venous insufficiency
- Drugs (calcium channel inhibitors)

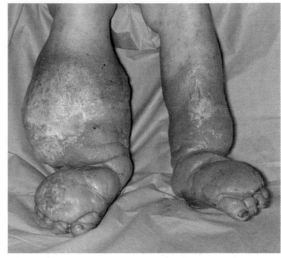

Fig 7.13 Bilateral lower limb swelling caused by primary lymphoedema.

Fig 7.14 Normal lymphoscintigraphy of the lower limbs.

7.11 Diabetic foot

Diabetic foot problems are the most common major end point in both type 1 and 2 diabetes mellitus. They cause significant morbidity and mortality, and are a major cost to the health service.

The cumulative lifetime risk of developing ulceration may be as high as 25%. The incidence is highest in men over 60 years old.

Aetiology

Diabetic ulceration is caused by neuropathy (35%), peripheral arterial occlusive disease (15%), or mixed neuroischaemia (50%).

Risk factors for diabetic foot ulceration

- Peripheral neuropathy
- Peripheral arterial occlusive disease
- Previous foot ulceration
- Living alone
- Visual impairment

Pathophysiology

The diabetic foot syndrome includes diabetic neuropathy, peripheral arterial occlusive disease, Charcot neuroarthropathy, foot ulceration, osteomyelitis, and amputation.

Neuropathy

Diabetic neuropathy tends to be a peripheral sensorimotor polyneuropathy. It is a consequence of nerve hypoxia caused by microvascular disease and persistent hyperglycaemia affecting neuronal metabolism. Sensory, motor, and autonomic nerves are all affected to varying degrees.

PAOD

Atherosclerosis follows the same pathological course as in non-diabetic patients but tends to affect more distal vessels.

Charcot neuroarthropathy

This is a devastating complication which is seen in 10% of patients with diabetic neuropathy. There is bone and joint destruction, fragmentation, and remodelling. The pathological process is not fully understood but the condition is likely to be caused by unrecognized trauma owing to loss of pain and proprioception.

Clinical assessment

The aim is to assess the severity of diabetes, risk factors and degree of neuropathy, ischaemia, and infection.

Neuropathy

- Symptoms include tingling, burning, and shooting pains which are often relieved by exercise
- The foot looks warm and has bounding pulses. Sensory disturbances are usually in a 'glove and stocking' distribution with reduced or absent ankle reflexes

PAOD

- First presentation is often with ulceration rather than a history of intermittent claudication
- The pain of intermittent claudication should be distinguished from neuropathic pain, which tends to be an ache in the foot or calf made worse by elevation and relieved by dependency

Examination of the foot

- Warm, red, swollen foot
- Ulceration (Topic 7.12)—deep ulcers may cause osteomyelitis
- Infection—cellulitis may be associated with ulcers. Paronychia is common
- Poor foot care (e.g. thick callus)

Investigations

- Wound swab sent for MC+S if infection suspected
- HbA1c assesses long-term glycaemic control
- Plain foot radiographs are required if osteomyelitis or Charcot neuroarthropathy suspected
- Non-invasive vascular assessment if no foot pulses are palpable

Management

A multidisciplinary team approach should be taken, with input of a diabetologist, nurse, podiatrist, orthotist, and vascular surgeon.

General (modification of risk factors)

- Smoking cessation
- Tight glycaemic control
- Tight blood pressure control (<130/80 mmHg)
- Statin to reduce cholesterol levels
- Antiplatelet agent

Foot care education

- Use well-fitting shoes with square toe boxes
- Daily foot inspections
- Keep feet covered and protected
- Avoid hazards such as hot water and radiators
- Regular podiatry
- Annual diabetic foot clinic review
- Early reporting of problems

Diabetic ulcers

The key to managing neuropathic ulcers is pressure relief. This is achieved by using appropriate shoes or a pressure-relieving plaster cast or scotch boot. Regular podiatry removes excess callus. Purely ischaemic ulcers rarely heal without revascularization.

Infection

Sepsis is a major risk factor for amputation and so necrotic tissue should be aggressively debrided at the earliest opportunity and the patient started on empirical broad spectrum IV antibiotics until microbiological cultures and sensitivities are available.

Arterial reconstruction

This is suitable in cases with clinically significant PAOD. There is a higher failure rate and many go on to need an amputation.

Amputation

In the UK, patients with diabetes mellitus make up ~30% of those undergoing amputation. It follows failure of arterial reconstruction or because reconstruction would be impractical or unsuitable due to poor peripheral vessels.

⊕ Lower limb amputation

Eighty per cent of amputations in the UK are a result of PAOD. Other reasons include severe pain, severe infection, malignancy, and trauma.

Choosing the level of amputation is dependent on: (1) the healing potential of the tissue; and (2) the patient's rehabilitation potential. Every attempt should be made to preserve the knee if the patient has the potential to walk again.

Transfemoral (above-knee) amputation is made 12 cm proximal to the knee joint and uses an equal anterior and posterior myocutaneous flap to give good cover of the distal femur.

Gritti–Stokes amputation is used in patients who will not be walking postoperatively but in whom a longer stump will be helpful with their nursing care. The femur is divided just proximal to the condyles and what remains of the patella is fixed to the cut surface, following removal of its articular surface. This procedure is more successful than a knee disarticulation.

Transtibial (below-knee) amputation makes up 70% of all amputations and offers the best prognosis for rehabilitation. The tibia is divided 15 cm distal to the knee joint and the fibula about 1.5 cm above this. The Burgess long posterior flap was traditionally used to form the stump; however, the skew flap technique is now favoured. It is based on the arteries that run with the short and long saphenous veins; it uses a long posterior muscle flap but equal skin flaps. It leaves a well-shaped stump that allows early prosthesis fitting. There is no difference in its healing rate when compared with the Burgess long posterior flap.

Distal amputations are usually only carried out if there is a good distal blood supply. Possible amputations include: Syme's amputation (ankle), Chopart's or Lisfranc's (forefoot), transmetatarsal, ray, and digit.

Complications

Early	**Late**
• Pain and psychological issues	• 'Phantom' limb pain
• Flap ischaemia	• Ischaemia
• Haematoma	• Infection
• Infection	• Ulceration
• DVT	• Neuroma

Prognosis

Amputation conveys a poor prognosis for patients with PAOD. It suggests that they have severe disease and so are also at high risk for ischaemic heart disease and cerebrovascular disease.

• 30% of unilateral amputees become bilateral amputees within 2 years
• 50% 5-year mortality rate

169

Chronic leg ulceration is very common and costs over £600 million per annum to manage in the UK. The point prevalence in the UK population is around 2% and it is most common in the elderly.

Aetiology

The main causes of chronic leg ulceration are venous insufficiency (70%) and arterial insufficiency (20%). In clinical practice, ulcers are often of mixed aetiology, e.g. neuroischaemic ulcers seen in diabetics.

Other, rarer, causes of leg ulceration include trauma, malignancy, infection, and inflammatory disorders (rheumatoid disease, SLE, polyarteritis nodosa).

Pathophysiology

Ulceration is a full-thickness break in the skin's epithelial surface. The pathophysiology depends on the underlying cause. This is discussed in the relevant topics earlier in the chapter.

Clinical assessment

Patients with complicated ulcers require an early referral for a specialist opinion. Indications include PAOD, diabetes, inflammatory disease, atypical distribution, and suspected malignancy.

General

- History of ulceration—pain, duration, recurrence
- Social history—independence and mobility
- Exclude peripheral arterial occlusive disease, diabetes mellitus, and rheumatoid disease

Leg

- Oedema
- Venous disease (insufficiency, DVT, varicose veins, venous dermatitis)
- Arterial insufficiency (check pulses and ABPI)
- Neuropathy

Ulcer (Table 7.2)

- Site, surface area, edges, depth, base
- Characteristics of surrounding soft tissues

Investigations

- ABPI should be performed on all legs to exclude arterial insufficiency (APBI <0.8)
- Wound swabs taken if infection is suspected
- Biopsy is indicated in non-healing or atypical ulcers
- Other investigations such as bloods, radiographs, and/or colour duplex ultrasound assessment are guided by the underlying aetiology

Management

A multidisciplinary team is often involved in managing patients with chronic leg ulceration. Hospital specialists often guide care that is delivered in the community.

General

- Mobility may need to be supported with occupational therapy and physiotherapy
- A social care package may be required for dependent patients with limited mobility
- Patients must be fully informed and helped in trying to comply with the recommended therapy to reduce complications and recurrence

Venous ulceration

Compression is the main factor in healing chronic venous ulcers. The type of wound dressing used appears to have a limited impact on speed of healing and should generally be simple and low adherent.

Graduated elastic compression stockings are the treatment of choice in uncomplicated healing venous ulcers, but multilayer bandaging is also used.

Skin grafting is considered in chronic ulcers to speed up skin coverage.

Arterial ulceration

Surgery or endovascular intervention is the mainstay of therapy. Without an improved blood supply, the ischaemic tissue is difficult to heal.

Diabetic ulceration

Neuropathic ulcers generally heal well once the pressure is relieved. Those with an ischaemic component need this addressed as above.

Complications and prognosis

Chronic ulcers require routine follow-up to ensure that they are making progress. Delayed healing may be caused by infection, undiagnosed arterial insufficiency, poor patient compliance, and malignancy.

Secondary prevention is important in healed ulcers to reduce the recurrence rates. In venous ulceration, this entails the continued use of compression stockings.

Table 7.2 **Characteristics of common leg ulcers**			
	Arterial	*Venous*	*Neuropathic*
Pain	Painful	Painful	Pain is dependent on extent of sensory neuropathy
Site	Located anywhere, but frequently seen on the dorsum of the foot	Commonly located in the 'gaiter' region, just above the medial malleolus	Located at points of high pressure (dorsum of toes or plantar aspect of metatarsal heads or heel)
Ulcer	Small, well circumscribed, punctate ulcers with a necrotic, poorly healing base	Shallow, irregularly-defined edges with sloughy, granulating base attempting to heal	Deep, well-defined edges with callused cuff. Base is healthy with granulation tissue (unless infected)
Leg	Surrounded by pale atrophic skin (shiny, thin, dry)	Surrounding skin pigmented with venous changes such as eczema, and lipodermatosclerosis. There may be surrounding varicose veins	The foot is normal or flushed. The ulcer is often surrounded by callus, suggesting an area of repetitive trauma
Temperature	Cool foot with a delayed capillary return >2 s	Warm foot with a normal capillary return <2 s	Warm foot with a normal or delayed capillary return
Pulses	No distal pulses	Distal pulses present	Bounding distal pulses are usually present unless co-existing PAOD
ABPI	ABPI <0.5	ABPI normal	ABPI normal (or reduced in PAOD)

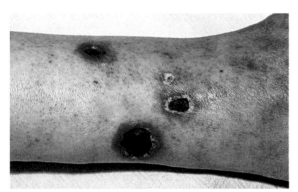

Fig 7.15 Arterial ulcer. Reproduced from Mackie (2003) *Clinical Dermatology: An Oxford Core Text*, 5e, with permission from Oxford University Press.

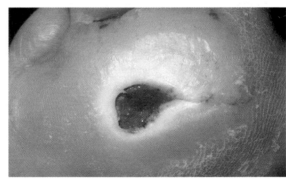

Fig 7.16 Neuropathic ulcer. Reproduced from Mackie (2003) *Clinical Dermatology: An Oxford Core Text*, 5e, with permission from Oxford University Press.

7.13 Miscellaneous vascular conditions

Vascular anomalies

Vascular tumours

Haemangiomas (strawberry naevae) are common benign self-limiting tumours which affect 10% of live births. They go through three phases—rapid proliferation, prolonged involution, and final involution. Large or multiple lesions should be imaged with ultrasound or MRI.

Management is generally expectant although active treatment may be indicated for very large tumours, frequent ulceration, compression of structures, and those associated with high output cardiac failure.

Options include steroid injection, embolization, and surgery.

Vascular malformations

Vascular malformations can be divided into capillary, lymphatic, venous, arteriovenous (AVM) or a combination.

- Capillary malformations (port wine stain) are the commonest. Histologically, they are ectatic capillaries in the dermis. They do not regress and can be treated with pulsed dye laser
- Congenital arteriovenous malformations are often aggressive. Superficial malformations present as warm, soft, pulsatile swellings which are compressible and have a palpable thrill and audible bruit on auscultation. Internal AVMs present with symptoms related to their location
- Acquired AVMs may be due to trauma or, more frequently, surgically created for high flow vascular access in renal dialysis patients (Bresca–Cimino technique is commonly used)

Associated syndromes

- Parkes–Weber syndrome: multiple AVMs, cutaneous capillary malformation, and bone and soft tissue hypertrophy
- Klippel–Trenaunay syndrome is a triad of varicose veins (no clinically apparent AVMs), cutaneous capillary malformations, and bone and soft tissue hypertrophy

Buerger's disease

Buerger's disease (thromboangiitis obliterans) is a non-atherosclerotic, segmental, inflammatory, occlusive disease that affects the small- and medium-sized arteries and veins of the upper and lower limbs. It is strongly associated with tobacco smoking. The aetiology is unknown but might involve an immunological phenomenon.

Clinical assessment

The majority of patients (>80%) present with distal ischaemic rest pain and/or ischaemic ulceration of the toes, feet, or fingers. They may also present with claudication of the feet, legs, hands, or arms and often describe Raynaud's phenomenon (see below).

Diagnostic criteria

- Age <45 years
- Current (or recent) history of tobacco use
- Presence of distal extremity ischaemia (claudication, rest pain, ischaemic ulcers or gangrene)
- Exclusion of autoimmune diseases, hypercoagulable states, and diabetes mellitus
- Exclusion of a proximal source of emboli
- Consistent angiograms showing disease in the clinically involved and non-involved limbs

Management

Patients must stop smoking, use protective footwear, and avoid cold environments. Reconstructive surgery is almost never attempted as it is rarely successful owing to the diffuse nature of the disease.

Raynaud's syndrome

Raynaud's syndrome is characterized by episodic digital ischaemia in response to cold or emotion, most common in women. Raynaud's disease is idiopathic (20%). Raynaud's phenomenon is associated with an underlying condition in 80%.

- Trauma (vibration)
- Arterial disease (atherosclerosis, Buerger's disease)
- Connective tissue disorders (scleroderma, SLE, rheumatoid disease)
- Blood disorders (cold agglutinins, cryoglobulinaemia)
- Drugs (oral contraceptive pill (OCP), beta-blockers)

Clinical assessment

The extremities pass through three distinct colour phases.

1. White—vasospasm
2. Blue—stagnation of anoxic blood
3. Red—build-up of metabolites results in a reactive hyperaemia

Investigations

Patients should be screened for underlying disease.

- FBC, U+Es, ESR, TFT
- Cryoglobulins
- Antithyroid antibodies, antimitochondrial antibodies, antinuclear factor

Management

Patients are advised to stop smoking and keep the extremities warm. Nifedipine and methyldopa are therapeutic in acute attacks. In cases with ulceration or gangrene, a prostacyclin (iloprost) infusion may avoid amputation. Cervical sympathectomy is used occasionally.

Renal artery stenosis

Renal artery stenosis is rare. In the young it is caused by fibromuscular dysplasia and in the elderly by atherosclerosis.

Stenosis reduces renal perfusion, resulting in hypertension (activation of the renin-angiotensin system) or renal dysfunction due to ischaemia. ACE inhibitors are contraindicated as they result in renal insufficiency. It is treated with percutaneous balloon angioplasty/stent or reconstructive surgery.

It is important to diagnose renal artery stenosis in patients undergoing aortovascular surgery as they are at risk of occlusion if it is not corrected before surgery.

Subclavian steal syndrome

Subclavian steal syndrome (SSS) is caused by proximal subclavian artery stenosis or occlusion which results in retrograde vertebral artery flow associated with transient neurological symptoms due to cerebral ischaemia.

The patient is usually asymptomatic until increased demand from the upper limb causes blood to be 'stolen' from the circle of Willis. Doppler USS has now superseded angiography as the diagnostic test of choice.

Percutaneous revascularization or bypass grafting restores antegrade vertebral artery flow to avoid cerebral hypoperfusion and improve perfusion to the upper limb.

Takayasu's arteritis

Takayasu's arteritis (Takayasu's aortitis, pulseless disease, aortic arch syndrome) is a chronic idiopathic arteritis. It is most prevalent in young female Asians. The aetiology is unknown but might involve an autoimmune phenomenon. The arteritis causes progressive scarring and stenosis.

Clinical assessment

Symptoms vary depending on the stage of the illness. Early symptoms include fever, fatigue, poor appetite, weight loss, night sweats, joint pain, and chest pain.

Later symptoms and signs are related to tissue ischaemia.

- Angina, shortness of breath, and fatigue (IHD and CCF)
- Fainting, dizziness, and changes in vision (TIA or CVA)
- Chronic renal failure and hypertension
- Intermittent claudication and muscle weakness

On examination, there are often weak or absent pulses in the arms, neck or legs, with a systolic pressure difference between the arms and legs. An ESR >40 mm/h suggests active disease. Investigations include duplex ultrasound, DSA, and MRA.

Management

Initial treatment is with prednisolone and antihypertensives. If there is no response, immunosuppressants (methotrexate) can be started. Prognosis is good (10-year survival >90%); however, if the disease becomes inactive the patient may be left with stenosed arteries, requiring percutaneous balloon angioplasty or stenting.

Thoracic outlet syndrome

The narrow space between the first rib and clavicle contains the subclavian artery, vein, and the brachial plexus. Compression of these structures may lead to neurological or vascular symptoms described as a thoracic outlet syndrome.

Compression may be caused by excess muscle development (swimmers), a healed fracture or a congenital cervical rib or fibrous band.

Clinical assessment

Patients normally present with upper limb 'claudication' made worse by raising their arm above their head and opening and closing their fist (Roo's test). Sometimes the artery becomes aneurysmal distal to the obstruction. This is prone to collect thrombus. Subsequent emboli may present as acute limb ischaemia. The neurological symptoms are usually in the distribution of the T1 nerve root. However, Horner's syndrome can result from compression of the sympathetic outflow from C8 to T2.

Diagnosis is difficult and often needs input from both radiologists and neurologists.

Management

Congenital cervical ribs or fibrous bands are excised and subclavian aneurysms are repaired; otherwise, management is conservative. The results for patients with vascular symptoms are better than those for patients with neurological symptoms.

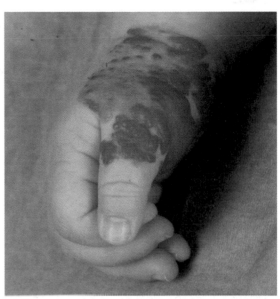

Fig 7.17 Haemangioma of the right hand.

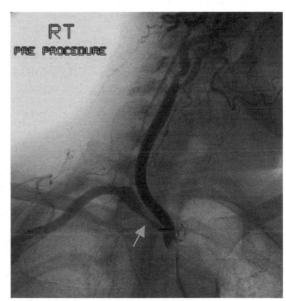

Fig 7.18 Arteriogram demonstrating a right subclavian stenosis (arrow), which is less common than left.

7.14 Case-based discussions

Case 1

A 27-year-old woman is referred by her GP with unilateral foot ulceration. She noticed a break in the skin over her left heel and first metatarsal head following a hot bath 3 days ago.

- Given this presentation, what questions would you specifically ask about her past medical history?

She is pain-free. Her temperature is 38.8°C and she has a sinus tachycardia. Her feet are warm, with bounding peripheral pulses. There is ulceration of her left foot.

- What else would you examine for?
- What is your differential diagnosis?

A wound swab is taken. An ECG is normal and her blood results are below.

Hb	11.2 g/dL	Na$^+$	135 mmol/L
WBC	14.3 x 10^9/L	K$^+$	5.0 mmol/L
Platelets	350 x 10^9/L	Creatine	300 umol/L
HCT	38%	Urea	25 mmol/L
Neut	15.1 x 10^9/L	CRP	45 mg/L
Lymph	2.0 x 10^9/L	Glucose	25 mmol/L

- Discuss her blood results.
- How are you going to manage her?

Discussion

She has type I diabetes mellitus with peripheral neuropathy. The ulcer looks infected and she is systemically unwell with elevated serum glucose. She requires admission, antibiotics, and careful wound management.

- What other complications are associated with diabetes?
- What features might distinguish a neuropathic ulcer from venous or arterial ulceration?
- What advice and follow-up would you give her?

Case 2

It is 21.00 and the emergency department refers you an 82-year-old man with an acutely ischaemic left leg. He has been getting cramping pains in both legs for some time.

This has deteriorated over the past 3 weeks and he is now woken at night by pains in his left leg. He had a heart attack 5 years ago and says he is on lots of medications.

- What other risk factors do you ask about?
- Define intermittent claudication.

He is in a lot of pain and looks dehydrated. You examine both lower limbs. The right leg is pale and cool. The nurse gives you his observations: temperature 36.5°C, HR 120 regular, BP 160/90 mmHg, SaO$_2$ 94% on room air.

- What is an ABPI and how would you measure it?
- Describe the pathological course of an acutely ischaemic limb.

His ECG shows left bundle branch block and the blood tests are normal, including his lipid profile. His ABPIs are 0.4 (left) and 0.7 (right).

- What is your initial management?
- Does he need to go to theatre as an emergency that night?

Discussion

He is a lifelong smoker, has hypertension, but is not diabetic. The history is of intermittent claudication with a recent deterioration which meets the criteria for chronic critical ischaemia. He should be resuscitated and started on IV heparin. The limb is threatened but there is time to fully investigate his arterial tree.

- What is the pathophysiology of atherosclerosis?
- How would you investigate him further?
- How could you calculate his future cardiovascular risk?

Case 3

You are fast-bleeped down to the resuscitation room in the emergency department. A 65-year-old man has been brought in by ambulance having collapsed at home with abdominal and back pain. His wife says he is waiting for an urgent operation to replace a tube in his tummy. He has just retired and walks the dog everyday.

- What is your initial approach?

He is maintaining an airway, is self-ventilating, and his heart sounds are normal. He has a large abdomen, is guarding on palpation, and the bowel sounds are quiet. The nurse shows you the observation chart: HR 115 regular, BP 90/60 mmHg, SaO$_2$ 92% on 5 L oxygen.

- Discuss the observations.
- What is 'shock' and what type might he be in?
- What are the aims of resuscitation in this circumstance?
- What investigations should be undertaken?

He is taken to theatre and undergoes an emergency AAA repair. Following this he is recovered to ICU.

- What early complications are associated with AAA repair?

Discussion

He had a leaking AAA and was a suitable candidate for an emergency repair. As in this case, if the clinical diagnosis is certain, there is no need for investigations which would delay emergency surgery.

- What are the indications for an elective AAA repair?
- What do you know about screening for AAA?

Chapter 8

Emergency surgery

⦿ Clinical skills

- CCrISP® system of assessment
- Management of a major transfusion reaction
- Imaging in head injury
- FAST scanning
- Interpreting a supine abdominal radiograph
- Interpreting the abdominal radiograph in possible bowel obstruction

⊕ Technical skills and procedures

- Emergency thoracotomy
- Diagnostic peritoneal lavage
- Emergency laparotomy in trauma
- Urethrography
- Principles of arterial repair
- Emergency diagnostic laparoscopy
- Video-assisted thoracoscopic surgery
- Emergency laparotomy
- Open appendicectomy
- Laparoscopic appendicectomy
- Segmental colectomy and end colostomy (Hartmann's procedure)
- Patch repair of perforated ulcer
- Incision and drainage of abscess/cyst
- Surgery for major soft tissue infection

8.1 Advanced Trauma Life Support™

Trauma is the leading cause of death in the first four decades of life and three times as many people are left permanently disabled. The Advance Trauma Life Support (ATLS) program is now the accepted standard for the first hour of trauma care of the injured patient.

The distribution of deaths is trimodal.

1. **Instant** death or within minutes of injury. The brain, high spinal cord or major blood vessels are the sites of injury. These patients are almost never salvageable owing to lack of rapid pre-hospital care

2. **Early** death, within minutes to several hours of injury. This period is often defined as the 'golden hour,' during which ATLS interventions can have a marked improvement on outcome

3. **Late** death occurs days to weeks after injury. It is often due to sepsis or multiple organ dysfunction. Good initial care reduces morbidity and mortality rates

Initial assessment and management

Seriously injured patients require prompt assessment and instigation of life-saving therapy. A systematic approach called the '**initial assessment**' has been developed and is outlined below.

1. Preparation
2. Triage
3. Primary survey
4. Resuscitation
5. Adjuncts to primary survey
6. Secondary survey
7. Adjuncts to secondary survey
8. Post-resuscitation monitoring and re-evaluation
9. Definitive care

1. Preparation

Preparation takes place as a **pre-hospital** and an **in-hospital phase**. During the pre-hospital phase, airway, immobilization, and control of major haemorrhage takes place. Communication with the receiving hospital (preferably a trauma centre) and fast transfer is key.

The in-hospital phase of preparation involves assembling the trauma team to receive the casualty and ensuring that all of the equipment is ready. Personnel must take universal precautions, with a minimum of eye protection, apron, and gloves.

2. Triage

Patients are triaged in the pre-hospital setting based on the need for treatment given the available resources. Priorities are usually based on ABC. It is also the responsibility of the pre-hospital team to allocate patients to the most appropriate hospital.

With **multiple casualties** that will not exceed the ability of the receiving centre to provide care, patients with life-threatening injuries are treated first.

In a situation with **mass casualties**, where the number of patients exceeds the ability of the receiving centre to provide care, patients with the greatest chance of survival are treated first.

3. Primary survey

Life-saving measures are initiated when a problem is identified. The primary survey is led by the team leader.

A Airway maintenance with cervical spine protection
B Breathing and ventilation
C Circulation with haemorrhage control
D Disability and neurological status
E Exposure and environmental control

4. Resuscitation

During the primary survey, aggressive resuscitation and management of life-threatening injuries take place. If the patient requires transfer to a different unit, this should be initiated at this point.

5. Adjuncts to primary survey

Monitoring

- Pulse oximetry
- Blood pressure
- ECG monitoring giving heart rate and rhythm
- Arterial blood gas

Urinary or gastric catheter

Urinary output reflects renal perfusion and is a sensitive indicator of circulating volume. Transurethral catheterization is contraindicated if urethral trauma is suspected (blood at penile meatus, blood in scrotum, perineal bruising, high-riding prostate, pelvic fracture).

A nasogastric tube reduces the risk of aspiration in patients with a distended stomach. It should be passed orally if there is a suspected cribriform plate fracture.

Radiographs and diagnostic tests

Radiological tests should not delay the resuscitation. They should be performed in the resuscitation area with a portable machine.

- Lateral cervical spine radiograph
- AP chest radiograph
- AP pelvis radiograph
- Diagnostic peritoneal lavage or abdominal USS

6. Secondary survey

The secondary survey starts once the patient is beginning to normalize and resuscitation is in full progress. The AMPLE history and a top-to-toe examination of the patient is completed.

- **A**llergies
- **M**edications
- **P**ast illness and **P**regnancy
- **L**ast ate or drank
- **E**vents and **E**nvironment related to injury

7. Adjuncts to secondary survey

Other specialized imaging and tests may be performed at this stage. The patient must be stable enough to be transferred to another area of the hospital.

- Further C-spine views (AP and odontoid peg views)
- CT scan
- Contrast radiographs
- Extremity radiographs
- Endoscopy and USS

8. Monitoring and re-evaluation

The injured patient must be constantly re-evaluated. This includes re-assessing ABC and ensuring that the results of blood tests, ECG monitoring, urine output, and imaging are not ignored. Also ensure at this point that the patient has had adequate analgesia.

9. Definitive care

Definitive care of a patient depends on the injuries. It may be the operating theatre, observation ward or transfer to another hospital.

Table 8.1 Primary survey

	Assessment	Management options
Airway and C-spine control	Look for signs of agitation (hypoxia), obtundation (hypercarbia), and accessory muscle use Listen for abnormal breath sounds (snoring, stridor, gurgling) Feel for tracheal deviation Suspect cervical spine injury	In-line immobilization of C-spine Oxygen therapy (saturations >95%) Chin lift and jaw thrust Oropharyngeal airway Nasopharyngeal airway Definitive airway—endotracheal Definitive airway—surgical
Breathing	Look for adequate and symmetrical chest wall movement. Asymmetry suggests flail chest or splinting. Listen for movement of air both on sides of chest. Decreased, altered or absent breath sounds suggests intrathoracic injury Pulse oximetry	Initiation of life-saving techniques (needle or tube thoracostomy) Continued oxygen therapy (face mask with reservoir bag) whilst self-ventilating Bag-valve-face mask ventilation Intubation and ventilation
Circulation and haemorrhage control	Look for obvious haemorrhage Assess pulse and blood pressure	Wide-bore peripheral access Initiate fluid resuscitation (warmed colloid/crystalloid/blood if required)
Disability	Determine level of consciousness with AVPU (A, alert; V, responds to voice; P, responds to pain; U, unresponsive) or GCS Assess pupils	GCS <8 is defined as a coma. These patients require a definitive airway
Exposure	Undress patient, removing soiled clothing to allow full assessment	Prevent hypothermia with warming device

Table 8.2 Secondary survey

	Assessment	Investigations to consider
Conscious level	Glasgow Coma Scale Score	CT brain
Pupils	Size Shape Reactivity	CT brain
Head	Scalp injury (lacerations) Skull injury (palpable fracture)	CT head
Maxillofacial	Soft tissue injury (lacerations) Bone injury (fracture) Teeth/mouth injury (malocclusion)	Facial bone radiographs or CT scan of facial bones
Neck	C-spine injury (pain/tenderness) Laryngeal/airway injury (subcutaneous emphysema) Neurological deficit Vascular injury (haematoma) Oesophageal injury	C-spine radiographs Endoscopy (OGD, laryngoscopy) Carotid angiography or duplex USS
Chest	Thoracic wall injury (subcutaneous emphysema, tenderness) Pneumothorax/haemothorax (altered auscultation) Bronchial injury Mediastinal injury (aortic disruption)	Chest radiograph CT chest Angiography Bronchoscopy Transoesophageal USS
Abdomen	Abdominal wall Intraperitoneal injury Retroperitoneal injury	DPL/FAST USS CT abdomen
Pelvis	Genitourinary tract injuries (inspect external genitalia + rectal and vaginal examination) Pelvic fracture (pelvic tenderness, widened symphysis)	GU contrast studies Contrast CT abdomen and pelvis Pelvic radiographs
Spinal cord	Cranial injury Cord injury Peripheral nerve injury	Spine radiographs MRI spine
Vertebral column	Column injury Vertebral instability Nerve injury	Spine radiographs CT vertebral column
Extremities	Soft tissue (compartment syndrome) Bone deformity Joint abnormality Neurovascular injury	Compartment pressures Extremity radiographs Angiography

8.2 Care of the critically ill surgical patient®

Critical illness may develop suddenly but usually evolves over a period of time.

Early detection is often difficult, but prompt treatment is critical to optimizing outcome in critically ill emergency and ward patients since treatment in the more obvious advanced stages is much more difficult and less successful.

Patients at risk

Preoperative assessment of surgical patients is important in identifying patients at greater risk of the development of critical illness and adverse responses to it. Particular risk factors for developing critical illness include:

- advanced age
- co-morbidities (e.g. renal failure, diabetes mellitus, smoking, occlusive vascular disease)
- major surgery
- multiple injuries
- malnutrition (starvation or obesity)
- massive blood transfusion
- immunosuppression (e.g. drug-induced, malignancy, malnutrition)

Early warning scoring systems

Scoring systems for vital signs are used on the ward as screening tools to identify unwell patients to prompt early review by experienced clinicians.

A score of between one and three is allocated for each of six parameters (respiratory rate, heart rate, systolic blood pressure, conscious level, temperature, and hourly urine output). The more abnormal a parameter is the higher the score. If the combined score exceeds a preset threshold it triggers the call for senior medical assistance.

CCrISP assessment

The Royal College of Surgeons of England has developed the Care of the Critically Ill Surgical Patient (CCrISP®) systematic approach for assessment and management of critically ill patients (see box). The ABCDE approach guides the initial assessment and management, and this is followed by a more detailed review of history and systematic examination.

Respiratory

Critical indicators

- High respiratory rate >20 per min
- Low oxygen saturations SaO_2 <95%
- High $PaCO_2$ >6.5 kPa

Aims

- Protect airway
- Maintain oxygenation
- Support ventilation (📖 Topic 15.12)

Cardiovascular

Critical indicators

- Poor peripheral perfusion (cool, reduce capillary return)
- Heart rate <45 bpm or >130 bpm
- Hypotension <100 mmHg
- Ischaemia or new onset arrhythmia on ECG

Aims

- Optimize fluid status
- Optimize cardiac output and oxygen delivery
- Appropriate perfusion pressure
- Treat arrhythmias; if possible maintain sinus rhythm

Renal

Critical indicators

- Urine output <0.5 mL/kg/h
- Raised urea and creatinine

Aims

- Optimize fluid status
- Normal blood pressure for individual patient to ensure good renal blood flow
- Avoid nephrotoxic drugs
- Consider renal replacement therapy

Gastrointestinal

Critical indicators

- Weight loss
- Low serum albumin
- Gastric ulceration

Aims

- Nutritional support to meet requirements (📖 Topic 4.2)
- Stress ulcer prophylaxis—early enteral feeding provides protection by maintaining a protective layer within the stomach. If there is any history of peptic ulcer disease or the patient is not being enterally fed, pharmacological prophylaxis should be started with a proton-pump inhibitor or histamine-2 antagonist

Neurological

Critical indicators

- AVPU and GCS used to score neurological status
- Pupillary reaction

Aims

- Exclude underlying causes—hypoxia, hypovolaemia, hypoglycaemia and drugs
- Improve cerebral perfusion by controlling mean arterial pressure and intracranial pressure (📖 Topic 10.1)
- Anxiolysis and appropriate sedation

Decision-making

The key question is: 'stable or unstable?' This will guide your decisions on further management, investigations, involvement of other specialists, and the level of care a patient needs (Table 8.3). Regular review ensures that the patient continues to progress rather than deteriorate.

Patients with two or more organ dysfunctions or respiratory failure unresponsive to non-invasive ventilation need to be managed in an intensive care setting.

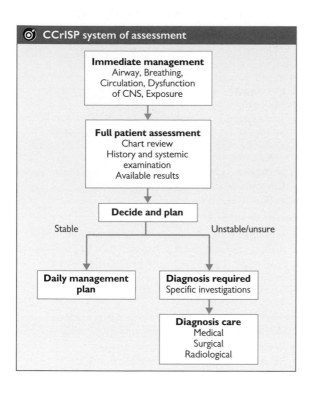

CCrISP system of assessment

Immediate management
Airway, Breathing,
Circulation, Dysfunction
of CNS, Exposure

Full patient assessment
Chart review
History and systemic
examination
Available results

Decide and plan

Stable   Unstable/unsure

**Daily management
plan**

Diagnosis required
Specific investigations

Diagnosis care
Medical
Surgical
Radiological

Table 8.3 Daily plan for stable patients	
Action point	**Options**
Investigations	Blood tests Radiology Special investigations
Specialist opinions	
Fluid balance	Maintenance Additional losses Target input and output
Nutritional requirements	Calorie requirement Supplementary feeding Route
Medications	Treatment of current condition Prophylaxis Regular medications
Occupational health and physiotherapy	Chest Mobility
Psychosocial needs	Psychology review
Level of care	Observations Move to lower level

8.3 Shock

Shock is an acute circulatory disturbance leading to inadequate end-organ perfusion and tissue oxygenation.

Aetiology

True hypovolaemia

- Blood loss (trauma, major surgery)*
- Dehydration*
- Burns

Relative hypovolaemia

- Sepsis*
- Anaphylaxis
- Neurogenic
- Adrenal insufficiency (Addisonian crisis)

Cardiogenic

- Myocardial infarction*
- Dysrhythmias (tachycardia or bradycardia)

Obstructive

- Cardiac tamponade
- Pulmonary embolus
- Tension pneumothorax

(*=common causes in surgical patients)

NB. 'Cellular shock' is the phenomenon of inadequate cellular utilization of oxygen owing to poisoning or cellular dysfunction but leads to the same cellular results.

Pathophysiology

Direct cellular effects

- Decreased tissue oxygenation results in low intracellular oxygen and a failure of mitochondrial oxidative phosphorylation
- Decreased production of high energy ATP leads to cellular dependence on low energy output via glycolysis
- Glycolysis increases the production of lactate, causing cellular acidosis and dysfunction. This results in membrane leakage and eventual cell death

$$ADP + P_i + H^+ + O_2 \text{ (energy)} \leftrightarrow ATP + H_2O$$

(ADP=adenosine diphosphate, ATP=adenosine triphosphate, P_i=inorganic phosphate, H^+=hydrogen ion)

Indirect tissue effects

- Cellular dysfunction increases intercellular gap junction leakage and membrane permeability (gut, capillary, lung alveoli, and general tissues)
- Increased permeability leads to interstitial oedema and organ dysfunction, leading to a spiral of decay (☐ Topic 8.4)

Principles of clinical assessment

Clinical assessment may go hand in hand with early management/resuscitation according to CCrISP protocols.

Identification of the cause

Some causes are obvious owing to the pattern or situation:

- Anaphylaxis—associated acute severe oedema, bronchospasm, vasodilatation, and collapse

In post-surgical patients there may be several causes or several factors together. There are general patterns but they are not always easy to spot:

- Hypovolaemia—cold peripheries, delayed capillary refill time, tachycardia, and hypotension (especially reduced pulse pressure). Clinical signs and observations can be used to estimate blood loss (Table 8.4)
- Cardiogenic—hypotension, tachycardia (unless due to brady-dysrhythmia), tachypnoea, raised CVP (JVP)
- Sepsis (☐ Topic 8.4)

Investigations—basic

- 12-lead ECG assesses cardiac dysrhythmias as a primary cause; *however*, remember 40% of all cardiac dysrhythmias occurring on a surgical ward are caused by underlying conditions, particularly sepsis
- Pulse oximetry may indicate need for HDU transfer for respiratory support
- Urinary catheter—hourly urine output (surrogate marker of GFR, renal blood flow, and hence systemic perfusion
- Bloods
- FBC, U+Es, G+S (cross-match if there is evidence of bleeding)
- Arterial blood gas to assess acid–base balance. Metabolic acidosis is common in any established cause of shock but raised lactate is the hallmark
- Blood cultures if sepsis is a possible cause

Investigations—selective/advanced

An indication for any of these suggests a patient who would best be managed in a critical care environment.

- Continuous ECG—to monitor rhythm or rate (usually done on HDU or ITU)
- CVP—to monitor fluid resuscitation status
- Arterial line—if continuous arterial pressure monitoring or repeated blood gas analysis required
- Radiology e.g. CT scan, if an underlying septic cause is sought; CXR if the suspected cause is cardiogenic or obstructive
- Transoesophageal Doppler—best non-invasive assessment of cardiac function, filling, and response to fluid resuscitation
- Pulmonary artery catheter (PAC)('Swan–Ganz catheter')—rarely used owing to complications and limited use, particularly in septic shock or MODS

Management

Emergency – resuscitation

All patients are likely to need basic manoeuvres whatever the cause of the shock:

- Oxygen—high flow via a non-rebreathing bag–mask with continuous pulse oxygen saturation monitoring
- IV fluid bolus—20 mL/kg isotonic crystalloid. Unless the cause is certainly cardiogenic shock, this limited volume fluid resuscitation is very rarely harmful and may be vitally important

Table 8.4 Classification of hypovolaemic shock

	Class I	Class II	Class III	Class IV
Blood loss (mL)	<750	750–1500	1500–2000	>2000
Blood loss (% volume)	<15 %	15–30 %	30–40 %	>40%
Pulse rate (bpm)	<100	>100	>120	>140
Blood pressure	Normal	Normal	Decreased	Decreased
Pulse pressure	Normal or increased	Decreased	Decreased	Decreased
Respiratory rate (/min)	14–20	20–30	30–40	>35
Urine output (mL)	>30	20–30	5–15	Negligible
Mental state	Slightly anxious	Mildly anxious	Anxious/confused	Confused/lethargic
Fluid replacement	Crystalloid	Crystalloid	Crystalloid and blood	Crystalloid and blood

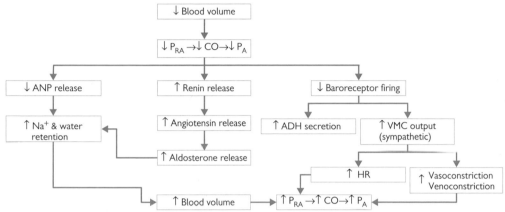

Fig 8.1 Physiology of the responses to hypovolaemia. P_{RA}, right atrial pressure; P_A, arterial pressure; CO, cardiac output; ADH, antidiuretic hormone; VMC, vasomotor centre; ANP, atrial natriuretic peptide, HR, heart rate.

Continuing management by cause

Hypovolaemic (including relative hypovolemia)

- Control ongoing blood loss by direct pressure or intervention (including laparotomy/thoracotomy)
- Maintenance of circulating volumes, e.g. initial rapid crystalloid infusion, blood transfusion
  - Assess response in terms of ↓HR, ↑BP, ↑ peripheral perfusion, ↑urine output
  - Rapid response = minimal loss with no need for further aggressive fluid resuscitation
  - Transient response = ongoing blood loss or inadequate fluid resuscitation. May need blood transfusion
  - Minimal response = critical hypovolemia and inadequate fluid resuscitation, possible ongoing haemorrhage. Almost certain to need blood transfusion
- Support of cardiac function

Anaphylaxis (adult)

- ABCDE, call for help
- IM adrenaline 500 mcg (0.5 mL of 1:1000 solution). Repeat after 5 mins PRN
- IV fluid challenge 500—1000mL (crystalloid)

- Slow IV or IM chlorphenamine 10 mg and hydrocortisone 200 mg

Sepsis—see Topic 8.4

Cardiogenic

- Optimization of rate and rhythm
- Optimization of fluid balance ('preload')
- Optimization of systemic vascular resistance ('afterload'), e.g. vasopressor, vasodilators
- Optimization of cardiac function, e.g. inotropes, chronotropes, lusiotropes

Special cases

Pregnancy causes maternal hypervolaemia which can lead to underestimation of the degree of shock

Athletes have ↑compensation due to hypervolaemia and improved cardiac output which can lead to underestimation of the degree of shock

Advanced age leads to ↓cardiac compliance and ↑organ sensitivity to hypoperfusion. Resuscitation needs to be carefully monitored to avoid fluid overloading

Hypothermia leads to ↓cardiovascular responses, ↑risk of coagulopathy, ↑'rewarming hypovolaemia'

8.4 SIRS and sepsis

Definitions

SIRS is a systemic inflammatory response characterized by the presence of two or more of the following.

- Core temp >38°C or <36°C
- Tachycardia >90 bpm
- Tachypnoea >20 bpm or $PaCO_2$ <4.3 kPa
- Neutrophil count >12x10^9/L or <4x10^9/L

Sepsis is the presence of SIRS with a proven source of infection.

Septic shock is sepsis with features of shock (see above).

MODS (multiple organ dysfunction syndrome) is the requirement for organ support of two or more organ systems in the presence of SIRS.

Aetiology

SIRS is a non-specific response to a range of injuries, including the following.

- Severe inflammation, e.g. acute pancreatitis, drug, and transfusion reactions
- Infection, e.g. pneumonia, peritonitis, severe colitis
- Injury—multiple trauma, major surgery, burns
- Immune reaction, e.g. severe type IV reactions
- Ischaemia–reperfusion injury

Thirty per cent of patients with SIRS will go on to be diagnosed with sepsis.

Pathophysiology

The underlying pathogenesis is a cellular response to inflammatory mediators:

- **iNOS (inducible nitric oxide synthase)**—activated by endothelial cell injury; NO massively increases capillary endothelial cellular leakage, activates neutrophils and macrophages, potent negative inotrope, and vasodilator
- **Interleukins IL-6, IL-1β**—released by neutrophils and macrophages, induce wideranging chemokine and cytokine release, activate complement
- **TNFα**—released by and potent activator of macrophages and neutrophils
- **PAF (platelet-activating factor)**—released in inflammation (e.g. pancreatitis), induces platelet degranulation

Primary insult

↓

Primary cytokine/chemokine activation

↓

Amplification of release (related to additional/ongoing insults, genetic profile, underlying co-morbidity)

↓

Failure of downregulation of cytokine release (genetic profile) ↓ release of IL-4, IL-10

↓

Reticuloendothelial cell activation, complement activation, and coagulation disorder development

↓

End-organ dysfunction

Endothelial cell dysfunction

- Activated by iNOS, TNFα, IL-6
- Activation results in capillary leakage, production of further mediators, induction of complement, and promotion of endovascular coagulation cascade

- Irreversible endothelial cell dysfunction is a major contributor to resistant SIRS/MODS and resulting mortality

Disorders of coagulation

- Pro-inflammatory mediators (e.g. PAF, IL-6) and exposed capillary subendothelium lead to activation of the coagulation cascade and ↑expression of tissue factor (TF). TF acts as a key mediator between the immune system and coagulation
- ↓Production of activated protein C (which acts to ↓ thrombin production, ↓endothelial cytokine release, ↓neutrophil activation) allows uncontrolled intravascular coagulation
- Fibrinolysis—↑fibrinolysis promoted by interleukins and complement activation
- The most pronounced manifestation of coagulation disorder is **disseminated intravascular coagulation (DIC)** with unchecked intravascular coagulation and associated unchecked fibrinolysis and haemolysis

Clinical assessment and management

Follow CCrISP guidelines. Immediate life-threatening problems should be identified and treated before definitive assessment and management of the underlying problems. Clinical deterioration is usually progressive, and early diagnosis improves survival.

Immediate

A—Airway

- Ensure the airway is open (jaw thrust, Geudel® airway). If the patient is so obtunded that the airway is compromised, put out a 'peri' arrest call—they are critically ill and will need intensive care treatment

B—Breathing

- Give high flow O_2 via a non-rebreathe mask
- Monitor peripheral oxygen saturations continuously

C—Circulation

- IV fluid bolus; 500 mL crystalloid repeated as necessary (📖 Topic 8.3)
- Central venous line (CVL) insertion is *not* part of the immediate resuscitation (it often takes too long and is only really useful once the patient has had first line treatment and is often best done on HDU/ITU)

Full assessment

- Investigations—take a full blood screen, including blood cultures, sample any available fluids for microbiology (e.g. urine, contents of drains, sputum, wound discharge). Specimens should be taken before administration of antibiotics if possible. CXR is helpful, AXR rarely is
- Examination/chart review—there may be multiple possible causes of SIRS. Some key areas to think about are:
- is there an untreated source of intra-abdominal or intrathoracic infection (undiagnosed leak, abscess/collection)?
- is there an atypical chest infection with minimal signs?
- is there a spreading deep soft tissue infection?

Table 8.5 Vasoactive and cardioactive drugs in SIRS/sepsis

	Actions/target receptor	Effects/uses
Epinephrine (adrenaline)	High affinity—β_1 and β_2 Low affinity—α_1	Primarily to augment cardiac contractility and rate Effects on SVR depend on dose and situation ($\uparrow$SVR in profound vasodilatation (e.g. sepsis), $\downarrow$SVR in cardiogenic shock)
Norepinephrine (noradrenaline)	High affinity—α_1 Low affinity—β_1 and β_2	Primarily to maintain SVR when inappropriately low (e.g. sepsis) Some $\uparrow$cardiac output
Dobutamine	β_1	Primarily to augment cardiac contractility in low cardiac output states
Milrinone	PDEI	$\uparrow$Cardiac contractility and relaxation in cardiogenic shock and cardiac dysfunction in SIRS/sepsis
Dopamine	High affinity—DA_1, β_1 and β_2 Low affinity—α_1	Limited uses. Most effects come via minor $\uparrow$in cardiac output due to β receptor effects

Target	Effects	Uses
PDE	$\uparrow$Cardiac contractility (inotropism) $\uparrow$Cardiac muscle relaxation (luistropy)	$\uparrow$Cardiac output $\downarrow$SVR
α_1	$\uparrow$Arteriolar/venous smooth muscle constriction	$\uparrow$SVR, $\uparrow$CVP
DA_1	$\uparrow$ Intrarenal vasodilatation $\uparrow$ Mesenteric vasodilatation	
β_1	$\uparrow$Cardiac contractility (inotropism) $\uparrow$Cardiac rate (chronotropism) $\uparrow$Cardiac muscle relaxation (luistropy)	$\uparrow$Cardiac output
β_2	$\downarrow$Smooth muscle tone	Splanchnic vasodilatation Bronchodilatation

PDEI, Phosphodiesterase inhibitor; SVR, systemic vascular resistance.

Ongoing diagnosis and management

Always think of these questions.

- **Does the patient need critical care?** Established SIRS can be managed on a surgical ward but the presence of shock, the need for respiratory, renal or cardiovascular support or more invasive monitoring indicate the need for transfer
- **Is there a source of sepsis to treat?** Consider changing vascular access lines, catheters, and management of superficial sepsis. For the role of advanced investigations see Topic 8.3
- **Is advanced radiological imaging needed?** CT scanning will identify sources of sepsis which need treatment (which may include radiological drainage), but the patient must be stabilized before transfer; CT scanners are often far from sources of support

Antibiotics

- Always give broad spectrum antibiotics IV; in SIRS there is little to be lost
- If the patient is already on treatment then consider changing or broadening the spectrum. If not, then give empirical treatment (e.g. IV Tazocin®, Impinenen®, Tigicil®)
- If the patient has been an inpatient for a while, consider adding antifungal treatment
- Always tailor treatment in response to microbiological sensitivities as soon as available
- Seek microbiological advice early on

Vasoactive treatments and inotropes (Table 8.5)

Vasoactive agents may be indicated when fluid resuscitation and additional boluses have not restored blood pressure.

Inotropes may be indicated in patients with a low cardiac output despite adequate filling.

The overall objective is to improve systemic blood pressure and blood flow resulting in restored tissue perfusion, but derangements of (micro)circulation in SIRS mean that pressure, flow, and perfusion do not always relate to each other as they do in health.

Advanced therapies

- Steroids are highly debatable in patients in septic shock unless there is an abnormal ACTH response
- Recombinant human-activated protein C has been used to give anti-inflammatory and anticoagulation effects but is unproven
- Close glycaemic control (serum glucose level <8.3 mmol/L using a continuous Insulin sliding scale). This should be combined with a nutrition protocol that preferentially uses the enteric route
- Thromboprophylaxis and stress ulcer prophylaxis should be given to all patients.

Complications and prognosis

SIRS and associated conditions are associated with significant morbidity and mortality rates:

- SIRS mortality = 7%
- sepsis mortality = 15%
- septic shock = 45%

Good communication is needed to keep the patient and the family aware of the care plan and likely prognosis.

Less aggressive care or withdrawal of support may be in the patient's best interest.

8.5 Blood products and transfusion

Whole blood = cells (red, white, platelets) + plasma.
Plasma = serum + clotting factors.

Serum = water, electrolytes, proteins, and suspended nutrients (e.g. LDL, HDL).

Group & save and cross-match

All blood cells (red, white, and platelets) have very many different antigens on their surface. The risk of a reaction to those antigens depends on the existence of preformed antibodies, previous exposure to those antigens, and the number and rate of antigens exposed.

ABO antigens—two alleles, each of which may code for protein 'tail' A, B or neither (O absent) or red cell surface antigens. All humans have pre-existing antibodies to those antigens which they do not possess (probably owing to in utero exposure to antigens).

Rh system—three pairs of alleles (C, D, and E), each of which code for either the presence (e.g. D +ve) or absence (e.g. D -ve) of cell surface antigen tails. Type D is the most prevalent (85%) and antigenic. Most humans do not possess preformed antibodies to RhD, RhE or RhC but they are formed readily by negative individuals on exposure to positive blood cells.

Minor antigens (e.g. Kell, Kidd, Duffy)—a near infinite range of pairs of alleles coding for the presence or absence of different surface antigenic tails. Humans only form antibodies to these antigens upon significant or repeated exposure.

Table 8.6 **ABO system**			
Genotype	**Phenotype**	**Antigens**	**Antibodies**
OO	O (47%)	None	Anti A and B
AA or AO	A (41%)	A	Anti B
BB or BO	B (9%)	B	Anti A
AB	AB (3%)	A and B	None

'Group and save'—means that the sample will be tested for the ABO and RhD status and the serum will be stored for possible further use. It is virtually never necessary to administer a blood transfusion using only the results of blood group analysis to match the blood. In extremis, type O RhD -ve blood (universal donor) can be given to recipients of any ABO/Rh group with a low risk of transfusion reaction.

Cross-match—means that the serum of the intended recipient is mixed with the red cells of the intended donor unit in the presence of activated complement to check if there is a reaction. This can be performed in less than 20 min if the lab is aware of the urgency.

Extended analysis (to identify the minor antigens responsible for a reaction) is a long and complex procedure only performed for patients in whom multiple transfusions give rise to problems of cross-matching blood.

Blood components

Blood components are produced from whole blood using centrifugation and require no further processing.

Whole blood (475 mL is added to 63 mL of anticoagulant), stored at 4°C, shelf-life of 5 weeks, rarely used

Packed red cells (1 unit = 280 mL) is a suspension of plasma-reduced red blood cells + preservative (e.g. SAG-M; saline, adenine, glucose, and mannitol) or CPD-adenine (citrate, phosphate, dextrose, and adenine).

- One unit of PRCs raises the haemoglobin by ~1 g/dL. Must be fully cross-matched
- Stored at 2–6°C, shelf-life of 35 days
- Used to increase the Hb (oxygen-carrying capacity) of the blood *not* as an intravascular volume expander without additional crystalloid infusions. Typically used if Hb <7g/dL (<9.5 g/dL in older patients and those with cardiorespiratory disease maintain)

Platelets (1 unit = 50 mL), pooled from 4 units of blood from a single donor. One unit of platelets increases platelet count by 100×10^9/L in a 70 kg adult.

- Do not need to be cross-matched but they should be ABO-compatible (and Rh-matched in women of childbearing age)
- Stored on an agitator at 22°C, shelf-life of 5 days
- Used for low platelet count or in active bleeding

Fresh frozen plasma (1 unit = 150–250 mL) contains all the coagulation factors except platelets. May be from a single donor or pooled. 1 mL of FFP per kg will raise most clotting factors by 1% in a 70 kg adult.

- Does not need to be cross-matched but should be ABO-compatible (and Rh-matched in women of childbearing age)
- Stored at −30°C, thawed over 20 min, shelf-life once thawed 2 h
- Used to counter the effects of massive blood transfusion or to temporarily reverse the effect of warfarin

Cryoprecipitate (1 unit = 20 mL) contains fibrinogen and factors VII, VIII, and XIII. Between five and ten pooled bags are normally given, but if cryoprecipitate is unavailable 5 units of FFP contain the same amount of fibrinogen as 10 units of cryoprecipitate.

- Ten bags of cryoprecipitate raise the fibrinogen 0.6–0.7 mg/L in a 70 kg adult
- Does not need to be ABO- or Rh-compatible

Blood products are derived from plasma and require complex steps to produce. They include human albumin solution, coagulation factor concentrate, and immunoglobulin solutions.

Pre-transfusion testing

All donated blood is routinely screened for hepatitis B, hepatitis C, HIV 1 and 2, HTLV, and syphilis. Other pre-donation processing includes:

- **Leukoreduction**—the further removal of stray white blood cells, reducing the chance of alloimmunization and febrile transfusion reactions. It is used in chronically transfused patients, transplant recipients, and patients with a history of febrile non-haemolytic transfusion reaction
- **Irradiated** blood is used in severely immunosuppressed patients and those at risk of transfusion-related graft-versus-host-disease
- **Cytomegalovirus** (CMV) infects leucocytes and many people are asymptomatic carriers. CMV-negative and leuko-reduced blood products are used in immunosuppressed patients to reduce CMV transmission and potential infection.

Complications of blood transfusion

Immunological

Acute haemolytic reaction

- This may be caused by ABO incompatibility as a result of clerical, bedside, sampling or laboratory error. It may also be caused by incompatibility within other antigen systems (Duffy/Kidd). Mediated by pre-formed recipient antibodies to donor erythrocytes, resulting in complement formation, membrane attack complex, and immediate haemolysis
- Cytokine and chemokine release mediates sympathetic inflammatory response characterized by sudden onset of hypotension, tachycardia, pyrexia, breathlessness, tachypnoea, and back pain. Haemolysis leads to anaemia, bilirubinaemia, and haemoglobinuria.

Non-haemolytic febrile reactions

- These reactions occur in 2% of transfusions. They are normally mild reactions caused by recipient antibodies directed against donor HLA and leucocyte-specific antigen on leucocytes and platelets
- Cytokine release mediates a mild pyrexia, typically over an hour after transfusion is started. Antipyrogens such as paracetamol 1 g po/pr limit pyrexia, but antihistamines are not helpful. Severe reactions feature high grade fever, rigors, nausea, and vomiting. The severity of symptoms is proportional to the number of leucocytes in the transfused blood and rate of transfusion. Leucocyte-depleted blood helps to prevent these reactions

Delayed extravascular haemolytic reaction

- Due to very low levels of pre-formed recipient antibodies to antigens (commonly Rhesus E, Kell, Duffy or Kidd), the production of which is enhanced on exposure to the antigen. There is accelerated destruction of transfused red blood cells 7–10 days following transfusion
- Pre-transfusion cross-match is unremarkable
- Haemolysis is extravascular, making haemoglobinaemia and haemoglobinuria uncommon. Characterized by an unexpected fall in haematocrit a few days post-transfusion, hyperbilirubinaemia and positive Coombs test

Anaphylaxis and allergic reactions

- Normally IgE-mediated histamine release reactions to plasma, platelets, and red blood cells. Mild allergic reactions are relatively common, and are characterized by erythematous papular rashes, wheals, pruritus, and pyrexia. These are treated by stopping the transfusion and administering chlorpheniramine. Anaphylaxis characterized by hypotension, bronchospasm, and angioedema occasionally occurs.

Transfusion-related acute lung injury

- Non-cardiogenic pulmonary oedema typically within 6 h of transfusion; mediated by recipient antibodies against donor HLA. Activated recipient leucocytes migrate to the lung, releasing proteolytic enzymes that cause a localized capillary leak syndrome and pulmonary oedema

Post-transfusion purpuric reaction

- Occurs a week following the transfusion and is a result of a reaction to platelet antigens

Graft-versus-host disease

- Rare complication in which donor lymphocytes mediate an immune response against the recipient

Infective

May be contamination of stored blood products with bacteria, although platelets, which are usually stored at room temperature, are at greater risk.

- Bacteria: *Staphylococcus* spp., *Enterobacter*, *Yersinia*, and *Pseudomonas* spp.
- Viral: CMV, EBV, HIV, HTLV, HCV, HBV
- Others: rickettsial diseases, protozoal disease (trypanosomiasis, malaria), filariasis, nvCJD

Contamination is difficult to detect. The recipient becomes pyrexial at above >40°C, and hypotensive. This may occur during the transfusion or hours after completion, and, unlike febrile transfusion reactions, is not self-limiting.

HIV can be transmitted by an infective but seronegative donor for about 15 days after infection. The HCV window is 20 days. CMV is common in the donor population (40–60%), and immunocompromised donors must receive leucocyte-depleted or CMV-negative blood.

Chronic blood transfusion

Iron overload can be seen in chronic blood transfusion.

Massive transfusion

Massive transfusion is defined as transfusion of a patient's total blood volume within 24 h. It is associated with a number of complications.

- Hypothermia if the blood is not warmed
- Hyperkalaemia owing to leakage of K^+ from red blood cells
- Hypocalcaemia as the citrate in the preservative binds Ca^{2+}
- Fluid overload resulting in pulmonary oedema
- Thrombocytopenia owing to dilution of functioning platelets
- Coagulopathy as PRCs are deficient in coagulation factors
- Reduced 2,3-diphosphoglycerate, leading to inadequate tissue oxygenation

---

Management of a major transfusion reaction

- Stop the transfusion
- 'ABC'
- Gain wide-bore IV access
- Give O$_2$ by mask, paracetamol 1 g IV, and consider hydrocortisone 100 mg IV
- Take a serum sample for storage
- Monitor BP, HR, RR, and SaO$_2$. Any deterioration should prompt consideration of referral to HDU
- Acute haemolysis may require forced diuresis, treatment of acute hyperkalaemia, and treatment of respiratory distress (on HDU/ITU)
- Non-haemolytic reactions may require IM adrenaline, nebulized salbutamol, and IV therapy (on the ward or HDU). Diagnosis of the cause is necessary
- Send the giving set and any remnant of the last unit to the lab for culture, and analysis/checking of grouping

8.6 Traumatic head injury

Head injuries are common. Most insults are trivial but a minority cause serious traumatic brain injuries (TBI).

There are approximately 100 000 admissions per year (UK) as a result of head injuries. Fifty per cent of emergency department attendances are children under 16 years old.

Aetiology

Commonest causes are:

- children up to age 7 years: falls, non-accidental injury, road traffic accidents (RTAs)
- young adults: RTAs, assaults, occupational injuries, sports injuries
- elderly: falls, RTAs

Pathophysiology

Primary brain injury

Occurs at or shortly after the time of trauma and is caused by bony, parenchymal, and vascular disruption and resulting acute bleeding.

Secondary brain injury

Ongoing neuronal injury owing to hypoxia, hypotension, altered intracerebral circulation, and/or raised intracranial pressure (ICP). These cause cellular ischaemia, oedema, inflammation, and cellular disorganization.

- **Skull fractures**—may be skull base or cranial vault. Fractures can be open or closed, linear or depressed.
- **Cerebral contusions**—focal intraparenchymal haematomas, located at the site of impact of brain on bony prominences of the inner surface of the skull ('coup' and 'contra-coup') (Fig 8.2)
- **Extradural (epidural) haematoma** secondary to disruption of meningeal arteries (e.g. middle meningeal) commonly due to skull fracture. Primary injury may or may not be associated with LOC; rapid expansion leads to rapid reduction in consciousness after a period of lucidity
- **Acute subdural/subarachnoid haematoma**—bleeding from cortical surface or arachnoid vessels.
- **Diffuse axonal injury (DAI)**—disruption of axons and neuronal integrity owing to high energy rotational shearing forces, often at the grey–white matter junction

Clinical assessment

Clinical assessment often runs concurrently with initial management and should follow ATLS guidelines.

Recognizing mechanisms and patterns of injury

- Loss of consciousness indicates a significant energy transfer and is important
- A period of lucidity following initial injury always indicates that the primary injury is potentially survivable and subsequent loss of function is likely to be caused by treatable intracranial bleeding
- The maximum energy transferred to the skull is the best guide to likely injury severity (kinetic energy of missiles, velocity of impact, rapidity of deceleration, associated multiple injuries or injuries typical of high energy transfer)
- Subsequent post-injury seizure, progressive headache or vomiting are all significant and may indicate major intracranial pathology

- Any focal neurology is always serious (including abnormal pupils)
- A decrease of 2 or more points on the Glasgow Coma Scale (GCS) is significant

Patterns of injury

- **Deceleration** (e.g. head on RTA)—mainly anterior and posterior cerebral contusions, DAI, and occasionally subdural haemorrhage. Secondary brain injury is common
- **Direct impact** (e.g. playground falls)—skull fractures common, at risk of acute extradural haemorrhage, acute subdural haemorrhage rare
- **Low velocity missile** (e.g. arrow, shotgun)—skull fractures common, local contusion/damage limited, secondary haemorrhage possible
- **High velocity missile** (e.g. modern military rifle)—extensive skull fractures common, DAI common owing to 'shock wave' local contusion/damage extensive, secondary haemorrhage possible

Investigations

- Trauma series of radiographs as indicated.
- C-spine series of radiographs (AP, lateral and peg) or CT C-spine if head being scanned
- Bloods and ECG
- Plain skull radiographs have limited indications and have been superseded by head CT

Management

- Initial approach follows ATLS guidelines
- Assume that all head injuries have an associated unstable spinal injury until proved otherwise
- Head injuries are also commonly associated with other injuries involving the chest and abdomen
- The National Institute for Health and Clinical Excellence (NICE) has published guidelines on the investigation and management of head injuries

Prevention of secondary brain injury

- Ensure hypovolaemia is avoided—it is better to ensure adequate fluid resuscitation than worry about developing cerebral oedema
- Ensure hypoxia is avoided—adequate control of the airway and supplemental oxygen are vital from site of injury to the ITU
- Prevent metabolic disturbances—keep blood sugars controlled in diabetics. Corticosteroids have no role to play in traumatic brain injury

Skull fractures

- Open fractures should be explored to reduce the chance of infection. Depressed fractures should be elevated if they are causing compression of the brain or will leave a significant cosmetic defect
- Skull base fractures which injure the dura (indicated by otorrhoea or rhinorrhoea) usually heal spontaneously; however, discussion with your local neurosurgical team is advised. Prophylactic antibiotics are not routinely used but patients should be advised on symptoms and signs of meningitis to look out for

Acute extradural haemorrhage

- The diagnosis should always be confirmed on CT scan
- Transfer to a neurosurgical unit is always required unless the patient is truly *in extremis* where ipsilateral cranial burr holes are exceptionally rarely required
- Optimal treatment is craniotomy, evacuation of the haematoma, control of the bleeding point, and restoration of skull vault anatomy

Intracerebral injury (DAI, intracerebral/subdural haemorrhage)

- Always manage in an ITU/specialist neuroITU where possible (📖 Topic 10.1)
- Control of ICP via invasive monitoring, control of ventilation, control of circulating volume, and use of osmotic diuretics require specialist care

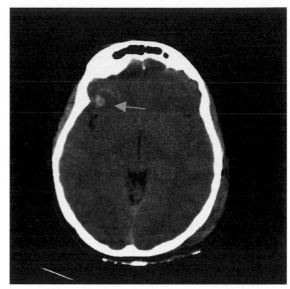

Fig 8.2 CT brain showing a right frontal contra-coup contusion (arrow). There is left parietal soft tissue swelling at the site of impact. The contusion has been caused by impact of the brain against the sphenoid ridge. There is no midline shift.

Table 8.7 Glasgow coma scale (GCS)

The GCS tests three categories which are each scored for the best response and then summed to give a total score of 3-15. Patients with a score of 8 or below are said to be in a coma.

Eye opening response

4	Spontaneous eye opening
3	Open in response to speech or noise
2	Open to painful stimulus
1	No eye opening

Verbal response

5	Orientated (normal conversation)
4	Confused conversation
3	Inappropriate speech (random words)
2	Incomprehensible speech (moaning)
1	No speech

Motor response

6	Obeys commands for movement
5	Localizes to pain (purposeful movement towards stimulus)
4	Withdraws away from painful stimulus
3	Abnormal flexor response to pain (decorticate posture)
2	Extensor response to pain (decerebrate posture)
1	No motor response

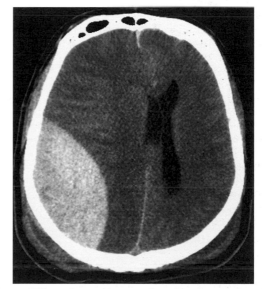

Fig 8.3 CT brain showing a bi-convex hyperdense lesion in the right parietal region representing an extradural haematoma. There is mass effect and midline shift to the left.

⊙ Imaging in head injury

CT head

Indications for a head CT scan (brain +/- cervical spine) are covered by the NICE head injury guidelines (CG4). They include:

- GCS <13 at initial assessment
- GCS 14 two hours post-injury
- any new neurological deficit
- any suspected skull base or depressed vault fracture
- post-traumatic seizure or vomiting

Spinal injuries may be classified into those that damage the bony and ligamentous spine and those that damage the spinal cord itself. Usually the latter is caused by instability from the former, although spinal cord injury without radiological abnormality (SCIWORA) exists.

Spinal cord injury

- There are ~500–700 traumatic spinal cord injuries (SCI) per year in the UK
- Peak age of incidence is 19 years

Aetiology

- Road traffic accidents
- Falls
- Workplace accidents
- Sporting activities (e.g. rugby, diving)
- Violent assaults

Pathophysiology

Primary injury

Direct disruption, vascular injury, and bleeding/contusion of the spinal cord. Neuronal injury and axonal disruption is almost always unrecoverable.

Secondary injury

Secondary injury is due to ischaemia, oedema, hypoxia, and loss of cellular and local circulatory homeostasis. This may be a vicious cycle owing to inflammation resulting in cord swelling within the bony spinal canal which may increase tissue pressure and reduce local tissue perfusion. In addition, spinal shock compromises tissue perfusion.

Patterns of SCI

Cord injuries may be **complete** (a loss of all function below the level of the lesion) or **incomplete** (distal sparing of motor or sensory function). Incomplete injuries may present in a variety of ways depending on the mechanism of injury:

- anterior cord
- posterior cord
- central cord
- Brown–Sequard (cord hemisection)
- cauda equina (Fig 10.21)

Spinal shock

This occurs after a SCI and may persist for up to 2 months. Damage to the spinal cord incites an inflammatory cascade. In this environment the highly sensitive neurons fail to conduct, and **neurological function below the level of the injury is significantly impaired**. Usually there is flaccid areflexia, priaprism, loss of anal tone, and loss of bulbocavernosus reflex.

Neurogenic shock

Neurogenic shock refers to the **cardiovascular effects of a loss of autonomic function below the level of a SCI**. (This is in contrast to spinal shock which refers to the neurological effects of the injury.) Loss of sympathetic tone causes a reflex dilatation of the arterioles controlling the major capillary beds. This rapid vasodilatation results in pooling of blood and an effective drop in circulating volume. This may precipitate cardiovascular crisis, especially in the case of a poly-trauma patient. The patient will be hypotensive with a paradoxical bradycardia. The skin will be erythematous, warm and dry.

Cervical spine injury

- Ten per cent of poly-trauma patients will have a cervical spine injury
- All major trauma or multiply-injured patients must be assumed to have a cervical spine injury until proven otherwise and managed by the ATLS protocol

Patterns of cervical spine injury

- *Jefferson's fracture*—compression injury causing a burst fracture of the ring of C1. The instability can be judged by the extent of outward displacement of the lateral masses of the atlas
- *Odontoid peg fractures*—classified by position of fracture line which indicates instability and risk of non-union
- *Hangman's fracture*—an extension injury causing bilateral fractures of the pedicles of C2 and potential dislocation of C1
- *Teardrop fracture*—fracture of the anterior–inferior aspect of a vertebral body which should be treated as unstable
- *Unilateral facet dislocation*—a flexion–rotation injury which may result in nerve root compression
- *Bilateral facet dislocation*—a flexion injury which is unstable and is often associated with neurological injury

Thoracolumbar spine injury

Two-thirds of thoracolumbar (T-L) spine injuries occur at the **T-L junction**. The majority of T-L injuries are not associated with neurological injury. However, they may cause significant deformity or functional impairment (e.g. pain).

Aetiology

These injuries are usually caused by high energy trauma but may be predisposed to by:

- osteoporosis
- ankylosing spondylitis
- malignancy

Pathophysiology

Patterns of T-L fractures

- Compression
- Burst (stable and unstable)
- Flexion distraction (e.g. a Chance fracture is a purely bony injury with the fracture extending from anterior to posterior). It is associated with intra-abdominal injuries and is often caused by the use of 'lap-belt' restraints)
- Fracture dislocation (involves ligamentous disruption)

Classification

The concept of the three column spine was developed to classify the stability of T-L fractures (Fig 8.4). It stratifies the risk of instability and thus neurological injury based on the columns disrupted.

There also exists a comprehensive AO classification system.

Clinical assessment

- Initial ATLS resuscitation and secondary survey
- The extent of SCI should be documented using a standardized rating scale (e.g. American Spinal Injury Association) Fig 10.4. This is only prognostic once acute spinal shock has resolved

Investigations

- In an alert cooperative patient who is not in pain and has no symptoms or signs of spinal injury, plain radiographs can be used to clear the spine
- Patients who have symptoms or signs of SCI require both CT and MRI imaging of the spine to determine the aetiology of the injury and optimal management

Management

Medical

- Optimize oxygenation and blood pressure to prevent tissue ischaemia
- All spinal injuries should be treated as unstable until they have been reviewed by a spinal surgeon
- The role of steroids is controversial; the only RCT (National Acute Spinal Cord Injury Study II - NASCIS II) study failed to show convincing evidence of clear benefit and any effective dose required would be very large

Surgical

- Decompression if there is neural compression from bone or intervertebral disc prolapse
- In some circumstances, even without compression it is appropriate to perform a decompressive procedure to allow anticipated swelling to occur
- Unstable injuries require either external stabilization (via traction or an orthosis) or internal fixation

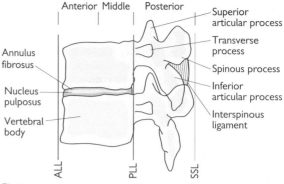

Fig 8.4 Three column concept of the spine. ALL – anterior longitudinal ligament; PLL – posterior longitudinal ligament; SLL – supraspinous ligament.

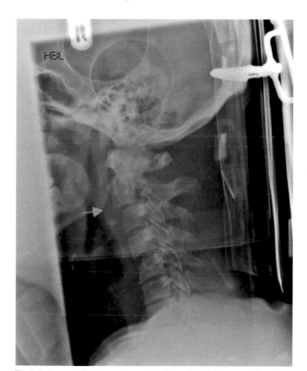

Fig 8.5 Lateral C-spine radiograph of a cyclist hit by a car. He was complaining of neck pain on arrival in the emergency department. There is an anterior slip of C2 on C3 and posterior slip of the posterior elements consistent with a fracture. There is a small amount of associated soft tissue swelling. A CT scan was arranged to evaluate the injury further.

8.8 Maxillofacial trauma

The maxillofacial skeleton is closely related to the eyes, brain, and airway. Trauma to the facial soft tissues and skeleton can have significant functional and aesthetic consequences.

Aetiology

- Interpersonal violence is the most common cause and the incidence is rising
- Trauma from road traffic collisions is declining owing to improved car safety such as crumble zones, airbags, and antilock brakes
- Other causes include falls from a height, sports injuries, and industrial accidents

Pathophysiology

Nasal fractures are the most common injury. Other fracture patterns depend on the mechanism of injury.

The airway is at particular risk in posteriorly displaced mandible and maxillary fractures, and with inhaled teeth. The face ad scalp are very vascular and so lacerations can result in significant blood loss.

Clinical assessment

Initial assessment and management often runs concurrently and follows ATLS principles.

History

- Mechanism of injury and forces involved
- Loss of consciousness
- Altered vision
- Tetanus status

Examination

- **Soft tissue** trauma to the face may injure nerves (e.g. branches of facial and trigeminal), salivary ducts, and lacrimal apparatus. Deformity and surgical emphysema may suggest underlying fractures
- **Scalp** wounds can bleed profusely. Check for boggy haematoma suggesting an underlying skull fracture
- **Nose** examination must exclude a septal haematoma which, if not drained, can result in septal necrosis. CSF rhinorrhoea suggests a base of skull fracture
- **Eyes** and surrounding structures should be assessed in all midfacial trauma. Check eye movements and visual acuity. Also examine eyelids, conjunctiva, and globe (rupture, lens dislocation, vitreous bleed), and for periorbital tenderness.
  Retrobulbar haemorrhage is an ocular emergency. Signs include severe pain, early loss of colour vision, relative afferent pupil defect ('swinging light test'), periorbital oedema, and bruising and proptosis
- **Pinna** haematomas should be drained if present. Battle's sign is bruising over the mastoid and suggests a fracture of the middle cranial fossa
- **Facial** skeleton should be palpated. Obvious deformity, step, crepitus, tenderness, and mobile bone are suggestive of fractures
- **Intraoral** examination is important in dentoalveolar and mandible fractures. Check for a step, malocclusion, and missing teeth

Investigations

Most injuries are diagnosed clinically. For instance, nasal fractures do not need routine investigations.

- **Plain facial radiographs** are indicated in suspected orbital, zygomatic, mandible, and dentoalveolar fractures. The view needed can be discussed with the radiographer

  15- and 30-degree views for orbital and zygomatic fractures; orthopantomogram (OPG), PA, lateral oblique, and reverse Towne's view for mandibular fractures
- **CT scan** gives the best views of orbital and midfacial trauma. It can be combined with a CT brain if indicated

Management

Maxillofacial trauma is often associated with other significant injuries (e.g. traumatic brain injury and C-spine injury). Follow ATLS guidelines and treat life-threatening injuries first.

Principal aims are to make an accurate diagnosis, and then to manage soft tissue and skeletal injuries definitively at the earliest opportunity at the same operation.

Soft tissue

- Clean and debride as necessary
- Assess need for antibiotics, e.g. dog bite
- Facial lacerations often need referral to plastic surgery to gain the best aesthetic and functional outcomes (e.g. facial nerve injury; laceration involving vermilion border of lip).

Nasal fracture

- Drain any septal haematoma
- Refer to ENT nasal fracture clinic for review in 7 days
- The nose can then be reassessed once the swelling has subsided and a decision on whether a manipulation under anaesthesia is needed to correct deviation. Severe unstable fractures may need wire fixation or open reduction with internal fixation (ORIF)

Orbit

- Patients with orbital fractures should be reviewed by an ophthalmologist urgently
- Medial wall fractures may be managed conservatively. Other fractures often have associated soft tissue injuries and facial fractures that require surgery

Midface fractures

- Most will need definitive early open reduction and internal fixation (with possibility of bone grafting)
- Skin incisions are placed in positions that allow good exposure and an aesthetic result (hairline, brow, eyelids, intraoral)

Mandible

- The aim is to restore occlusion
- Fractures of the body and ramus generally undergo ORIF. Condylar fractures and stable fractures with normal occlusion can be managed conservatively

Complications and prognosis

Soft tissue infections are uncommon. Most complications arise from poor diagnosis and initial definitive treatment. This is especially true of orbital fracture management resulting in enophthalmus. Facial scarring can also cause significant psychological morbidity.

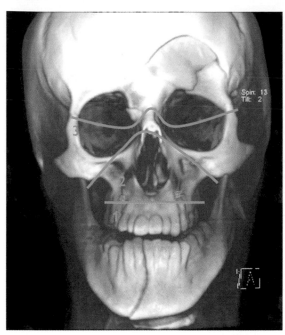

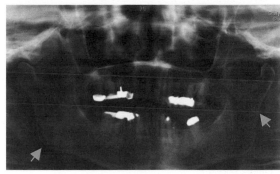

Fig 8.7 Orthopantomogram showing fractures across the left ramus of the mandible and the right mandibular body. There is no significant displacement and no dislocation of the temporomandibular joints.

Fig 8.6 Surface rendered CT reconstruction showing multiple facial fractures following an assault. These include fractures of the left lateral orbital wall, roof of orbit, frontal sinus, nasal septum, and mandible. The division of the Le Fort classification of facial fractures is also shown.

- Le Fort 1—transverse fracture with two segments. The floating palate contains alveolus, palate, and pterygoid plates
- Le Fort 2—pyramidal fracture across nasal bones, medial wall of orbit, and down in to maxilla
- Le Fort 3—craniofacial dysfunction with detachment of the midfacial skeleton from the skull base

8.9 Cardiothoracic trauma

- Cardiothoracic injuries account for 25% of deaths from trauma
- Fifty per cent of patients who die from multiple injuries have a significant thoracic injury

Aetiology

Causes are divided into penetrating (knife, gunshot (high and low velocity)) and blunt (blasts, RTA: deceleration (shearing and rotational) and compression)

NB. Features of penetrating injuries often coexist in severe blunt injuries owing to the effects of bony fractures

Pathophysiology

Injuries tend to follow distinct patterns according to the mechanism of injury, for example:

- restrained passenger in a high speed RTA: rib and sternal fractures, aortic and tracheobronchial disruption, cardiac and pulmonary contusion
- chest stab wounds: pneumo(haemo)thorax, haemopericardium, cardiac injury

Clinical assessment and management

- Manage all major injuries of the chest by ATLS protocol
- Cardiothoracic injuries from the bulk of critical injuries identified and managed in both the primary and secondary surveys
- Learn to recognize patterns and deal with each injury as it is discovered. Many primary survey injuries are not diagnosed by radiology or scanning but clinical signs and features

Investigations

- Mandatory: CXR
- Consider ECG (especially for blunt cardiac injuries), cardiac echo; thoracic CT (often combined with abdominal CT) most sensitive for most non-critical thoracic injuries

Life-threatening injuries (primary survey)

Tension pneumothorax

- Pattern—may occur in penetrating and blunt injuries. Commonly associated with major rib fractures
- Features—ipsilateral hyperresonance and absent breath sounds, contralateral tracheal and cardiac displacement, progressive tachycardia, and hypotension with pulsus paradoxus
- Emergency Rx—stab needle thoracostomy (14G cannula, ipsilateral second intercostal space mid-clavicular line)
- Definitive Rx—open tube thoracostomy (fifth intercostal space mid-axillary line)

Sucking pneumothorax

- Pattern—exclusively in sharp penetrating injuries or compound rib fractures, causing a pleurocutaneous fistula. Clinically significant if the wound diameter is greater than two-thirds of the tracheal cross-section
- Features—open wound 'sucking' in association with respiratory cycle, ipsilateral tracheal and cardiac deviation
- Emergency Rx—simple occlusive dressing over the wound
- Definitive Rx—wound exploration, toilet/debridement, tube thoracostomy and closure

Massive haemothorax

- Pattern—commonly in blunt compression/crush injuries but also sharp penetrating (knife)
- Features—ipsilateral stony dullness, absent breath sounds, distended neck veins with peripheral hypoperfusion (tachycardia and hypotension), contralateral cardiac displacement ('white out' or 'pleural effusion' on supine CXR)
- Emergency Rx—resuscitation room tube thoracostomy
- Definitive Rx—thoracotomy indicated if tube drains >1500 mL immediately or >200 mL per hour

Flail chest

- Pattern—exclusively in blunt compression injuries causing rib fractures in both anterior and posterior portions of the ribs. Main injury is *not* paradoxical chest movement but underlying severe lung contusion
- Features—tachypnoea, hypoxia (low oxygen saturations), tachycardia, asymmetrical/paradoxical chest movement
- Emergency Rx—oxygen supplementation
- Definitive Rx—respiratory support (PEEP or IPPV) and close monitoring on critical care

Cardiac tamponade

- Pattern—may be caused by sharp penetrating injuries (stab wounds) causing underlying ventricular laceration or blunt injury with associated major vessel rupture. Blunt injuries often associated with underlying myocardial injury
- Features—profound hypotension, ↑JVP, and muffled heart sounds ('Beck's Triad'), tachycardia, and reduced pulse pressure. Dysrhythmias, including SVT, VF, and pulseless electrical activity (PEA), may occur as pre-terminal events. Diagnosis may be aided by emergency echosonography if time permits
- Emergency Rx—needle pericardiocentesis (14G cannula, 2 cm below left edge of xiphisternum towards left scapula apex)
- Definitive Rx—according to underlying cause may require thoracotomy/sternotomy

Aortic disruption

- Pattern—usually caused by severe deceleration injuries causing 'rotation avulsion' injury to the aortic arch or aortoventricular junction. May have associated coronary artery origin injuries
- Features—asymmetrical brachial artery pressures, peripheral hypoperfusion, widened mediastinum on supine CXR. Definitive investigation is thoracic CT scan
- Emergency Rx—control of blood pressure (permissive, controlled mild hypotension)
- Definitive Rx—aortic repair

Significant injuries (secondary survey)

Rib fractures

- Pattern—fourth to ninth ribs most frequently fractured; associated with underlying lung contusion and simple pneumothorax. Lower rib fractures are primarily injuries of the abdomen and are associated with liver, splenic or renal injuries
- Features—pain on inspiration and palpation (often with crepitus)
- Definitive Rx—analgesia (± regional nerve block) and early chest physiotherapy

Sternal fracture

- Pattern—usually the upper or middle one-third fractured as a result of an RTA. Associated with underlying cardiac contusion
- Features—deformed or 'stepped' sternum, lateral CXR—visible fracture. Dysrhythmias (ECG) indicate cardiac injury
- Definitive Rx—analgesia and early mobilization

Simple pneumothorax/haemothorax

- Pattern—often diagnosed only on 'trauma series' CXR
- Definitive Rx—treat (tube thoracostomy) if larger than 20%, symptomatic or in any patient likely to undergo a general anaesthetic

Pulmonary contusion

- Pattern—mostly associated with overlying chest wall injuries and massive deceleration injuries. Most common potentially lethal chest injury. Risk of worsening associated consolidation and local pulmonary oedema
- Features—progressive hypoxaemia, tachycardia, tachypnoea
- Definitive Rx—analgesia, physiotherapy, and oxygenation. Consider respiratory support for a patient with significant hypoxia

Tracheobronchial tree injury

- Pattern—high speed deceleration/crush injury
- Features—surgical emphysema of the neck, acute severe stridor, persistent large air leak from chest tube
- Definitive Rx—requires emergency cardiothoracic assessment since it may rapidly become life-threatening

Oesophageal rupture

- Pattern—upper abdominal blunt trauma resulting in a linear tear or penetrating injury can result in mediastinis or empyema
- Features—confirmation of injury can be made by CT, OGD or contrast studies
- Definitive Rx—surgical repair if diagnosed early and patient stable enough for surgery, or TPN (or gastrostomy) feeding and antibiotics

Cardiac contusion

- Pattern—severe crush or deceleration injury. Penetrating injuries (stabs) may cause acute infarction owing to coronary vessel laceration
- Features—progressive tachycardia, hypotension, ↑CVP, dysrhythmias
- Definitive Rx—cardiac support (fluid restriction, control of blood pressure, careful inotropic support, ventricular assist devices in severe cases)

Diaphragmatic rupture

- Pattern—violent abdominal compression (restrained RTA)
- Features—right-sided may show only a 'raised hemidiaphragm' (liver displacing the right lower lobe), left-sided may show a stomach bubble in left hemithorax. Accurate diagnosis on thoracoabdominal CT
- Definitive Rx—repair if respiratory function compromised or in young (to prevent late lung sequelae)

⊕ Emergency thoracotomy

Indications

- Cardiac arrest after penetrating trauma
- Cardiac tamponade after penetrating trauma
- >1500 mL or 200 mL/h blood from chest drain

Access

- Anterolateral thoracotomy: very fast, needs only a scalpel, very limited access but can be extended, difficult to carry out internal cardiac massage, bleeding from the internal mammary artery can be problematic
- Bilateral extended anterior thoracotomy ('clamshell'):– fast, needs heavy scissors and scalpel, gives excellent access to the mediastinum and both pleural cavities
- Median sternotomy: fast, gives excellent exposure to heart and great vessels, requires a sternal saw and power source
- Subxiphoid approach: fast, but limited access to pericardium

Procedures

- Direct repair of ventricular and atrial lacerations is possible
- Evacuation of pericardial haematoma and drainage
- Control of intrathoracic bleeding point
- Aortic repairs

Survival

The survival following emergency thoracotomy for penetrating trauma is about 10%, and less than 1–2% for cardiac arrest following blunt trauma

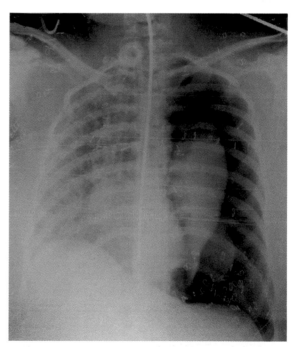

Fig 8.8 Supine chest radiograph showing a left-sided tension pneumothorax (tracheal deviation, left lung collapse, translucent left hemithorax, relatively dense right hemithorax, flattened left hemidiaphragm, right-shifted heart.

8.10 Abdominal trauma

Aetiology

Causes are divided into penetrating (knife, gunshot (high and low velocity)) and blunt (blasts, RTA: deceleration (shearing and rotational) and compression)

NB. Features of penetrating injuries often co-exist in severe blunt injuries owing to the effects of bony fractures

Pathophysiology

Injuries tend to follow distinct patterns according to the mechanism of injury.

- Gas-filled viscera (stomach, duodenum, and small bowel) are susceptible to burst injuries due to compression
- Solid viscera (liver, spleen, kidneys, and pancreas) are susceptible to fracture/rupture due to compression and laceration owing to rotational forces
- Major vessels may be torn in rapid deceleration

Injuries often occur in patterns. For example:

- restrained passengers in a high speed RTA: direct compression injuries (lower rib fractures, pancreatic rupture, small bowel contusions), deceleration rotational injuries (liver laceration), pelvic visceral injuries (urethral disruption, rectal laceration) owing to pelvic compression fractures
- abdominal stab wounds: small bowel laceration, mesenteric vascular injuries, liver laceration
- blunt assault: renal contusions, splenic rupture, rib fractures, mesenteric haematoma

Low velocity gunshot wounds cause direct penetration and lacerations limited to the trajectory which is often short owing to limited kinetic energy.

High velocity gunshot wounds typically cause severe injuries in the abdomen because of high energy transfer, pressure wave-induced extensive tissue cavitation (in both solid and hollow viscera), projectile 'tumbling', and projectile fragmentation.

Clinical assessment and management

- Manage all major injuries of the abdomen by ATLS protocol
- Abdominal injuries may be identified during the primary survey as life-threatening; consider if emergency laparotomy is required for resuscitation in these cases

Investigations

- Mandatory—CXR, pelvic XR
- Optional
  - Diagnostic peritoneal lavage (DPL)
  - Focal assessment by sonography in trauma (FAST)
  - CT abdomen–pelvis (often with thorax): the diagnostic investigation of choice for all suspected intra-abdominal injuries in the stable or responding patient. Patients must always be accompanied to the CT scanner by the trauma team unless they are fully stable
  - Contrast studies—rarely, for possible UGI ruptures
  - Diagnostic laparoscopy—occasionally for uncertain penetrating injuries

Life-threatening injuries (primary survey)

Liver laceration

- Pattern—may occur in penetrating and blunt injuries. Commonly associated with major rib fractures

- Features—unresponsive hypotension, abdominal distension, pain, and peritonitis in the conscious patient
- Emergency Rx—laparotomy. Most liver bleeding will stop with packing and liver repair/resection should be avoided
- Definitive Rx—may include transfer to a major liver unit if possible once stabilized

Splenic rupture

- Pattern—may occur in penetrating and blunt injuries. Commonly associated with major rib fractures
- Features—unresponsive hypotension, abdominal distension, pain, and peritonitis in the conscious patient, left flank bruising. Delayed rupture may occur up to 1 week post-injury with left upper quadrant and subscapular pain
- Emergency Rx—laparotomy if unstable
- Definitive Rx—usually splenectomy, splenorhaphy/splenic wrap/partial splenectomy is occasionally possible

Major vessel laceration

- Pattern—commonest in deceleration injuries but gunshot wounds that are potentially lethal are usually so because of vascular injury
- Features—unresponsive hypotension, abdominal distension, back and flank pain, flank bruising, CT diagnosis
- Emergency Rx—laparotomy: these are the only critical injures that require immediate definitive repair. May require vascular grafting

Significant injuries (secondary survey)

Duodenal rupture

- Pattern—almost always due to compression seat belt injury
- Features—positive DPL (bile-stained), features of peritonitis (immediate or developing over first 24 h of admission), may be associated with pancreatic or lumbar injury ('Chance' distraction fracture), CT scan diagnosis
- Emergency treatment—if part of multiple injuries, close all defects with surgical staples and plan delayed definitive management
- Definitive Rx—early diagnosis, primary repair (or excision of injured segment with anastomosis), peritoneal lavage

Small bowel lacerations

- Pattern—mostly caused by sharp penetrating trauma
- Features—positive DPL (bile-stained), features of peritonitis (immediate or developing over first 24 h of admission), features of sepsis
- Emergency treatment—if part of multiple injuries close all defects with surgical staples and plan delayed definitive management
- Definitive Rx—early diagnosis, primary repair (or excision of injured segment with anastomosis), peritoneal lavage

Pancreatic disruption

- Pattern—compression/deceleration injury
- Features—back pain, flank bruising, hyperamylasaemia not always present, mostly diagnosed on CT scanning
- Definitive Rx—analgesia, TPN or jejunostomy feeding, drainage of pancreatic collections

Large bowel lacerations

- Pattern—mostly caused by sharp penetrating trauma
- Features—positive DPL (faecal contamination), features of peritonitis (immediate or developing over first 24 h of admission), features of sepsis
- Definitive Rx—early diagnosis, primary repair, peritoneal lavage, +/- defunctioning proximal stoma. Late diagnosis, excision of injured section and end-colostomy formation, peritoneal lavage, and drainage

Splenic laceration

- Pattern—may occur in penetrating and apparently low velocity blunt injuries
- Features—usually diagnosed on CT scanning. Delayed rupture may occur up to 1 week post-injury with left upper quadrant and subscapular pain
- Definitive Rx—may be managed conservatively for stable patients with low grade (non-hilar) injuries diagnosed on CT scanning. Injuries graded from 1 (minor subcapsular tear or haematoma) to 4 (shattered spleen)

Renal laceration and other urological injuries are covered in Topic 8.11.

⊕ Diagnostic peritoneal lavage

This method has been the standard initial investigation for over 20 years and is regarded as both safe and highly sensitive; it does, however, have a significant false-positive rate.

Indications

- Equivocal physical examination in trauma
- Unresponsive hypotension in trauma
- explained shock (including that unresponsive to resuscitation) in trauma
- Clinical peritonitis

Contraindications (relative)

- Advanced cirrhosis
- Coagulopathy

Procedure

- Ensure gastric and bladder decompression with nasogastric tube and catheterization
- Infraumbilical incision of the peritoneum (either open or closed) under local anaesthetic
- Insert peritoneal catheter and aspirate. Free blood, bile, chyme or faeces is an immediate positive result and the procedure halted in preparation for laparotomy
- Infuse 1000 mL warmed 0.9% saline, leave for 3–4 min, drain via gravity
- Positive results: red cell count >100 000/mL, white cell count >500/mL

⊙ Fast scan

- 2D greyscale ultrasonography
- Focused to left and right subphrenic spaces (and occasionally pelvis and subhepatic spaces) looking for large amounts of 'free fluid' (blood)
- Advantages—speed, available in the resuscitation room
- Disadvantages—non-specific, modest sensitivity, no assessment of closed solid organ injury

⊕ Emergency laparotomy in trauma

Indications

- Unexplained shock (including that unresponsive to resuscitation) in trauma
- Clinical peritonism
- Positive DPL
- Evisceration
- Gunshot wounds (traversing the peritoneal cavity or visceral/vascular retroperitoneum)
- Bleeding from the rectum, stomach or genitourinary tract from penetrating trauma

Access

- Midline laparotomy: very fast, needs only a scalpel, offers good access to all areas, enables access from pelvis to diaphragms, more limited access to liver and spleen
- 'Roof top' subcostal laparotomy: fairly fast, offers optimal access to liver and spleen, may be extended into the lower chest across the costal margin, offers very limited access to the lower abdomen and pelvis

Procedures—principles

- The aim is to stop bleeding, **stop visceral leakage, clean the peritoneal cavity, and return the patient to ITU** before they become acidotic and cold ('damage limitation surgery')
- Massive haemorrhage should be controlled by packing until haemodynamic stability is restored
- Liver bleeding is best controlled by packing (above and below)
- Splenic conservation should only be considered by experienced surgeons; splenic trauma discovered at laparotomy is usually best treated by splenectomy
- Multiple bowel injuries should be closed as quickly as possible (e.g. stapling devices); definitive resection and anastomosis is rarely the best treatment
- Abdominal closure is not required for ventilated patients; the abdomen can be covered by waterproof infusion bags ('Bogota bag') or moist packs
- Always consider 're-look' laparotomy at 24–48 h

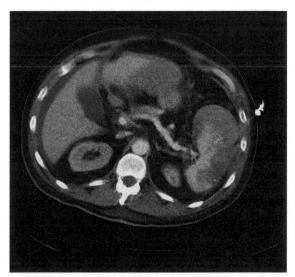

Fig 8.9 Abdominal CT showing a ruptured spleen surrounded by blood.

8.11 Urological trauma

Aetiology

Causes are divided into penetrating (knife, gunshot (high and low velocity)) and blunt (blasts, RTA: deceleration (shearing and rotational) and compression)

Pathophysiology

Injuries tend to follow distinct patterns according to the mechanism of injury. For example:

- restrained passengers in a high speed RTA: direct compression injuries (renal parenchymal contusions or, rarely, avulsion of the vascular pedicle)
- crush injuries or vehicle versus pedestrian injuries; pelvic fractures (bladder laceration, urethral laceration), spinal injury (renal contusion), deceleration rotational injuries (liver laceration), pelvic visceral injuries (urethral disruption, rectal laceration) caused by pelvic compression fractures
- abdominal stab wounds: small bowel laceration, mesenteric vascular injuries, liver laceration
- blunt assault: renal contusions
- low velocity gunshot wounds cause direct penetration and lacerations limited to the trajectory which is often short owing to limited kinetic energy
- high velocity gunshot wounds typically cause severe injuries in the abdomen owing to high energy transfer, pressure wave-induced extensive tissue cavitation, projectile 'tumbling', and projectile fragmentation

Clinical assessment and management

- Manage all major injuries of the abdomen and pelvis by ATLS protocol
- Renal tract injuries are very rarely life-threatening and are mostly identified on secondary survey or subsequent imaging
- Urethral injuries may be identified during the primary survey and must be correctly managed to prevent making the injury worse

Investigations

Mandatory investigations

- Chest and pelvic radiographs, urinalysis, pr examination

Optional investigations

- CT abdomen–pelvis (often with thorax) is the diagnostic investigation of choice for all suspected intra-abdominal injuries in the stable or responding patient. Patients must always be accompanied to the CT scanner by the trauma team unless they are fully stable
- IVU is the most useful investigation for determining functionality and urine leak (pelvi-ureteric laceration)
- Retrograde cystourethrogram is performed in cases of suspected urethral disruption or bladder laceration
- Microscopic haematuria after trauma is a common finding in the emergency department. This does not require imaging unless the patient has had a period of shock (BP <90 systolic) or if associated with a penetrating injury

Renal injuries

- Pattern—5–10% of abdominal injuries affect the kidneys. Commonest causes in the UK are road traffic collisions, sports injuries, falls, and assaults

- Features—macroscopic haematuria, loin and back pain (thoracolumbar spinal injuries have a high predictive value for associated renal injury), hypotension, and features of shock are rare, usually diagnosed on CT scanning

Table 8.8 American Association for surgery of trauma classification of renal injuries	
1	Contusion
2	<1 cm laceration not affecting medulla/collecting system
3	>1 cm laceration not affecting medulla/collecting system
4	Laceration involving medulla/collecting system
5	Shattered kidney or avulsed renal artery or vein

- Emergency treatment—emergency nephrectomy is extremely rarely required for major vascular injury
- Definitive Rx—conservative for grades 1–3; observation, possible serial imaging (CT, US, and IVU), Hb monitoring, can usually be managed conservatively. Grade 4/5 injuries may require exploration/nephrectomy (partial or total)
- Complications—secondary haemorrhage, perinephric abscess, and intrarenal arteriovenous fistula development
- Long term follow-up—IVU, BP, creatinine

Ureteric injuries

- Pattern—rare, mostly caused by sharp penetrating trauma (excluding iatrogenic trauma)
- Features—immediate presentation, contrast extravasation on CT scan or IVU. Delayed presentation, flank pain, fever, perinephric 'urinoma' on CT
- Definitive Rx—early diagnosis, primary repair over ureteric stent if isolated or defunctioning nephrostomy if part of polytrauma

Bladder injuries

- Pattern—major pelvic fractures owing to crush or RTA (also occasionally iatrogenic)
- Features—suprapubic pain, frank haematuria, inability to void urine, extravasation of contrast on CT scanning, IVU or retrograde cystogram
- Definitive Rx—intraperitoneal leakage, primary repair with catheter; extraperitoneal leakage, catheterization (urethral or suprapubic)

Urethral injuries

- Pattern—major pelvic fractures owing to crush or RTA (also occasionally iatrogenic)
- Features—suprapubic pain, blood at the urethral meatus, inability to void urine, perineal swelling/bruising (blood and urine), high riding prostate on rectal examination, extravasation of contrast on retrograde cystogram
- Emergency Rx—do not attempt urethral catheterization; ultrasound-guided suprapubic catheterization or catheterization by a senior urologist if the diagnosis is seriously suspected. Open cystostomy is rarely required
- Definitive Rx—incomplete laceration, conservative management with a urethral catheter. Complete transection, primary repair with catheter

Genital injury

Common traumatic injuries include:

- penile fracture—acute pain and detumescence; Mx—immediate surgical repair
- penetrating penile/scrotal injuries (including scrotal testicular 'degloving'—exploration and debridement
- testes injury—most haematomas settle with simple analgesia and support. Large haematocele/suspicion of rupture may require exploration

---

⊕ Urethrography

Procedures

- Aseptic technique
- Insert size 12F catheter 2 cm into urethra
- Gently inject 5–10 mL of water-soluble contrast solution
- Ideally should be performed under screening control. Alternatively, a single oblique radiograph can be taken to delineate the urethra

---

8.12 Vascular trauma

Aetiology

There are a number of modes of injury.

- Penetrating—gunshot, stabbing, fracture/fragment laceration
- Blunt—fracture/dislocation (direct compression/injury by the bony fragments or compression caused by the resulting haematoma/oedema)
- Iatrogenic—minimal access procedures, intra-arterial drug injection)
- Cold injury—frostbite

Pathophysiology

Injury to the vascular tree has three main consequences:

1. Haemorrhage if the vessel is lacerated or divided (worst in open 'compound' injuries), may cause hypovolaemic shock
2. Distal ischaemia of the organ/tissue supplied in arterial injuries (depends on the organ/tissues involved, the degree of collateral circulation, completeness of arterial injury)
3. In situ thrombosis in the vessel at and distal to the injury)

Classification of vascular injuries

Arterial lacerations

- Incomplete mural injury—associated with intimal disruption, vasospasm, and in situ thrombosis with no extravasation. Common in fractures, e.g. brachial artery in displaced supra-condylar fracture in children, popliteal artery is displaced in distal femoral fractures in adults
- Incomplete laceration—length of vessel involved depends on mechanism of injury, often results in major haemorrhage owing to incomplete vasospasm, characterized by periarterial haematoma and false aneurysm formation, e.g. common femoral artery after transarterial interventional procedures
- Complete division—usually caused by penetrating injury; initial bleeding is profound but often self-limiting owing to vasospasm and thrombosis; severed ends often widely separated due to retraction

Venous lacerations

Often associated with severe progressive bleeding if major veins are involved owing to high flow rates in the veins and limited vasospasm to control the luminal diameter; thrombosis leads to a risk of proximal embolization, e.g. pelvic venous bleeding after displaced pelvic fractures.

The majority of arterial injuries will require exploration. Damage to small or medium sized veins can usually be managed conservatively; however, larger veins will also need to be repaired.

Clinical assessment and management

- Manage all major vascular injuries by ATLS protocol
- Open bleeding injuries are controlled by direct pressure; avoid tourniquets or attempts at direct suture or clip haemostasis in the resuscitation room
- Closed vascular injuries of the limbs, pelvis or abdomen can lead to severe hypotension and shock with no obvious blood loss
- Always assess the perfusion of the affected limb, distal pulses, and venous return in limb vessel injuries
- Vascular compromise may occur late after the injury because of critical loss of lumen by subsequent swelling or progressive thrombosis; repeated observations are vital; be prepared to change from conservative management if the situation deteriorates

Investigations

- Bloods—FBC, clotting, G+S (cross-match if active bleeding)
- Doppler USS adds little—the absence of pulses is the most important indicator for intervention
- Intra-arterial digital subtraction angiography (iaDSA) provides the most accurate delineation of arterial injury but is invasive and may not be readily available in unstable patients. May be used intra-operatively
- CT angiography is best for large vessel injuries

Conservative management

- Incomplete injuries or iatrogenic partial lacerations may be managed conservatively
- If there is no evidence of a transmural injury then anti-coagulation may reduce the risk of in situ thrombosis owing to intimal disruption. IV heparin should be used since it is easiest to reverse its effect quickly when there is a significant chance of surgical intervention being required

Operative management

- The arrest of life-threatening haemorrhage takes precedence over limb-threatening injuries
- Major vascular injury is rarely isolated. Soft tissues and bones may also be involved. Vascular reconstruction needs to take this into account
- Primary amputation should be considered if revascularization will lead to a life-threatening reperfusion syndrome or further haemorrhage

Complications and prognosis

The return of blood flow to tissue following prolonged ischaemia can induce a reperfusion syndrome. Other complications of vascular injury include arteriovenous fistula and stenosis.

Cold injury

Prolonged cooling to temperatures <10°C causes peripheral vasoconstriction, and reduced intracapillary and intravenular flow.

At temperatures <2°C there is a risk of in situ thrombosis or small vessels and freezing of tissue fluid.

Extremities such as digits, nose, and ears are most at risk.

Management

- Affected extremities should be rewarmed slowly. Rapid rewarming risks worsening tissue trauma because of thermal injury and rapid cellular changes
- Amputation should be delayed for as long as possible until the potential tissue loss can be fully assessed; the extent of tissue which is actually non-viable is often much less than appears at first inspection
- Early amputation should only be considered for the development of infection ('wet gangrene')
- Tissue autoseparation often occurs spontaneously

⊕ Principles of arterial repair

- Primary sutured closure of arterial lacerations is theoretically ideal but rarely possible; even in stab lacerations there is almost always disruption to the wound edges and a stenosis almost inevitable with closure
- Vein patching (using saphenous or median cubital vein) is best for limited injuries
- Vein interposition grafting is usually required for complete division of an artery; it has the best long-term patency
- Arterial interposition grafting is rarely used
- Synthetic material (e.g. Dacron) interposition grafting should be avoided unless vein is not available because of the risk of infection and long-term risk of graft failure
- Temporary intraluminal shunts can be used to maintain perfusion during complicated repairs

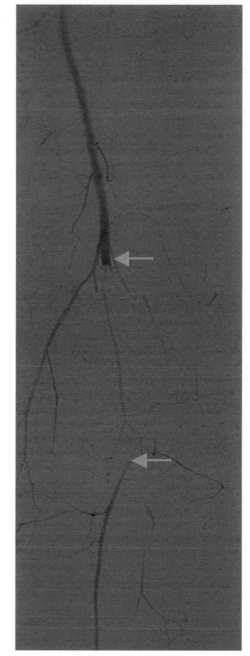

Fig 8.10 A selective DSA of the left femoral artery showing a sharp cut-off of the popliteal artery at the level of the femoral condyles. The posterior tibial artery reconstitutes at the level of the proximal third of the leg. The anterior tibial artery is totally occluded. The posterior tibial artery shows poor retrograde flow. This injury was sustained during a traumatic dislocation of the left knee in a road traffic collision.

8.13 Assessment of the acute abdomen

The 'acute abdomen' can be the presentation of one or more of a range of symptoms (including nausea, vomiting, bloating, and change in bowel habit), but the commonest is pain.

Acute abdominal symptoms may be entirely *de novo* or an acute exacerbation of a longstanding problem—do not underestimate patients with a pre-existing history; they too can have serious acute intra-abdominal disease.

Clinical assessment

There are many ways to assess the acute abdomen, but the commonest is to aim to determine the following.

- Is the apparent pathology confined to one zone of the abdomen or is it generalized?
- If it is confined to one zone, what are the possible anatomical explanations?
- Is there evidence of peritonitis (localized or generalized)?
- Does the patient have any features of systemic involvement in the underlying process (e.g. sepsis, jaundice)?

History

Abdominal pain should always have key features documented:(mnemonic SOCRATES)

- **S**ite
- **O**nset
- **C**haracter (sharp, dull, 'pressure')
- **R**adiation
- **A**lleviating factors
  Motion—suggests hollow visceral colic
  Topical heat—suggests inflammatory origin
- **T**iming (constant, colicky)
- **E**xacerbating factors
- **S**everity

Always document associated symptoms or possible directly relevant factors.

- Nausea or vomiting
- Anorexia
- Bowel habit (diarrhoea or constipation)
- Stools (colour, smell, pus, blood, mucus)
- Micturition (colour, frequency, pain)
- Menstrual cycle and likelihood of pregnancy
- Gynaecological symptoms (pv discharge)
- Previous episodes
- Previous investigations
- Foreign travel

Examination

Look for patterns—examination findings should be grouped in an attempt to clarify the underlying situation in the peritoneal cavity/organs. They very rarely directly indicate the exact pathological diagnosis but tend to confirm the history findings in terms of a clinical diagnosis which will give rise to a possible differential diagnosis:

- distension, central abdominal tympanism, increased, hyperactive bowel sounds = intestinal obstruction (may be small or large bowel)
- localized tenderness, guarding (muscle contraction in response to light pressure) and pain elicited on movement or coughing during palpation = localized peritoneal irritation

- diffuse extreme tenderness, abdominal rigidity, sparse or absent bowel sounds = established diffuse peritoneal irritation (may be pus, blood or bile)

Common pitfalls during examination

- Generalized peritonitis is often maximal in the zone of origin of the pathology—check carefully in the other zones to demonstrate a generalized pathology
- Full signs of peritoneal irritation may not be present in the elderly, very young or those on immunosuppression; findings may be subtle in these groups

At the end of the examination the objective is to have:

- a clear differential diagnosis
- a limited set of targeted investigations most likely to achieve a diagnosis

Investigations

Investigations should be targeted, especially more sophisticated and costly ones.

Basic investigations

Always or very frequently requested.

- Urinalysis (dipstick and MC+S)
  - Nitrites are highly sensitive and specific for the presence of a UTI
  - Blood, protein, and ketones have a low sensitivity and lower specificity for any one diagnosis
- Blood tests
  - FBC, U+Es, creatinine, LFTs
  - Amylase—modest rises are common in many inflammatory, ischaemic or septic processes in the abdomen or elsewhere, but rises three times the upper limit of normal (usually >1000 iu) are diagnostic of pancreatic pathology
  - CRP—moderate sensitivity (not all inflammatory processes are associated with a rise in CRP) and very low specificity for intra-abdominal pathology. Best to monitor the progress of treatment if raised at diagnosis
- Erect chest radiograph—primary use is to look for free intra-abdominal gas but also assesses basal lung pathology
- Supine abdominal radiograph—only a few diagnoses can be truly reached on the 'plain film':
  - gallstone 'ileus': small bowel dilatation, air in the biliary tree, and a radio-opacity in the RLQ (gallstone)
  - large bowel volvulus: gross dilatation of one segment of large bowel, characteristic orientation (RLQ–LUQ in caecal, LLQ–RUQ in sigmoid)
  - renal colic: extrapelvic stones in the distribution of the ipsilateral renal tract

Second line investigations

- USS abdomen (always specify which area should be assessed, e.g. biliary/liver, renal tract, pelvic)
  - Investigation of choice for suspected biliary tract, ovarian, and some renal tract pathology
  - Transvaginal US is superior to transabdominal in the assessment of the adenexae
- CT abdomen—often the diagnostic investigation of choice for suspected abdominal pathology. Where possible, should be with IV and oral contrast (and rectal contrast if a leak from the distal large bowel is suspected)

- Intravenous urogram (IVU)—most sensitive and specific investigation for renal tract pathology, especially stone disease
- Gastroscopy—most useful for the diagnosis of acute gastritis, ulceration, and oesophageal pathology
- Colonoscopy—occasionally indicated in acute colonic bleeding and the diagnosis of acute colitis, but should be used with care for possible inflammatory or infective pathologies in the colon since there is an increased risk of perforation or bleeding
- Diagnostic laparoscopy—see below
- Diagnostic laparotomy—see below. Do not forget that a laparotomy may be diagnostic and therapeutic

◎ Interpreting a supine abdominal radiograph scan

Key features which are always pathological and should be looked for with care:

- thickened, irregular mucosal outlines indicate oedema due to inflammation or ischaemia of the affected loops
- generalized 'greyness' and paucity of gas-filled loops indicates free fluid (serous, blood or pus)
- small volumes of extraluminal air may appear as crescents, slivers or stellate shapes of gas between bowel loops, under the liver or along the falciform ligament

Common pitfalls

- Not all apparently dilated loops of bowel are pathological, especially in the elderly or chronically bedbound where the large bowel is often 'capacious'
- 'Sentinel loops' of air-filled bowel are often incidental findings
- The 'unremarkable' radiograph excludes nothing! Always rely on clinical assessment

⊕ Emergency diagnostic laparoscopy

Common indications

- Possible acute appendicitis/gynaecological pathology
- Possible perforated ulcer
- Possible acute biliary pathology

Procedure—principles

- Consider placing the patient's legs in stirrups to allow Lloyd–Davis or lithotomy position (especially for women): both allow access to the rectum and vagina in women for assessment or manipulation
- Initial port should be 10/12 mm periumbilical
- An alternative occasionally used is the left upper quadrant when there has been previous surgery and access cannot be achieved centrally
- Port insertion should be under direct vision ('Hassan technique') to minimize risk of inadvertent injury
- Subsequent ports are determined by the pathology encountered and may be 5 or 10/12 mm
- Ports should be placed well away from suspected pathology, in pairs which allow the instruments to 'triangulate' on the area of interest (📖 Topic 8.14)
- Always have wash and suction available
- Use atraumatic forceps to handle bowel or delicate structures (e.g. ovaries); 'Petelin's' forceps are *not* atraumatic
- Close 10/12mm port sites with suture(s)

⊕ Emergency laparotomy

Procedure—principles

- A midline laparotomy should be used unless there is a high degree of certainty about the diagnosis and the procedure to be undertaken and the exposure needed
- Periumbilical incisions are best where the diagnosis is unknown; they can be extended up or down as required
- Send samples of any free fluid encountered initially for MC&S (and cytology if clear ascites)
- Smell the abdomen! Purulent but odourless fluid is often UGI in origin. Foul 'faeculent' smell is LGI or pelvic organ in origin
- Assess the abdomen methodically and slowly; once the bowel loops are disturbed it may become less clear where the source of infection arose and this is particularly true for sites of small bowel obstruction
- Start quadrant by quadrant
- Always complete the assessment; there may be more than one origin or trouble
- In sepsis, make sure *all* collections are drained or dealt with; try to ensure the peritoneal cavity is free of contamination as far as is safely possible
- In obstruction, make sure all sites are dealt with, bypassed or defunctioned

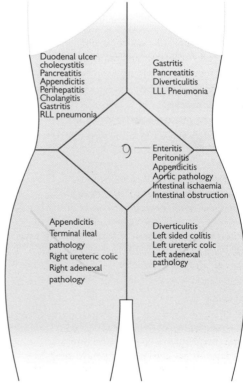

Fig 8.11 Differential diagnosis of abdominal pain arising in different areas.

8.14 Acute appendicitis

Acute appendicitis is the most common provisional diagnosis and most common acute procedure in UK general surgical take. Peak incidence is 10–15 years of age (rare <2 and >80 years of age) and it is slightly more common in males (M:F 1.4:1).

Aetiology

Obstructive appendicitis

- Paediatric appendiceal obstruction may be caused by lymphoid hyperplasia, faecoliths, and worms
- Adult appendiceal obstruction may be due to faecoliths, appendiceal adenomas or caecal tumours. It tends to progress with the classic, short clinical history and always requires surgery

Phlegmonous appendicitis

- Possibly associated with URTI
- Caused by primary bacterial or viral infection in the appendiceal wall
- It often runs a slower, more variable clinical course and may resolve spontaneously or with 'blind' antibiotic treatment

Pathophysiology of obstructive appendicitis

Obstructive appendicitis is caused by occlusion of the appendiceal lumen, causing stasis and infection, increased pressure, and resulting avascular necrosis of the wall.

1. Obstruction of the lumen increases intraluminal pressure. This is caused by mucus secreted by mucosa, proliferation of bacteria, and white cells/pus
2. Intraluminal pressure then exceeds that of the appendiceal veins, causing congestion and thrombosis
3. Appendiceal wall ischaemia causes ulceration and necrosis
4. Bacterial translocation and appendiceal perforation causes intraperitoneal inflammation

Clinical assessment

Acute appendicitis is a clinical diagnosis, but radiological investigations should be considered in certain groups.

History

- Abdominal pain is characteristically vague, central abdominal pain, which worsens and migrates/localizes to RIF; pain typically precedes accompanying symptoms
- Anorexia, nausea or vomiting are important features suggesting an organic cause for the symptoms
- Useful guides as to the presence of 'true' peritonism are: pain reproduced by laughing, coughing, during travel into hospital in the car
- History of foreign travel or abnormal food intake may be helpful
- Fever is typically low grade (37.5–38.5°C)

Examination

General

- Flushed and febrile (typically <38.5°C). A high fever (>39°C) suggests perforation or an alternative diagnosis
- Dry coated tongue and fetor oris (foul breath)

Abdomen

- Restricted anterior abdominal wall movement on deep respiration
- Maximal tenderness in right iliac fossa at McBurney's point (one-third along the line from the anterior superior iliac spine to the umbilicus)
- Peritonism (localized, generalized) as evident by percussion tenderness and/or guarding (i.e. involuntary anterior abdominal wall contraction)
- Gaseous distension (localized ileus) or fullness (mass) may be palpable in RIF

- Digital rectal and pelvic examinations are almost never informative in children with abdominal pain and should not be performed. In adults they should always be done to exclude occult rectal pathology

Eponymous signs in acute appendicitis

- **Rovsing's sign**: palpation in the left iliac fossa causes maximal pain in the right iliac fossa
- **Psoas stretch sign:** painful hip flexion with the patient supine, indicating inflammation of the psoas sheath (i.e. posterior lower abdominal wall)
- **Obturator sign**: painful hip rotation, indicating inflammation of the obturator internus muscle (i.e. posterior lower abdominal wall)

Common differential diagnoses according to age

- Children <16 years: non-specific abdominal pain (NSAP), 'viral' infections, acute constipation, ovulation
- Adults <50 years: Crohn's disease, acute enteritis, tubo-ovarian pathology, gallstones
- Adults >50 years: acute diverticulitis, caecal tumours, intestinal ischaemia

Investigations

Investigations are primarily to exclude alternative diagnosis and to support the diagnosis in children, but should be considered with increasing frequency with increasing age of the patient as the differential diagnosis widens.

- Urinalysis helps to exclude a UTI. Any appendicitis may cause pyuria and microscopic haematuria
- Bloods: ↑ WCC ↑ CRP are non-specific
- Pregnancy test—serum βHCG is always required in any woman of childbearing age
- Plain abdominal radiograph—should be performed in adults unless the diagnosis has been made clinically with confidence. Non-specific radiological signs suggestive of appendicitis are: faecolith; blurred right psoas margin; abnormal right iliac fossa gas pattern (localized ileus); scoliosis (pained posture)
- Ultrasound scan—pelvic scans may be useful in women of childbearing age where gynaecological pathology is suspected. Biliary ultrasounds may be useful where biliary colic is a suspected differential
- Abdominopelvic CT scan should be considered for:
  - all adults where the diagnosis is unclear after observation
  - when there is a suspicion of an appendix mass
  - in the elderly where the differential diagnosis is wide and has a significant impact on the choice of surgery
- Laparoscopy may be used as a diagnostic procedure as well as offering the opportunity to proceed to treatment

Management

Initial

- Fluid resuscitation
- Analgesia—opiate analgesia never masks the clinical signs and should never be withheld prior to senior review
- Antiemetics if required (e.g. prochlorperazine 12.5 mg IV)

Conservative

- Observation and repeated examination ('watchful waiting') should be considered where the patient has significant symptoms or signs but is well and where a clear diagnosis of appendicitis cannot be made sufficiently certainly to justify urgent surgery

- 'Blind' antibiotics should never be used until a diagnosis has been reached unless the patient has frank peritonitis
- Uncomplicated acute appendicitis may be treated by intravenous antibiotics in the very elderly or those unfit for surgery

Antibiotics in acute appendicitis

- **Prophylaxis** (single dose IV) is given on induction prior to diagnostic or therapeutic surgery. Established non-perforated appendicitis does not need further antibiotic treatment
- **Established therapeutic antibiotics** (5-day course IV → oral) are given if perforated appendicitis with peritoneal soiling (pus or faeces) is found at operation. Proven appendiceal mass or appendicitis on CT is managed conservatively
- **Blind therapeutic antibiotics** (open-ended IV) are given in suspected appendicitis booked for surgery and possible appendicitis with diffuse peritonitis or features of severe systemic sepsis awaiting investigation

Operative

Appendicectomy is the treatment of choice and should be undertaken at the earliest opportunity. The rate of perforation is 15–40% in the first 36 h but increases with time.

Complicated appendicitis

Complicated appendicitis is defined as gangrenous or perforated appendix with free intraperitoneal pus.

Appendix mass

An appendix mass without diffuse peritonitis (other than diagnosed under GA) may be managed in two ways:

- IV antibiotics and observation followed by delayed appendicectomy (after 3 months or so). This may reduce the risk of a difficult acute appendicectomy but risks failure of antibiotic treatment, may involve a prolonged recovery from the initial attack, and includes the risk of recurrent inflammation
- Acute appendicectomy—this may be an extensive procedure involving a laparotomy or even ileocaecal resection but avoids the risk of failed primary treatment and may speed overall recovery

⊕ Laparoscopic appendicectomy

Additional points (🕮 Emergency laparoscopy, Topic 8.13)
- Appendiceal vessels may be secured by diathermy, endoclips or endovascular staples
- The appendiceal base is secured by an 'endoloop' or endovascular staples
- Deliver the appendix via one of the ports in an 'endobag' to reduce the risk of port site infection
- Lavage the abdomen (especially the pelvis)

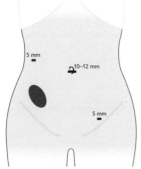

Fig 8.12 Port positions for a laparoscopic appendicectomy.

⊕ Open appendicectomy

Preoperative

- Check the patient for the presence of an appendix mass prior to starting—it may indicate a difficult procedure
- Consider a midline laparotomy for patients over the age of 60 years or where the diagnosis is uncertain (ideally will have had a preoperative CT scan)

Operative

- RIF grid iron incision or Lanz; aim for the lateral border of the rectus sheath if possible
- Muscle splitting approach and incision of peritoneum
- Send any peritoneal fluid for MC&S (or swab)
- If the appendix is not obvious, locate it by following the caecal teniae to their confluence. Careful digital manipulation is useful where there are significant periappendiceal acute adhesions
- Divide the mesoappendix and secure the appendicular vessel(s) (ties, clips or diathermy)
- Ligate the base of the appendix and excise it, sending the specimen to histology
- Burying of the appendiceal stump is unnecessary
- A formal caecal or even ileocaecal resection may be necessary where there is severe necrosis and sepsis damaging the adjacent colon
- Drains are not indicated unless there is a pre-formed paraappendiceal abscess
- Purulent or faeculent fluid in the peritoneal cavity should be thoroughly lavaged, including the paracolic gutters and pelvis
- Abdominal wall is closed in layers with emphasis on closure of the external oblique aponeurosis (only layer to impart strength to closure)

Postoperative

- Oral diet should be started as soon as tolerated
- Nasogastric tubes should not be used routinely

Complications

Intraoperative and early	Late
• Ileus	• Adhesions (bowel obstruction)
• Intra-abdominal abscess (e.g. pelvic)	
• Wound infection (5% or more where there is severe acute appendicitis)	
• Adhesional small bowel obstruction	

8.15 Acute upper gastrointestinal haemorrhage

Acute upper gastrointestinal haemorrhage (UGIH) is a relatively common emergency with an incidence of 1 per 1000 adults per year in the UK and is highest in economically deprived areas.

Although 70% of UGI haemorrhages stop spontaneously, 10% bleed continuously and about 20% re-bleed.

This results in 75% of cases requiring a blood transfusion and 25% of cases needing endoscopic or operative intervention. Mortality rate is 5–7%.

Aetiology
A cause of bleeding is found in approximately 80% of patients. Most common causes are:

- peptic ulcer (35–50%)
- acute gastric erosions (~15%)
- oesophagitis (~10%)
- oesophageal or gastric varices (5–10%)
- Mallory–Weiss tear (~10%)
- upper gastrointestinal malignancy (<5%) (gastric>>oesophageal)
- rare causes: vascular malformations, Dieulafoy lesion, aortoduodenal fistula (<2%)

Clinical assessment
Clinical assessment often runs concurrently with resuscitation and active management.

Assessment of haemodynamic status
- Immediate assessment for signs of general haemodynamic compromise—peripheral temperature, capillary refill time, central pallor, tachycardia, low blood pressure (reduced pulse pressure and postural drop most sensitive), low O_2 sats
- Always send blood for G&S (or cross-match if transfusion is needed or looks likely)

Identification of cause
Melaena is common but according to rate of bleeding and GI transit blood passed pr may be melaena, dark red, clotted or occasionally bright and dark.

Haematemesis is commonest with oesophagogastric lesions.

Alcohol use/abuse, smoking, and NSAID use are common risk factors and are too non-specific to be of diagnostic use.

Bleeding diatheses do not cause UGIH but exacerbate the course and make surgical intervention more likely.

- **Peptic ulcer/acute gastric erosions**—prodromal history of dyspepsia common; back pain made worse by hunger suggests an underlying posterior duodenal ulcer
- **Oesophagitis**—history of GORD symptoms is common; dysphagia suggest an underlying stricture or malignancy
- **Mallory–Weiss tear**—there is always some form of vomiting or retching prior to the passage of any blood but not all patients give a clear history; blood is characteristically bright red and only in the vomitus with no melaena
- **Oesophageal or gastric varices**—often copious or catastrophic dark red haematemesis; history of alcohol use or liver disease relatively common
- **Upper gastrointestinal malignancy**—prodromal weight loss, anorexia, and dyspepsia are suggestive of malignancy

Investigations
- Bloods—low Hb (chronic bleed), raised urea (large 'blood meal'), clotting studies (deranged in liver disease), abnormal LFTs (liver disease)
- OGD may be an acute emergency but should always be within 24 h of admission if possible; may be diagnostic and therapeutic. In severe bleeds or unstable patients this requires an experienced endoscopist and dedicated 'bleeding' scope suitable for advanced endoscopic measures
- Upper GI angiography is very rarely required except in obscure causes of recurrent bleeding

Management
Resuscitation
- Ensure large calibre peripheral venous access is available from admission—a central venous catheter is not the best access for resuscitation fluids
- If shocked on admission, catheterize, give supplemental O_2, and consider fluid resuscitation; synthetic colloids are usually adequate, uncross-matched blood should be avoided unless *in extremis*
- Continued active haemorrhage requires simultaneous diagnosis and treatment. This should be performed in theatre or the anaesthetic room with senior surgical, anaesthetic, and critical care personnel

Non-variceal haemorrhage
Continue appropriate fluid resuscitation and blood transfusion (cross-matched) where needed with close monitoring.

Endoscopic therapy
- Vasopressor injection—1:10 000 adrenaline in saline; effective for ulcers, bleeding erosions, bleeding vascular malformations
- Thermal coagulation
- Haemoclips

Satisfactory control of active bleeding should be achieved at the end of the procedure; if not, surgical intervention will be required.

Twenty per cent will re-bleed despite successful first treatment

Repeat endoscopic therapy is possible for stable patients with suitable pathology

Drug therapy
- Acid suppression—IV PPI (blood clot stability is reduced in acid environment). Proven to reduce the risk of re-bleeding, requirement for blood transfusions and duration of hospital stay
- Somatostatin—IV high dose. May reduce splanchnic blood flow in critical cases and inoperable cases
- Antifibrinolytic drugs, e.g. tranexamic acid. There is equivocal evidence in support of reduction in mortality rates and the need for surgical intervention

Surgery
Indicated for:
- massive haematemesis likely to be caused by aortoenteric fistulation
- acute bleed not controlled/uncontrollable by endoscopic therapy

- after failed endoscopic therapy (re-bleed after first or second time)
- continued slow bleeding despite endoscopic therapy evidenced by ongoing transfusion requirement

Principles
- Ulcers, erosion—ulcer suture (duodenal) or excision (gastric)
- Malignancy—partial gastrectomy

Mortality rates are 8–14%. Mortality and the probability of re-bleeding can be predicted.

Variceal haemorrhage
Ninety per cent of patients with portal hypertension have varices and, of these, 30% will have an UGI bleed, carrying a mortality rate of 50%.

Endoscopic therapy
- Banding of varices (oesophageal—less effective than for gastric)
- Paravariceal sclerotherapy

Drug therapy
- Acid suppression—IV PPI
- Reduction in portal venous pressure/blood flow—vasopressin/glypressin/terlipressin IV infusion, β-blockers
- Reduction in consequences of 'blood meal'—lactulose (reduces ammonia absorption and decreases GI transit). Metronidazole to reduce bowel flora

Surgical
- Sengstaken–Blakemore tube provides tamponade, salvage procedure, effective in 90%, but 50% re-bleed within 24 h of tamponade removal
- Oesophageal transection almost universally fatal
- Portocaval or mesentericocaval shunting (e.g. transjugular intrahepatic portosystemic shunting—TIPSS) may be considered

Since 70% of patients with a variceal haemorrhage will re-bleed, secondary prevention measures should be considered. These include β-blockers (possibly with isosorbide mononitrate), TIPSS, surgical shunting, sclerotherapy, and endoscopic ligation.

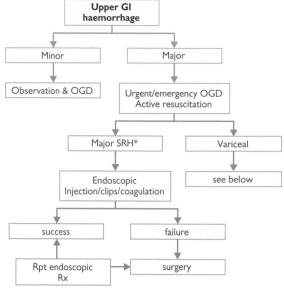

*stigmata of recent or active haemorrhage

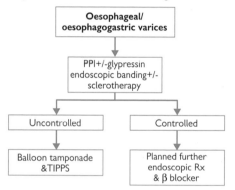

Fig 8.13 Guidelines for managing upper GI haemorrhage. Adapted with kind permission of the British Society of Gastroenterology (www.bsg.org.uk)

Table 8.9 Rockall score for predicting mortality rates of acute upper GI bleeding			
	0	**1**	**2**
Age (years)	<60	60–79	>80
Shock	None	HR>100 bpm	Systolic BP<100 mmHg
Co-morbidities	None	Cardiac	Hepatorenal disease Carcinoma

Percentage mortality rates for scores: 0 = <1%; 1 = 3%; 2 = 6%; 3 = 11%; 4 = 25%; 5 = 40%; 6 = >80%.

8.16 Lower gastrointestinal haemorrhage

Lower gastrointestinal haemorrhage is bleeding arising anywhere from the ligament of Treitz to the anal canal. Eighty per cent stop spontaneously, while 30% requires in-hospital investigation or treatment.

Aetiology

A cause of acute significant bleeding is found in approximately 80% of patients. Most common causes are:

- diverticular disease
- acute colitis (ulcerative, infective, neutropenic)
- colorectal tumours (cancer>adenoma)
- colonic angiodysplasia
- NSAID-induced colonic ulceration
- anorectal causes: internal haemorrhoids, solitary rectal ulcer
- rare causes: vascular malformations, Meckel's diverticulum-related bleeding, post-radiotherapy colorectal neovascularization, Crohn's colitis, small intestinal tumours

Clinical assessment

Clinical assessment often runs concurrently with resuscitation and active management.

Assessment of haemodynamic status

- Immediate assessment for signs of general haemodynamic compromise—peripheral temperature, capillary refill time, central pallor, tachycardia, low blood pressure (reduced pulse pressure and postural drop most sensitive), low O_2 sats
- Always send blood for G&S or cross-match

Identification of cause

The colour of the blood is unhelpful as a guide to origin (either pathology or level); ileal bleeding may appear fresh pr.

- **Diverticular disease**—commonly entirely unheralded, no prodromal symptoms, frank blood passed unexpectedly, initially often mixed with stools, then frank blood and clots with no faeces. May be copious volumes with collapse, especially in the elderly
- **Acute colitis**—usually a history of loose stools and frequency prior to the appearance of blood and mucus mixed with the stools. Often accompanied by abdominal pain, nausea, and malaise
- **Colonic tumours**—often some prior history of small 'herald' bleeds mixed with stools. Change in bowel habit may be minor or go unreported

Investigations

- Bloods—low Hb and ferritin (chronic bleed), clotting (deranged in liver disease), abnormal LFTs (liver disease)
- Stool samples for infective causes of colitis
- Rigid sigmoidoscopy—should be performed wherever possible to exclude simple anorectal causes
- Acute urgent flexible sigmoidoscopy/colonoscopy—indicated for bleeding which does not resolve spontaneously, must be done unprepared, often difficult, requires an experienced endoscopist and plenty of time. Locates a cause in around 60% of cases where bleeding is continuing

- Helical CT angiography—often preferred over conventional invasive visceral angiography, non-invasive but lower yield and non-therapeutic
- On-table colonoscopy/enteroscopy—may be required for occult but ongoing bleeding

Management

Resuscitation

- ABC
- Ensure large-calibre peripheral venous access is available from admission—a central venous catheter is not the best access for resuscitation fluids
- If shocked on admission, catheterize, give supplemental O_2, and consider fluid resuscitation; synthetic colloids are usually adequate, uncross-matched blood should be avoided unless *in extremis*
- Continued active haemorrhage requires simultaneous diagnosis and treatment. This should be done in theatre or the anaesthetic room with senior surgical, anaesthetic, and critical care personnel

Endoscopic therapy

- May be conducted colonoscopically
- Vasopressor injection—1:10 000 adrenaline in saline; effective for isolated ulcers, bleeding angiodysplasia, rarely possible in bleeding diverticular disease

Endovascular therapy

- Coil or plug embolization of feeding vessels is possible for active colonic or small bowel bleeding not suitable for endoscopic or surgical treatment, but risks ischaemic injury to affected bowel

Surgery (emergency)

Indicated for:

- acute ongoing colitic bleed
- acute ongoing tumour-related bleeding
- acute diverticular, angiodysplastic or other (including undiagnosed) bleeding with failed or impossible non-surgical treatment

Principles

- Resection of the affected segment
- Primary anastomosis only in stable patients with definite control of bleeding; if there is doubt, twin stomas should be made of the ends
- May require synchronous on-table endoscopy to identify the bleeding source
- Extensive or 'blind' colonic resection should only be used where all attempts at localization have failed

⊕ Segmental colectomy and end colostomy (Hartmann's procedure)

Preoperative

- If left-sided pathology is seriously suspected prior to theatre, review by the stoma specialist for marking may be invaluable
- Place the patient in low Lloyd–Davis position especially if the diagnosis is uncertain—access to the rectum
- Laparoscopy is sometimes performed to confirm the diagnosis prior to laparotomy and may very rarely be used to assist the resection

Operative

- Send any peritoneal fluid for MC&S (or swab)
- Assess the abdomen for collections of infected/faeculent fluid—these must all be dealt with by drainage or lavage during the procedure
- Ensure that the pathology is isolated and not multifocal
- A decision is required on the operative strategy for resection if the underlying pathology is unknown preoperatively. If malignancy is seriously considered, then a radical resection should be attempted, including a high mesenteric excision/tie; otherwise, a conservative resection may be undertaken
- The distal colon/rectum may be closed by staples or sutures or left open with a drain if it cannot be closed
- A proximal colostomy is formed where marked or appropriate; a small spout is often used
- Pelvic drains (low pressure suction or tube drains) are used where there is significant pelvic sepsis

8.17 Gastrointestinal obstruction

Gastrointestinal obstruction is often referred to as mechanical or functional, but the division is of little practical use. All true obstruction has the same basic management and possible complications.

The distinction between small or large bowel obstruction only relates to the differential diagnosis.

Gastrointestinal ileus should be considered as a separate condition.

- 5% acute surgical emergencies

Aetiology
Small bowel
- Adhesions and 'internal hernias' (60–70%)
- Acute (strangulated) hernia (20%)
- Malignancy (small bowel carcinoma, lymphoma, carcinoid, caecal carcinoma, peritoneal carcinomatosis) (5%)
- Strictures (Crohn's, NSAID, radiotherapy) (5%)
- Foreign bodies (gallstones, bezoars) (<5%)
- Intussusception
- Volvulus (true) (<1%)

Large bowel
- Primary malignancy (60%)
- Strictures (diverticular>Crohn's) (20%)
- Volvulus (sigmoid, caecal) (5%)
- Luminal bodies (impacted faeces>perianal inserted items) (5%)

Pathophysiology
- Proximal dilatation above the obstruction causes fluid, electrolyte, and gas accumulation and decreased absorption
- Stasis increases bacterial growth, gaseous distension and increased production of hypertonic products of digestion
- Initial response is increased peristaltic activity (colicky pain and visible peristalsis)
- Distension leads to mural oedema, reduced venous and capillary blood flow, cellular hypoxia, and translocation of bacterial products and eventually whole bacteria. This results in systemic features of bacteraemia and eventually septicaemia
- Progressive distension and increased intramural pressure reduces arterial flow and leads to mural ischaemia with eventual infarction if unrelieved. This is greatly exacerbated in causes which constrict or impair blood supply (e.g. severe adhesions, strangulated hernia)
- Vomiting exacerbates fluid and electrolyte loses

Types of obstruction
- **Closed loop** obstruction develops as a result of obstruction to both inlet (afferent) and outlet (efferent) ends of a single segment of bowel; it is commonest in adhesions, hernia, and volvulus. Large bowel obstruction with a competent ileocae-cal valve is a form of closed loop obstruction. It has a much higher risk and rate of progression than complicated obstruction
- **Simple obstruction** is obstruction without ischaemia or secondary septic features
- **Complicated obstruction** is ischaemia, perforation or systemic sepsis

Clinical assessment
History
All causes tend to demonstrate the cardinal symptoms:
- colicky, central abdominal pain. The development of constant pain strongly suggests the presence of ischaemia
- vomiting (early feature, initially gastric/bilious, progressing to faeculent with intestinal stagnation and bacterial overgrowth)
- abdominal distension (greater the more distal the obstruction)
- absolute constipation (late and unreliable feature)

Ask for a possible history of previous abdominal operations or herniae.

Examination
The cardinal features are:
- distended abdomen (hyperresonant percussion note)
- hyperactive bowel sounds (may be 'tinkling' or 'crescendoic'). Absence of bowel sounds suggests the development of peritonitis associated with ischaemia

Features of peritonism are strongly suggestive of bowel infarction or perforation.

Features of hypovolaemia and shock are common and do not always indicate complicated obstruction.

Always look carefully for a possible cause—scars and all hernial orifices.

Investigations
- Bloods—FBC (microcytic anaemia suggests a pre-existing tumour), U+Es (features of dehydration and electrolyte imbalance), ABGs (presence of metabolic acidosis suggests intestinal ischaemia)
- AXR (plain supine)—always taken to identify a possible cause, assess probable level (small or large bowel)
- erect CXR—to assess for free gas; indicative of perforation
- CT (abdominal multislice) is the investigation of choice in all but obvious causes which require surgery, or simple obstruction which is apparently resolving spontaneously. Even if the diagnosis of adhesions is likely, other diagnoses should be excluded by urgent scanning. It has a high sensitivity for complications (ischaemia and perforation)
- Gastrografin follow-through—rarely used acutely in adults
- Gastrografin enema—occasionally used to confirm suspected distal large bowel obstruction not confirmed on CT scanning

Management
Initial resuscitation
- ABC
- Fluid resuscitation (IV fluids, hourly urine output, daily U+Es). Remember to replace pre-existing losses, ongoing losses and basic requirements
- 'Bowel rest' (NBM, NG decompression and antiemetics). Reduces the risk of aspiration and may decompress partial adhesional obstruction sufficiently to allow spontaneous resolution
- Analgesia
- Antibiotics have no role unless there are signs of peritonism, when theatre is indicated

Conservative

- Consider in those with incomplete obstruction, where adhesions are suspected on CT scan or those with peritoneal carcinomatosis. Contraindications include peritonism, features of sepsis, high-grade obstruction or definite pathology on CT scan
- Watchful waiting must be reviewed at least twice a day and a further decision regarding surgery made after 48 h
- Palliative care (conservative management with no intention to reconsider surgery) should be considered for peritoneal carcinomatosis and terminal malignancy (extensive metastases with very short life expectancy) or patients considered unfit for general anaesthesia/intervention

Surgery/interventional endoscopy

Active intervention should be the default treatment after resuscitation unless a conservative trial or palliative care has been chosen.

Interventional endoscopy

This includes endoluminal stent placement and laser recanalization. It is used for obstructing distal (left-sided) colonic tumours. It may be used as a 'bridge to surgery.'

Surgery—principles

- Patients should be placed in the Lloyd–Davis position to allow access to the rectum
- Identify all sites of obstruction (there may be several, particularly in adhesions)
- Where possible, release, remove or resect the causative pathology
- Where there has been a resection, primary anastomosis should be avoided in the presence of severe sepsis, diffuse malignancy, chronic malnutrition, and seriously ill patients. Proximal obstruction may be relieved by 'on-table lavage' in colonic obstruction
- A proximal defunctioning loop stoma is an alternative in critically ill patients and may allow subsequent definitive surgery once the patient is better

Gastrointestinal 'paralytic' ileus

A condition of loss of functional inhibition of the propulsive activity of the bowel.

It usually affects the stomach (gastric ileus) or colon (often termed 'pseudo-obstruction'). Small bowel ileus is rare even after surgery and is usually caused by metabolic or drug effects.

Causes:

- metabolic disturbances ($\uparrow$ or $\downarrow$ Na^+, K^+, Ca^{2+}, Mg^{2+}, $\uparrow$ Ur, $\uparrow$ or $\downarrow$ T_4, hypothermia)
- drug side effects (e.g. anticholinergics, antipsychotics, opiates)
- central nervous system abnormalities (e.g. spinal injury, Parkinson's, neurodegenerative disorders)
- local inflammation (e.g. acute pancreatitis, peritoneal sepsis)

Investigations

As for obstruction—CT scanning is usually preferred to ensure there is no mechanical cause. Per rectal contrast enema may be used if there is suspected distal large bowel obstruction.

Management

- All complications of obstruction may occur in ileus but are much less common
- Conservative management is usual
- Surgery is very rarely indicated unless for complications
- Prokinetics (e.g. metoclopramide) may be helpful
- Parasympathomimetics (e.g. neostigmine) should be used with great caution owing to occasional severe autonomic side effects

---

⊙ Interpreting the abdominal radiograph in possible bowel obstruction

- Not all obstructed loops are either dilated or fluid-filled. Normal calibre loops do not exclude obstruction
- 'Ground glass' appearance may be caused by extensive fluid-filled obstructed loops
- Look at the areas of the hernial orifices for 'non-anatomically placed' loops of small bowel
- Small bowel loops are characteristically centrally placed, have complete transverse lines (valvulae conniventes), may be fluid-filled ('string of bubbles', 'ladder pattern')

Diagnoses which may be 'made' on AXR

- Gallstone ileus—distal small bowel obstruction, radio-opacity in the RLQ, air in the biliary tree
- Caecal volvulus—'bean' sign apex to LUQ
- Sigmoid volvulus—'bean' sign apex to RUQ
- foreign body

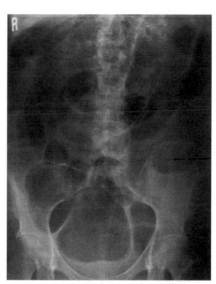

Fig 8.14 Supine abdominal radiograph showing multiple loops of dilated small bowel and a deflated colon suggestive of intestinal obstruction.

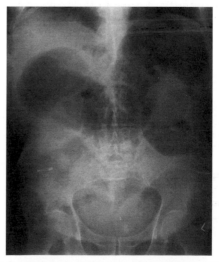

Fig 8.15 Supine abdominal radiograph showing dilatation of the transverse colon. There is no air seen in the rectum.

8.18 Gastrointestinal perforation

Perforation of the gastrointestinal tract may occur anywhere from the upper oesophagus to the anorectal junction.

The majority of causes in the UK are caused by intrinsic pathology of the GI tract, but trauma (usually violent penetrating trauma) and iatrogenic (e.g. during surgery or instrumentation of the GI tract) perforations also occur.

Perforation may occur in association with obstruction. This is not directly covered here although the basic management is the same.

Aetiology (intrinsic)
Oesophagus
- Spontaneous rupture during forceful vomiting ('Boerhave's syndrome')
- Carcinoma (usually fistulation)
- Impacted foreign body (late presentation)

Stomach/duodenum
- Peptic ulcer**
- Carcinoma (stomach)*

Small bowel
- Ulceration (NSAID, Meckel's diverticulum)
- Tumour (carcinoma, lymphoma)
- Crohn's disease*
- Foreign bodies

Colon
- Diverticular disease (diverticulitis)**
- Carcinoma*
- Stercoral (faecal) ulceration*
- Colitis (ulcerative, infective, ischaemic)

** = most common
* = common

Pathophysiology
- Perforation into a visceral cavity or space (peritoneum, pleura, mediastinum) is almost always associated with features of acute shock owing to autonomic activation +/- bacterial contamination or release of pus
- Autonomic activation leads to tachycardia, tachypnoea, cold peripheries, and moderate hypotension owing to central vasodilatation
- Good initial response to fluid resuscitation is typical because of the correction of relative hypovolaemia associated with vasodilatation
- Untreated release of enteric content or pus/bacterial products leads to progression to septic shock

Clinical assessment
History
Intraperitoneal perforation
- Rapid onset of abdominal pain ('kicked in the stomach') is classic but often not described and the onset may be more progressive
- Pain becomes established and remains constant, exacerbated by movement, coughing
- Modest distension is common
- Features indicative of a cause should be sought but are often lacking or non-specific:

- peptic ulceration—dyspepsia, PPI use, hunger pain, truly instantaneous onset of pain
- Malignancy—dysphagia (oesophagus), dyspepsia, weight loss (stomach), change in bowel habit, rectal bleeding (colon)
- Crohn's disease—diarrhoea, weight loss, abdominal pain
- Diverticular disease—gradual onset LLQ pain, fever, anorexia
- Stercoral perforation—constipation (longstanding and recent), distension

Retroperitoneal/extraperitoneal perforation
- Frequently gradual onset, with vague symptoms and predominant features of sepsis/inflammation
- Upper retroperitoneal pathology (posterior duodenal ulcer)—back pain, interscapular pain
- Lower retroperitoneal pain (diverticulitis, Crohn's disease)—lower quadrant and loin pain, limp, pain on hip movement

Intrathoracic perforation
- Acute oesophageal rupture is always related to a history of vomiting
- Chest pain, back pain, interscapular pain, inspiratory pain

Examination
Features of free intra-abdominal perforation may not always all be present but are typical.
- Moderate distension
- Generalized board-like rigidity (profound guarding)
- Absent or very scanty bowel sounds

Specific features may be present which suggest a cause and are much commoner in retroperitoneal perforation.
- Palpable mass (e.g. diverticulitis mass, tumour)
- Localization of tenderness and guarding to one quadrant of the abdomen

Investigations
- Urinalysis
- Bloods—FBC (microcytic anaemia suggests possible underlying tumour), ↑WCC, U+Es
- Erect CXR—only 80% of intraperitoneal perforations show free gas under one or other hemidiaphragm
- Plain AXR—of little value
- CT (multislice)—the investigation of choice in suspected perforations where a decision to take the patient to theatre has not yet been made
- Gastrografin swallow—occasionally used for possible oesophageal perforation where the CT is uncertain

Management
Initial resuscitation
- ABC
- Fluid resuscitation (IVI, hourly urine output, daily U+Es). Initially a bolus of fluid is required to correct the features of shock, but ongoing major fluid tranfusion requirements suggest another pathology (e.g. leaking aortic aneurysm or intra-abdominal bleeding)
- The patient should be NBM but NG decompression is unhelpful

- Analgesia, supplemental oxygen
- Antibiotics (e.g. cefuroxime and metronidazole) may be used 'blind' in ill patients awaiting theatre or urgent CT scanning

Conservative

- A trial of supportive care, PPI, and limited oral intake has been used for gastroduodenal ulcer-related perforations but only where the patient is entirely stable with no features of ongoing peritonism and, ideally, where a dilute Gastrografin swallow has shown the perforation to have self-sealed
- Contraindications include peritonism, features of sepsis, age, and co-morbidity (making a failed trial more risky)
- Palliative care may be considered for terminal malignancy (extensive metastases with very short life expectancy) or patients considered unfit for general anaesthesia/intervention
- Radiologically-guided drainage of collections is only useful in retroperitoneal perforations which are contained

Surgical

- All patients should be considered candidates for surgery once the diagnosis of perforation is made
- Laparoscopy may be helpful to locate the cause and occasionally perform the repair (e.g. simple perforated peptic ulcer)
- A midline laparotomy is the usual choice of access

The principles of surgery are:

- close perforations where the underlying disease will heal spontaneously (e.g. perforated peptic ulcer)
- resect perforated bowel which is intrinsically diseased— primary anastomosis should be avoided in the presence of established sepsis, diffuse malignancy, chronic malnutrition, and seriously ill patients. A stoma should be formed in these circumstances (📖 Topic 8.15)

⊙ Patch repair of perforated ulcer

Emergency laparotomy 📖 Topic 8.13

Procedure

- Closure of the ulcer is by patch and *not* approximation of the ulcer edges
- A strip of omentum is separated (pedicled)
- Sutures are placed into the bowel wall adjacent to either side of the perforation
- The omental patch is laid over the perforation and the sutures tied over the patch to hold it in place
- May be performed laparoscopically

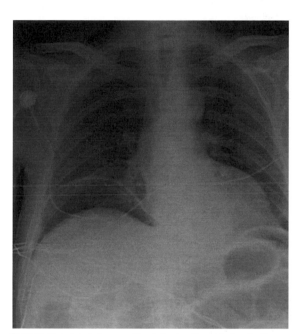

Fig 8.16 Pneumoperitoneum. Erect chest radiograph showing free air under the diaphragm. The right hemidiaphragm is elevated and separated from the liver. There are also dilated loops of small bowel seen in the upper abdomen.

8.19 Acute pancreatitis

This condition is an acute inflammatory condition of the pancreas typified by a local and systemic reaction. The incidence is 150–420 cases per million in the UK (and rising). The condition is associated with increased latitude (Scotland>England).

Aetiology

Aetiologies are remembered by acronym GET SMASHED. **G**allstones (40%), **E**thanol (40%), **T**oxins and drugs (e.g. steroids, diuretics), **S**urgery or trauma, **M**etabolic (e.g. hyperlipidaemia), **A**utoimmune and inherited, **S**corpion sting and infections, **H**ypothermia and hereditary, **E**RCP, **D**uodenal obstruction.

Pathophysiology

Local

Oedematous (phlegmonous) (80% of cases).

- Primary pathology disrupts pancreatic enzyme secretion, causing intrapancreatic enzyme activation (trypsin, lipase, amylase). This results in acinar cellular disruption and interstitial oedema
- Progressive pancreatic inflammation results in peripancreatic inflammation (phlegmon formation)
- During resolution, pockets of protein-rich serous fluid may form in the phlegmon. They may combine to form peripancreatic fluid collections. Persistence of these collections causes pseudocyst formation
- This condition is occasionally confined to areas of the pancreas when mild

Haemorrhagic (15%)

- Progressive inflammation causes disruption of intrapancreatic and peripancreatic blood vessels (especially veins). This may lead to peripancreatic bleeding
- Major vessel disruption may cause extensive retroperitoneal haemorrhage (blood in flank tissues—Grey–Turner's sign; blood in periumbilical tissues—Cullen's sign)
- Rarely confined to part of the pancreas

Necrotizing (5%)

- Extensive vascular disruption causes pancreatic ischaemia and tissue necrosis. This may also affect vessels supplying adjacent organs, e.g. transverse colon, spleen, stomach
- Necrotic tissue may become infected through haematogenous seeding. This may cause 'infected necrosis' and pancreatic abscess formation

Systemic

Acute pancreatitis is a potent cause of SIRS and related conditions (MODS)(📖 Topic 8.4).

Typical system organ effects/dysfunctions are:

- lungs—interstitial fluid (ARDS), effusions, disordered gas transfer
- kidneys—acute glomerular dysfunction, acute tubular dysfunction/necrosis, acute cortical necrosis
- GI tract—gastric ileus, liver dysfunction, ascites
- blood—neutrophilia, thrombosis, DIC,
- cardiovascular—myocardial depression, vasodilatation

Systemic effects specific to pancreatitis include:

- hypocalcaemia—owing to sequestration of Ca^{2+} by necrotic fat and low albumin

Clinical assessment

History

- Constant, progressive, severe epigastric pain radiating to the back
- Nausea, vomiting, upper abdominal bloating
- Aetiological factors (previous gallstones, alcohol intake, family history, medications, viral exposure, previous attacks)

Examination

- Epigastric tenderness, possible guarding
- Abdominal distension (gastric ileus, peripancreatic phlegmon or ascites)
- Features of SIRS—shock/pyrexia/tachycardia
- Grey–Turner's or Cullen's sign (rare)

Investigations—diagnostic

Guidelines for the UK Working Party on Acute Pancreatitis recommend that aetiology should be determined in at least 80% of cases.

- Serum amylase is readily available but non-specific (raised in acute inflammatory conditions, tissue infarctions), may not rise at all, and is transitory. Over 1000 iu is diagnostic of pancreatitis or hyperamylasaemia. Urinary amylase persists longer than serum amylase
- Serum lipase is more specific and sensitive for diagnosis as it has a long serum half-life and is exclusively produced by the pancreas
- Abdominal ultrasound is the first line diagnostic investigation of choice and should be performed in all cases within 48 h and more urgently in severe cases
- The objective is to assess for the presence of gallstones and identify the presence of CBD dilatation
- The diagnosis of CBD stones has a sensitivity of 25–50% in acute pancreatitis; this is greater if combined with biochemical measurements (bilirubin and alanine transaminases)
- Fasting glucose, plasma calcium and lipids, and viral antibody titres are usually performed once acute attack has settled

Investigations—severity/complications

- Bloods—FBC, U+Es, LFTs
- Erect CXR and plain AXR
- Contrast-enhanced abdominal CT—main indications
- Within 48 h for acute severe pancreatitis to assess severity and early necrosis
- Within 7 days for patients failing to improve with effective therapy and for suspected pancreatic necrosis
- Delayed for suspected pseudocyst formation
- Radiologically-guided aspiration—indicated to prove the presence of infected necrosis

Management

Supportive

- High flow supplemental oxygen and saturation monitoring
- IV fluid resuscitation (may require multiple boluses); monitor by urinary catheter, hourly urine volumes, and fluid balance monitoring
- Analgesia—may require PCA

- Nutritional support—early enteral feeding is ideal (via nasojejunal tube if necessary); it preserves the gut mucosal barrier and thus limits bacterial translocation. In severe cases with small bowel dysfunction, parenteral feeding may be required

Treatment of cause/process

- Routine antibiotics have no proven role. They have a proven role in infected necrosis and should be broad spectrum
- Urgent therapeutic ERCP including sphincterotomy; indicated in proven CDB stones with obstruction and failure to resolve/severe cases
- Infected necrosis has an extremely high mortality rate; combination IV antibiotics, radiological drainage, and surgical debridement (necrosectomy)
- Cholecystectomy (laparoscopic)—'same stay' surgery may be used or delayed for 6 weeks post-recovery

Complications and prognosis

Mortality rates increase according to the severity of the pancreatitis. Overall mortality remains at 5–10% and, if complications develop, this may increase to ≥35%.

Pseudocyst

A pseudocyst is defined as a localized collection of pancreatic secretions that lack an epithelial lining and is persistent for more than 4 weeks.

- Treatment—drainage should be considered if the pseudocyst is ≥5–6 cm, causes gastric outlet obstruction or pain, becomes infected or haemorrhages. Drainage can be either surgical, percutaneous or endoscopic (cystogastrostomy and cystoenterostomy being the commonest)

Fistulas

Fistulas result from pancreatic duct disruption; they should be suspected in patients who develop a large ascites or pleural effusion.

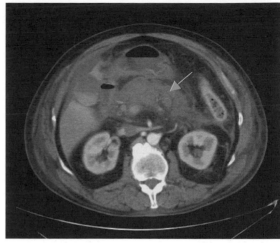

Fig 8.17 CT abdomen showing significant pancreatic necrosis (arrow) secondary to acute pancreatitis. There are extensive inflammatory changes of the pancreas with no enhancement of the body and most of the tail of the pancreas. The head has normal enhancement.

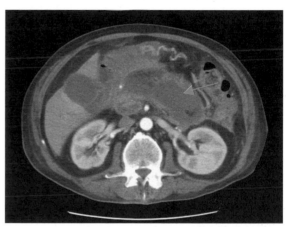

Fig 8.18 CT abdomen with contrast showing a pancreatic pseudocyst (arrow) 8 weeks after the scan in Fig 8.18 was taken. This went on to be drained endoscopically as it was causing obstruction of the common bile duct.

Table 8.10 **Modified Glasgow (Imrie) severity scoring in acute pancreatitis**		
P O₂	Arterial pO₂	<8 kPa
A ge	Age	>55 years old
N eutrophils	WCC	>15 × 10⁶/L
C alcium	Corrected calcium	<2.0 mmol/L
R enal	Urea	>16 mmol/L
E nzymes	AST >125 mmol/L	LDH >600 u/L
A lbumin	Albumin	<32 g/L
S ugar	Glucose	>10 mmol/L

Scored at 48 h following admission. A score of >3 is graded severe and patients should be considered for higher dependency unit admission.

APACHE II (acute physiology and chronic health evaluation) scoring or Atlanta criteria may also be used to determine the severity of pancreatitis (these have the benefit of a more rapid determination of prognosis than modified Glasgow criteria.)

Cellulitis

Cellulitis is a diffuse infection/inflammation of the skin and subcutaneous tissues.

Aetiology

- Usually *Staphylococcus aureus* or Group A beta-haemolytic streptococci (*Streptococcus pyogenes*) (erysipelas is an acute *Strep. pyogenes* dermal infection in children)
- Anaerobic cellulitis (mixed organisms, Gram-negative rods and fungi) may occur particularly in immunocompromised patients
- There is usually a preceding breach of the skin through either trauma or surgery. Patients with chronic wounds and foreign bodies passing through the skin are at particular risk

Features

- Signs of inflammation (induration, tenderness on palpation, spreading erythema, warm to palpation (best differentiation between underlying infected and inflammatory causes). There may also be local lymphangitis and reactive lymphadenopathy
- Fever, malaise, and anorexia suggests a systemic response/ bacteraemia

Investigations

- Not required in simple cases
- Local wounds should be swabbed
- Take blood cultures if systemically unwell
- The extent, spread, and response to treatment can be monitored by a line demarcating the limit of the erythema

Treatment

- Empirical antibiotic treatment (e.g. flucloxacillin or benzylpenicllin) is started IV until a response is achieved and is then converted to oral therapy
- Analgesia and elevation of a dependent limb help to control the associated pain and swelling
- Over 90% of cases will respond to antibiotics

Complications

- Local abscess formation is uncommon
- Superinfection with Gram-negative or anaerobic organisms may lead to necrotizing fasciitis or gangrene

Gangrene

Gangrene is necrosis of body tissues, either as a result of infection (wet) or ischaemia (dry).

Wet gangrene can be subdivided:

- **clostridial** (spore-forming Gram-positive rods predominate— *C. perfringens, C. novyi, C. septicum*). Gas formation is prominent
- **non-clostridial (progressive synergistic bacterial)**— non-gas-forming with mixed anaerobic and microaerophilic organisms, often of GI tract origin, are a common cause

Both cause gross blue/purple discoloration of the overlying skin owing to intradermal haemorrhage and necrosis.

Treatment follows the same principles as for necrotizing fasciitis (NF).

Dry gangrene is caused by ischaemic necrosis. It may be patchy in peripheral tissues such as digits (e.g. due to frostbite,

vasopressor therapy, diabetic angiopathy) or whole limb (e.g. caused by arterial occlusion). Many affected parts will eventually autoamputate.

If extensive, secondarily infected or causing complications because of tissue lysis, necrotic tissue should be surgically debrided or limbs amputated.

Furuncles, carbuncles, and infected sebaceous cysts

- A furuncle (boil) is an abscess which develops in a hair follicle. Multiple boils clustered together form a network of sinuses and boils which is termed a carbuncle. *Staphylococcus aureus* is the most common pathogen
- Sebaceous cysts contain inspissated sebum and skin oils. Infection may occur after trauma or be spontaneous, usually with skin organisms

The face, neck, back, armpits, and buttocks are the most common sites for both conditions.

Treatment

- Boils tend to be self-limiting. They will come to 'a head', discharge, and heal by repair. This can be hastened by applying warm compresses
- Infected sebaceous cysts may take longer to resolve and are more likely to require surgical toilet
- Surgical incision/drainage and debridement is used to hasten this process
- Antibiotics are only used to hasten resolution of persisting soft tissue infection after surgical treatment or discharge

---

⊕ Incision and drainage of abscess/cyst

Operative principles

- Small lesions may be treated under local anaesthetic; be wary since the surrounding skin is often hypersensitive and may require more LA than normal
- Large abscesses are best treated under GA
- Place the incision over the 'head', anatomical centre or point of maximum fluctuance if these are not obvious
- A cruciate incision or even excision of the central overlying skin helps maintain early postoperative drainage
- Curette or debride the underlying tissue to remove infected or necrotic elements. The wall of an infected sebaceous cyst may be hard to remove completely but doing so will reduce the risk of cyst reformation
- Only pack the lesion when there is a large cavity—use adsorbant material (e.g. Sorbsan®)

Postoperative

- Remove the pack prior to discharge. Arrange district nurse review/repacking if required

Necrotizing fasciitis

Fasciitis is infection tracking in normally anatomically preserved subcutaneous planes (e.g. deep fascia of the skin, myofascial planes).

Aetiology/pathology

- Always a synergistic, spreading infection
- Commonly involves *Staphylococcus aureus*, *Streptococcus pyogenes*, enterococci *(Strep faecalis/milleri)*, mixed Gram-negative rods, and *Bacteroides* spp.
- There is usually a preceding breach of the skin but it may be too small to detect
- More common and more rapidly progressive in the immuno-compromised (especially diabetics)

Features

- Signs of inflammation are late since the infection spreads widely in the subcutaneous fascial planes before the skin becomes involved by necrosis secondary to extensive arteriolar thrombosis
- Pain out of proportion to the physical signs in a susceptible patient should always raise the question of this diagnosis
- Fever, malaise, and anorexia is common and develops rapidly into SIRS/sepsis syndrome (📖 Topic 8.4)

Investigations

- Surgical exploration may be required to confirm the diagnosis
- Culture all available samples (blood, pus, tissue)

Treatment

- Start high-dose broad spectrum IV antibiotics as soon as the diagnosis is made or seriously considered (must include anaerobic and wide Gram-positive as well as negative cover)
- Always explore surgically

> ➕ **Surgery for major soft tissue infection**
>
> *Operative principles*
> - Excise all dead tissue, however extensive
> - Where the skin is apparently viable (bleeds on cutting), keep it (soft tissue coverage may be very difficult)
> - Open tissue planes to check for evidence of advancing infection, incise muscle to check for bleeding (none or dark venous bleeding indicates impending necrosis and the need for excision)
> - Plan a repeat procedure in 24 h whatever the patient's response

Complications

- Extensive tissue loss is common and may need plastic surgical reconstruction
- SIRS and MODS are common and death possible

Ingrowing toenail

Aetiology

- Chronic irritation and secondary infection of the paronychial tissues owing to disruption by the edge of the nail
- Commonest in the great toe in teenage boys

- Beware of the new diagnosis in adults—it may represent a subungual skin tumour
- Aggravated/precipitated by poor-fitting shoes, frequent sports activity, poor cutting of the toenail (too close and angled, giving rise to an in-turned 'leading edge')
- Secondary bacterial and fungal infection common
- May result in a paronychial abscess (typically chronic relapsing)

Investigations

- Nail clippings if fungal infection is suspected

Treatment

- Chiropody, careful attention to foot hygiene, shoe fitting, nail care
- Antibiotics for acute bacterial infections
- Nail wedge excision in acute subungual infection to allow drainage
- Surgical procedures for failed conservative management:
- Wedge excision—removal of lateral one-third of nail in an attempt to allow repair of the nail fold as the new nail grows in
- Nail avulsion—as above with the whole nail
- Nail avulsion and destruction—phenol injection, curettage or diathermy ablation of nail bed epithelium in an attempt to prevent nail regrowth (if incomplete, can cause problems with patchy nail regrowth)

Breast sepsis

Breast abscesses are most commonly associated with lactation but can occur at other times. An abscess forms when the ducts become blocked and then infected. In lactating women, the organism is usually *Staphylococcus aureus* but in non-lactating women they are caused by streptococci or anaerobes. Rare organisms include *Mycobacterium tuberculosis* and actinomycosis.

In non-lactating women, the main differential diagnosis is inflammatory breast cancer (aggressive tumour presenting with a solid mass and local inflammatory signs), and so this needs to be excluded during the assessment

Features

- Breast shows signs of inflammation and is very tender. A fluctuant abscess is most commonly palpable in the areolar or periareolar area. There may be associated nipple inversion, fever, and axillary lymphadenopathy
- ↑CRP, ↑WCC
- Breast USS to assess for a collection which can be aspirated under local anaesthetic and exclude a coincident mass

Management

- Aspiration (repeated daily in necessary) is the treatment of choice
- Incision; drainage may be used if very large or failing to respond to aspiration
- Oral antibiotics are usually safe even in breastfeeding women

Complications

- May cause a periareolar fistula (rare)
- Chronic or recurring infection and scarring (commonest in smokers)

8.21 Case-based discussions

Case 1

A 29-year-old female pedestrian is knocked down by a van travelling at 40 mph. On arrival in the resuscitation room the paramedic crew handover note that she is maintaining her airway but has poor saturations on 15 L O_2 and is haemodynamically unstable. They have placed a 20G venflon in the back of her right hand through which they are running a bag of 0.9% normal saline.

- Describe the steps of a primary survey

Her airway is clear but she is not maintaining it. The trachea is central. There is poor chest expansion on the right side with dullness on percussion and quiet breath sounds. There is no external bleeding.

HR 15 regular, BP 89/40 mmHg, RR 28, sats 91% on 15 L O_2 with a reservoir.

- What injuries might explain these findings and how are you going to manage them?
- Describe how you would insert a chest drain

She now has a Geudel airway. Her right chest is decompressed with a chest drain which drains 800 mL of blood. She has widebore IV access in both antecubital fossa and has received 1000 mL of gelofusin. HR 50 regular, BP 95/55 mmHg, RR 20, sats 98% on 10 L O_2.

- What are the indications for an emergency thoracotomy?

During painful sternal stimulation she opens her eyes and all limbs extend abnormally. Only incomprehensible verbal sounds are audible. The diameter of the left pupil is 7 mm and has a sluggish response to light; the right pupil is 4 mm and has a normal light reflex. She suddenly has a self-terminating grand mal seizure lasting 1 min.

- What is her GCS? Should she be intubated?
- What are the possible causes of her coma?
- Describe the essential investigations in a patient with a coma. How do you account for the pupil reflexes?
- Describe the anatomy of an extradural haematoma
- What further interventions might she receive on NICU to optimize her neurological outcome?

During the primary survey, life-threatening problems must be treated in order of ABC. Once the airway was protected she had a chest drain placed to decompress the right-sided haemothorax. She had a left extradural haematoma and the associated swelling had caused a third cranial nerve neuropraxia over the tentorium.

Case 2

A 16-year-old girl is admitted to the surgical assessment unit. She is complaining of abdominal pain which started 24 h ago around her umbilicus and has now moved to the right iliac fossa. It is associated with a loss of appetite but no nausea or vomiting.

- What other questions would you ask when taking a history?

She has no urinary symptoms, is sexually active, and her periods are normal. She takes the oral contraceptive pill.

On examination she is mildly febrile and looks unwell. There is tenderness across her lower abdomen which is maximal in the right iliac fossa where she is guarding. Urinalysis shows leucocytes +, blood +.

Your provisional diagnosis is acute appendicitis.

- Name some other differential diagnoses that might fit with this girl's symptoms

She has a senior review and is booked for an emergency appendicectomy (open or laparoscopic).

- How would you consent her for the procedure?
- What prophylactic treatment would you instigate pre-operatively?
- Name three possible early complications of appendicectomy.

Case 3

You are referred a 79-year-old man by his GP. He has a 2 day history of colicky abdominal pain, worse across his lower abdomen. It has been associated with anorexia. He has not opened his bowels for 4 days. He has previously had an appendicectomy but is otherwise well.

- What other questions would you ask when taking a history?

You think he might have an intestinal obstruction.

- What examination findings would support this?

He has distension with central tympanism and flank dullness. Bowel sounds are intermittent but active when present.

- What investigations would you to request?
- What initial steps are you going to take before a senior review takes place?

The diagnosis of intestinal obstruction is confirmed on CT scanning with a probable location in the distal sigmid colon.

- What additional tests would be available to confirm the diagnosis and prepare the patient for theatre?

The patient goes to theatre later that day and has a Hartmann's procedure with resection of an obstructing sigmoid tumour. You are called by the nursing staff that evening because his EWS score is triggered: HR 105 regular, RR 24, sats 94% on room air, and temperature 38°C.

- What is your differential diagnosis?
- How would you assess the patient and what plan would you make for his care?

Chapter 9

Trauma and orthopaedic surgery

Basic principles

Knowledge

◎ Clinical skills

- Describing a fracture
- Compartment syndrome
- Paediatric fractures
- Open fractures
- Reduction of shoulder dislocation

➕ Technical skills and procedures

- Closed reduction and plastering
- Knee arthroscopy
- Hemiarthroplasty of the hip joint
- Dynamic hip screw
- Total hip replacement
- Joint aspiration

9.1 Musculoskeletal physiology

Bone

Anatomy

Macrostructure

Mature bone has two main types of bone structure (Fig 9.1).

- Compact bone (cortical, dense bone) forms the outer layer. It is very hard and heavy, and makes up over 80% of the total bone mass
- Trabecular bone (cancellous, spongy bone) is central. It has an open structure with a large surface area. It makes the bones lighter and contains blood vessels and marrow

Bone shapes

1. Long bones make up the appendicular skeleton. They have the most complex structure (Fig 9.1)
2. Short bones are roughly cuboid in shape (e.g. carpal and tarsal bones). Cancellous bone is surrounded by a thin layer of cortical bone and periosteum
3. Flat bones (e.g. skull, scapula, sternum) have a thin inner and outer table of cortical bone with central cancellous bone (diploë)
4. Sesamoid bones are similar to short bones but sit in tendons (e.g. patella). They move the tendon away from the joint and improve its mechanical properties
5. Irregular bones do not fit into any of the above categories; they include facial bones and vertebrae

Microstructure

- Osteoblasts secrete organic bone matrix (osteoid). They become osteocytes when surrounded by bone matrix
- Osteoclasts are multinucleated cells derived from monocytes. They actively resorb bone
- Bone matrix has both organic and inorganic components. The organic (osteoid) matrix is composed of type I collagen and proteoglycans. The inorganic matrix is mainly calcium and phosphate salts
- Periosteum covers bones and contains blood vessels, nerves, and lymphatics. Its inner surface is osteogenic and contains osteoblasts and osteoclasts

Physiology

Ossification

Bone undergoes either intramembranous or endochondral ossification; both result in the same microstructure.

- **Intramembranous ossification** is directly from mesenchyme and occurs in flat bones such as the skull
- **Endochondral ossification** is the development of bone from mesenchyme but with an intermediate cartilage stage that acts as a model. It occurs in long bones

Remodelling

Immature (woven) bone is produced during development and initial bone healing. It has an irregular array of collagen fibres which are remodelled by osteoclast resorption and osteoblast deposition to form mature (lamellar) bone which is either compact or trabecular.

Function

- Calcium homeostasis—bone stores 99% of total body calcium as calcium hydroxylapatite. Stimulation by parathyroid hormone (PTH) increases osteoclast activity and release of calcium

- Haemopoiesis occurs in the medullary cavities of bones. In adults, red bone marrow is mainly found in flat bones and at the proximal ends of long bones. Yellow bone marrow is inactive and contains a high percentage of adipocytes
- Structure and protection of internal organs
- Movement—the skeleton is required for muscles to act on to create movement

Cartilage

Anatomy

Structure

- Matrix makes up over 80% of cartilage. It is primarily made of proteoglycans. These large molecules have a protein backbone with glycosaminoglycan (GAG) side chains
- Chondrocytes are mature cartilage cells that are scattered through the cartilage matrix which they secrete and maintain
- Fibres are found within the matrix which define the different types of cartilage (type I or II collagen or elastin)

Types of cartilage

- Hyaline cartilage is the most common form and contains mainly type II collagen. It functions both as articular cartilage in synovial joints and as the centre of ossification in growing bones
- Elastic cartilage has a similar structure to hyaline cartilage but also contains elastin bundles. It is found in the pinna of the ear, Eustachian tubes, and epiglottis, all structures that require stiffness and flexibility
- Fibrocartilage is a tougher form of cartilage that contains types I and II collagen. It is found in intervertebral discs and symphyses (e.g. pubic symphysis).

Function

Cartilage is a dense avascular connective tissue. Its main function is to act as a framework for bone growth during development and to provide smooth articular surfaces.

Joints

Anatomy

Types of joint

- Fibrous joints have fibrocartilage uniting two bones, allowing very little movement
- Cartilaginous joints are either primary or secondary. Primary cartilaginous joints have hyaline cartilage uniting two bones, allowing no movement
  Secondary cartilaginous joints have fibrocartilage uniting two bones, but with a thin layer of hyaline cartilage on the articular surface of each bone
- Synovial joints have a thin layer of hyaline cartilage on each articular surface which are separated by a joint space and surrounded by a joint capsule lined with synovium. They are subdivided by the direction of movement possible in the joint

Physiology

There are rich arterial plexuses surrounding synovial joints which penetrate the joint capsule along with veins and lymphatics. Articular nerves are derived from the ones supplying the overlying skin (Hilton's law) and are both for pain and proprioception.

Tendons and ligaments

Tendons and ligaments are tough fibrous connective tissues. Tendons connect muscle to bone whereas ligaments connect a bone or cartilage to another bone. Ligaments have limited elasticity and act to reinforce and stabilize joints.

Skeletal muscle

Skeletal (striated) muscle is one of three types of human muscles, the others being cardiac and smooth muscle.

Anatomy

Structure

Skeletal muscle is made of many parallel muscle fibres arranged in bundles or fascicles. Connective tissue surrounds the whole muscle (epimysium), the bundles (perimysium), and the individual muscle fibres within them (endomysium). Each muscle fibre contains myofibrils which are divided into sarcomeres.

Types of muscle fibre

There are two main types of human skeletal muscle fibres: they are determined by their ATP use which itself is dependent on the type of myosin isoenzyme (fast or slow).

- Slow fibres (type I) perform continuous slow sustained contraction and use oxidative phosphorylation as their main energy source. They have relatively high endurance under aerobic conditions and a red appearance owing to high concentration of myoglobin and capillaries
- Fast fibres (type II) perform infrequent but intense fast contractions and use anaerobic glycolysis as their main energy source. They have relatively low endurance owing to rapid depletion of intramuscular glycogen stores and a white appearance caused by relative paucity of myoglobin and capillaries

Physiology

Neuromuscular junctions (NMJ)

Each muscle fibre is innervated by one motor neuron and so has one NMJ. However, a motor neuron can innervate multiple muscle fibres.

Excitation–contraction coupling

- An end-plate potential generated by a single motor neuron action potential (AP) is enough to depolarize the muscle fibre and initiate a muscle AP
- Muscle AP is propagated in both directions along the sarcolemma and through the T tubule system
- T tubule system communicates with the sarcoplasmic reticulum where voltage gated L-type calcium channels open, releasing calcium into the sarcoplasm around the myofibrils
- Calcium binds to troponin C on the actin filament where they interact with tropomyosin and troponin. The resulting complex moves to reveal the sites on the actin where the myosin heads will bind
- Cross-bridge cycling begins (see sliding filament theory below)
- Relaxation is prompted by a reduced calcium concentration as it is pumped out of the sarcoplasm into the sarcoplasmic reticulum

Muscle contraction

The sliding filament theory suggests force generation in a skeletal muscle fibre occurs when myosin cross-bridges bind to actin filaments, resulting in the relative sliding of thin and thick filaments. This is known as the **sliding filament theory** and produces muscle shortening with no change in filament length.

The tension (the amount of force produced) of a muscle is a function of the proportion of active cross-bridges. It depends on calcium concentration and the initial length of the contracting muscle.

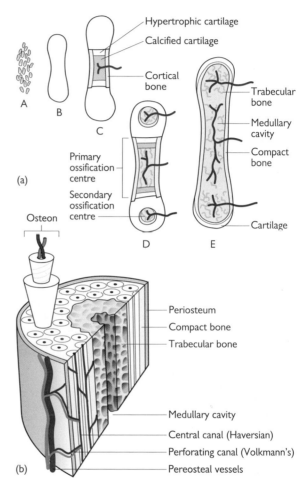

Fig 9.1 (a) Endochondral ossification. (A) Condensation of mesenchymal cells. (B) Mesenchymal cells differentiate to become chondrocytes and lay down a cartilage template. (C) Hypertrophic cartilage calcifies and is remodelled to become secondary bone and bone marrow (D) Secondary ossification sites develop in the epiphyses. (E) Following puberty the ossification centres fuse and no further growth occurs. (b) Microstructure of a mature long bone. The osteon (Haversian system) is the functional unit of compact bone. Concentric layers (lamellae) surround a central canal containing nerves and vessels. Osteocytes are scattered throughout in small spaces (lacuna), communicating with each other via canaliculi.

9.2 Fracture assessment

A fracture is the local separation of a bone into one or more pieces.

Aetiology

- **Trauma**—violent force exceeds the strength of normal bone
- **Fatigue**—repetitive normal force exceeds the strength of normal bone over a period of time (e.g. 'march' fracture)
- **Bone pathology**—normal force exceeds the strength of abnormally weak bone (e.g. osteoporosis, tumours)

Fracture terminology

The type of fracture sustained is dependent on many factors related to the cause of the injury and type of bone.

- **Open** fractures can be 'in–out' where bone fragments penetrate the skin, or 'out–in' where the injury causes soft tissue loss over the fracture site. Most fractures are closed with intact soft tissue
- **Hairline fractures** result from minimal trauma and are often difficult to detect. They may be complete or incomplete and there is no displacement
- **Torus fractures** are the compression failure of one cortex which appears 'buckled' on a radiograph. **Greenstick fractures** are fractures of one cortex with the bones hinged on the periosteum of the opposite side. These only occur in children
- **Simple fractures** have one fracture line and can be transverse (perpendicular to the axis of the bone), oblique (angle of 30° or more), or **spiral** (result of indirect twisting force)
- **Multifragmentary (comminuted) fractures** result in multiple bone fragments and can be wedge or complex
- **Impacted fractures** have one bone driven in to the other (e.g. impacted femoral neck fracture)
- **Compression or crush fractures** result from compression of cancellous bone (e.g. vertebral wedge fracture)
- **Avulsion fractures** result from sudden muscle contraction or traction on a ligament or capsule attachment
- **Depressed fractures** have a localized segment of depressed cortical bone (e.g. skull fractures)
- **Intra-articular fractures** involve the joint surface and can lead to stiffness and post-traumatic osteoarthritis
- **Fracture-dislocation** is a dislocation of a joint associated with a fracture
- **Complicated fractures** involve damage to surrounding structures such as nerves or blood vessels

Bone healing

There is a spectrum of bone healing processes. Primary (direct) healing is very similar to normal bone remodelling and occurs in simple undisplaced or impacted fractures where there is no gap.

When there is a bigger gap, bone heals via callus formation (secondary healing). This can be divided into three main phases. Clinical union can occur within a month, although remodelling and return of full strength takes longer.

Reactive phase

- Haematoma forms immediately and the associated inflammatory response leads to an influx of polymorphonuclear leucocytes, macrophages, and lymphocytes

Repair phase

- Haematoma organized into granulation tissue
- Osteoclasts resorb non-viable bone

- Pluripotent mesenchymal stem cells, osteoblasts, and fibroblasts proliferate and lay down a new matrix of fibrous tissue and cartilage
- This is mineralized to form fracture callus. Hard callus forms at the periphery and is via intramembranous ossification; soft callus is formed centrally before endochondral ossification. Eventually these tissues bridge the fracture gap
- Various growth factors and proteins regulate the healing process. Bone morphogenic proteins (BMP) derived from the bone matrix are particularly important

Remodelling phase

- The initial woven bone is converted to lamellar bone. This process can take many months. Radiographically there is restoration of the trabecular and cortical lines as well as the original bone contour

Fracture assessment

Fractures are mostly traumatic and the initial approach should follow ATLS® guidelines if appropriate.

History

- Mechanism of injury, including direction and magnitude of forces involved
- Associated medical conditions
- Consider non-accidental injury

Examination of suspected fracture site

- Look for swelling, deformity, asymmetry, abnormal posture, and signs of vascular compromise
- Feel for tenderness over a fracture site and distal neurovascular status
- Movement of the fracture site should be avoided as it will cause pain but is helpful if the diagnosis is in doubt

Investigations

- Plain radiographs should be carefully requested with the clinical question and views required clearly stated (usually a minimum of two views at right angles)
- CT scans often provide additional information to plain radiographs in the acute setting (e.g. cervical spine) and when planning fracture management (e.g. tibial plateau)
- MRI and ultrasound have a place in assessing soft tissues but are rarely used in the acute setting of fracture management
- MRI or isotope bone scan are helpful in detecting suspected fractures over 48 h old not seen using plain films

Fracture classification

There are many different fracture classification systems, often with eponymous names. The Müller AO Classification is now commonly used in clinical practice. It is organized according to the morphological complexity, difficulty of treatment, and prognosis. The alpha-numeric code describes the location and type of fracture (see below).

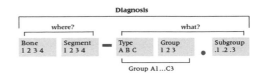

◎ Describing a fracture

The following points will help to communicate the details of a fracture clearly to colleagues.

- Bone and side
- Open or closed
- Level of fracture—is a distinct part (e.g. greater trochanter) within an anatomical division of a long bone (e.g. proximal diaphysis)?
- Type of fracture (simple or multifragmentary)
- Displacement is the movement of the bone ends in relation to one another and is described in terms of the distal segment
- Angulation of the distal fragment
- Rotation of the bones
- Complications, e.g. neurovascular injury

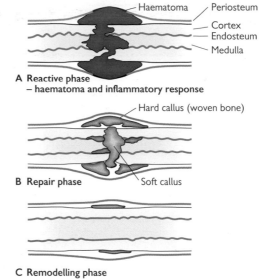

A **Reactive phase**
– haematoma and inflammatory response

B **Repair phase**

C **Remodelling phase**

Fig 9.3 Secondary bone healing.

221

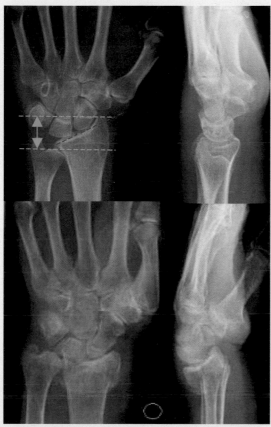

Fig 9.2 A Plain PA and lateral left wrist showing normal anatomy. Key features are the radial inclination (red), palmar (volar) tilt (blue), and increased radial height (green).
B Fractured left distal radius before reduction.
'This 42-year-old lady has sustained a closed fracture of her left distal radius. It is a transverse fracture with impaction, dorsal displacement, and angulation. The hand is neurovasularly intact'.

9.3 Fracture management

The aims of fracture management are bony union without deformity, and restoration of function and return to normal daily activities and employment.

Non-operative

The approach is to reduce, immobilize, and rehabilitate. The immobilization can be achieved using casting (see box), functional bracing, and traction.

Casts

A cast acts as a splint to hold the fracture reduced; it improves bone healing and patient comfort.

They are usually used with a small amount of padding to reduce the risks of pressure sores. Traditionally, plaster of Paris is used, although other materials such as fibreglass provide strong light-weight casts, often in funky colours.

Functional bracing

Functional bracing relies on the soft tissues and brace to control fracture alignment. It allows earlier mobilization of surrounding joints.

Traction

Traction holds a fracture out to length. It can be fixed or balanced depending on how the counterbalance is designed. Traction can be achieved using plaster, skin or skeleton. It is becoming 'old fashioned'.

Operative

Internal fixation

Internal fixation may follow open or closed reduction and utilizes different types of implant, including screws, plates, and intramedullary nails. There is often debate surrounding their indications and technical use.

External fixation

External fixation allows stabilization of a fracture remote from the site of injury. This is particularly useful in open and peri-articular fractures. It also allows adjustment of the alignment and fixation during healing.

There are many different constructs (simple, ring and hybrid) used for different fracture patterns and sites.

Percutaneous fixation

Kirschner wires (K-wires) can be drilled across a fracture site following closed reduction. They are then removed, often in out-patients, once healing is complete. They can also be used to apply skeletal traction and in the design of some external fixation devices.

Fracture complications

Early complications

Neurovascular injury

Significant blood loss can be associated with both the fracture (femoral shaft) and by interruption of local blood vessels (pelvis). In the limbs, vascular injuries can lead to ischaemia. Peripheral nerve injury is often associated with a vascular injury.

Fat embolism

Release of bone marrow fat into the systemic circulation occurs in 50% of long bone fractures although is clinically detectable in only a small number of cases. It presents 24–72 h after injury, with hypoxia, restlessness, and confusion. It can lead on to ARDS and coma. Management is supportive.

Compartment syndrome

A rise in pressure within a fascial compartment can lead to ischaemic necrosis (see box).

Infection

External fixation pins and percutaneous K-wires can develop pin site infections. They usually affect only the soft tissues and can be managed with good pin site hygiene and antibiotics.

Osteomyelitis is relatively rare but there is an increased risk in open fractures and those treated by open reduction and fixation.

Late complications

Malunion

Union of the bone ends is achieved but with an abnormal anatomical outcome, i.e. shortening, angulation, and rotation.

Delayed union

This is a slower healing period than would normally be expected for a particular bone. It may progress to non-union.

There are many factors that can delay healing, including fracture variables, nutritional status, immune status, and drugs.

Delayed union in internally fixed fractures can often be improved by allowing loading of the fracture site (e.g. removing locking screws from an intramedullary nail).

Non-union

Non-union is failure of bone healing to progress over a period of 3 months. It can be hypertrophic (hypervascular) with abundant callus formation, or atrophic (hypovascular) with local bone resorption. It can also result in a pseudarthrosis where there is cartilaginous tissue and fluid between the fracture ends.

The aetiology is similar to delayed union, with additional factors such as infection, implant failure, and soft tissue interposition.

Management often entails bone grafting and improved fixation of the fracture site.

Avascular necrosis

Fracture may disrupt the blood supply to part of a bone, leading to avascular necrosis (AVN). An example is the scaphoid bone, in which the principal blood supply enters through the dorsal waist. A fracture through the waist leaves the proximal segment prone to AVN.

Amputation

A number of scoring systems are used to grade limb injuries. Limbs with significant bone, soft tissue or vascular injury may require amputation.

The mangled extremity severity score (MESS) was designed for the lower limb but can also be applied to the upper limb. A score of 7 or above is usually an indication for amputation.

◎ Compartment syndrome

Compartment syndrome is an orthopaedic emergency. It may occur in any fibro-osseous compartment, e.g. hands, feet, thigh, forearm. However, it is most common in the leg.

Aetiology

- Trauma—fracture or soft tissue crush, burns
- External compression—splints and casts
- Lithotomy position
- Internal increase in compartment pressure—haemorrhage
- Reperfusion injury

Pathophysiology

Perfusion of muscle and nerves relies on adequate capillary perfusion pressure (CPP). Blood flow through tissue relies on the difference between CPP and interstitial fluid pressure. All muscle groups are arranged in compartments surrounded by a rigid fascial sheath. As fluid leaks into a compartment as a result of injury, the interstitial fluid pressure rises. Once this exceeds CPP, capillary blood flow ceases and ischaemia develops.

As muscle necroses, myocytes break down and release more osmotically active particles. These attract water from arterial blood and lead to a further rise in compartment pressure. This vicious cycle propagates, although some compensation occurs by autoregulation.

Clinical assessment

In conscious patients pain is the earliest and most reliable symptom of the 6 Ps (pain, paraesthesia, perishingly cold, pallor, paralysis, pulselessness). Severe pain on passive stretch of an involved muscle group should raise suspicion. Waiting for other signs to become evident means it is usually too late to save the compartment.

Compartment pressures can be measured using a needle and transducer. A difference of 30 mmHg or less between diastolic pressure and intracompartmental pressure has been suggested as a threshold for fasciotomies.

Management

- Relieve any external compression. This may involve removing bandages or splitting a cast
- Elevate the limb to the level of the heart; any higher will reduce arterial pressure
- Emergency surgical decompression should be performed within 4 h of the onset of symptoms
- Fasciotomy of the affected compartments should be full length and the wounds left open
- A second look is required once the swelling has subsided and the wound closed directly or with SSG

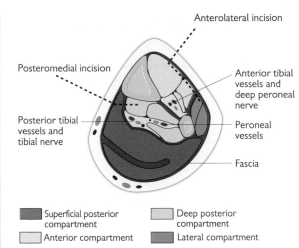

Superficial posterior compartment

Deep posterior compartment

Anterior compartment

Lateral compartment

Fig 9.4 Cross-section of leg showing the four compartments and placement of two skin incisions to gain access for decompression of all the compartments.

✚ Closed reduction and plastering

Many fractures can be managed conservatively with closed reduction and plaster fixation. This can be performed in the emergency department or in theatre. A Colles' fracture reduction is used as an example.

Closed reduction of Colles' fracture

- Assess radiographs and clinical appearance of fracture
- Analgesia as required
- Apply traction to disimpact the fracture and then increase the deformity, dorsiflexing the distal fragment
- Reduce the fracture back into anatomical position by pronation and palmar flexion
- Correct rotation and then lock the reduction with further pronation
- Assess the quality of reduction by clinical appearance and palpation of the fracture site
- Maintain the reduction whilst applying an appropriate plaster

Plastering

Generally a plaster-of-Paris back slab is applied acutely to achieve three-point fixation and then completed once the swelling has subsided within a few days.

1. Protect skin with a stockinette
2. Protect bony prominences with a layer of Velband
3. Measure the length and width of plaster required. Six layers are usually sufficient for a child; use 12 in an adult
4. Trim the plaster to fit the limb
5. Hold the plaster at both ends and submerge in tepid water. Remove and squeeze out excess water and then smooth the layers together
6. Position the plaster carefully and smooth out any wrinkles. The plaster may be reinforced with additional slabs
7. Arrange a check radiograph and review at 24–48 h for application of a full circumferential cast (often changed to fibreglass cast)

9.4 Congenital and developmental conditions

Developmental dysplasia of the hip

Developmental dysplasia of the hip (DDH) covers a range of conditions in which there is abnormal growth of the hip. DDH encompasses both dislocations developing *in utero* and postnatally.

Incidence is 2 per 1000 live births and there is a female preponderance (F:M 6:1). It is classified as either early (neonatal) or late (>6 months).

Aetiology and pathophysiology

Risk factors include female sex, family history, and decreased intrauterine space (breech position, first born, oligohydramnios).

The three main factors are excessive capsular laxity, a shallow acetabulum with abnormal slope, and rotation of the proximal femur.

The femoral head gradually moves away from the medial wall of the acetabulum, subluxes, and then dislocates. The acetabulum becomes flattened and dysplastic owing to lack of stimulus to grow around the femoral head. The muscles around the hip joint become short and contracted.

Clinical assessment

Early (neonate)

- Galeazzi sign assesses limb length discrepancy caused by unilateral DDH. Bilateral DDH gives a false-negative
- Barlow's test identifies potential for passive dislocation of the hip and is combined with Ortolani's manoeuvre, which is the palpable reduction of a dislocated hip

Late

- Limited abduction
- Trendelenberg gait
- Asymmetrical skin folds are not accurate

Investigations

- Hip ultrasound has a high sensitivity and is used for Graf's classification of DDH in neonates
- Plain AP and frog radiographs are used in patients >6 months
- Hip arthrogram may show rose thorn sign, hour glass constriction of capsule, capsule distension, medial pooling of dye, and confirms the reduction of the joint following manipulation

Management

The aim of treatment is to obtain a concentric reduction and promote early acetabular development. It is based on age.

- Newborn—Pavlik harness holds the hips in a stable position of flexion with some abduction allowed
- Infant—Pavlik harness or closed reduction and hip spica for 3 months
- Child—open reduction, femoral shortening, and acetabuloplasty

Complications and prognosis

Ninety per cent of cases diagnosed at birth resolve within 3 months. The most devastating complication is avascular necrosis of the femoral head.

Legg–Calvé–Perthes disease

Legg–Calvé–Perthes disease is idiopathic avascular necrosis of the proximal femoral head in a growing child.

It most commonly affects boys (M:F 4:1) aged 4–8 years old.

Aetiology and pathophysiology

The condition is thought to be caused by transient vascular compromise or synovitis. The femoral head goes through four pathological stages: (1) ischaemia/necrosis, (2) fragmentation/resorption, (3) reossification/resolution, and (4) remodelling.

Clinical assessment

A painful intermittent limp is the main symptom. On examination there is often limited internal rotation and abduction (worse on hip flexion). Passive hip flexion causes external rotation (Catterall's sign).

Investigations

- Plain AP and frog lateral hip radiograph
- Bone scan and MRI detect early disease
- Hip arthrogram determines hip position for splint and to plan osteotomy

Classification

The Column classification is commonly used in clinical practice; others include Waldenström, Catterall, and Salter–Thompson.

Management

The aim of treatment is a spherical, well covered femoral head with a near-normal range of movement. This can be achieved by containing the head in the acetabulum, either using physiotherapy and braces or surgery.

Operative management is considered in more severe cases and in older children.

- Varus osteotomy of the proximal femur (centres the femoral head deep in the acetabulum)
- Inominate osteotomy rotates the acetabulum for better containment of the femoral head

Complications and prognosis

Early presentation of the disease (~5 years) has a better prognosis. Most children see a complete resolution although this may take a few years. The main complication is a deformed femoral head, resulting in early secondary osteoarthritis.

Slipped upper femoral epiphysis

Slipped upper femoral epiphysis (SUFE) is a condition where the femoral neck 'slips' off the femoral head which stays in the acetabulum. Subsequent development of the femoral head and function of the hip joint is impaired.

It most commonly affects boys (M:F 3:2) aged 12–15 years old. It is bilateral in 25% of cases.

Aetiology and pathophysiology

Risk factors for SUFE include rapid growth, obesity, and endocrine diorders.

During the adolescent growth spurt the epiphysis is vulnerable to shear stresses. It is also believed that the slope of the epiphysis increases in some individuals.

Clinical assessment

- Pre-slip: pain in hip, thigh or knee, limited internal rotation
- Acute slip: symptoms <3/52 and usually follows trauma (Salter–Harris type 1 fracture)
- Chronic slip (60%): symptoms >3/52 with pain and fixed flexion deformity of hip. Flexion makes hip go into external rotation and there is decreased internal rotation

Investigations

- Plain AP and frog lateral radiographs of both hips. The slip is graded as mild, moderate or severe based on the degree of displacement and slip angle (Fig. 9.6)
- Isotope bone scan detects pre-slips and avascular necrosis

Management

The aim is to stabilize the femoral epiphysis on the femoral neck. Operative internal screw fixation is most successful. Severe slips may need an osteotomy.

Complications and prognosis

Reduced range of motion in hip joint, gait abnormalities, chondrolysis, avascular necrosis, and osteoarthritis.

Irritable hip

Irritable hip or transient synovitis of the hip is a very common condition in children, especially boys under 10 years old. Its aetiology is unknown although it may follow a viral URTI.

Clinical assessment

Children present with a limp and pain radiating to the knee. There is often a reduced range of hip movement.

Investigations

- Bloods—FBC, ESR and CRP are normal
- Plain AP and frog lateral hip radiographs are normal
- Hip ultrasound may show a joint effusion

Management

Most cases resolve over a few days following analgesia and rest. It is important to exclude other differential diagnoses such as DDH, Perthes disease, SUFE, and arthritis (septic or juvenile).

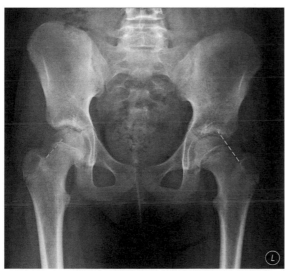

Fig 9.6 Plain AP hip radiograph showing left-sided SUFE. The Klein lines drawn along the superior border of the femoral neck should pass through part of the femoral head as happens on the right side.

Paediatric fractures

During childhood the skeleton is growing and the bones have a more elastic quality and are able to remodel following injury. Torus and greenstick fractures are classically seen in childhood (Topic 9.1). As the growth plates are still open they are prone to injury.

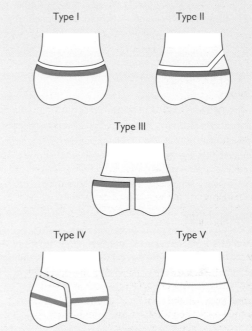

Type I   Type II

Type III

Type IV   Type V

Fig 9.5 Salter and Harris classification of physeal fractures.

Salter and Harris classification of physeal injuries

Type I	Separation of the epiphysis from the metaphysis through the physis
Type II	Fracture through the physis into the metaphysis, creating a triangular fragment
Type III	Fracture through physis extending into the joint, dividing the epiphysis
Type IV	Fracture through the epiphysis, physis, and metaphysis
Type V	Compression of the physis

Management

Type I injuries undergo closed reduction and plaster stabilization. Type II injures may require K-wire fixation following closed reduction. Type III and IV almost always need ORIF. Type V present late with growth arrest.

Complications

The main complications are overgrowth as a result of a diaphyseal injury or growth arrest as a result of physeal injuries.

Hallux valgus

Hallux valgus is lateral deviation and/or rotation of the hallux (big toe) often associated with medial deviation of the first metatarsal (metatarsus primus varus). It is often associated with soft tissue swelling (bunion) over the medial surface of the first metatarsal head, and leads to difficulty wearing normal footwear and painful movement.

It is a common condition, with a bimodal age distribution and female preponderance. It is often familial in young adults.

Aetiology

- Trauma (intra-articular damage, dislocation)
- Inflammatory (psoriatic, rheumatoid, and gouty arthritis)
- Neuromuscular (MS, Charcot–Marie–Tooth)
- Biomechanical and structural abnormalities (abnormal metatarsal length, genu valgum)
- Poor footwear is probably a risk factor rather than a cause of hallux valgus

Pathophysiology

Once the valgus deformity has developed it progressively worsens because of the pull of extensor and flexor hallucis longus. This causes stretching of the medial capsule of the joint and bone proliferation over the medial side of the metatarsal head, forming a bunion.

Clinical assessment

Patients complain of medial pain around the first metatarsophalangeal joint (MTPJ) associated with walking and improved by removing footwear.

Examination

The foot is examined during walking, weightbearing, and non-weightbearing.

- Look—hallux position; medial prominence (bunion); plantar keratosis under the interphalangeal joint (IPJ) or MTPJ, widening of the foot
- Feel—medial bursa; pain around MTPJ during movement
- Move—the deformity should be passively correctable without pain. Crowding of toes with second toe overriding and being displaced by first toe eventually results in dislocation

Investigations

- Weightbearing plain AP and lateral radiographs of the foot allow assessment of severity of disease, degenerative changes, and bone quality

Management

Conservative

- Footwear with wider and deeper toe box and padding
- Analgesia

Operative

The aim of surgery is to reduce pain and improve function; it is unlikely to improve cosmesis. There are numerous procedures.

- Metatarsal osteotomy (Chevron or Mitchell's)
- Distal soft tissue release (modified McBride procedure)
- Excision arthroplasty (Keller's procedure)
- Arthrodesis of the first MTPJ
- Exostectomy to remove medial bony swelling

Complications and prognosis

Over 75% of patients gain improvement in their symptoms. Operative treatment should avoid replacing a mildly symptomatic hallux valgus with a stiff MTPJ.

Hallux rigidus

Hallux rigidus literally means 'stiff great toe' and is caused by degeneration of the first MTPJ.

Clinical assessment

Movement becomes severely limited in dorsiflexion and patients take shorter steps to avoid extension of the great toe or roll their weight round the lateral aspect of the foot when walking. Pain is related to osteophyte impingement and worn cartilage. It usually improves at rest.

Management

Conservative management includes analgesia and stiffened sole inserts to reduce the movement at the first MTPJ during walking. Manipulation under anaesthetic with or without steroid injection may be useful in early stages.

Surgical options include excision of osteophytes, excision arthroplasty (Keller procedure), arthrodesis, and joint replacement.

Lesser toe deformities

Claw/hammer/mallet toes

These deformities of the lesser toes are common in advanced age. Most are idiopathic. Rarer causes include neurological disorders (MS, Charcot–Marie–Tooth, cerebral palsy, stroke), diabetes mellitus, and inflammatory arthropathies.

Clinical assessment

Patients complain of pain due to callosities on the dorsal aspect of the toes where they rub against the shoe. They may also complain of nail deformities and callosities at the tips of the toes.

Management

Conservative

- Shoe insoles and large toe boxes relieve pressure on the metatarsal heads

Operative

- Lengthening of extensor tendons
- Flexor to extensor tendon transfers
- IPJ fusion

Metatarsalgia

This is pain under the metatarsal heads. The commonest cause is a change in foot function, resulting in increased weight being transferred through the lesser metatarsal heads, e.g. shortened first ray, hallux valgus, pes cavus, inflammatory arthritis.

Conservative management with insoles is usually successful. Surgery can be used as a last resort to shorten the metatarsal necks (Weil's osteotomy).

Morton's neuroma

Morton's neuroma (intermetatarsal neuroma) is a condition caused by inflammation of the common digital nerve as it passes between the metatarsal heads; the third then second interdigital spaces are most commonly affected. It typically affects middle-aged women.

Inflammation of the nerve as it passes under the transverse metatarsal ligament makes it enlarge and become very sensitive. Patients complain of pain and tingling on weightbearing, like having a pebble in the shoe.

Management options include footwear modification, insoles, steroid injection or surgical excision of the neuroma.

Foot arch conditions

Pes cavus

Pes cavus is a foot with an abnormally high longitudinal arch which does not flatten during weightbearing. This is usually caused by an imbalance in the musculature creating the foot arches. The underlying cause is neurological in 60% of cases.

The spectrum of problems include clawing of the toes, dorsiflexion of the calcaneus, and contraction of the plantar fascia.

Conservative management with shoe modifications is usually successful. Operative options involve soft tissue releases/tendon transfers and osteotomies.

Pes planus

Pes planus (flat foot) is the loss of the medial longitudinal arch. It is classified as either flexible or spastic/rigid. Flexible flat foot generally does not need treatment. Rigid cases, such as those seen in cerebral palsy, often need surgery.

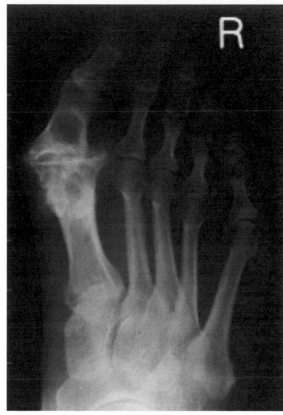

Fig 9.8 Plain AP radiograph of right foot showing hallux rigidus. There is significant joint degeneration with loss of joint space, metatarsal head cysts, osteophyte formation, and subchondral sclerosis.

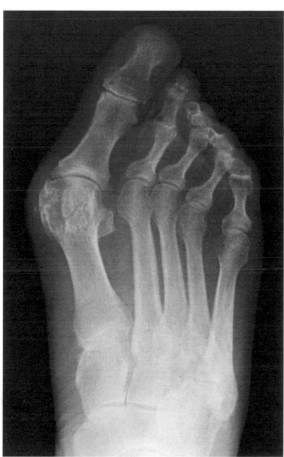

Fig 9.7 Plain AP radiograph of right foot showing hallux valgus. There is medial deviation of the first metatarsal and lateral deviation of the hallux. It is important to establish whether the first MTPJ is congruent or not. Congruent joints, as above, are less likely to progress.

Calcaneal fractures

The calcaneus (os calcis) has a complex shape. It articulates on three surfaces with the talus (subtalar joint) and cuboid. It is commonly injured by axial loading from a fall from a height or road traffic collision (RTC). A wedge fracture of the spine is associated with 5% of cases.

Classification

Calcaneal fractures can be either intra-articular (75%) or extra-articular, and displaced or undisplaced. CT scan classification systems are used to guide surgical management of complex fractures.

Clinical assessment

1. Look—the heel is tensely swollen, and may appear wider and flatter with some valgus tilt
2. Feel—tender over heel
3. Move—unable to weightbear due to pain

Investigations

- Plain radiographs—lateral view is the most important; axial view shows the heel, sustentaculum tali, anterior talocalcaneal joint, and posterior talocalcaneal joint; AP view shows the calcaneocuboid joint; oblique views may be helpful if no fracture is identified with standard views
- Ankle CT scan is used to assess the degree of comminution and extent of intra-articular fractures

Management

Extra-articular fractures are usually managed conservatively in a short leg cast for 4–6 weeks.

Undisplaced intra-articular fractures are managed conservatively with early non-weightbearing mobilization. Displaced fractures are more complex. Low performance patients can be managed conservatively. Open or closed reduction and fixation are performed once the swelling has subsided (7–10 days). Occasionally, primary arthrodesis is indicated.

Complications

Approximately 60% of patients have a good outcome. Common problems include widened heel, chronic pain, and ill-fitting footwear. Sural nerve injury and peroneal tendon impingement can complicate surgery.

In the longer term, subtalar joint stiffness and pain may require subtalar fusion.

Tarsal dislocations

The mechanism of injury varies. Historically, a Lisfranc injury was sustained when a horse rider fell with their foot caught in the stirrups leading to twisting of the forefoot. Now the injuries are often a result of high-energy trauma.

Classification

1. Subtalar dislocation involves both the talocalcaneal and talonavicular joints. The majority are medial dislocations as a result of forced inversion of the foot. The talar head is pushed dorsolaterally
2. Midtarsal dislocation is rare as this joint is fairly stable

3. Total talar dislocation is very rare and often an open injury. There is a high risk of infection
4. Tarsometatarsal fracture-dislocation (Lisfranc injury) is rare

Clinical assessment

1. Look—swelling of the mid foot. Frank dislocations are usually detectable but a high index of suspicion is required for minimally displaced dislocations
2. Feel—assess neurovascular status; tenderness over the mid-foot
3. Move—ankle joint movement intact; reduced inversion and eversion with pain on movement

Investigations

- Plain AP radiograph should detect both the dislocation and any associated fractures
- Foot CT scan aids assessment of fractures

Management

- Closed reduction under GA
- Fixation with K-wires or small fragment screws may be required if the reduction is unstable.

Complications

Subtalar stiffness is the main problem. Post-traumatic osteoarthritis may be treated with an arthrodesis.

Metatarsal and phalangeal fractures

The forefoot is vulnerable to injury. Most fractures and dislocations can be managed conservatively once reduced.

Classification

- Fifth metatarsal fractures—avulsion fracture of the base of the fifth metatarsal is the commonest fracture of the lower limb and is sustained during sudden inversion of the foot
- March fracture is a fatigue fracture of the neck of the second metatarsal often not detected until callus is seen. Walking plaster helps to control pain
- Phalangeal fractures commonly result from a crush

Clinical assessment

- Look—localized swelling. Check for dislocations
- Feel—point tenderness over fracture site
- Move—pain on movement. Weightbearing through heel

Investigations

- Plain AP and lateral radiograph centred on the injury

Management

- Analgesia, elevation, and observe circulation in toes
- Reduce displaced fractures or toe dislocations under LA
- Support bandage or buddy strapping sufficient for most phalangeal fractures
- Multiple displaced metatarsal fractures need ORIF as do unstable toe dislocations

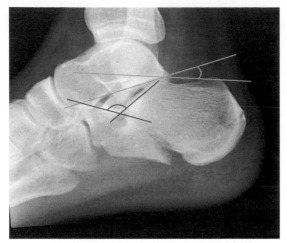

Fig 9.9 Plain lateral radiograph showing a partially displaced intra-articular fracture of the os calcis.

- Bohler's salient angle is formed by the intersection of two lines at the posterior articular surface originating from the anterior articular process and superior angle of the tuberosity (green). Normal angle is 20–40° but this is reduced following a fracture
- The crucial angle of Gissane is marked in red. A reduced angle suggests disruption of the subtalar joint

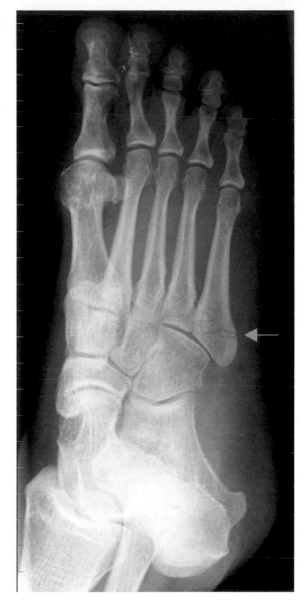

Fig 9.10 Plain AP radiograph of the fifth metatarsal of the right foot. A minimally displaced intra-articular fracture runs perpendicular to the axis of the metatarsal. A Jones fracture is more distal to the joint.

The tibia, fibula, and talus form the ankle joint. It is a modified mortise and tenon joint, allowing flexion and extension as well as a small degree of rotation. The tibia and fibula are joined by strong anterior and posterior tibiofibular ligaments to form the mortise and the talus is the tenon.

The talus is held in position laterally by three ligaments forming the lateral ligament complex (anterior talofibular ligament, the calcaneofibular ligament, and the posterior talofibular ligament). On the medial side the strong deltoid ligament fans out from the tibia to attach to the talus.

Acute ankle sprain

A sprained ankle is an injury to the lateral ligament complex of the ankle. It is a common injury and forms at least 15% of all sports-related injuries. It is usually caused by sudden inversion and adduction of a foot whilst in plantar flexion.

Clinical assessment

The injury is characterized by pain, swelling, and tenderness over the ligament complex. The anterior draw test or talar tilt test may be positive if there is abnormal laxity. The patient is able to weightbear carefully.

Investigations

- Plain AP and lateral radiographs (Ottawa ankle rules)
- Stress views are not normally required
- MRI scan may be indicated in chronic instability after recurrent sprains when planning surgical reconstruction

Classification

- Grade I—mild stretching with no instability
- Grade II—partial rupture with mild instability
- Grade III—complete rupture with instability

Management

Initial management is symptomatic relief with ice, analgesia, elevation, and ankle support (e.g. Tubigrip®). Early protected mobilization rather than immobilization improves outcome.

Recurrent sprains are an indication for specialist referral. Chronic pain may be the result of an osteochondral defect. Operative management is rarely indicated. Complications include chronic ankle pain and instability, stiffness, and swelling.

Achilles tendon rupture

Achilles tendon rupture is usually sustained playing sport during push-off (e.g. squash). It is most common in men aged 30–50 years old.

Clinical assessment

- Sudden pain in the Achilles tendon region, often with an audible snap and difficulty walking owing to inability to plantar flex with power (e.g. climb stairs)
- Lower calf may be swollen and a gap on palpation of the tendon is noted 2–6 cm above the calcaneal insertion
- Simmond's test is positive if there is no movement of the foot when the calf is squeezed with the patient prone
- Ultrasound or MRI can be used to confirm the diagnosis

Mangement

Conservative

Cast immobilization is often favoured in less functionally demanding patients. The foot is held in equinus by cast immobilization for 4 weeks and then may be put in a more neutral position for another 4 weeks. Physiotherapy to improve leg strength and ankle range of movement should be started after cast removal.

Operative

Surgical repair of the tendon is considered in the young and athletic. In an acute rupture the two ends can be approximated and the paratenon closed. A percutaneous approach is not as strong as an open repair initially but reduces the wound complications. A similar cast immobilization regime is used postoperatively.

Complications and prognosis

Cast immobilization has a lower complication rate but higher re-rupture rate (5–15%) than surgical repair (2–5%). Operative complications include infection, skin necrosis, and fistula.

Ankle fractures

Ankle fractures are the most common lower limb fracture. High-energy impact or low-energy twists can lead to fractures, commonly by causing rotation of the talus. This occurs if the foot is externally or internally rotated by an external force or abduction and adduction of the foot.

Classification

- Weber classification is based on the level of the fibula fracture in relation to the syndesmosis. It does not take account of other injuries (e.g. medial malleolus)
  - Type A—below
  - Type B—at the level (often spiral or oblique)
  - Type C—above
- Descriptive classification is based on the malleoli involved and the presence of displacement
- Lauge–Hansen classification is based on the position of the foot and the direction of the deforming force

Clinical assessment

- Look—ankle grossly swollen. Check the skin viability which may be compromised in fracture-dislocations
- Feel—location of pain will give a clue to ligamentous injury
- Move—reduced movement and inability to weightbear. Stress testing is usually not possible

Investigations

- Plain AP and lateral ankle radiograph show fracture/dislocation. A mortise view (10–20°) in line with the intermalleolar line may show diastasis (widening of the gap between the tibia and fibula)

Management

Initial approach should follow ATLS guidelines. Suspected ankle fractures should be promptly assessed and fracture-dislocations reduced and stabilized in the emergency department to prevent overlying skin ischaemia.

Conservative or operative management depends on the patient, fracture type, and stability.

Undisplaced fractures

- Type A injuries are stable fractures and can be treated with minimal splintage. Tubigrip or a below-knee cast for pain control is adequate
- Type B injuries confined to the lateral part of the ankle are stable. A below-knee cast for 6–8 weeks is usually sufficient. Regular review must be arranged to exclude talar shift
- Type C injuries may often look undisplaced but there is a significant ligament injury and these should be considered for examination under anaesthesia +/- fixation

Displaced fractures

The majority of these fractures need ORIF. However, if reduction and cast stabilization is chosen, regular review of fracture healing is essential.

The medial and posterior malleoli are fixed with lag screws and the fibula with a plate.

Complications and prognosis

Conservative management carries the risk of poor reduction or displacement. Internally fixed fractures are at risk of delayed wound healing, infection, malunion, non-union, joint pain, instability, and stiffness. Less than 5% require arthrodesis.

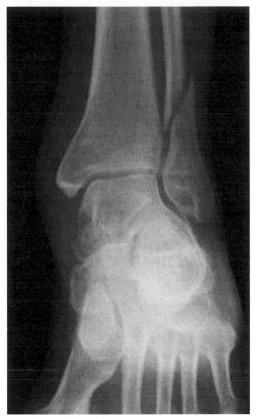

Fig 9.11 Weber type B ankle fracture (Müller 44-B1).

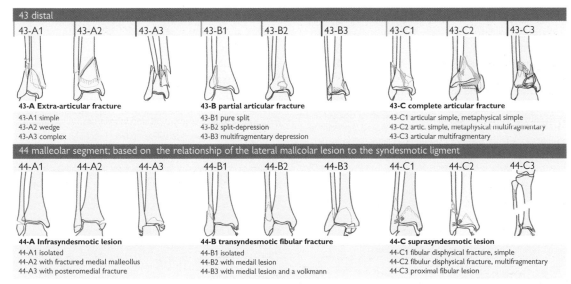

Fig 9.12 Müller AO classification of ankle fractures. Weber A = 44-A1, B = 44-B1, C = 44-C1. Reproduced from the *Müller Classification of Fractures* with kind permission of Springer–Verlag Ltd.

Collateral ligament injuries

The medial collateral ligament (MCL) is the most commonly injured ligament of the knee. Injury is often sustained during sporting activities and results from either a direct valgus force or an indirect force during unusual pivoting.

Clinical assessment

MCL injuries are often associated with injuries to other structures in the knee. On examination there is point tenderness over the medial aspect of the knee and occasionally a joint effusion. The injury is graded I–III (grade I, stretching but no instability; grade II, stretching, end point to laxity; grade III, complete disruption of fibres with instability and no end point to laxity). Over 20% of cases are associated with anterior cruciate ligament and other injuries. Attempt to exclude these during the examination.

Investigations

- Plain AP and lateral knee radiographs exclude a fracture
- MRI is the criterion standard for non-invasive assessment of collateral ligament injuries

Management

In the acute phase rest, ice, compression, and elevation is recommended. The current trend is to manage most injuries conservatively with a hinged brace. Grade III injuries or those associated with other conditions may require surgery if there is significant instability.

Lateral collateral ligament injuries are less common. Severe injuries are more likely to require surgery.

Cruciate ligament injuries

Anterior cruciate ligament (ACL) injuries occur during hyperextension or rotational injuries with the knee flexed. They are often associated with other injuries (MCL and medial meniscus) especially following direct trauma. The posterior cruciate ligament is stronger and less frequently injured.

Clinical assessment

A joint effusion develops quickly in up to 70% of cases. This is accompanied with severe knee pain and reduction in the range of movement. The Lachman test is sensitive for acute ACL rupture. The knee is placed in 30° of flexion and the femur held with a non-dominant hand. The other hand applies anterior force to the calf and the amount of displacement is noted. Anterior and posterior draw tests are other useful diagnostic tests.

Investigations

- Plain AP and lateral knee radiographs exclude a fracture
- MRI is very sensitive at detecting cruciate injuries

Management

Initial management is conservative before consideration of delayed intra-articular reconstruction. Active rehabilitation programmes following surgery are very successful.

Meniscal injuries

Two menisci (medial and lateral) sit on the flat tibial plateau and act to deepen the articular surface. The medial meniscus is C-shaped and attached at its periphery to the joint capsule as well as the deep portion of the MCL. The lateral meniscus is an incomplete O-shape; it is also attached peripherally to the joint capsule but not to the lateral collateral ligament. The menisci play an important role in loadbearing and distribution, stability, and proprioception.

Meniscal injuries are very common in young adults (medial >lateral). The typical mechanism of injury is twisting or sudden change of direction whilst the knee is weightbearing. The two main types of tear are longitudinal and radial (horizontal) although there are many descriptions of more complex types.

Clinical assessment

Symptoms include acute knee pain usually localized to the joint line of the affected compartment. Locking, clicking, and instability with the joint giving way are also common.

Approximately 50% of patients will develop a joint effusion which is often delayed by a few hours. Pain and swelling cause a reduced range of movement with displaced tears causing locking of the joint. McMurray's test is positive if there is a click heard or felt as the knee is gradually extended from a position of being flexed and externally rotated.

Investigations

- Plain knee radiographs exclude degenerative joint changes and fractures
- MRI is the criterion standard for non-invasive assessment of meniscal and intra-articular pathology
- Arthroscopy allows definitive diagnosis and treatment

Management

In the acute phase rest, ice, compression, and elevation is recommended. An active rehabilitation programme is suitable for most injuries although the patient's level of activity must be considered. Surgical intervention is indicated in severe cases or if there is locking of the knee.

Arthroscopy is the standard approach. Partial meniscectomy benefits injuries in the avascular region. Meniscus repair is considered if the injury is in the peripheral vascular region, is longer than 1 cm, or if over 50% of the meniscus is involved. Total meniscectomy should be avoided owing to the risk of secondary osteoarthritis and rotational instability.

Knee fractures

Fractures about the knee include fractures of the femoral condyles, patella, and proximal tibia. Their aetiologies vary but they are generally caused by a direct high-energy trauma or through axial loading following a fall from a height.

Clinical assessment

Symptoms include pain, joint swelling, reduced weightbearing, and range of movement. The joint may be unstable if there are associated ligament injuries.

Investigations

- Plain knee radiographs including oblique views
- CT scan is used for detailed assessment of tibial plateau fractures to help plan surgery

Management

Generally, undisplaced fractures can be managed conservatively with immobilization of the knee and non-weightbearing. Displaced fractures require internal fixation to improve articular alignment, joint stability, mobility, and reduce the risk of secondary osteoarthritis.

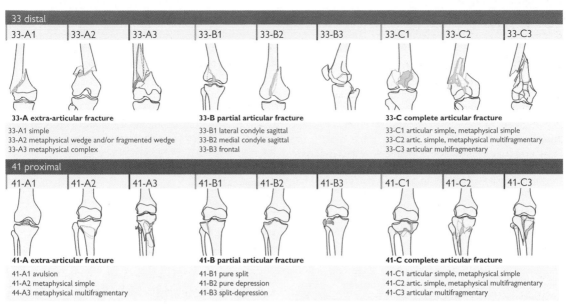

33 distal								
33-A1	33-A2	33-A3	33-B1	33-B2	33-B3	33-C1	33-C2	33-C3

33-A extra-articular fracture

33-A1 simple
33-A2 metaphysical wedge and/or fragmented wedge
33-A3 metaphysical complex

33-B partial articular fracture

33-B1 lateral condyle sagittal
33-B2 medial condyle sagittal
33-B3 frontal

33-C complete articular fracture

33-C1 articular simple, metaphysical simple
33-C2 artic. simple, metaphysical multifragmentary
33-C3 articular multifragmentary

41 proximal								
41-A1	41-A2	41-A3	41-B1	41-B2	41-B3	41-C1	41-C2	41-C3

41-A extra-articular fracture

41-A1 avulsion
41-A2 metaphysical simple
44-A3 metaphysical multifragmentary

41-B partial articular fracture

41-B1 pure split
41-B2 pure depression
41-B3 split-depression

41-C complete articular fracture

41-C1 articular simple, metaphysical simple
41-C2 artic. simple, metaphysical multifragmentary
41-C3 articular multifragmentary

Fig 9.13 Müller AO classification of distal femoral fractures and proximal tibial fractures. Reproduced from the *Müller Classification of Fractures* with kind permission of Springer–Verlag Ltd.

233

➕ Knee arthroscopy

Knee arthroscopy is usually performed under general anaesthetic but regional anaesthesia can also be used.

Procedure

- Patient supine
- Thigh tourniquet is often used. It reduces bleeding and gives a better image
- Knee flexed to 90°
- The first port is placed laterally for the scope and then a second medially for instruments. Additional sites are used depending upon the procedure
- A continuous flow of sterile water is pumped through the joint
- Each structure is systematically examined
- Therapeutic procedures include washout of the joint in septic arthritis, excision of meniscal tears, removal of loose bodies, and debridement of articular surface lesions
- The instruments are removed and port sites closed

Complications

Intraoperative and early	*Intermediate and late*
• Bleeding (haemarthrosis) (1%)	• DVT
• Septic arthritis (0.1%)	
• Wound infection	
• Nerve injury (rare)	
• DVT	

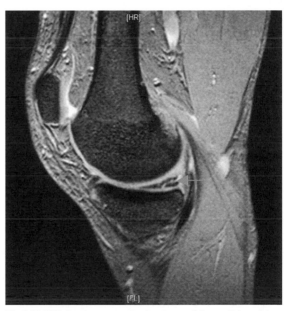

Fig 9.14 MRI showing a posterior horn tear of the medial meniscus.

Femoral shaft fractures

Femoral shaft fractures are frequently sustained during high-energy trauma (e.g. fall from a height or RTC). Pathological fractures may result from osteoporosis, tumour (usually subtrochanteric region) or osteomyelitis; stress fractures are rare.

Classification

The femoral shaft extends from 2.5 cm below the lesser trochanter to 8 cm above the knee joint and is subdivided into proximal, middle, and distal thirds. The AO system is used for classification.

Clinical assessment

Initial assessment and management should follow ATLS guidelines.

- Localized pain and inability to weightbear
- Shortened thigh length caused by overlap of the bone ends
- External rotation of the distal segment of the limb
- Adduction of the distal limb but abduction of the proximal pieces by the hip abductors

Associated injuries

- Fractures of proximal femur (5%), pelvis, patella
- Knee ligament injury (5%)
- Rare: neurovascular injury, dislocation of the hip

Investigations

- Bloods—FBC, U+Es, cross-match 2 units
- Plain AP and lateral radiographs of the entire femur
- Plain AP and lateral hip radiograph owing to risk of associated hip fracture
- Lower limb arteriography is indicated in penetrating injuries (e.g. gunshot)

Management

Immediate

Following ATLS assessment the fracture is reduced and the limb put in traction (10–15 lb) to limit blood loss and need for transfusion.

Conservative

Flexible IM nails (Nancy nails) are now generally used in children. Those under 4 years old can be placed in a hip spica. Balanced skin or skeletal traction using a Thomas splint is still occasionally used in children, periprosthetic, and osteoporotic fractures.

Operative

- Internal fixation with an IM nail is now the preferred choice in adults. The nail can be inserted through the proximal or distal femur and may be reamed or unreamed. It is locked into position to prevent rotation and provides stability of the fracture pieces in all planes, allowing early mobilization.
- External fixation is used in open fractures where decontamination is necessary or where the fracture is unstable
- Dynamic compression plate fixation is rarely indicated

Complications and prognosis

Complications include infection (5% open nailing, <1% closed nailing), fat embolus syndrome, malrotation of the distal limb, delayed union, and non-union.

Traction involves a prolonged hospital stay, poor control of length and alignment and an increased risk of DVT, stiffness, and pressure sores.

Tibial shaft fractures

The tibia and fibula can fracture from direct trauma (e.g. car bumper), transmitted trauma through the feet (e.g. fall from a height) or torsional stresses (e.g. football).

Owing to its ring structure, the leg tends to break in two or more places. Tibial shaft fractures are more likely to be open as the shaft lies subcutaneously. Isolated fractures of either bone are rare and tend to be from direct injuries.

Classification

The AO system is used for classification (Fig. 9.15).

Clinical assessment

- Severe pain and inability to weightbear
- Deformity of the leg
- Assess vascular supply (popliteal, dorsalis pedis, and posterior tibial)
- Assess neurology (common peroneal nerve commonly injured in proximal fibula fractures)

Associated injuries

- Knee ligament injury (20%)
- Compartment syndrome
- Neurovascular injury

Investigations

- Bloods—FBC, U+Es, G+S or cross-match
- Plain AP and lateral radiographs of the leg, including the knee and ankle joints
- DSA may be indicated if a vascular injury is suspected or to plan free flap reconstruction

Management

Immediate

Stabilize the leg in a splint and elevate to the level of the heart with the patient lying supine. Admission is usually required for analgesia and regular observations for compartment syndrome. Open fractures are an orthopaedic emergency (see box). They are best managed by lower limb trauma units with orthoplastic teams

Conservative

Undisplaced and minimally displaced stable tibial fractures are managed with a long leg cast for 6–8 weeks. The knee is held in 15° flexion and the ankle at 90°.

Isolated fibula fractures are managed with a walking cast for pain relief.

Operative

- IM nailing is very successful for managing closed displaced fractures. Plates and screws are rarely used
- External fixation may take the form of monolateral, multiplanar, or circular frames. It is indicated in open fractures although some surgeons use an unreamed IM nail
- Amputation rates for type IIIC injuries are >50%

Complications and prognosis

Compartment syndrome of the anterior compartment is particularly common in mid-shaft tibial fractures. If compartment syndrome is diagnosed, all four fascial compartments of the leg should be decompressed via full length longitudinal medial and lateral incisions.

Altered bone healing (delayed union, non-union, malunion) is common in open and more complex fractures. Anterior knee pain is commonly seen following nailing.

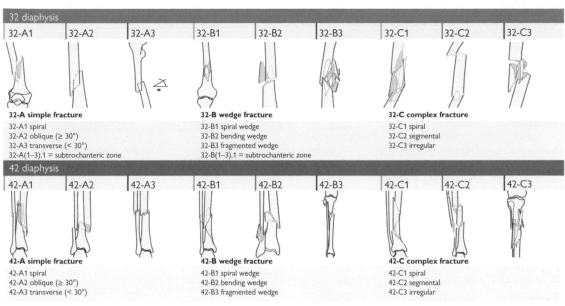

32 diaphysis								
32-A1	32-A2	32-A3	32-B1	32-B2	32-B3	32-C1	32-C2	32-C3

32-A simple fracture

32-A1 spiral
32-A2 oblique (≥ 30°)
32-A3 transverse (< 30°)
32-A(1–3).1 = subtrochanteric zone

32-B wedge fracture

32-B1 spiral wedge
32-B2 bending wedge
32-B3 fragmented wedge
32-B(1–3).1 = subtrochanteric zone

32-C complex fracture

32-C1 spiral
32-C2 segmental
32-C3 irregular

42 diaphysis								
42-A1	42-A2	42-A3	42-B1	42-B2	42-B3	42-C1	42-C2	42-C3

42-A simple fracture

42-A1 spiral
42-A2 oblique (≥ 30°)
42-A3 transverse (< 30°)

42-B wedge fracture

42-B1 spiral wedge
42-B2 bending wedge
42-B3 fragmented wedge

42-C complex fracture

42-C1 spiral
42-C2 segmental
42-C3 irregular

Fig 9.15 Müller AO classification of femoral and tibial shaft fractures. Reproduced from the *Müller Classification of Fractures* with kind permission of Springer–Verlag Ltd.

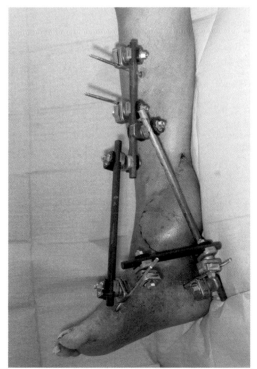

Fig 9.16 External fixation of an open tibial fracture and soft tissue reconstruction with an anterior lateral thigh (ALT) free flap.

⊙ Open fractures

Open fractures are orthopaedic emergencies. They often result from high-energy trauma and are associated with other injuries.

Gustilo–Anderson classification

Type	Description
I	Wound <1 cm long, clean, low-energy trauma
II	Wound >1 cm long, more extensive soft tissue damage, low energy
III	High-energy trauma, extensive soft tissue damage and contamination. Subdivided into A, B, and C

- A Segmental or severely comminuted open fracture; adequate soft tissue to cover the skeleton
- B Large high-energy wound with significant contamination, periosteal stripping, and bone exposure; needs soft tissue cover
- C Fracture with arterial injury requiring repair irrespective of soft tissue injury

Management

- Follow ATLS guidelines
- Assess neurovascular status of limb
- Intravenous antibiotics and analgesia
- Swab wound for microbiology
- Establish tetanus status and give prophylaxis as required
- Photograph and then dress wound with povidone-iodine or normal saline-soaked gauze
- Formal surgical debridement under GA should be carried out by senior surgeons. Remove all devitalized tissue and foreign material, and irrigate wound with a large volume of warm normal saline
- Fracture stabilization depends on the injury but is often a form of external fixation
- Wound is left open and reviewed at 48 h for further debridement or closure/soft tissue reconstruction

Complications

Early problems include compartment syndrome and inadequate surgical debridement. Infection and delayed bone healing are common.

9.10 Proximal femur

Fractures of the proximal femur are common and are an increasing problem worldwide because of ageing populations.

The incidence is 10 per 1000 population (UK) per year, with a mean age of 80 at presentation (F:M 4:1).

Aetiology

Femoral neck fractures are sustained in three main populations.

- Elderly women usually following a fall
- Elderly population with pre-existing bone pathology
- Younger adults following high-energy trauma

Risk factors

- Osteoporosis
- Excessive alcohol intake
- Visual impairment
- Dementia
- Previous hip fracture

Classification

Proximal femoral fractures are classified as either intracapsular or extracapsular. The importance of this is related to the blood supply to the femoral head which comes from three main sources:

1. retinacular (capsular) vessels which arise from the medial and lateral circumflex arteries circling the base of the neck
2. artery of the ligamentum teres entering the tip of head
3. nutrient artery of the femoral shaft

Displaced fractures of the femoral neck disrupt the retinacular and endosteal blood supply to the head which has then to rely solely on the ligamentum teres. Possible complications include avascular necrosis and healing problems. The blood supply may be preserved in undisplaced or impacted fractures.

Intracapsular

Intracapsular neck fractures can be either displaced or undisplaced. Other descriptive terms can be used such as subcapital and transcervical. The Garden classification of femoral neck fractures is not very helpful.

Extracapsular

Extracapsular fractures are divided into stable or unstable (three or more parts). Descriptive terms such as basicervical, intertrochanteric, and subtrochanteric are also used. Extracapsular fractures do not tend to disrupt the blood supply to the femoral head.

Garden classification of subcapital femoral neck fractures

This is based on a plain AP radiograph of the hip.

Type	Description
I	Partial fracture with impaction. Medial cortical trabeculae intact but angulated
II	Complete fracture, no displacement. Medial cortical trabeculae intact and aligned
III	Complete fracture with partial displacement. No trabecular alignment
IV	Complete fracture with full displacement. The proximal fragment is free and lies correctly in the acetabulum so that the trabeculae appear normally aligned

Clinical assessment

History

- Mechanism of injury—mechanical or medical fall
- Social circumstances and mobility
- Head injury and other associated injuries must be excluded

Examination

- Full systems examination
- Mental test score in elderly
- Groin pain radiating down medial thigh which is increased on hip rotation and attempted weightbearing
- Displaced fractures may make the lower limb shortened, abducted, and externally rotated
- Undisplaced fractures result in a reduced range of hip movement. Patients can rarely weightbear

Investigations

- Bloods—FBC, U+Es, G+S
- ECG and chest radiograph
- Plain AP pelvis and lateral hip radiograph
- MRI is used if diagnosis is uncertain, although CT or bone scintigraphy are alternatives

Management

The majority of patients are elderly, and initial management must address pain, fluid balance, and medical co-morbidities. Early intervention (<24 h) is associated with better outcomes.

Intracapsular femoral neck fractures

Patients with undisplaced or impacted fractures who are managing to mobilize can be treated conservatively with analgesia and physiotherapy. However, operative fixation with cannulated screws is usually preferred as it reduces the risk of fracture displacement.

Displaced fractures are likely to disrupt the blood supply to the femoral head and so are traditionally managed with a hemiarthroplasty, but a total hip replacement should be considered in those over 60 years of age with rheumatoid arthritis or pre-existing degenerative joint disorders.

In some centres and in younger patients these fractures are reduced and fixed with cannulated screws as there is increasing evidence that avascular necrosis is not as common as previously reported.

Extracapsular femoral neck fractures

Whether stable (30%) or unstable, the majority are managed with closed reduction and internal fixation. This is either extramedullary (dynamic hip screw) or intramedullary (femoral nail).

Complications and prognosis

The mortality rate in the elderly population rises following a fracture but returns to normal after 1 year. Mortality rate in the first year is up to 30%.

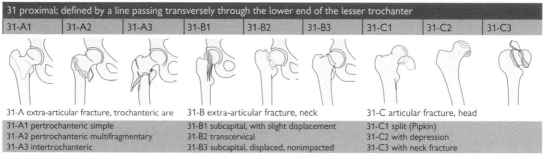

31 proximal; defined by a line passing transversely through the lower end of the lesser trochanter								
31-A1	31-A2	31-A3	31-B1	31-B2	31-B3	31-C1	31-C2	31-C3

31-A extra-articular fracture, trochanteric are | 31-B extra-articular fracture, neck | 31-C articular fracture, head

31-A1 petrochanteric simple
31-A2 petrochanteric multifragmentary
31-A3 intertrochanteric

31-B1 subcapital, with slight displacement
31-B2 transcervical
31-B3 subcapital, displaced, nonimpacted

31-C1 split (Pipkin)
31-C2 with depression
31-C3 with neck fracture

Fig 9.17 Müller AO classification of proximal femoral fractures. Reproduced from the *Müller Classification of Fractures* with kind permission of Springer–Verlag Ltd.

➕ Hemiarthroplasty of the hip joint

Hemiarthroplasty involves replacing the femoral head with a prosthesis. Where possible it is performed under regional anaesthesia (spinal or epidural).

Procedure
- Lateral approach is preferred as it reduces the risk of dislocation. Anterolateral and posterior approaches can also be used
- Incision centred over greater trochanter
- Divide fat, fascia lata, detach gluteus medius +/-minimus, and incise capsule
- Dislocate hip
- Cut neck of femur near base and ream medulla. Size the head
- An uncemented Austin Moore prosthesis is the standard choice of device although cemented devices are becoming more popular
- Insert prosthesis and reduce hip
- Wound closed in layers

Complications
- Infection occurs in up to 20% cases (hip, UTI, chest)
- Medical conditions (VTE, AMI, CVA)
- Femoral shaft fracture rate is 5% and occurs at reduction of the prosthesis
- Dislocation (4%)

➕ Dynamic hip screw

A dynamic hip screw is an implant with a large screw that is placed up the neck into the femoral head. The shaft of the screw passes through a plate that is fixed with screws to the lateral side of the proximal femoral shaft.

Procedure
- Patient supine on fracture table
- Fracture reduced by closed technique
- Lateral approach to the proximal part of the femur
- Image intensifier used to position a guidewire in the head of the femur—centrally and as close to the subchondral bone as possible. The lag screw and then plate are inserted
- Wound closed in layers

Complications
- Infection
- Medical conditions (VTE, AMI, CVA)
- Device failure
- Malunion (shortening and rotation)

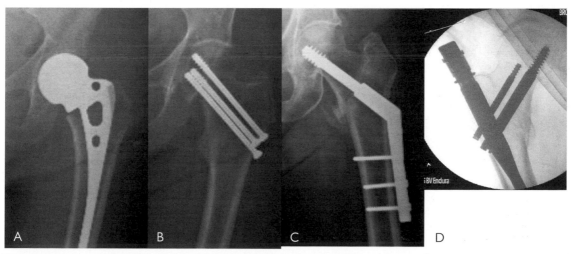

Fig 9.18 Plain AP radiographs of left hips showing: **A** Austin Moore hemiarthroplasty; **B** cannulated screws; **C** dynamic hip screw; and **D** a right proximal femoral nail seen on intraoperative screening.

9.11 Pelvis

The sacrum and the left and right inominate bones form the pelvis. They are held together posteriorly by the strong sacroiliac ligaments and anteriorly at the weaker symphysis pubis. Like breaking a Polo mint, fractures of the pelvic ring usually occur in two places.

Pelvic fractures

Fractures usually occur because of high-energy trauma. They are of varying severity, from simple stable fractures requiring nothing more than analgesia to severely displaced, unstable, and life-threatening fractures.

Classification of pelvic ring fracture

The Tile classification (below) or Young and Burgess are commonly used.

Type A Stable fractures

A1   Fractures not involving the pelvic ring
A2   Stable and minimally displaced fractures of the pelvic ring

Type B Rotationally unstable but vertically stable

B1   Anterior–posterior compression fracture (open book)
B2   Lateral compression (ipsilateral)
B3   Lateral compression fracture (contralateral)

Type C Rotationally and vertically unstable

C1   Unilaterally vertically unstable
C2   Bilaterally vertically unstable
C3   Associated with acetabular fracture

Clinical assessment

Initial approach follows ATLS guidelines and life-threatening injuries should be treated first.

- Look for deformity and limb length discrepancy
- Bimanual compression and distraction of iliac wings assesses pelvic stability
- Digital rectal examination (high-riding prostate), blood at urethral meatus, and vaginal examination may indicate a urological injury

Investigations

- Bloods—FBC, U+Es, cross-match 4 units
- Plain AP pelvic radiograph is part of a trauma series and is usually diagnostic. Plain oblique pelvic radiographs with pelvis tilted 45° internally and externally (Judet views)
- CT scan

Management

Immediate

Unstable widely displaced fractures often cause major haemorrhage and, in the haemodynamically unstable, they need to be reduced with external wrapping in the emergency department or with the application of an external fixator.

Conservative

- Type A fractures (e.g. pubic rami fractures and avulsion fractures of the iliac crest) can be managed with analgesia and mobilization with protected weightbearing. Large avulsions may require ORIF with screw fixation

Operative

- Type B and C fractures are often complex and require the input of pelvic surgeons to decide on the appropriate internal fixation
- Type C3 fractures involving the acetabulum are a priority, as a good reduction reduces the risk of osteoarthritis

Complications and prognosis

Pelvic fractures can cause injury to local blood vessels (sacral venous plexus, superior gluteal artery), and death from haemorrhage is 20%. The urethra, bladder, and lumbosacral plexus are also at risk of injury.

Traumatic hip dislocation

The hip joint is generally stable and in the adult a direct high-energy force is required to dislocate it (e.g. fall from a height and RTC). Children's hips dislocate more easily.

Hip dislocations are often associated with acetabular rim, femoral head or nerve injuries (femoral or sciatic).

Classification

- Anterior dislocations can be superior or inferior (Epstein classification)
- Posterior dislocations (Thompson and Epstein classification)
- Central dislocations are caused by direct force to the lateral aspect of the hip. The head of the femur is pushed through the acetabulum into the pelvis to cause a central fracture-dislocation

Clinical assessment

- Anterior dislocations—hip pain with the lower limb externally rotated, abducted, and extended at the hip. Femoral nerve injury may result in muscle weakness and numbness in its distribution. Femoral artery injury also needs to be excluded
- Posterior dislocations—hip pain with the lower limb usually shortened, adducted, and internally rotated. Sciatic nerve injury may result in muscle weakness (plantar or dorsiflexion) or numbness of the posterior leg and foot

Investigations

- Bloods—FBC, cross-match
- Plain AP pelvic radiograph is part of the trauma series and is usually diagnostic. A lateral radiograph should also be performed and both are repeated post-reduction
- Plain oblique (Judet) pelvic radiograph can be helpful if the dislocation is not clear on an AP

Management

Initial approach follows ATLS guidelines and life-threatening injuries should be treated first.

- Closed reduction is performed within 4–6 h of injury, either in the emergency department under sedation or under GA. The neurovascular status should be documented before and after reduction
- Open reduction is needed if closed reduction fails, the joint is unstable or if there are associated fractures that need open reduction and internal fixation
- Stable hip reduction is followed by 2 weeks of hip traction (2.5–5 kg) and gradual mobilization non-weightbearing as appropriate
- Hip CT scan is needed post-reduction in all cases

Complications and prognosis

Complications of the dislocation include vascular injury, avascular necrosis, post-traumatic osteoarthritis, neurological deficit, and heterotopic ossification.

Prognosis is related to the severity of injury and time taken to reduce the dislocation. Anterior dislocations do better than posterior dislocations, and those with associated fractures do worse.

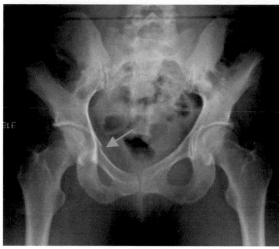

Fig 9.20 Plain portable AP radiograph of the pelvis showing a fracture through the superior and inferior pubic rami on the right (arrow). There is disc incontinuity of the arcuate foramina in the right side of the sacrum, suggesting a second pelvic fracture in this region extending up into the right sacral ala.

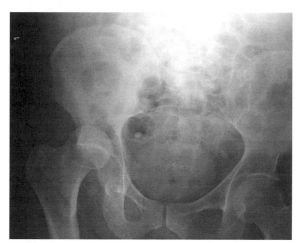

Fig 9.19 Plain AP hip radiograph showing a posterior dislocation of the right hip. The femur is adducted and internally rotated. The head of the femur is lying lateral and superior to the acetabulum. In an anterior dislocation, the femur is abducted and externally rotated. The head of the femur lies medial and inferior to the acetabulum.

Clavicle fractures

Clavicle fractures are very common and usually result from a direct blow to the shoulder or forces transmitted through the arm when falling.

Classification

The Allman classification divides the fractures in to inner (5%), middle (80%), and outer thirds (15%). The outer third fractures are subdivided depending on their relationship to the coracoclavicular ligament complex.

Clinical assessment

The bone lies subcutaneously and so the diagnosis can often be made clinically. There is tenderness, swelling, and sometimes deformity at the fracture site.

In middle third fractures the outer fragment is pulled down by the weight of the arm and the inner part pulled up by the sternomastoid muscle (Fig 9.21).

The subclavian and axillary vessels, brachial plexus, and lung pleura are closely related to the clavicle. Injuries to these structures must be excluded.

Investigations

- Plain AP radiograph is usually sufficient. Ensure that joints at both ends are included; additional 45° cephalic and caudal views may be helpful
- Weightbearing views of the shoulders to assess the ligament complex are not routine

Management

Conservative

The majority of fractures can be managed with a broad arm sling, analgesia, and early mobilization once there is clinical union (4–6 weeks).

Operative

Indications for surgery include open fractures, severe skin tethering, neurovascular injury, and significant medialization of the upper limb.

Complications and prognosis

- Malunion leaving a visible deformity is common. Conservative management usually outweighs the benefits of surgery
- Non-union is most common with distal third fractures and in those treated with operative fixation

Scapula fractures

Scapula fractures are uncommon. Those involving the blade of the scapula usually occur because of direct trauma and may be associated with significant rib injuries. Conservative treatment is usually successful with a broad arm sling and analgesia.

Fractures of the glenoid can also usually be treated conservatively but a CT scan to assess the fracture pattern may show that open reduction and internal fixation would be a better option. Displaced glenoid fractures, scapular spine fractures, and acromial fractures need ORIF as deltoid pulls them out of place.

Shoulder dislocation

The shoulder is particularly prone to dislocation owing to its large range of movement and shallow glenoid fossa.

It is regularly put under physical stress and is particularly susceptible to dislocating if there is underlying ligamentous laxity. Anteroinferior dislocations are by far the most common, but the shoulder may also dislocate postero-inferiorly or, rarely, inferiorly (luxatio erecta).

Classification

Anterior dislocation (97%)

This is the most common dislocation, often resulting from a fall on an outstretched hand. The humeral head externally rotates out of the glenoid and lies inferior to the clavicle and anterior to the scapula, often causing damage to the glenoid labrum or the anterior joint capsule. Facture of the humeral head is rare.

Posterior dislocation (3%)

Epileptic convulsions or electric shocks are the classic mechanisms involved, although this can also occur after a fall on an adducted arm or after a direct blow to the shoulder. The head of the humerus lies directly posterior to the glenoid.

Inferior dislocation

This is a rare dislocation which is usually sustained by hyperabduction of the shoulder. The humeral head lies in a subglenoid position, and the joint capsule and rotator cuff tendons are nearly always injured. The axillary artery and brachial plexus are at risk of injury.

Clinical assessment

The patient is usually in severe pain and supports the elbow with the good arm to prevent any movement.

Examination

- Anterior dislocation—the normal rounded contour of the shoulder is lost, being more squared off, and the arm may be held in slight abduction. The humeral head is usually palpable inferior to the clavicle
- Posterior dislocation—the arm is held locked in medial rotation. The shoulder looks flat and has a bulge posteriorly and a prominent coracoid anteriorly
- Inferior dislocations—the patient's arm is held in full abduction and the humeral head can be felt in the axilla
- Neurovascular status of the upper limb must be assessed before reduction, especially the axillary nerve which passes round the neck of the humerus. This supplies sensation to the 'regimental badge' area over the deltoid

Investigations

- Plain AP shoulder radiograph usually shows an anterior dislocation with the humeral head lying in a pre-glenoid, subcoracoid or subclavicular position.
  A posterior dislocation is often missed, but the humeral head may have a more rounded shape owing to medial rotation—'light bulb' sign
- Scapular lateral (Y-view) or axillary view should also be performed to confirm the diagnosis

Management

Most patients are treated with closed reduction (see box). Operative intervention is rarely indicated.

⊙ Reduction of shoulder dislocation

Most patients tolerate shoulder reduction with analgesia and sedation in the emergency department. Some can manage without and some require a GA.

Anterior reduction techniques

- **Kocher's** is the most popular method. The elbow is held at 90° close to the body. The arm is very slowly externally rotated up to 90°, keeping the elbow close to the chest wall. Reduction will normally occur during external rotation but once at 90° it may be necessary to adduct the arm, bringing the elbow across the chest wall.
  Once reduced, internally rotate the shoulder, placing the hand on the opposite shoulder
- **Hippocratic**—traction is applied to the arm in slight abduction, with countertraction to the body usually with a towel slung under the axilla
- **Stimson's**—the patient is prone with their arm dependent. A weight is applied to the arm or the patient holds a sandbag and is left for 10–15 min. During this time the shoulder will usually reduce

Posterior

Traction is applied to the arm at 90° of abduction whilst externally rotating. Most can then be managed as for an anterior dislocation. Unstable reductions need to be immobilized in a shoulder spica with the arm held abducted and externally rotated for 3–4 weeks.

Inferior

Prompt reduction reduces any neurovascular compromise. Traction to the abducted arm is usually successful, but open reduction may be necessary.

Follow-up

Once reduced, the neurovascular status should be reassessed. The arm should be placed in a body bandage to support it and prevent external rotation; check radiographs are reviewed.

In the young, support in the sling should continue for 3–4 weeks. In the elderly this can be reduced to 1 week as the risks of re-dislocation are lower. Patients should be followed up in fracture clinic to assess for rotator cuff injuries and to start physiotherapy. Patients who recurrently dislocate should be considered for reconstructive surgery.

Complications

A long-term complication is recurrent dislocation: 80%+ if first time is aged <18, dropping to 25% if aged 18+. The older you are, the more likely you are to have a cuff tear: obtain an ultrasound within a few weeks if repair is considered.

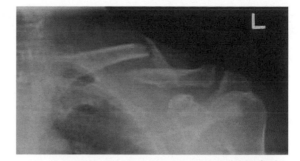
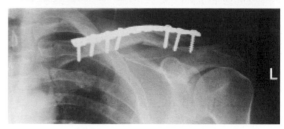

Fig 9.21 Plain AP radiograph of a left clavicle showing a displaced middle third fracture. This underwent ORIF with a plate and screws.

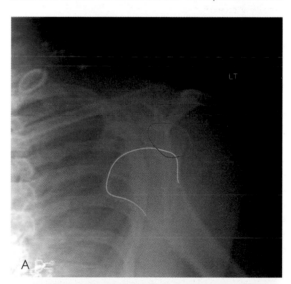

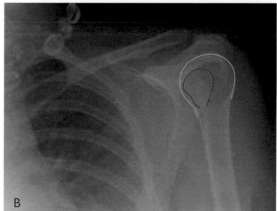

Fig 9.22 Plain Y view of the left shoulder showing an anterior shoulder dislocation and then AP view post-reduction. Red line indicates glenoid fossa and the green line is the head of the humerus.

Soft tissue disorders

Supraspinatus tendonitis

Supraspinatus tendonitis usually occurs in the over 40s. The supraspinatus tendon passes from the greater tuberosity over the head of the humerus and under the coracoacromial ligament. The tendon becomes inflamed over the head of the humerus owing to repetitive movements (e.g. a weekend of painting) and causes pain as it passes through the narrow subacromial space.

The patient experiences pain in a small arc between 60 and 120° of abduction. However, on passive abduction this movement can be pain-free.

The pain often settles with physiotherapy and simple anti-inflammatory drugs. An injection of steroid and local anaesthetic around the tendon is also effective in 50% of cases.

Acute calcific tendonitis

This is characterized by acute onset of shoulder pain and is most common in 30–50-year-olds. A similar condition may occur in other tendons or ligaments around other joints. In the shoulder, the supraspinatus tendon is most commonly affected. It is thought that local ischaemia causes fibrocartilage metaplasia and deposition of calcium hydroxyapatite crystals. These lie dormant for a period of time. Then invasion by inflammatory cells attempts to remove the calcium, producing an acute inflammatory reaction in the tendon, causing pain and swelling.

The symptoms are often of acute agonizing shoulder pain and the patient is very reluctant to allow movement or palpation of the joint. Plain radiographs of the shoulder usually reveal an area of calcification in the tendon above the greater tuberosity.

Symptoms will usually resolve over weeks to months. Analgesia is necessary. If in severe pain, an injection of steroid and local anaesthetic can be helpful.

Ruptured biceps tendon

Rupture of the long head of biceps from its origin on the superior labrum usually occurs in the over 50s. The patient feels a snap, usually on minimal exertion and the detached muscle belly forms a prominent ball in the lower part of the upper arm (Popeye sign).

If the tear is in the elderly and causes no loss of function, simple reassurance is all that is needed. If the patient is young, biceps tendon tenodesis may be necessary.

Adhesive capsulitis (frozen shoulder)

This condition is characterized by a progression through pain, stiffness, and resolution over a period of a year to 18 months. The cause is unknown, but is thought to be autoimmune and histologically appears to resemble Dupuytren's disease with the presence of proliferating myofibroblasts. It is particularly prevalent in diabetic patients.

The patient is usually aged 40–60 years old. The pain in the shoulder gradually increases over several months and is worse on all movements (distinguishing it from supraspinatus tendonitis). After about 6 months the pain begins to subside but the joint becomes increasingly stiff and eventually painless. This frozen shoulder lasts for approximately 6–12 months and severely limits daily activities. Gradually, movement will slowly return but the patient will usually be left with some lasting limitation.

Radiographs are usually normal and the diagnosis is a clinical one based on the history through the successive phases.

Treatment is mainly with physiotherapy. Glenohumeral cortisone injections, manipulation under anaesthetic, and arthroscopic capsular release may also be considered.

Instability

Shoulder instability is the tendency to subluxation or complete dislocation of the shoulder joint.

It often follows traumatic dislocation of the shoulder which results in laxity of the anterior capsule or tear of the glenoid labrum. Non-traumatic causes include laxity of the capsule or consequence of a movement disorder.

Diagnosis is usually based on the history and examination. Stress tests may cause the sensation of impending dislocation (e.g. apprehension test). Shoulder arthroscopy may be used to confirm the diagnosis.

Specialist physiotherapy is often successful at strengthening the rotator cuff. Surgical options include the Bankart procedure which repairs the anterior capsular attachments, and capsular shift which tightens the capsule. Postoperative rehabilitation is crucial to a good outcome.

Proximal and shaft humeral fractures

Fractures of the proximal humerus usually occur because of a fall onto an outstretched hand. The majority are in postmenopausal women with osteoporosis.

Classification

Fractures may be through the anatomical neck, surgical neck, greater tuberosity or lesser tuberosity, and are usually described according to the site and the number of displaced parts (e.g. two-part, three-part or four-part) and whether the humeral head is dislocated or not.

Neer classification refers to the number of segments displaced >1 cm or angulated >45° (four primary segments: greater tuberosity, lesser tuberosity, humeral head, and humeral shaft).

Clinical assessment

Pain and swelling around the shoulder after a fall. Check for signs of brachial plexus or vascular injury.

Investigations

- Two views should be performed to assess accurately and in complex cases a CT of the shoulder is helpful

Management

For simple fractures with minimal displacement, conservative management with a collar and cuff until pain has subsided, followed by active mobilization and physiotherapy.

In fractures of the anatomical neck there is a high risk of avascular necrosis and these patients should be considered for either a hemiarthroplasty or fixation by screw if young. Complex three- or four-part fractures with or without dislocation will usually require open reduction and internal fixation or prosthetic replacement.

Humeral shaft fractures can be transverse, oblique or spiral. The majority are managed conservatively with a U slab, hanging cast or a humeral brace. Pathological fractures may require intramedullary nailing.

Complications and prognosis

Vascular and nerve injuries, particularly in multipart fractures with displacement. Malunion, joint stiffness, and avascular necrosis of the humeral head.

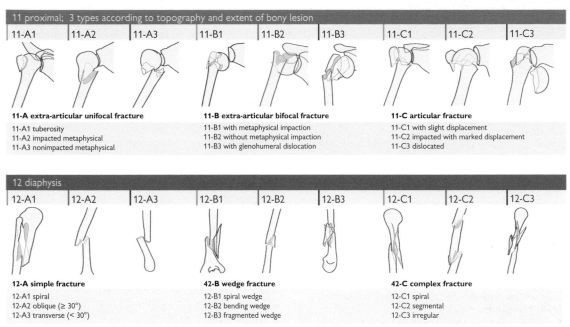

Fig 9.23 Müller AO classification of proximal and diaphyseal fractures of the humerus. Reproduced from the *Müller Classification of Fractures* with kind permission of Springer–Verlag Ltd.

Epicondylitis

Medial epicondylitis (golfer's elbow) and lateral condylitis (tennis elbow) are overuse syndromes often seen in active people.

They present with pain on the medial or lateral side of the elbow which radiates into the forearm and is exacerbated by activity. A plain radiograph is often performed to exclude other joint pathology. Most cases resolve with rest and NSAIDS.

Elbow fractures

Fractures about the elbow joint (distal humerus and proximal radius/ulna) are often complex. Extra-articular supracondylar fractures are often seen in children following a fall onto an extended arm.

Classification

Distal humerus

- Children's supracondylar fractures classified by Gartland
  Type I—undisplaced
  Type II—displaced with intact posterior cortex
  Type III—completely displaced (posteromedial or postero-lateral)
- Adult distal humeral fractures are complex and are best classified by Müller classification

Proximal radius/ulnar

These fractures involve the radial head (Mason classification), coronoid process or olecranon.

Clinical assessment

- The elbow is painful, swollen, and often deformed with no movement
- Brachial artery compression, spasm or rarely rupture is uncommon but must be excluded. Early reduction is important
- Nerves are often injured (radial>median (anterior interosseous branch)>ulnar)

Investigations

- Plain AP and lateral elbow. Anterior 'fat pad' is suggestive of a fracture

Management of supracondylar fractures

Conservative

Undisplaced fractures are stabilized in a plaster cast with the elbow flexed at 100° with a check radiograph at 1 week.

Operative

Displaced fractures require closed reduction. Unstable fractures also benefit from K-wire fixation. Type III supracondylar fractures or evidence of neurovascular comprise need emergency ORIF.

Complications and prognosis

Over 90% of cases have an excellent result with a comfortable range of movement. Complications include cubitus varus, cubitus valgus, and myositis ossificans. Brachial artery injury leading to Volkmann's ischaemic contracture is rare.

Forearm fractures

The radius and ulna bones are held together by the annular ligament proximally, the interosseous membrane along their diaphyses, and the radio-ulnar ligament distally.

This close approximation means that isolated fractures of one bone are uncommon. Similarly, if one bone is fractured but its proximal and distal attachments are intact then the other bone must be dislocated.

Classification

- **Monteggia injury**—fracture of the ulna shaft with dislocation of the radial head
- **Galleazzi injury**—fracture of the radial shaft with dislocation of the distal radio-ulnar joint
- **Nightstick injury**—isolated fracture of the ulna shaft
- **Greenstick fractures** are childhood injuries. One cortex buckles and the other remains intact. The bone remodels but can angulate owing to differential growth of the two cortices

Clinical assessment

- Localized pain and deformity
- Second most common open fractures
- Examine both elbow and wrist joint
- Exclude neurovascular injury
- Exclude compartment syndrome

Investigations

- Plain AP and lateral radiographs of the forearm which must include the elbow and wrist joints

Management

Isolated undisplaced fractures are rare and can be managed in an above-elbow cast for 6 weeks with weekly reviews.

Operative

Both Monteggia and Galleazzi fractures need to have the dislocations reduced and ORIF of the fractures with a dynamic compression plate.

Complications and prognosis

Neurovascular injury and compartment syndrome are uncommon. Union rates and functional outcome are excellent.

Volkmann's contracture

This is the end-stage of an ischaemic injury to the muscles and nerves of the limb following a compartment syndrome. Fibrous scar tissue replaces the muscle, which contracts, producing a contracture in the muscle compartment affected. It is most commonly due to trauma to the brachial artery.

Distal radius and ulna fractures

Fractures of the distal radius and ulna are very common. The age distribution is bimodal. Younger patients sustain them following high-energy trauma and elderly osteoporotic patients following a fall.

Classification

The Frykman classification differentiates between intra- and extra-articular fractures and is in common use. The AO classification is comprehensive but unreliable.

- Extra-articular fracture of the distal radius within 1 inch of the wrist joint (**Colle's fracture**). There is dorsal angulation and displacement of the distal fragment. It is sustained by falling on an outstretched hand with the wrist extended
- **Smith's fracture** is a fracture of the distal radius with volar angulation of the distal fragment. It is sustained following a fall on outstretched arm with wrist flexed

- **Barton's fracture** is a complete displacement of an intra-articular fracture involving the volar lip of the distal radius, taking the carpus with it

Clinical assessment

Localized pain and deformity of the wrist with reduced range of movement. The classic 'dinner fork' deformity is associated with a distal radius fracture.

Investigations

- Plain AP and lateral wrist radiograph
- Normal values are: volar tilt 11°, radial inclination 22°, radial length 11 mm longer than ulnar length

Management

Closed reduction and plaster fixation with a below-elbow cast is the treatment of choice for stable extra-articular fractures. A reduction with >20° dorsal angulation, > 5 mm shortening or comminution should be considered for internal fixation.

Operative

Most Barton's and Smith's fractures need ORIF using volar locking plates. K-wiring and external fixation are other surgical options and their use depends on the fracture pattern.

Complications and prognosis

Acute vascular injuries are rare. Median nerve injury occurs in up to 10% of cases and can present as an acute carpal tunnel syndrome. Acute tendon injuries are uncommon but late EPL rupture is a classic finding.

Complex regional pain syndrome and chronic stiffness occurs in up to 25%.

Hand fractures

Scaphoid

Violent hyperextension of the wrist can fracture the waist of the scaphoid. On examination there is no deformity or bruising but may be tenderness and swelling in the anatomical snuff-box. Pinch grip or hyperextension of the thumb may cause pain.

Plain radiographs should include four views. Patients with a suspected fracture are placed in a back slab POP and have repeat radiographs at 10 days.

Bennett's fracture

Fracture of the base of the first metacarpal extending into the carpometacarpal joint. It can be held with a POP but is unstable and the best option is internal fixation.

Phalangeal fractures

Stable fractures can be managed with buddy strapping. Unstable or intra-articular fractures require reduction and K-wire fixation.

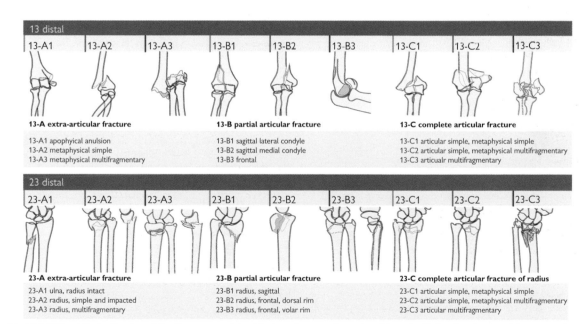

Fig 9.24 Müller AO classification of distal humerus and distal forearm fractures. Reproduced from the *Müller Classification of Fractures* with kind permission of Springer–Verlag Ltd.

Osteoarthritis

Osteoarthritis (OA) is a common progressive, non-inflammatory degeneration of articular cartilage accompanied by subchondral bone changes.

It is very common and incidence increases with age. There is variability between ethnic groups. Hip OA is most commonly in those of western origin; knee OA is most common in Afro-Caribbean patients.

Aetiology

Primary OA is idiopathic, although both genetic susceptibility and environmental factors play a role.

Secondary OA is associated with joint trauma, obesity, endocrine disorders (diabetes mellitus), abnormal articular surface, malalignment of the joint, joint instability, inflammatory disorders (gout, septic arthritis), neuropathies (Charcot joints), and congenital or developmental disorders (Perthes disease, SUFE).

Pathophysiology

Hyaline joint cartilage initially becomes swollen, leading to stretching of the collagen network in the matrix. This softens the cartilage and makes it susceptible to further damage. Fibrillations form in the superficial layer and gradually become deeper and perpendicular to the joint surface.

The chondrocyte population diminishes and with them the matrix. The subchondral bone undergoes substantial remodelling in response to these mechanical and metabolic events. The radiological changes are seen well before clinical presentation and do not correlate with pain.

Clinical assessment

History

- Gradual onset of joint pain, swelling, and stiffness with limitation of movement
- Joint stiffness is worse after a period of rest
- Restriction of activities of daily living
- Severe disease may lead to joint instability

Examination

- Generalized OA affects at least three joints or groups of joints and is often subdivided into nodal and non-nodal.
- Hands—nodal OA is characterized by Heberden's nodes at the DIPJ of the fingers. Bouchard's nodes are at PIPJ. OA of the first carpometacarpal joint causes loss of dexterity and pinch grip
- Hip—pain and restriction of internal rotation and flexion. Antalgic gait
- Knee—pain worse on weightbearing. Knee effusion and crepitus is almost universal

Investigations

- Blood tests—FBC, U+Es, bone profile. CRP may be mildly raised in early disease
- Plain AP and lateral of the involved joints. OA is graded on radiographic rather than clinical features

Management

The aim is to reduce pain and improve function. This is usually achieved with conservative management. Operative intervention may be considered in patients with uncontrolled pain or functional impairment.

Conservative

- Advice on modifying activities and lifestyle (e.g. weight loss and self-management programmes)
- Occupational therapy and physiotherapy
- Paracetamol is the first line analgesia
- Supplements such as glucosamine may help

Operative

Hip and knee arthroplasties are very common procedures, with 90% lasting over 10 years. Options include:

1. arthroscopic debridement and washout
2. arthroplasty: joint replacement or resurfacing
3. arthrodesis is used in smaller joints and those with no option for athroplasty
4. osteotomy (rarely done but often successful)

Complications and prognosis

The disease is progressive and causes considerable morbidity due to pain and restriction of function.

Rheumatoid arthritis

Rheumatoid arthritis is a systemic autoimmune inflammatory disease that primarily affects synovium and associated tissues. Its incidence is declining although it remains common (F:M 3:1).

Aetiology

Immunological factors (HLA–DRB1) are important in the development and progression of disease. Hormonal factors may also play a role. The incidence amongst women reduces following the menopause, and pregnancy often leads to remission of disease.

Pathophysiology

Plasma cells and lymphocytes invade the affected synovium. The synovium becomes swollen and inflamed, forming a pannus. This damages surrounding tissues such as the articular cartilage. Patients with a clinical diagnosis of rheumatoid arthritis but with negative rheumatoid factor or agglutination tests are said to have seronegative RA.

Clinical assessment

History

- Insidious onset over weeks to months
- Polyarthritis mainly affecting small joints
- Morning joint stiffness
- Fatigue and diffuse musculoskeletal pain

Examination

- Joint thickening with effusion
- Tendon rupture (hands)
- Extra-articular: rheumatoid nodules, dry eyes, dry mouth, lymphadenopathy, nerve entrapment (e.g. carpal tunnel syndrome), airway obstruction, pericardial effusion

Investigations

- Bloods—FBC (raised WCC, normocytic anaemia), raised ESR and CRP
- Positive antinuclear test
- Positive rheumatoid factor

Management

Conservative

- Simple analgesia—NSAIDs (first line)
- Corticosteroid therapy
- Disease-modifying drugs: methotrexate, anti-TNF
- Occupational therapy (aids and appliances)

Operative

- Synovectomy is rarely indicated, but in the hand extensor tenosynovectomy is performed to prevent extensor tendon rupture
- Joint arthroplasty or arthrodesis

Complications and prognosis

RA causes significant morbidity owing to joint deformity and systemic complications. Fifty per cent of patients are unable to work at 10 years. Life expectancy is also reduced.

⊕ Total hip replacement

There are many types of implant and approaches to the operation. The principles are outlined below.

Procedure

- Posterior or anterolateral incision followed by minimally traumatic approach to hip capsule
- Femoral head is excised
- Medullary canal is reamed out to accept a stem that has an articulating surface on top. This can be cemented, or not, into the femur
- Acetabulum is reamed to make it hemispherical and a cup is inserted
- The implants are made from a variety of materials
- Close in layers

Complications

Intraoperative and early	Late
• Femoral shaft fracture	• Infection
• Sciatic nerve injury	• Dislocation
• Infection	• Failure/loosening
• Venous thromboembolism	
• Leg length discrepancy	
• Dislocation	
• Medical complications	

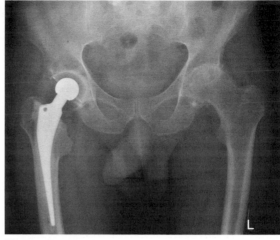

Fig 9.25 Plain AP radiograph showing both hips. There is severe OA of the left hip, including joint space narrowing, subchondral sclerosis, and bone cysts, osteophytes. The right hip has already been treated with a total arthroplasty.

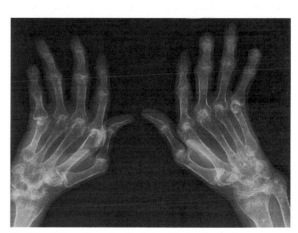

Fig 9.26 Plain radiograph of both hands in a patient with rheumatoid arthritis. There is joint space narrowing, subluxation, and erosions. The bones are osteopenic. Clinically the patient may have a Boutonnière deformity of their left thumb, subluxation, and ulnar deviation at the MCP joints.

Osteomyelitis

Osteomyelitis is infection of bone. It can be acute or chronic. The incidence is falling in developed countries, especially in the paediatric population.

Aetiology

Risk factors include diabetes, peripheral occlusive arterial disease, sickle cell disease, HIV/AIDS, intravenous drug abuse, and immunosuppression.

Haematogenous osteomyelitis is usually from a single organism. Contiguous spread often leads to multiple organisms. *Staphylococcus* spp. followed by *Streptococcus* are most common. *Haemophillus influenzae* is now less common in infants due to vaccination. Atypical organisms are seen in immunosuppressed patients.

Pathophysiology

Routes of spread

- Haematogenous spread is most common in children
- Direct trauma, e.g. open fractures, puncture wounds, joint replacement surgery
- Contiguous spread from nearby focus of infection, e.g. diabetic ulcer

Sequence of changes

1. Transient bacteraemia
2. Focus of inflammation in metaphysis of long bone
3. Necrosis of bone leading to formation of sequestrum
4. Formation of reactive new bone or involucrum
5. Formation of sinuses draining pus to skin via cloacae

Clinical assessment

History

- Commonly long bones (50% in tibia)
- Fever with inability to use or guarding of affected limb

Examination

- Localized inflammation
- Look for sinuses draining pus
- Assess movement of joints above and below for joint involvement
- Assess for focus of infection (e.g. ulcers, fractures) and predisposing conditions (e.g. PAOD, needle tracks)

Investigations

- Bloods—FBC (50% show elevated WBCs), ESR, and CRP (commonly raised in the acute stage); U+Es, LFTs, serum glucose, and bone profiles
- Blood cultures (50% positive in acute osteomyelitis)
- Bone and joint fluid needle aspirate for Gram stain
- Plain radiographs are generally insensitive in acute osteomyelitis as bone changes take >2 weeks. Look for the triad of soft tissue swelling, bone destruction, and periosteal reaction. May show evidence of fractures or tumours underlying the infection
- CT, MRI, and technetium-labelled bone scans are all available to assist in radiological diagnosis. None are able to give an absolute diagnosis
- Open bone biopsy for histopathological diagnosis is needed if high clinical and radiological suspicion

Management

Conservative

General supportive measures include analgesia and intravenous fluids. Splinting of the affected limb may aid pain control.

Start empirical antibiotics and then tailor them to microbiology results for a prolonged course of ~4 weeks. Longterm antibiotics can usually be administered orally.

Operative

Required in almost all cases unless the history is very short (1–2 days) and there is a rapid response to antibiotic therapy. Surgical management should follow the same principles as that for any infection with:

- drainage of the abscess
- debridement of necrotic tissue
- restoration of blood supply
- coverage of bone with soft tissues

The extent of the surgery depends on the individual case and some will only require drainage of the subperiosteal abscess, others extensive debridement with soft tissue flaps and split-skin grafts. If the bone is unstable due to bone necrosis or fracture, then fixation will be required.

Complications

- Septic arthritis from local spread into joints
- Growth plate failure with reduced bone growth in children
- Metastatic abscesses, e.g. brain, kidney, lung
- Amputation
- Chronic osteomyelitis is longstanding and difficult to eradicate, usually caused by relapse of primary infection; hallmarks include sequestrum, involucrum, and cloacae

Septic arthritis

Septic arthritis is inflammation of a synovial membrane causing a purulent effusion into the joint space. It is an orthopaedic emergency as it can lead to rapid joint destruction.

Aetiology

Septic arthritis is almost exclusively caused by bacterial infection. Risk factors for septic arthritis include immunosuppression, chronic joint disease, rheumatoid arthritis, intravenous drug abuse, joint prosthesis, and recent joint surgery.

Eighty per cent of cases are caused by Gram-positive aerobes (*Staphylococcus aureus* and streptococci), with the rest being Gram-negative anaerobes (e.g. *Neisseria gonorrhoeae*).

Atypical infection with pseudomonas, mycobacteria, fungi, and spirochaetes should be suspected in more indolent cases in immunosuppressed patients.

Pathophysiology

Bacterial seeding of the synovium may occur via haematogenous spread, contiguous spread from overlying cellulitis or local osteomyelitis, traumatic joint injury or iatrogenic inoculation during surgery or joint aspiration.

Infection of the synovial membrane and release of proteolytic enzymes into the synovial fluid by bacteria leads to destruction of the articular cartilage and pannus formation.

Clinical assessment

Septic arthritis is usually acute and monoarticular (90%). However, it can also become chronic and may be polyarticular in certain cases.

History

- Acute onset of pain and swelling in a single joint with a reduced range of movement
- Ask about a history of trauma, underlying joint disease, steroid use or chronic illness
- Ask about symptoms of sexually transmitted diseases. If they have fever, tenosynovitis, dermatitis, and a migratory polyarthralgia then suspect gonorrhoea

Examination

- Fever
- Hot, swollen, tender monoarthritis (50% hip, 20% knee)
- Reduced range of movement

Investigations

- Bloods—FBC (↑WCC), ↓CRP
- Blood cultures
- Joint aspiration with synovial fluid sent for urgent Gram staining, microscopy, and cultures
- Plain joint radiographs are usually normal in the acute phase
- Ultrasound of the joint is cheap and very sensitive in diagnosing joint effusions, but is unable to differentiate the cause
- CT and MRI are expensive and are not necessary if the clinical suspicion is high and the joint easily aspirated
- Urethral, cervical, pharyngeal, and rectal swabs for microbiology if gonococcal infection suspected

Management

General approach

Urgent administration of empirical broad spectrum intravenous antibiotics following collection of a specimen until organisms and sensitivities are available. The course usually lasts for 6 weeks. Antibiotics are switched to oral once there has been a significant clinical improvement.

Analgesia and splinting of the affected joint helps to relieve pain.

Operative

Drainage and washout of joint is essential. This can be via arthroscopy for subcutaneous joints (knee) or arthrotomy for deep joints (hip). The initial drainage of the effusion may need to be repeated. Once specimens are obtained in theatre, high-dose intravenous antibiotics are commenced.

Complications and prognosis

Delay in diagnosis leads to destruction of the articular surface and early degenerative arthritis. Septic arthritis of a child's hip can cause necrosis of the capital epiphysis and disastrous consequences for the hip joint.

If treated promptly, full recovery can be anticipated.

⊕ Joint aspiration

There must be an effusion within the joint to aspirate a joint easily. Each joint has a standard approach for the needle.

Procedure

- Aseptic technique
- Infiltrate the skin with local anaesthetic
- Insert large-bore needle attached to 20 mL syringe
- Aspirate as much fluid as possible
- Send for immediate microscopy and Gram staining
- Can be repeated if fluid reaccumulates

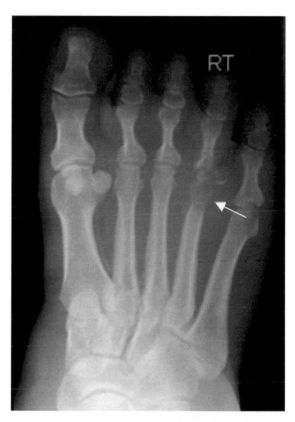

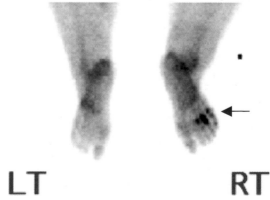

Fig 9.27 A Plain radiograph of the right foot showing destruction of the head of the fourth metatarsal and proximal phalanx of the fourth toe. **B** Bone scintigraphy shows increased uptake in that region. This confirmed the clinical suspicion of osteomyelitis associated with a foot ulcer in a patient with type II diabetes.

9.17 Crystal arthropathies

Crystal arthropathies are characterized by the deposition of crystals in joints and soft tissues. This leads to inflammation and destruction of the affected joints. Monosodium urate monohydrate (gout) and calcium pyrophosphate dehydrate deposition are the two most common conditions.

Gout

Gout is caused by the deposition of monosodium urate monohydrate crystals. Incidence is 16 per 1000 population (UK) and rising. Onset is usually 30–60 years (postmenopausal in women) and it is much more common in men (M:F 9:1) owing to higher urate levels.

Aetiology

Primary gout is idiopathic. Secondary causes are related to increased production, altered metabolism or decreased excretion of uric acid.

- Decreased renal clearance—hypertension, diuretics, ciclosporin, CRF, dehydration, low dose aspirin, excess organic acids (exercise, starvation, ketoacidosis)
- Altered metabolism—glucose-6-phospate deficiency
- Increased production—cytotoxic drugs, lymphoproliferative and myeloproliferative disorders

Risk factors

- Advanced age
- Family history
- Diets high in purines—red meat, oily fish, yeast, and alcohol. Dairy products are lower in purines
- Dehydration following trauma or major surgery

Pathophysiology

Humans are deficient in uricase and so are unable to degrade uric acid which is the end product of purine nucleotide metabolism. A small amount is also acquired from the diet. Excretion is 70% renal, 30% GI tract.

In patients who develop gout, the concentration of monosodium urate in the blood becomes very high, and urate crystals are deposited from a supersaturated solution.

Urate crystals deposited in the joints are phagocytosed by polymorphs which release lysosomal enzymes and indigestible crystals, resulting in an acute inflammatory synovitis.

Clinical assessment

Four stages have been described—asymptomatic hyperuricaemia, acute gouty arthritis, intercritical gout, and chronic tophaceous gout.

Acute gout

- History of a provoking event (e.g. trauma, surgery, drugs)
- Hot, red, swollen, and tender monoarthritis although can be polyarticular (10%). Metatarsophalangeal joint of the great toe is most common. Other joints include ankle, wrist, and knee
- Tenosynovitis, bursitis or cellulitis are less common presentations
- Fever, chills, and malaise can be present and are therefore not useful in distinguishing from septic arthritis

Chronic tophaceous gout

- History of recurrent attacks
- Asymetrical joint swelling
- Tophi are large accumulations of uric acid and urate crystals surrounded by inflammatory cells and fibrosis. They develop in tendon sheaths, bursae, and periarticular tissue.

Investigations

- Bloods—WCC and ESR usually elevated. Check for hyperuricaemia (>0.5 mmol/L). Note this is not diagnostic as 5% of population have a raised serum urate, and only 5% of these will develop gout
- Joint aspiration—synovial fluid for microscopy, WCC, Gram stain, and MC+S (Gram stain and culture negative)
- Microscopy shows needle-shaped crystals negatively birefringent under polarized light
- Plain radiographs may show soft tissue swelling but are usually normal in acute gout. Chronic gout causes changes similar to other types of degenerative arthritis

Differential diagnosis of acute gout

- Septic arthritis
- Other crystal arthropathy (e.g. pseudogout)
- Traumatic arthritis and haemarthrosis
- Rheumatoid arthritis
- Reactive arthritis
- Psoriatic arthritis

Management

The clinical course is often very variable. Many patients will not have another attack for many months or years. Others have progressive shortening of the intercritical periods and develop deterioration of joint function.

Asymptomatic hyperuricaemia does not need treatment.

Acute gout

- NSAIDS (indomethacin)—aspirin should be avoided as it can increase uric acid levels unless in very high doses
- Intra-articular or short course of systemic corticosteroids can be used if NSAIDs are contraindicated

Chronic gout

- Allopurinol is the mainstay of therapy. It is a xanthine oxidase inhibitor which reduces the production of uric acid. It should only be started after an acute attack has subsided and is contraindicated in patients with renal disease
- Lifestyle advice includes keeping hydrated, weight loss, and reducing dietary purine and alcohol intake

Operative

There is no indication for surgery in acute gout. It may be indicated in chronic gout to debride large tophi or to correct joint deformity.

Complications and prognosis

Joint destruction is the main complication. Renal tract stones are now found in <10% of patients.

Calcium pyrophosphate deposition

Calcium pyrophosphate dehydrate crystal deposition arthropathy (pseudogout) is most prevalent in women. It commonly affects the knee, wrist, and shoulder joints. It tends to develop more insidiously than gout and is associated with many metabolic abnormalities.

Microscopically, crystals are shorter and often rhomboidal. They exhibit weakly positive birefringence to polarized light. Treatment is with simple analgesia and intra-articular steroid injections.

Table 9.1 Synovial fluid findings in different arthropathies				
Parameter	Normal range	Non-inflammatory	Inflammatory	Septic
Viscosity	High	High	Low	Variable
Colour	Light yellow	Straw/yellow	Yellow	Variable
Clarity	Clear	Clear	Clear	Cloudy and opaque
WCC (µL)	<200	200–2000	2000–75 000	>100 000
Culture	Negative	Negative	Negative	85% positive
Glucose	Same as serum	Same as serum	Low	Very low

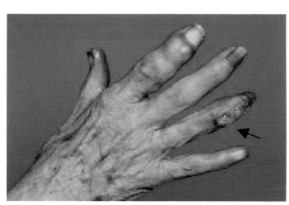

Fig 9.28 Chronic tophacious gout of the interphalangeal joints. Notice the ulceration over the ring finger DIPJ (arrow). Reproduced with kind permission from *The Oxford Handbook of Clinical Medicine*, 7th edn.

Bone tumours

Primary tumours of the bone are rare and account for less than 1% of malignancies and less than 0.5% of all cancer deaths.

Pathophysiology

Benign

- Osteochondroma (exostosis) is the most common benign bone tumour. It often grows on long bones at the epiphyseal plates. Malignant change is rare
- Chondroma (enchondroma) develops in the metaphysis of long bones from small deposits of cartilage within the medullary cavity
- Osteoid osteoma and osteoblastoma develop as small deposits of osteoid tissue in the diaphysis of long bones. They are often very painful
- Chondroblastoma is rare. It develops in the epiphysis of long bones

Malignant

- Multiple myeloma is the most common primary bone tumour. There is a monoclonal proliferation of B cells which replaces the normal bone marrow. Plasma electrophoresis shows high levels of plasma proteins and urinalysis shows light chains (Bence–Jones proteins)
- Osteosarcoma is the second most common bone malignancy
- Chondrosarcoma
- Ewing's sarcoma is common in children; it is highly malignant and metastasizes early

Metastatic deposits

Metastatic carcinoma of the bone is the most common bone tumour overall. Common primary sites include breast, thyroid, kidney, lung or prostate.

Clinical assessment

- Pain—usually unremitting even at rest and can be a dull ache to severe in nature
- Swelling—either due to tumour size, effusion in nearby joint or haemorrhage into tumour
- Tenderness
- Overlying erythema
- Loss of function—nerve compression
- Pathological fractures

Investigations

- Plain radiographs demonstrate site of tumour, bone destruction, and periosteal reaction
- Biopsy—FNA, core, incision or excision biopsies are crucial for diagnosis and should be performed after imaging as they can distort the anatomy. They should also be planned so that the technique used compliments the future treatment, i.e. the biopsy track positioned so that it can be excised with the tumour
- CT scan good for bone imaging
- MRI better for soft tissue imaging
- Isotope bone scan detects lesion but does not identify aetiology

Management

Bone tumours should be managed in regional centres by a multidisciplinary team. Following diagnosis and staging, options available include surgery as well as chemotherapy and radiotherapy. The treatment plan varies depending on the patient and the type, site, and stage of tumour.

Operative

Surgery aims to remove the tumour and prevent it from recurring. Resection can be:

- local curettage of benign lesions
- wide resection of tumour, capsule, and reactive surrounding tissue
- radical excision of entire bone with reconstruction (e.g. endoprosthesis)
- amputation is used if extensive tumour and reconstruction not possible

Conservative

Non-surgical treatment consists of chemotherapy and radiotherapy which can be used in combination with surgery ether to reduce the size of the tumour prior to excision or after to prevent recurrence.

Soft tissue tumours

Soft tissue is supportive tissue not of epithelial, skeletal or lymphohaematopoietic origin. Embryologically, most of it is derived from mesoderm.

Benign tumours are at least ten times more common than malignant tumours (sarcomas). They tend to grow centripetally, displacing or compressing local tissue and respecting tissue boundaries and compartments. They have a high chance of local recurrence but rarely metastasize.

Clinical assessment

Clinically, soft tissue tumours present as a discrete mass. This is usually soft and non-painful. Examination determines its characteristics and extent.

Investigations

- Simple lipomas do not require imaging
- Suspicious lesions need imaging before biopsy (CT/MRI)
- Biopsy all soft tissue masses >5 cm in diameter and enlarging or symptomatic lesions

Staging

Histological grading is an important prognostic indicator in sarcomas and guides further management.

Management

Benign soft tissue tumours can be excised. Limb sarcomas are excised with adjuvant radiation therapy or chemotherapy.

Table 9.2 Musculoskeletal tumours		
	Benign	**Malignant**
Bone	Osteoid osteoma Osteoblastoma	Osteosarcoma
Bone marrow		Lymphoma Myeloma
Cartilage	Chondroma Chondroblastoma	Chondrosarcoma
Fibrous tissue	Fibroma	Fibrosarcoma
Fat	Lipoma	Liposarcoma
Vascular	Angioma	Angiosarcoma
Miscellaneous	Giant cell tumour	Ewing's sarcoma Adamantinoma

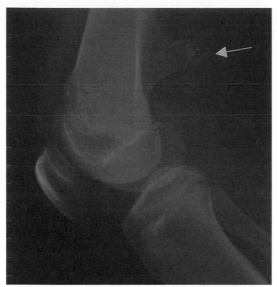

Fig 9.29 Exostosis (arrow) on the posterior surface of the distal femur.

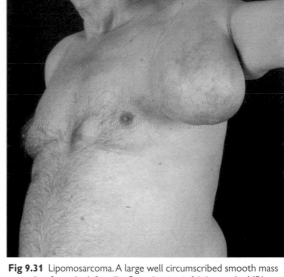

Fig 9.31 Lipomosarcoma. A large well circumscribed smooth mass extending from the left axilla. On palpation it felt lumpy. An MRI was arranged to define its anatomical relationship with the structures of the axilla further before surgical excision and reconstruction.

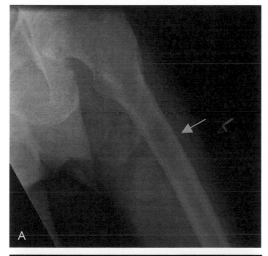

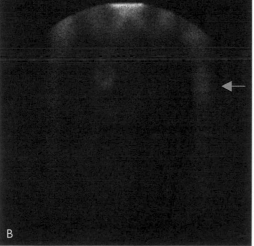

Fig 9.30 Metastatic bone deposit (osteolytic). **A** Plain AP radiograph of the left femur showing a subtle radiolucent area in the proximal femur. **B** It is clearly visible on bone scintigraphy.

Osteoporosis

Osteoporosis is increased porosity of bone owing to loss of bone mass. The World Health Organization defines it as bone mineral density 2.5 standard deviations below the mean for a young, white adult woman.

Aetiology

Primary osteoporosis is idiopathic, postmenopausal or age-related. Risk factors include increased age, female sex, Caucasian origin, family history, smoking, and a low BMI.

Secondary osteoporosis can be caused by:

- malnutrition/malabsorption (vitamin C and D deficiency)
- drugs (corticosteroids, anticoagulants, alcohol)
- neoplasia (multiple myeloma)
- endocrine disorders (thyroid disorders, hyperparathyroidism, Addison's disease, and diabetes mellitus)

Pathophysiology

Bone production and bone resorption are tightly coupled; imbalance leads to osteoporosis. There are three main mechanisms.

1. Low peak bone mass during skeletal growth
2. Increased bone resorption (low oestrogen levels following the menopause)
3. Decreased bone production (e.g. abnormal calcium metabolism)

Clinical assessment

The symptoms and signs are related to the affected bones. Bone pain, loss of height, kyphosis, and fractures are common with vertebral column disease.

Investigations

- Blood tests—normal ALP and calcium
- Dual energy X-ray absorpitiometry (DEXA scan) is the criterion standard; quantitative ultrasound can also be used

Management

By the time the condition is diagnosed it is usually too late for treatment to have an impact on disease progression.

Conservative

- Drugs
- Calcium
- Vitamin D
- Bisphosphonates
- Hormone replacement therapy
- Exercise and weight training—general low level exercise is not protective

Operative

Osteoporotic fractures may require fixation and are often challenging owing to the poor quality bone.

Complications and prognosis

Pathological fractures are the main complication. Treatment reduces the total number within a population.

Rickets and osteomalacia

Osteomalacia is the incomplete mineralization of osteoid bone after closure of the growth plates. Rickets is a similar disease process but occurs in growing bone prior to closure of the growth plates. A lack of vitamin D in the diet or deficit in its metabolism is usually responsible.

Incidence in western society is low, but is widespread in developing countries. By definition, rickets is a disease of children, occurring in the growth phase.

Aetiology

- Vitamin D deficiency related to poor dietary intake, inadequate sunlight exposure or malabsorption (coeliac disease, or following gastrectomy or bowel resection)
- Renal disease—chronic renal failure, renal tubular acidosis
- Cirrhosis
- Anticonvulsant therapy

Clinical assessment

Ricketts may develop early in life and is characterized by:

- failure to thrive and 'growing pains'
- widening of epiphyses
- prominent costochondral junctions ('rickety rosary')
- thin deformed skull (craniotabes)
- valgus or varus deformities of long bones

Osteomalacia may present with fairly vague symptoms:

- bone pain and tenderness
- myopathy
- weight loss and malnutrition
- pathological fractures

Investigations

- Bloods—rickets: low or normal serum calcium, low phosphate, high alkaline phosphatase; osteomalacia: low serum calcium and phosphate levels, high ALP
- Plain radiographs—rickets: widening and cupping of the epiphyses and bowing of long bones; osteomalacia: ostopenic bones, crush fractures or tension fractures (Looser's zones)

Management

Underlying cause needs to be corrected and supplementary vitamin D is added to the diet.

Osteotomies are considered for correction of limb deformities. Fractures require appropriate fixation.

Paget's disease

Paget's disease is a metabolic bone disorder characterized by abnormal bone remodelling. It was first described by Sir James Paget in 1877 as osteitis deformans.

Aetiology

The aetiology of Paget's disease is unknown. Recent theories suggest that a viral infection by the paramyxovirus family may be implicated. There is support for a genetic predisposition, with clustering found in families.

Pathophysiology

The axial skeleton (pelvis, sacrum, spine, ribs, and skull) is the most commonly affected. Three stages of the disease process have been described.

1. Lytic phase—excessive osteoclastic activity with bone resorption. A less intense osteoblastic reaction with deposition of disorganized woven bone. Characterized by high bone turnover

2. Mixed phase—osteoclastic activity becomes less intense whilst osteoblastic activity continues to be disorganized. New bone forms abnormally with islands of lamellar bone in abnormal woven bone
3. Sclerotic phase—osteoblastic activity also reduces. Previously laid down woven bone converts to lamellar bone

Clinical assessment
Many patients are asymptomatic and are only diagnosed through incidental findings on radiographs.

History
- Bone pain is the most common symptom
- Headache if disease involves the skull
- Deafness and tinnitus—from cranial nerve compression or ossicle involvement
- Neurological symptoms if bone compresses nerves. Common in the vertebra
- Bowing of limbs, curvature of spine, increased head size
- Pathological fractures
- Secondary osteoarthritis

Investigations
- Bloods—high ALP, normal serum calcium and phosphate. Bone-specific ALP can be measured and is used in patients with familial predisposition
- Plain radiographs—lytic lesions in the early phase followed by sclerotic lesions later. Enlargement of the bones distinguishes from metastases
- Bone scan assesses the extent of the disease process

Management
Conservative
Medical management must control symptoms of pain, but also slow disease progression to prevent complications.
- Analgesia
- Bisphosphonates are stable analogues of pyrophosphate. They stabilize bone by binding and inhibiting osteoclastic activity
- Calcitonin inhibits osteoclastic activity and promotes osteoblastic activity
- Physiotherapy, as well as supportive measures introduced by occupational therapists, enables patients to maintain strength and mobility

Operative
Surgical intervention is usually only required for management of complications. Fractures and nerve compression may need urgent surgery. Bone deformities may require joint replacement or osteotomies to realign limbs. It is often challenging as the bone is very hard and bleeds excessively owing to the increased bone blood flow.

Complications and prognosis
The vast majority of patients have a benign clinical course.
- Pathological fractures are caused by ineffective mineralization of the bone
- Neurological—cranial and spinal nerve lesions
- Osteoarthritis
- Cardiac failure—in patients with extensive disease owing to increased bone vascularity
- Paget's sarcoma—complicates less than 1% of patients with Paget's disease. Commonly the femur is involved. This condition has a poor prognosis, with 5% 5-year survival

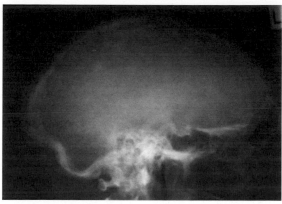

Fig 9.32 Paget's disease of the skull showing a typical 'cotton wool' appearance owing to areas of increased sclerosis and lucency.

9.20 Cased-based discussions

Case 1

It is 0200 and your trauma bleep goes off: '17-year-old male, high speed road traffic collision, ETA 10 minutes.' In the resuscitation room the trauma team assembles. You have been designated as team leader.

- What do you do before the casualty arrives?
- What is the sequence of a primary survey?

The paramedics bring him in on a scoop board, with three-point cervical spine protection. ABCDE is completed. He is talking and has good bilateral air entry in his chest. His initial cardiovascular observations are HR 120 bpm, BP 110/85 mmHg, peripherally he is cool. He is complaining of severe pain in his left leg.

- Does he need fluid resuscitation and, if so, what is your initial approach?
- What primary survey imaging are you going to request?
- What is a secondary survey?

Following a trauma series and secondary survey the cervical spine is clinically cleared. There is a 1 cm x 1.5 cm wound over his medial shin at the midpoint. There is some bruising surrounding the wound but it looks relatively clean. It is very tender to palpate.

- What must be assessed when examining the limb?
- Describe a system for classifying open fractures

Plain radiographs of his left leg show a minimally displaced transverse fracture of the midshaft of the tibia. He is now back in the resuscitation room and is cardiovascularly stable. He is still in considerable pain.

- What is your general approach to his management?
- What do you specifically do in relation to his leg?

He is now on the ward and is due to go to theatre in the morning. The nurse looking after him is concerned about his continuing pain.

- What is compartment syndrome and how would you assess for it?
- What are the potential complications of fractures?

Case 2

You see an 88-year-old partially sighted woman in the emergency department. She has had multiple attendances because of falls and this time appears to have fractured her right hip.

- What are the risk factors for proximal femoral fractures?
- Describe your clinical assessment and the potential findings?

Plain radiographs show an extracapsular fracture of her right hip.

- What is the difference between an intracapsular and extracapsular fracture of the proximal femur and how might it affect management?
- What is your initial approach to her management?

She needs a dynamic hip screw. She seems a little confused.

- How do you assess her confusion? Is she competent to give consent?
- How would you consent a patient for a DHS?

Case 3

A 43-year-old man presents to your emergency department with a painful swollen right knee joint. He is usually fit and well, apparently drinks 30 units of alcohol per week and fell over playing football a few days ago.

- What else should your history cover?
- Describe the typical examination findings of the differential diagnoses

He says it has developed over night and is getting worse. On examination, the joint looks swollen and is held partially flexed. It is warm and there is a tense effusion.

- What investigations do you request and how might they help the diagnosis?
- How would you aspirate his knee joint and what tests would you send the samples for?

The diagnosis of septic arthritis is made and he is due to go to theatre for an emergency washout of the joint.

- What is your initial management?
- Briefly describe the steps in knee arthroscopy and its potential complications

Case 4

You are in the emergency department and see an elderly woman who has fallen over. She has a painful and deformed right wrist.

- How would you assess and investigate her problem?
- Describe fractures of the distal radius and ulna.

She said she felt dizzy and had some chest pain just before the fall but feels fine now. She did not lose consciousness or suffer any other injuries. She is generally fit and healthy and is not on any medications.

- Does this change your assessment and management?
- How would you perform closed reduction and application of a back slab in this case?
- Describe the sequence of events in bone healing

Case 5

A 65-year-old retired man who is a keen golfer is seen in the preadmission clinic to be admitted for an elective left hip replacement. He has osteoarthritis causing severe pain and functional limitation.

- What is osteoarthritis?
- What are the classic radiographic features of a joint with osteoarthritis?

He is fit and well and takes no medications. He has already had a right total hip replacement and that went well.

- What investigations would you request?
- How would you assess his risk of venous thromboembolism?
- What thromboprophylaxis would be appropriate?
- What complications would you mention when consenting?
- Briefly outline the surgical steps in a total hip replacement

Chapter 10

Neurosurgery

Basic principles

Knowledge

Covered elsewhere

◎ Clinical skills

- Raised intracranial pressure
- Algorithm for the management of acute onset low back pain

✚ Technical skills and procedures

- Insertion of ICP monitor
- Burr hole drainage of chronic subdural haematoma
- Diagnostic lumbar puncture
- Insertion of external ventricular drain

Dedicated neuroscience high dependency care units have the experience and protocols to provide focused management of patients with serious central and peripheral nervous system diseases.

Indications for admission

- Primary brain injury (reduced conscious level/raised intracranial pressure (ICP)/impaired airway protection)
- Spinal cord injury (to optimize tissue perfusion and manage neurogenic shock)
- Ventilatory support for neuromuscular respiratory failure
- Status epilepticus
- Medical co-morbidity in neuroscience patient, e.g. cardiorespiratory dysfunction and sepsis
- Elective perioperative management of neurosurgical procedures, e.g. tumour resection or aneurysm clipping

Aetiology

The most common neurosurgical conditions admitted to NICU are:

- traumatic brain injuries
- subarachnoid haemorrhages
- spontaneous intracerebral haemorrhages
- acute hydrocephalus
- spinal cord injuries

Pathophysiology

The consequences of inadequate tissue perfusion are similar for both the brain and spinal cord.

Cerebral perfusion

Most secondary brain injury results from cerebral ischaemia. Cellular hypoxia prevents sufficient energy generation. This causes the normal membrane ion pumps to fail and the cells rapidly depolarize. Large quantities of glutamate, the predominant excitatory neurotransmitter in the brain, are released. This stimulates excess calcium uptake, which produces mechanical cell damage owing to osmotic swelling. Excess calcium also causes disruption of cell and tissue homeostasis.

Cerebral blood flow

Energy delivery in the brain is tightly linked to cerebral blood flow (CBF). In the non-injured brain, CBF averages 50 mL per 100 g per minute and represents 15% of total resting cardiac output. Local CBF is tightly coupled to local changes in cerebral metabolic rate by several mediators. One of the most potent of these is CO_2, which causes vasodilatation. Changes in $PaCO_2$ owing to hypoventilation or hyperventilation profoundly affect overall CBF (Fig 10.1).

Cerebral perfusion pressure

To maintain perfusion of the brain, the mean arterial pressure (MAP) must be greater than the ICP. This difference is the cerebral perfusion pressure (CPP).
CPP = MAP − ICP

Pressure autoregulation

A reflex mechanism exists within the cerebral arteriole wall that keeps CBF constant across a wide range of CPP (Fig 10.2). Rapid decompensation occurs above or below this range, leading to raised ICP or hypoperfusion. In the injured brain this mechanism fails. In these circumstances, changes in CPP have a linear effect on CBF and the range of CPP providing optimal tissue perfusion is very narrow.

Intracranial pressure

The skull is rigid and has a fixed internal volume. The Monroe–Kellie doctrine states that increases in volume of any of its contents (blood, CSF or brain) without reduction of the others will increase ICP.

Decreases in CSF and venous blood volume can buffer small (100–120 mL) increases in volume owing to brain swelling or an intracranial mass lesion. Beyond this level, ICP rises rapidly (Fig 10.3).

Management

The goal of neuroscience intensive care is to minimize the effect of the primary damage and to prevent secondary injury to the brain and spinal cord.

- Adequate oxygenation (PaO_2 >12 kPa)
- Maintain cerebral perfusion pressure >70 mmHg
- Normalize intracranial pressure <25 mmHg
- Monitoring of nutrition, fluid, and electrolyte balance
- Maintain stable blood glucose levels to avoid increasing cerebral lactic acidosis
- Thromboembolic prophylaxis with TEDS and pneumatic compression boots, and low molecular weight heparin is used cautiously because of the risk of intracerebral haemorrhage

Complications and prognosis

The complications of neuroscience intensive care are similar to those of general intensive care.

- Nosocomial infection, e.g. pneumonia, urinary tract, vascular access sites
- CNS infection via multiple intracranial procedures, e.g. external ventricular drains, ICP monitors
- Lung consolidation and barotrauma
- Pressure sores
- Stress gastric ulceration
- Damage to mucosal/conjunctival surfaces
- Venous thromboembolism (VTE)

After discharge, patients may be left with multiple complications related to prolonged immobilization, intubation, and ventilation.

- Impaired cardiac and respiratory function (breathlessness and fatigue)
- Autonomic disturbance (postural hypotension)
- Neuropathy/myopathy
- Joint contractures
- Tracheal stenosis
- Psychological disturbance (depression, anxiety)

Prognosis

Public health measures, such as improved car design, and advances in initial trauma resuscitation have led to an increasing number of patients surviving their primary brain or spine injury.

Despite resuscitation, some of these survivors will have major neurological damage. In these circumstances, intensive care support is ultimately futile and treatment will usually be withdrawn after brainstem testing has been performed. Other patients may be left with devastating neurological injuries and show little evidence of neurological recovery. Discussions about withholding or withdrawing treatment in these cases are often necessary.

The majority of patients admitted to neuroscience intensive care units are eventually able to be discharged to lower dependence care settings. These patients often require prolonged rehabilitation (📖 Topic 10.2).

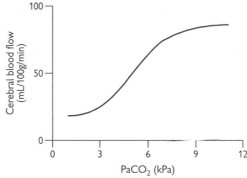

Fig 10.1 Relationship between $PaCO_2$ and cerebral blood flow. Increased $PaCO_2$ (i.e. hypoventilation in reduced consciousness) causes increased CBF and raised ICP. Management aims to control $PaCO_2$ in the low normal range, but hyperventilation to lower $PaCO_2$ is avoided as it causes vascular constriction, hypoperfusion, and hypoxia.

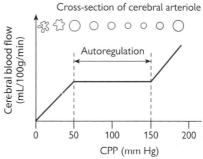

Fig 10.2 Myogenic pressure autoregulation maintains CBF for perfusion pressures between 50 and 150 mmHg. Outside this range, the arteriole is unable to compensate for the extremes of CPP. Brain injury may lead to autoregulation being lost, resulting in suboptimal CBF.

◎ Raised intracranial pressure

Normal adult ICP when supine averages 10–20 mmHg (14–27 cmH$_2$O). Rises in ICP can be controlled by an escalating range of interventions that either reduce the intracranial volume or decrease the cerebral metabolic demands and reduce cerebral swelling.

- Raise head of bed (gravitational effect decreases ICP)
- Remove compression of jugular veins (improves venous drainage)
- Increase patient sedation and/or analgesia (reduces cerebral metabolic demand)
- Paralysis (prevents increased ICP owing to coughing/straining and allows accurate control of ventilation)
- Fix end-tidal CO_2 in low normal range (4.0–4.5 kPa) (NB. Hyperventilation to reduce CO_2 is contraindicated as it causes vasoconstriction and cerebral hypoxia)
- Anticonvulsants to treat occult seizures
- 'Triple-H-therapy'—hypertension, haemodilution, hypervolaemia improves cerebral perfusion
- Diuresis using boluses of mannitol (osmotic diuretic that also affects red cell rheology), furosemide or hypertonic saline
- Insertion of external ventricular drain (reduces CSF volume)
- Controversial therapies include thiopentone coma, mild hypothermia and decompressive craniectomy

---

➕ Insertion of ICP monitor

- Normally inserted at Kocher's point on the right (non-dominant hemisphere): this is the intersection of the sagittal mid-pupillary line and a coronal line passing through the midpoint between the external auditory meatus and the lateral canthus of the orbit
- Prep and drape the right side of the head
- 1 cm linear incision
- Twist drill craniostomy or burr hole
- Pressure monitor calibrated to atmospheric pressure
- Dura pierced with stylet or opened in cruciate fashion
- ICP wire inserted 1–2 cm into brain parenchyma (ICP may also be measured via subdural or intraventricular probes)
- ICP waveform examined to check appropriate position

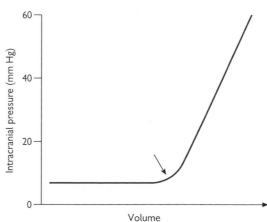

Fig 10.3 Pressure–volume curve showing the effect of increases in intracranial volume on intracranial pressure and the point of decompression (arrow).

Neurological impairment is the largest cause of disability in patients living in the community. The two most common neurosurgical conditions that require rehabilitation services are traumatic brain injury (TBI) and spinal cord injury (SCI).

Clinical assessment

Multidisciplinary assessment of the illness should be undertaken in terms of the WHO International Classification of Functioning (WHO ICF). The model considers the pathology, the impairment it causes, changes in the patient's activity (i.e. disability), and limitations of their participation (i.e. handicap). These are put in the context of the patient's personal, physical, and social circumstances.

Assessment tools

- The Glasgow outcome score (GOS) categorizes outcome following TBI (Table 10.1) The extended Glasgow outcome score (GOS-E) has eight categories, assessed by a structured interview.
- The American Spinal Injuries Association (ASIA) impairment scale classifies neurological status following SCI (Fig 10.4)
- The Barthel activities of daily living (ADL) index documents a patient's independence in personal self-care
- The Rivermead mobility index (RMI) records a patient's mobility

Table 10.1 Glasgow Outcome Score (GOS)	
Outcome	Score
Good recovery—resumes normal life	1
Moderate disability—able to cope with all activities of daily living but is unable to participate in previous social or work activities	2
Severe disability—partially or totally dependent on carers to aid activities of daily living, unable to engage in most of previous social or work activities	3
Persistent vegetative state—does not respond to external stimuli and not aware of environment	4
Dead	5

Management

Comprehensive rehabilitation requires a multidisciplinary team-based approach:

- appropriate neurosurgical, neurological, and/or radiological follow-up to monitor for and prevent sequelae (e.g. hydrocephalus following TBI or spinal syrinx following SCI)
- rehabilitation (education) of patient and carers
- nutrition, bladder, and bowel care
- environmental adaptation (e.g. wheelchair, hoists)
- neuropsychological management (including cognitive behavioural therapy and life management strategies)
- facilitate the use of appropriate community services

Complications

The complications of TBI and SCI may include:

- pressure sores
- venous thromboembolic events
- urinary tract damage
- constipation
- contractures
- secondary psychological problems such as depression and anxiety

Neuropsychology

A clinical neuropsychology service may be available to assist with differential diagnosis, preoperative screening, e.g. prior to epilepsy surgery or deep brain stimulation, outcome evaluation, outpatient case management, and/or inpatient rehabilitation. Psychological therapies may also be employed as necessary.

A neuropsychological evaluation should include a multiaxial DSM (Diagnostic and Statistical Manual of Mental Disorders) assessment and/or psychological formulation, together with an appropriate battery of neuropsychometric tests and questionnaire measures (i.e. quality of life). It is employed to characterize, monitor, and manage any cognitive, emotional or behavioural sequelae associated with neurological injury or illness. Cognitive domains of interest include:

- estimated pre-morbid ability and current level of general intellectual skills
- remote memory and day-to-day memory/new learning ability
- expressive, receptive, and pragmatic language skills
- visuoconstructive and spatial skills
- attention
- executive skills (i.e. organization, planning, behavioural self-regulation)
- processing speed
- psychomotor speed and dexterity
- literacy and numeracy

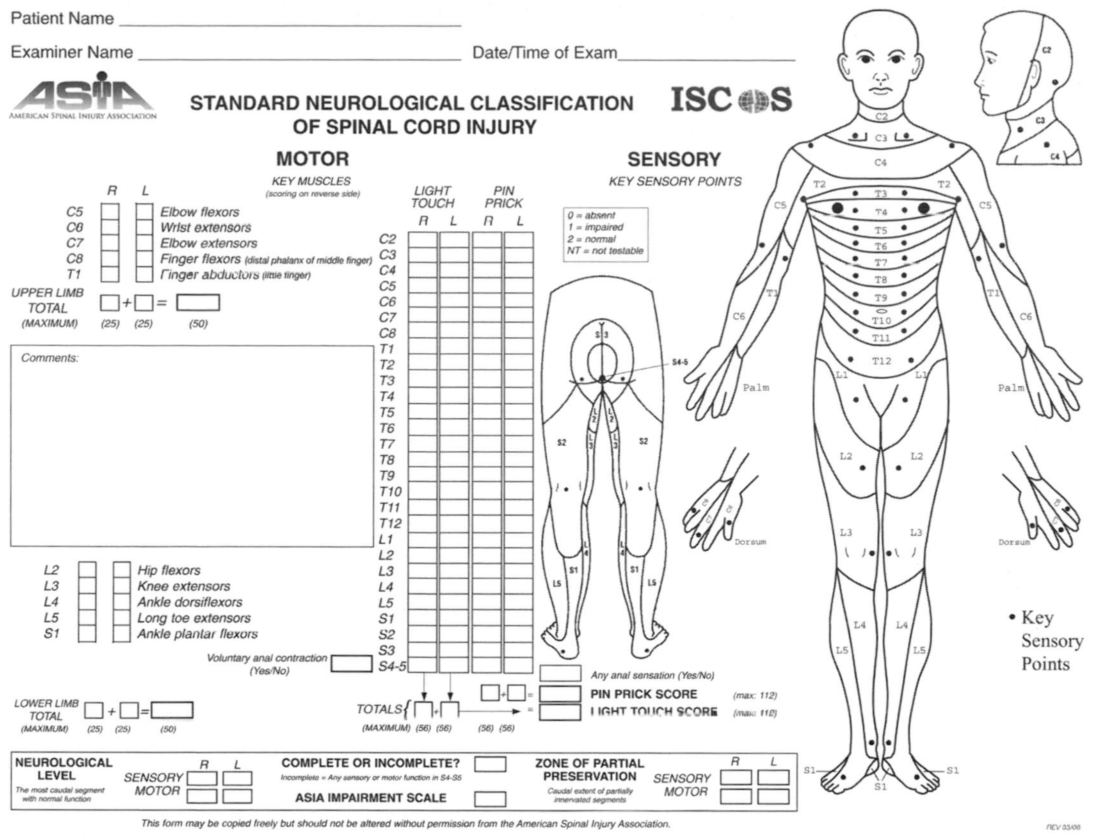

Patient Name _____

Examiner Name _____ Date/Time of Exam_____

ASIA AMERICAN SPINAL INJURY ASSOCIATION

STANDARD NEUROLOGICAL CLASSIFICATION OF SPINAL CORD INJURY

ISC◉S

MOTOR
KEY MUSCLES (scoring on reverse side)

	R	L	
C5			Elbow flexors
C6			Wrist extensors
C7			Elbow extensors
C8			Finger flexors (distal phalanx of middle finger)
T1			Finger abductors (little finger)

UPPER LIMB TOTAL ☐ + ☐ = ☐
(MAXIMUM) (25) (25) (50)

Comments:

L2			Hip flexors
L3			Knee extensors
L4			Ankle dorsiflexors
L5			Long toe extensors
S1			Ankle plantar flexors

Voluntary anal contraction (Yes/No)

LOWER LIMB TOTAL ☐ + ☐ = ☐
(MAXIMUM) (25) (25) (50)

SENSORY
KEY SENSORY POINTS

LIGHT TOUCH / PIN PRICK

0 = absent
1 = impaired
2 = normal
NT = not testable

C2 C3 C4 C5 C6 C7 C8 T1 T2 T3 T4 T5 T6 T7 T8 T9 T10 T11 T12 L1 L2 L3 L4 L5 S1 S2 S3 S4-5

Any anal sensation (Yes/No)

TOTALS { ☐ + ☐ } ☐ + ☐ = ☐
(MAXIMUM) (56) (56) (56) (56)

PIN PRICK SCORE (max: 112)
LIGHT TOUCH SCORE (max: 112)

NEUROLOGICAL LEVEL	R	L		COMPLETE OR INCOMPLETE?		ZONE OF PARTIAL PRESERVATION	R	L
The most caudal segment with normal function	SENSORY			Incomplete = Any sensory or motor function in S4-S5		Caudal extent of partially innervated segments	SENSORY	
	MOTOR			**ASIA IMPAIRMENT SCALE**			MOTOR	

This form may be copied freely but should not be altered without permission from the American Spinal Injury Association.

REV 03/06

• Key Sensory Points

Fig 10.4 ASIA International Standards for Neurological Classification of SCI, revised 2002; Chicago, IL. (Copies of this chart may be freely downloaded from www.asia-spinalinjury.org.)

MUSCLE GRADING

0 total paralysis

1 palpable or visible contraction

2 active movement, full range of motion, gravity eliminated

3 active movement, full range of motion, against gravity

4 active movement, full range of motion, against gravity and provides some resistance

5 active movement, full range of motion, against gravity and provides normal resistance

5* muscle able to exert, in examiner's judgement, sufficient resistance to be considered normal if identifiable inhibiting factors were not present

NT not testable. Patient unable to reliably exert effort or muscle unavailable for testing due to factors such as immobilization, pain on effort or contracture.

ASIA IMPAIRMENT SCALE

☐ **A = Complete:** No motor or sensory function is preserved in the sacral segments S4-S5.

☐ **B = Incomplete:** Sensory but not motor function is preserved below the neurological level and includes the sacral segments S4-S5.

☐ **C = Incomplete:** Motor function is preserved below the neurological level, and more than half of key muscles below the neurological level have a muscle grade less than 3.

☐ **D = Incomplete:** Motor function is preserved below the neurological level, and at least half of key muscles below the neurological level have a muscle grade of 3 or more.

☐ **E = Normal:** Motor and sensory function are normal.

CLINICAL SYNDROMES (OPTIONAL)

☐ Central Cord
☐ Brown-Sequard
☐ Anterior Cord
☐ Conus Medullaris
☐ Cauda Equina

STEPS IN CLASSIFICATION

The following order is recommended in determining the classification of individuals with SCI.

1. Determine sensory levels for right and left sides.

2. Determine motor levels for right and left sides.
   Note: in regions where there is no myotome to test, the motor level is presumed to be the same as the sensory level.

3. Determine the single neurological level.
   This is the lowest segment where motor and sensory function is normal on both sides, and is the most cephalad of the sensory and motor levels determined in steps 1 and 2.

4. Determine whether the injury is Complete or Incomplete (sacral sparing).
   If voluntary anal contraction = No AND all S4-5 sensory scores = 0 AND any anal sensation = No, then injury is COMPLETE. Otherwise injury is incomplete.

5. Determine ASIA Impairment Scale (AIS) Grade:

   Is injury **Complete?** If YES, AIS=A Record ZPP
   NO → (For ZPP record lowest dermatome or myotome on each side with some (non-zero score) preservation)

   Is injury motor **incomplete?** If NO, AIS=B
   YES → (Yes=voluntary anal contraction OR motor function more than three levels below the motor level on a given side.)

   Are **at least** half of the key muscles below the (single) **neurological** level graded 3 or better?
   NO → AIS=C   YES → AIS=D

   If sensation and motor function is normal in all segments, AIS=E
   Note: AIS E is used in follow up testing when an individual with a documented SCI has recovered normal function. If at initial testing no deficits are found, the individual is neurologically intact; the ASIA Impairment Scale does not apply.

10.3 Chronic subdural haematoma

Chronic subdural haematoma (SDH) is one of the commonest neurosurgical conditions. It occurs when blood has collected and expanded in the subdural space over the course of days to weeks.

Incidence is 1–13 per 100 000 per year (depending on the age profile of the population). It increases with age and peaks >50 years (M:F 2:1).

Aetiology

The majority of chronic SDHs form slowly and progressively after an initial minor head injury, usually in an elderly patient. Approximately 40% of patients are unable to recall a head injury. Up to 30% are bilateral. A minority form as the result of a conservatively managed acute subdural haematoma.

Risk factors

- Cerebral atrophy (age-related white matter change associated with vascular disease and alcoholic degeneration)
- Anticoagulation and coagulation disorders
- Other conditions that predispose to minor head injuries, such as epilepsy or cardiovascular disease
- Arachnoid cysts (seen in younger patients)

Pathophysiology

Rupture of small bridging veins between the dura and the cortical surface causes bleeding. The blood initiates an inflammatory reaction. This releases angiogenesis factors which lead to the formation of small friable capillaries. In addition, both the coagulation and fibrinolytic systems are overactivated, producing a vicious cycle of continued bleeding.

The subdural space is progressively enlarged by the slowly extravasated blood. The liquefied haematoma has a high protein content and therefore oncotic pressure which leads to osmotic swelling. With time, the haematoma may become sufficiently large to cause a mass effect, resulting in raised ICP.

Clinical assessment

The classic presentation is of an elderly patient with a history of a trivial head injury followed by several weeks of insidious deterioration in neurological function.

- Raised ICP: headache, confusion/deterioration in memory, decreased conscious level
- Focal mass effect: hemiparesis, dysphasia

Investigations

- Brain CT scan shows a crescent-shaped mass between the inner table of the skull and the outer surface of the cortex. Most chronic SDH are located over the fronto-parietal convexity (Fig 10. 6). The natural history is for the clot to be hyperdense relative to brain in the first week following injury, isodense in the second and third weeks, and hypodense in the fourth week following liquefaction. Bilateral isodense subdurals can be missed
- Brain MRI may detect isodense chronic SDH missed by CT
- Basic coagulation screen (more detailed clotting studies are indicated in the case of recurrent presentations).

Management

Conservative

- Observation if the haematoma is small without significant mass effect
- Steroids have been suggested to limit the inflammatory reaction

Operative

- Burr hole (or twist drill) craniostomy (see box). Recent evidence suggests a subdural drain should be carefully inserted at the end of the procedure
- Craniotomy is indicated if the clot has not completely liquefied or has become loculated and the patient is still symptomatic

Complications and prognosis

Over 90% of operated cases show residual blood on early postoperative imaging, and up to 20% of cases require a further operation. Some surgeons start prophylactic anticonvulsants to prevent seizures. Rarely, a subdural empyema can develop postoperatively.

✚ Burr hole drainage of chronic subdural haematoma

- Position the patient supine with head rotated away from side of SDH or neutral if bilateral SDH
- Two incisions are usually planned—one frontal and one parietal (this is guided by the imaging findings). They are usually placed in the line of a 'trauma craniotomy' incision so the burr holes can be converted to a craniotomy if necessary
- Minimal shave of incisions, sterile prep and drape of scalp on side(s) to be operated upon, give prophylactic antibiotics at induction
- Infiltrate local anaesthetic
- 3 cm linear incision through scalp down to skull
- Burr holes fashioned with pneumatic perforator
- Dura cauterized with bipolar diathermy and opened in cruciate fashion. The dural leaflets are shrunk back with bipolar diathermy
- Usually chronic SDH drains under pressure but occasionally a membrane has formed which needs to be opened carefully with bipolar diathermy
- Copious irrigation with warmed saline or Ringer's solution through both burr holes until fluid is running clear
- Incision closed in layers with absorbable sutures to galea and non-absorbable sutures to skin

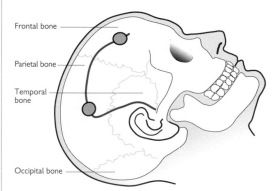

Fig 10.5 Burr hole positions for drainage of chronic SDH placed on the trauma craniotomy line.

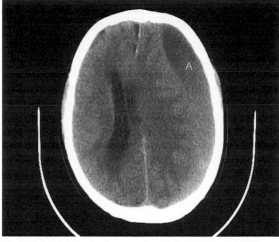

Fig 10.6 Axial CT brain showing a large left-sided chronic SDH causing significant mass effect and midline shift. The frontal part of the haematoma is hypodense (A) to normal brain, but with patient lying in the scanner the denser fresher blood has settled in the parietal region which appears isodense (B).

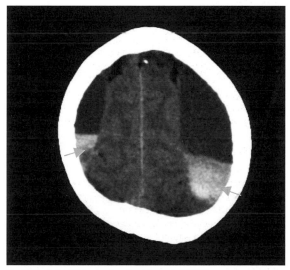

Fig 10.7 Axial CT brain showing bilateral SDH. There is hyperdense acute blood layering posteriorly on both sides (arrows) because of an acute bleed into existing chronic SDH which is the hypodense area above.

10.4 Subarachnoid haemorrhage

Subarachnoid haemorrhage (SAH) is extravasation of blood into the subarachnoid space. It is the cause of 5% of all strokes. Incidence is 10–15 per 100 000 per year, with a median age of 56 years (risk increases with age). Overall, it is more common in women (M:F 2:1), although before 40 years of age, it is more common in men.

Aetiology

Eighty-five per cent of all spontaneous SAH are caused by aneurysm rupture. Other causes include arteriovenous malformations and dural fistulae.

Risk factors

Genetic and environmental factors have a role in the development of cerebral aneurysms and their risk of rupture.

- Family history of intracranial aneurysms
- Smoking and hypertension both independently increase the risk of developing cerebral aneurysms
- Several rare connective tissue disorders are associated with cerebral aneurysms, including autosomal dominant adult polycystic kidney disease, Ehlers–Danlos type IV, neurofibromatosis type I, and Marfan's syndrome.

Pathophysiology

Intracranial aneurysms usually develop at the branching points of large cerebral arteries of the Circle of Willis. Eighty five per cent of aneurysms are found in the anterior circulation. The most common point is the junction of the distal internal carotid artery and the posterior communicating artery (Fig 10.10).

They are thought to be caused by a degenerative process initiated by haemodynamic stress on the vessel wall. Loss of internal elastic lamina and thinning of the tunica media allows small outpouchings to develop which are subsequently expanded by hydrostatic pressure. The lack of an external elastic lamina makes cerebral vessels particularly vulnerable to aneurysmal dilatations. Most cerebral aneurysms are saccular ('berry') although they can have other morphologies.

When the ruptured blood is extravasated into the basal cisterns (enlarged subarachnoid spaces), the force and extent of rupture can force blood into the brain parenchyma, ventricular system, and occasionally the subdural space.

Clinical assessment

History

- Sudden onset of severe headache without warning ('thunderclap'). Any patient describing this must have a SAH excluded
- SAH can present in less obvious ways. A patient may present with a first seizure or after an accident caused by them losing consciousness transiently at the time of the ictus
- Delayed presentation may be with symptoms of meningeal irritation (neck stiffness and photophobia)

Examination

The majority of patients are neurologically intact at presentation, although a spectrum of neurological dysfunction can be seen up to and including coma. Many patients die before reaching hospital.

Classification

Severity is graded using the World Federation of Neurological Surgeons (WFNS) grading system (Table 10.2). When assessed at initial presentation it predicts outcome. Those in grades IV and V have a high mortality rate (>85%).

Investigations

- Non-contrast CT brain scan (Fig. 10.8) should be performed as soon as possible after the ictus. When performed within 24 h it has a sensitivity of 95%
- A negative CT with a suggestive history is a mandatory indication for a lumbar puncture. It should be delayed until at least 12 h following the ictus. This allows time for the breakdown of blood products
- A positive CT scan or lumbar puncture will prompt investigation of the cause of the bleed. The first line investigation is usually a high resolution CT angiogram (CTA) (Fig 10.9). Patients with negative or equivocal CTAs will require four-vessel digital subtraction angiography (Fig 10.10).

Management

Immediate

Initial approach follows ABC resuscitation. The aim is to prevent secondary brain injury. Those patients with higher WFNS grades will need high dependency care (📖 Topic 10.1).

- Maintain slight hypervolaemia. Hypotension and excessive hypertension should be avoided
- Regular antiemetics and analgesia (avoid sedatives)
- Nimodipine (calcium channel blocker) improves outcome probably by limiting vasospasm and hence preventing cerebral infarction. It is given at an oral dose of 60 mg every 4 h and continued for 21 days from the ictus

Exclusion of the aneurysm

Following resuscitation, the aim is to exclude the aneurysm from the circulation. Most centres now advocate early intervention for low grade bleeds. There are two options to secure the aneurysm:

1. surgical craniotomy and clipping of the neck of aneurysm under direct vision
2. endovascular coiling with platinum Guglielmi detachable coils which are deployed in the aneurysm and induce thrombosis

Most UK centres are now preferentially opting for coiling.

Complications and prognosis

- Re-bleed—an unsecured aneurysm that has bled has a risk of 1–2% per day for the first fortnight of bleeding again
- Mass effect—caused a large SAH may result in an intracerebral haemorrhage (ICH) which may increase ICP and require surgical evacuation
- Posthaemorrhagic hydrocephalus—blood within the subarachnoid space disrupts the usual circulation and absorption of cerebrospinal fluid (CSF), producing hydrocephalus. This may require placement of an external ventricular drain or regular lumbar punctures to relieve the pressure
- Hyponatraemia is common following SAH and requires liaison with your endocrinology team to determine the cause and appropriate treatment (usually cerebral salt wasting).

Clip or coil

The recent shift in management of aneurysms from clipping to coiling was promoted by the International Subarachnoid Aneurysm Trial (ISAT). It concluded that, for the trial population, clipping should be reserved for aneurysms that are not possible to coil. Not all neurosurgeons accept its conclusions.

Table 10.2 WFNS grading system for SAH

Grade	GCS	Major focal signs*
I	15	Absent
II	13–14	Absent
III	13–14	Present
IV	7–12	Present or absent
V	3–6	Present or absent

*Major focal signs = aphasia, hemiparesis or hemiplegia.

➕ **Diagnostic lumbar puncture**

A CT scan must be performed before a LP if the patient has symptoms or signs of raised ICP or focal neurological deficits.

Procedure

- The patient is positioned in lateral decubitus 'fetal' position (knees to chest, spine flexed) or sitting with spine flexed
- Strict aseptic technique is employed. Prepare and drape lumbar region and iliac crests
- Identify intercrestal line which intersects the spinous process of L4 in midline, palpate L4/5 interspace inferiorly
- Infiltrate skin and subcutaneous tissue with 1% lidocaine, taking care not to enter epidural space
- Assemble manometer while anaesthetic is taking effect
- Puncture the skin in the midline using a 19–22G spinal needle. The needle is aimed slightly cranially in line with the angle of the adjacent spinous processes
- Resistance is felt as the needle passes through the ligamentum flavum which then gives way on entering the thecal sac
- Withdraw the stylet and check for CSF flow; immediately connect the manometer and record the opening pressure
- Collect three 1 mL samples in sterile tubes for spectrophotometry (oxyhaemoglobin and/or bilirubin), biochemistry (glucose and protein), and microbiology (Gram stain and cell count). The spectrophotometry sample needs to be transported to the laboratory by hand to be immediately centrifuged to prevent a false-positive result from red cell lysis
- Reconnect the manometer and record the closing pressure before inserting the stylet and removing the needle

Complications

- Headache lasting for up to a week is seen in 25% of cases. It is due to low CSF pressure owing to CSF leak. It can be reduced by using a blunt-tipped needle
- Brain herniation may occur if there is raised ICP (contraindication for LP)
- CSF infection is rare

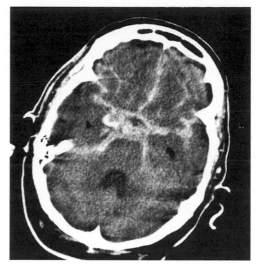

Fig 10.8 CT brain showing a SAH with blood outlining the basal cisterns and subarachnoid spaces.

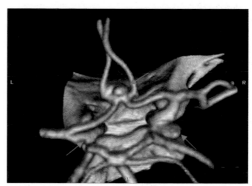

Fig 10.9 3D reconstruction of a CTA showing the circle of Willis with bilateral posterior communicating artery aneurysms and a bilobed anterior communications artery aneurysm (red arrow).

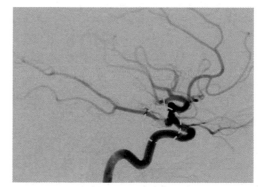

Fig 10.10 DSA following injection of the left internal carotid artery showing a partially treated left posterior communicating artery aneurysm. The majority of the aneurysm has been filled with coils. However, this follow-up angiogram shows that a remnant persists the neck (arrow).

10.5 Hydrocephalus

Hydrocephalus [G. *hydór* water, *kephale* head] is an excessive volume of CSF, leading to an increased ICP. It is the result of impaired absorption, altered flow or increased formation of CSF.

Aetiology

Impaired absorption
- Inflammatory (e.g. meningitis)
- Following subarachnoid haemorrhage or intraventricular haemorrhage (often seen in pre-term infants)

Altered flow
- Intraventricular lesion blocking CSF circulation or intracranial lesion compressing ventricular system (e.g. posterior fossa haematoma or tumour)
- Congenital: stenosis of the aqueduct of Sylvius, Dandy–Walker malformation, Arnold–Chiari malformation

Increased formation
- Choroid plexus tumour (rare)

Pathophysiology

CSF is produced by a combination of ultrafiltration and active ion transport. Eighty per cent is secreted by the choroid plexus of the lateral ventricles. It is produced at a rate of 20 mL/h. The total volume of CSF in an adult is approximately 150 mL. This means the total CSF volume is recycled over three times per day.

The fluid circulates throughout the ventricles and subarachnoid space of the brain and spine before the majority is absorbed into the superior sagittal venous sinus via the arachnoid villi (Fig. 10.11).

- **Communicating hydrocephalus** is caused by impaired absorption. The CSF can freely circulate from the ventricular system into the subarachnoid space, but reabsorption is impaired owing to a blockage in the subarachnoid space or dysfunction of the arachnoid villi
- **Non-communicating hydrocephalus** is caused by a blockage preventing circulation of CSF from the ventricles into the subarachnoid space. This process causes ventriculomegaly (increased size of ventricles) proximal to the blockage
- **Normal pressure hydrocephalus** is characterized by enlarged ventricles and normal LP opening pressure with intermittent transient increases in ICP

Ex vacuo ventriculomegaly is a passive increase in ventricular size owing to cerebral atrophy or focal loss of brain parenchymal volume (e.g. following an infarct). This is not classified as hydrocephalus.

Clinical assessment

The symptoms and signs of hydrocephalus depend on the speed of its onset and the age of the patient. Acute obstruction (e.g. haemorrhage or with some tumours/cysts) will cause a rapid rise in intracranial pressure (ICP). This can lead swiftly to coma and death. In contrast, elderly patients with normal pressure hydrocephalus may only show a subtle deterioration in function over several years.

History

This should be focused on eliciting symptoms of raised ICP.
- Headache—worse when lying and straining, eased by standing, often wakes the patient in the early morning (due to vasodilation from increased $PaCO_2$ as a result of hypoventilation during sleep)

- Nausea and vomiting
- Drowsiness and confusion
- Visual disturbance
- Slow gait, incontinence, and cognitive decline in normal pressure hydrocephalus

Examination
- Tense fontanelles in infants prior to closure (20 months)
- Increasing head circumference in children prior to completed fusion of sutures (12 years old)
- Papilloedema
- Decreased visual acuity
- Enlarged blindspot
- Impaired upgaze (eventually 'sun-setting' of eyes)

Investigations
- CT scan or MRI may show ventriculomegaly. There may be an obvious obstructive lesion or pattern of ventricular enlargement indicating the position of a blockage
- Lumbar puncture opening pressure is a good approximation of the ventricular pressure. It should *not* be performed in cases of non-communicating hydrocephalus. In these circumstances, reducing the pressure in the spinal subarachnoid space may lead to caudal herniation of the medulla through the foramen magnum, damaging the cardiovascular and respiratory centres and resulting in death ('coning')
- ICP monitoring is often used in equivocal cases and, in most centres, a continuous ICP trace is recorded for at least 24 h.

Management

Acute hydrocephalus is a surgical emergency. It requires the temporary insertion of an external ventricular drain (EVD) or definitive CSF diversion via a shunt or ventriculostomy.

Shunt insertion requires insertion of a proximal catheter into the lateral ventricle via either a frontal or parieto-occipital burr hole. This is connected to a valve which regulates the pressure or flow of CSF that is drained. The valve drains into a distal catheter which is tunnelled subcutaneously and most commonly enters the peritoneum. Shunts may also drain into the pleural space or into the right atrium.

In appropriate elective cases, and occasionally in emergencies, shunt insertion is being replaced as the procedure of choice by endoscopic third ventriculostomy. In this procedure, an endoscope is used to create a CSF fistula through the floor of the third ventricle into the prepontine subarachnoid space.

Complications
- Infection owing to colonization of the shunt during insertion usually presents within the first 6 months following surgery. Rates between 0 and 30% have been reported. It requires exteriorization or removal of the shunt, temporary CSF diversion, and reinsertion when the infection has been cleared. An EVD is a temporary measure owing to the high risk of infection
- Blockage can occur at any point during the lifetime of a shunt. This may be due to cellular debris, choroid plexus obstructing the ventricular catheter, or breakdown of the shunt tubing. Most shunts have a lifespan of 5–10 years
- Seizures are common and occur in up to 30% of cases
- Overdrainage of CSF can lead to 'low pressure headaches' and the development of chronic subdural haematomas

⊕ Insertion of external ventricular drain

Procedure

- Preferentially inserted at Kocher's point on the right (non-dominant hemisphere). This is the intersection of the sagittal mid-pupillary line and a coronal line passing through the midpoint between the external auditory meatus and the lateral canthus of the orbit
- Prep and drape the right side of the head, give prophylactic antibiotics (based on local guidelines)
- 3 cm linear incision in the sagittal plane
- Fashion a burr hole using a pneumatic perforator
- Diathermy and open the dura with a small cruciate incision
- Insert the drain angled towards the ipsilateral medial canthus in the sagittal plane and the ipsilateral tragus in the coronal plane (this is usually perpendicular to the brain surface). CSF flow should be obtained by a depth of 6 cm (never go deeper)
- If no CSF is obtained, then the trajectory should be re-evaluated
- The tunnelling needle is attached and the tubing tunnelled subgaleally as far as possible from the entry site
- The incision is closed in two layers (the galea and skin), and the drain is sutured to the skin to prevent accidental removal
- The catheter is connected to a sterile, sealed drainage system, with strict instructions about volume and/or rate of CSF drainage

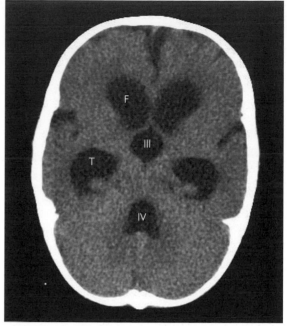

Fig 10.12 CT scan showing communicating hydrocephalus with dilatation of all four ventricles. III, third ventricle; IV, fourth ventricle; F, frontal horn of right lateral ventricle; T, temporal horn of right lateral ventricle.

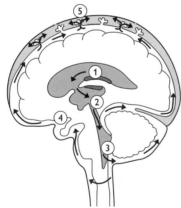

Fig 10.11 Diagram showing the flow of cerebrospinal fluid from production in the ventricles to absorption into the circulation (midline sagittal view).

1 CSF produced by the choroid plexus in the lateral and third ventricle
2 CSF passes from the third ventricle via the aqueduct of Sylvius into the fourth ventricle
3 From the fourth ventricle CSF enters the subarachnoid space through the two lateral foramina of Luschka and central foramen of Magendie
4 CSF circulates through the basal cisterns
5 CSF absorbed by the arachnoid villa into the venous blood of the superior sagittal sinus

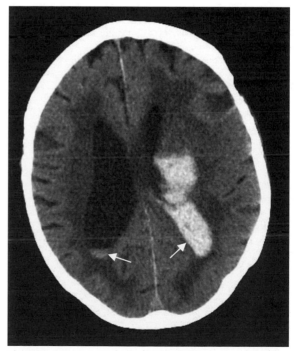

Fig 10.13 CT scan showing obstructive hydrocephalus with dilatation of the lateral ventricles caused by an intra-ventricular extension (arrows) of a hypertensive basal ganglia haemorrhage.

10.6 Intracranial tumours

The overall incidence of brain tumours is 20 per 100 000 people per year in the UK. Of these, 60% are metastases. In childhood, brain tumours are the most common solid tumour. The proportion of tumours that arise from the brain decreases with age. In children, most tumours are infra-tentorial (i.e. arise in the posterior fossa of the skull).

Aetiology

- Intrinsic brain tumours can develop from many different cell types
- Metastases commonly arise from lung, breast, kidney, thyroid or skin (melanoma)

Pathophysiology

Intracranial tumours are often described as either benign or malignant. The definition of these terms differs from other tumours as it is extremely rare for a primary brain tumour to metastasize to elsewhere in the body. The malignant potential of an intrinsic brain tumour refers to its potential to invade through the adjacent brain parenchyma. Benign tumours still have the potential to cause devastating neurological injury or death owing to local compression of structures within the limited volume of the skull.

Classification

The World Health Organization classifies brain tumours based on the tissue of origin and histological grade.

- *Astrocytomas* are the commonest primary tumour. They arise from glial cells, and are separated into grades I–IV
- *Glioblastoma multiforme (GBM)* is a grade IV astrocytoma. This is a very poorly differentiated aggressive tumour, with a median survival of <1 year
- *Oligodendrogliomas* are slow-growing tumours, typically with calcification seen on CT imaging
- *Ependymomas* arise from the lining of the ventricles
- *Medulloblastomas* are the most common tumour in children, arising from the cerebellar vermis
- *Meningiomas* are normally benign tumours arising from the arachnoid layer of the meninges, causing compression of adjacent brain; they may progress to invade the overlying cranium and scalp
- *Nerve sheath tumours* are slow-growing tumours arising from Schwann cells, commonly affecting cranial nerve VIII (acoustic neuroma)
- *Germ cell tumours* are rare, and include germinomas and teratomas. They form in the pineal region
- *Pituitary region* tumours: micoadenomas (<10 mm) usually present because of endocrine disturbance; macroadenomas (>10 mm) are usually noticed owing to compression of the optic chiasm
- *Lymphomas* are typically steroid-sensitive, and are therefore difficult to biopsy if steroids have been commenced previously

Clinical assessment

Patients usually present with features of raised ICP or focal neurological deficit. Occasionally tumours are discovered incidentally, e.g. when abnormalities are discovered during routine ophthalmological or auditory examinations.

All patients should have a systemic review, focused on eliciting symptoms and signs which might suggest the presence of an extracranial primary tumour.

Investigations

- Cross-sectional imaging (CT/MRI) with contrast will usually demonstrate the lesion. In some cases, the radiological features will enable a WHO grade to be assigned. In all cases, serial imaging is used to monitor for tumour recurrence or progression
- Screening investigations will be needed to identify a primary tumour if the intracranial lesion is suggestive of a metastasis

Management

Treatment is planned to control the neurological symptoms (raised ICP or focal structural damage) and to establish a tissue diagnosis.

Conservative

- Vasogenic oedema responds to high-dose glucocorticoids (e.g. dexamethasone 4 mg qds)
- If the patient has had a seizure, antiepileptic medications are started; in some centres they are also commenced prophylactically prior to intracranial surgery

Operative

The operative management is decided based on the patient's symptoms, imaging findings, and co-morbidities.

- Biopsy provides a tissue diagnosis alone. This is often the intervention of choice in low grade cases that may be suitable for radiotherapy or radiosurgery. It can be performed either freehand or stereotactically (using a frame or image-guidance system). Stereotactic surgery has the advantage of a lower false-negative rate; however, it is more complicated and time-consuming to perform, especially if the tumour is large
- Debulking: a subtotal resection can be performed if the tumour is causing mass effect but cannot be totally removed either due to its relationships to eloquent areas of brain or because of its inevitable extensive microscopic invasion
- Resection is performed for benign tumours or metastases. Some centres perform multiple intraoperative frozen sections to achieve maximal resection of malignant tumours

Adjuvant therapy

Every tumour case should be discussed at a multidisciplinary team meeting involving neurosurgeons, neuro-oncologists, neuroradiologists, and neuropathologists. These meetings decide the appropriateness of adjuvant therapies such as chemotherapy or radiotherapy.

Some cases will be suitable for further resection, and a few cases with appropriate tumours may be offered stereotactic radiosurgery (the most common form being 'gamma-knife') which uses high-energy radiation to cause irreparable molecular damage to the tumour. The extent of adjuvant therapy is partially decided by the patient's 'performance status' (Karnofsky score, Table 3.2).

Palliative care

Unfortunately, many patients with high-grade tumours will not tolerate extensive surgery or adjuvant therapies. They require a support network to help with their terminal care.

Complications and prognosis

Prognosis is based on the tissue type and histological grading. It can range from a median survival of 9 months (and in many cases only a few weeks) for a GBM to a cure following complete microscopic resection of a grade 1 meningioma.

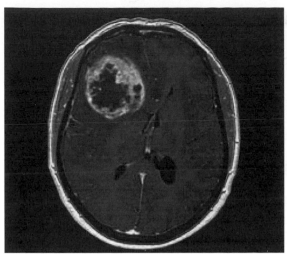

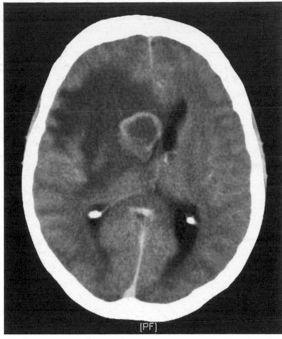

Fig 10.14 T1-weighted contrast-enhanced axial MRI showing a right frontal lesion with central low density surrounded by avid enhancement. It is causing mass effect and midline shift. Its location in the non-dominant right frontal lobe in a young patient allowed a frontal lobe resection. The histology confirmed a GBM.

Fig 10.16 Contrast-enhanced CT scan showing a large peripherally enhancing lesion with central necrosis and extensive surrounding oedema, causing compression of the right lateral ventricle and a moderate degree of midline shift to the left. This lesion is a metasasis from a primary breast tumour.

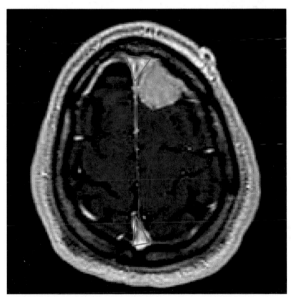

Fig 10.15 T1-weighted contrast-enhanced axial MRI showing a durally based left convexity lesion with homogenous enhancement. This is a typical image finding of a meningioma. It was resected but clear dural margin was not possible owing to the adjacent superior sagittal sinus (approximate boundaries marked with triangles), so adjuvant radiotherapy would usually be considered.

The most common infections of the central nervous system are diagnosed and managed by physicians. It remains important for surgeons to recognize the symptoms and signs of both medically and surgically treated CNS infections in view of their high morbidity and mortality rates.

Intracerebral abscess

An intracerebral abscess is a localized collection of pus within the parenchyma of the brain.

Aetiology

Intracerebral abscesses can develop because of haematogenous dissemination from a peripheral focus, or can be due to contiguous spread (typically from frontal sinusitis or mastoiditis owing to *Streptococcus milleri*), or following a penetrating head injury. Common pathogens are aerobic streptococci, anaerobes and *Staphylococcus aureus*.

Risk factors include AIDS, immunosuppression, and intravenous drug abuse.

Pathophysiology

Histologically, an abscess begins as an area of cerebritis which undergoes central necrosis. This forms a fibrous capsule which produces the classical spherical 'ring-enhancing' lesion on contrast imaging. There is usually extensive surrounding vasogenic oedema.

Clinical assessment

Clinical signs can develop rapidly but, if diagnosed early, patients are not usually systemically unwell. Sudden deterioration may occur if the abscess ruptures into a ventricle.

Presentation is with raised ICP or focal neurological deficit. General examination should attempt to exclude sources of infection (e.g. heart murmurs and peripheral stigmata of bacterial endocarditis).

Investigations

- CT brain will show a 'ring-enhancing lesion' that is sometimes difficult to differentiate from a metastasis or some astrocytomas (compare Figures 10.14 and 10.17)
- Diffusion-weighted MRI can differentiate between an abscess and a tumour
- Peripheral inflammatory markers
- Blood cultures
- Chest radiograph and further imaging may be indicated to identify primary infection

Management

- Resuscitation if the patient is septic
- Steroids to treat cerebral oedema
- Prophylactic anticonvulsants
- Antibiotics should be delayed until a sample is sent for microbiology if possible

Operative

- A lesion suspicious of being an abscess needs emergency aspiration to obtain microbiological samples and reduce mass effect
- Pus should be sent for urgent Gram stain, culture, and sensitivity tests

Complications and prognosis

Although intracranial abscesses often have an insidious course they can lead to serious complications, including seizures, venous infarction, ventriculitis, meningitis, or herniation due to raised ICP.

With early diagnosis and management, mortality rates are less than 5%. Delay in diagnosis can lead to a mortality rate of 50%.

Subdural empyema

Subdural empyemas are a rare but serious condition. They usually form because of direct venous spread of bacterial sinusitis or mastoiditis. Pus collects underneath the dura and spreads over the entire convexity of the hemisphere and adjacent to the falx.

If left untreated, thrombosis of the cortical veins or cavernous sinus can lead to cerebral infarction.

Management involves emergency craniotomy and drainage of the pus. One-third of patients are left with permanent seizures, 20% have a residual deficit, and up to 20% die.

Epidural abscess

The epidural space is a potential space between the dura mater and inner table of the skull. Suppurative infection here is usually iatrogenic but can also be from direct spread from the paranasal sinuses, middle ear, and orbit.

Postoperative meningitis

Postoperative meningitis is often difficult to diagnose in the context of a patient who has recently undergone neurosurgery, as many have symptoms and signs of meningeal irritation and raised inflammatory markers related to their recent surgery. It should be suspected in any postoperative patient who is failing to progress or is deteriorating. It is usually associated with pyrexia. The most common pathogens are skin flora. Diagnosis is made by microbiological analysis of CSF samples, showing elevated or rising polymorph cell counts or the presence of organisms. Brain imaging should be performed to exclude an abscess or empyema.

Management

Antibiotic therapy should be guided by culture sensitivities—occasional empirical treatment will be started. Many cases will require intrathecal administration of antibiotics to achieve maximal tissue penetration. A craniotomy bone flap is at risk of colonization and osteomyelitis owing to its lack of blood supply. It should be removed in the presence of confirmed infection. A cranioplasty to replace the flap can be performed when the infection has been cleared.

Spinal infections

Discitis is uncommon following spinal surgery since the advent of prophylactic antibiotics. Pain exacerbated by movement is usually the primary symptom. MRI of the spine is the investigation of choice. Metastatic disease has a similar appearance but can be distinguished as tumour does not usually cross the disc space.

Spinal epidural abscesses are usually due to haematogenous spread, secondary to discitis or iatrogenic. Symptoms are those of spinal cord or nerve root compression, back pain, and fever.

Osteomyelitis of the vertebral body can lead to collapse and spinal instability. Patients present with severe back pain.

Spinal infections are treated initially with antibiotics but they may also require surgical debridement, decompression, and stabilization.

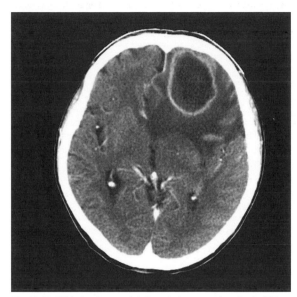

Fig 10.17 CT brain showing left frontal abscess with a classical thin 'rim-enhancing' capsule, necrotic centre, and surrounding oedema.

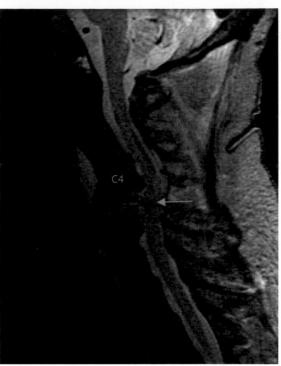

Fig 10.18 Sagittal MRI of the cervical spine showing osteomyelitic collapse of C5 with adjacent discitis; this is causing significant cervical spine deformity and is compromising the spinal cord (arrow).

10.8 Degenerative spinal conditions

The spine is the main weightbearing structure of the skeleton. It gives protection to neural structures whilst allowing considerable flexibility of movement.

Pathophysiology

The combination of compressive loading, repeated movement, and ageing inevitably leads to spondylosis (degeneration of the spine). The lumbar and cervical regions are usually most affected by spondylosis as they have more dynamic mobile segments than the thoracic spine, which is splinted by the ribcage. In the cervical spine, the C3/4, C4/5, and C5/6 levels are most commonly affected. In the lumbar spine, L4/5 and L5/S1 are affected most.

Dehydration of the intervertebral discs (seen as decreased signal on a T2-weighted MRI) leads to increased wear of the vertebral body end-plates. Osteophytes form and narrow the spinal canal. This is accentuated by compensatory hypertrophy of the posterior longitudinal ligament and the ligamentum flavum.

Degeneration of the annulus fibrosus of the intervertebral disc may lead the nucleus pulposis to herniate—a prolapsed intervertebral disc (PID). This will narrow the spinal canal still further.

In the context of spinal canal stenosis, it is probable that repeated flexion–extension movements cause chronic ischaemia of the spinal cord and nerve roots, further exacerbating symptoms.

Clinical assessment

The majority of patients with degenerative spine disease present with isolated low back pain which can be managed in a primary care setting. 'Red-flag' symptoms of serious spinal pathology listed below warrant specialist referral.

- Age <20 or >55 years
- Fever and night sweats
- Weight loss
- History of malignancy
- Non-mechanical back pain
- Spinal tenderness or neurological signs

Neurological symptoms and signs are related to compression of the cord (myelopathy) or the nerve roots (radiculopathy). Narrowing in the lumbar region causes spinal claudication or cauda equina syndrome if acute.

Spinal canal stenosis

Spinal canal narrowing in the cervical spine (Fig 10.19) may cause myelopathy (numbness, clumsiness, upper motor neuron weakness), affecting the arms and legs. It may progress to loss of bladder control.

Stenosis in the thoracic spine will only cause myelopathic symptoms in the legs and bladder.

Spinal canal stenosis in the lumbar region leads to the syndrome of spinal claudication (pain radiating to both legs upon standing and walking, relieved by bending forwards or sitting). This is due to relative narrowing of the spinal canal diameter when in extension versus flexion.

Nerve root compression

Narrowing of the neural exit foramina impinges the nerve roots, causing radicular symptoms (unilateral referred pain, dermatomal sensory changes, and myotomal lower motor neuron symtoms). This is called brachalgia in the upper limb and sciatica in the lower limb.

Disc prolapse

An acute PID (Fig 10.20) will cause rapid onset of symptoms. The position of the disc (central, posterolateral or far lateral) will affect which neural structure is compromised (respectively, cord/cauda equina, nerve root or nerve root from level above). The most common PID occurs laterally at L4/5 and thus compresses the L5 nerve root.

Cauda equina syndrome

Compression of the cauda equina presents with bladder, bowel or sexual dysfunction with perineal/perianal sensory disturbance.

Investigations

- Plain radiographs will show bony degenerative changes and spondylolisthesis
- MRI will show the extent and position of neural compression. It is indicated in all patients presenting with low back pain associated with symptoms of serious spinal pathology or neurological signs. Patients presenting with cauda equina compression or new motor deficits warrant immediate scans

Management

- Acute onset low back pain can be managed according to the algorithm
- Cauda equina compression requires emergency decompression via a wide laminectomy plus discectomy at the affected level
- Radicular symptoms may in the first instance be managed conservatively as the majority resolve with non-operative management
- Persistent/severe cervical radiculopathy is usually treated with anterior cervical discectomy (with or without graft) or posterior foraminotomy. In the lumbar spine, microdiscectomy is the gold standard operation for uncomplicated posterolateral PID causing sciatica
- Progressive myelopathy requires urgent decompression to prevent further deterioration
- Lumbar canal stenosis can be treated successfully by laminectomy at the affected level
- Isolated back or neck pain does not respond well to surgery except in the cases of spondylolisthesis (slip of one vertebral body on another) or spondylolysis (congenital or traumatic defect of the pars interarticularis). If symptomatic, these conditions may be treated with a fusion procedure

→ Extra

Disc replacement

In many spinal operations, the intervertebral disc is removed and the adjacent vertebrae are encouraged to fuse via a graft or fixation. Some spinal surgeons now advocate the use of prosthetic intervertebral discs rather than fusion. They argue that disc arthroplasty maintains segmental motion. This preserves 'natural' spinal dynamics and prevents the development of adjacent level disease. However, artificial discs are expensive and the majority of patients do not seem to experience problems following fusion procedures.

◎ **Algorithm for the management of acute onset low back pain**

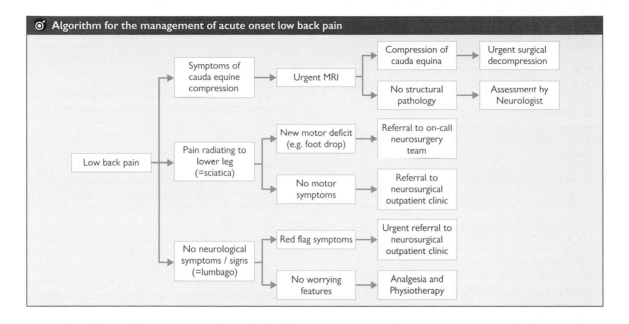

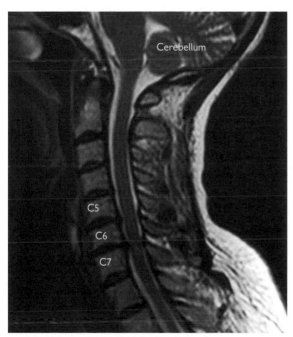

Fig 10.19 Sagittal T2 MRI of the cervical spine showing disc bulges and oestophytes narrowing the canal at C5/6 and C6/7.

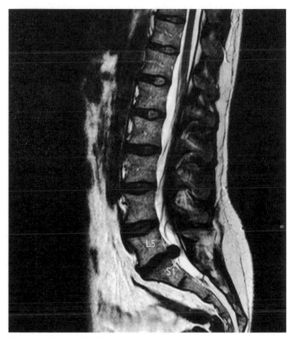

Fig 10.20 Sagittal T2 MRI of the lumbar spine showing a massive disc prolapse at L5/S1 compressing the cauda equina.

10.9 Case-based discussions

Case 1

A 65-year-old man is brought to the emergency department by his wife. She found him at home behaving unusually and complaining of a severe headache.

- How would you assess this patient?
- What is your differential diagnosis of confusion and headache?

You take a history and then examine him. He opens his eyes when you speak to him, mutters incomprehensibly but recognizes his wife and will follow simple commands.

- What is his GCS?
- What investigation would you perform first?

His initial CT is shown in Fig 10.13.

- Does he need a neurosurgical referral?
- What is the most likely cause of this haemorrhage?
- Are any further investigations indicated? What if this was a 20-year-old woman?

Discussion

His acute confusional state and headache point to a neurological cause, but the differential diagnosis is wide and includes infective and metabolic causes. You should consider the fact that he may have had a seizure.

The neurosurgical conditions to exclude with an acute presentation like this are a spontaneous haemorrhage or a traumatic brain injury.

A CT should always be performed prior to a lumbar puncture in a patient with a reduced conscious level to exclude an intracranial mass lesion.

His scan shows a haemorrhagic stroke, commonly due to hypertension. There is no evidence to support evacuating the haematoma; however, he has blood within his ventricles and is developing hydrocephalus. This may require insertion of an EVD and therefore he requires careful observation. The advice of local neuroradiologists should be sought regarding further investigations. In a young person, the presence of an underlying arteriovenous malformation should be excluded.

Case 2

A 29-year-old man is seen in the emergency department at midnight following an alleged assault outside a pub. His friends report he was knocked unconscious for a couple of minutes. He appears to be drunk.

- Why is it unsafe to discharge him with head injury advice?

He is moved to the observation ward. The nurses are busy with an acutely confused patient and only manage to do the first set of neurological observations at 2 am. He does not open his eyes, is mumbling incoherently, and pulls his hand away when his nail bed is pressed firmly. His right pupil is significantly larger than the left and does not constrict to light.

- What is his GCS?
- Is the difference in pupil size (anisocoria) significant?
- Which cranial nerve is being compressed and where?
- What and where is the most likely intracranial lesion?
- Describe your initial management of this patient.

The on-call anaesthetist arrives and intubates the patient. The on-call neurosurgeon's phone is engaged.

- Should you take the patient directly to theatre and prepare him for the neurosurgeon or should you organize an urgent CT scan?

Discussion

This patient is not suitable for discharge because he has a reduced conscious level (he appears drunk but may be suffering the effects of a head injury) and has undergone a significant force head injury making him lose consciousness. According to the current NICE guidelines, he warrants a CT scan in the emergency department.

An expanding intracranial lesion may cause compression of the ipsilateral third cranial nerve. This is traditionally considered to occur as it crosses the free edge of the tentorium.

The most likely explanation for his deterioration is an extradural haematoma. He presented with the classic lucid interval. However, there are alternative explanations, such as a seizure, and therefore a CT scan is mandatory. Initial management should follow ATLS guidelines. His low GCS is an indication for intubation to protect his airway.

Case 3

A 42-year-old woman is brought to the emergency department after being involved in a minor road traffic accident. She drove into the back of a stationary car at low speed and is complaining of head and neck pain.

- How would you initially assess and manage this patient?

On examination she complains of pain in her mid-cervical region and you organize for cervical spine radiographs to be performed. Whilst you are reviewing the films she collapses and is unresponsive. She is resuscitated but has a GCS of 3. A CT of the brain is performed (Fig 10.8).

- What has occurred?
- How would you communicate the severity of her condition to the local neurosurgeon? What is her prognosis?

She is taken to the NICU, intubated, and ventilated.

- What causes raised ICP and how can it be measured?
- Her ICP is 31 mmHg and her MAP is 75 mmHg. What is her CPP? Describe the consequences of this.
- How might you improve her CPP?

Discussion

This patient has had a small SAH followed by a large re-bleed. She was initially WFNS grade 1 which became grade 5 following her collapse. This has a very poor prognosis—many neurosurgical centres would not admit this patient.

Medical management on the NICU will be guided by insertion of an ICP monitor. In this case, a combination of extravasated blood and cerebral oedema will cause an increase in ICP. Her CPP is poor. This will cause brain hypoperfusion unless it is corrected by reducing the ICP and/or increasing the blood pressure. ICP control can be achieved by an escalating series of measures. A difficult decision needs to be made as to how aggressively to treat her condition given it has such a poor prognosis.

Chapter 11

Otolaryngology and head and neck surgery

◎ Clinical skills
- Paediatric hearing assessment
- Auditory rehabilitation
- Vestibular function tests
- Otalgia
- Stertor and stridor

✚ Technical skills and procedures
- Insertion of grommets
- Tonsillectomy
- Drainage of peritonsillar abscess (quinsy)
- Functional endoscopic sinus surgery
- Superficial parotidectomy
- Panendoscopy
- Total laryngectomy
- Neck dissection

Audiology is the study of hearing and balance. This topic outlines some of the methods used to assess hearing. Vestibular assessment is discussed in Topic 11.3.

Tuning fork tests

Tuning fork tests are basic tests of hearing that help to discriminate between conductive and sensory hearing loss. The Rinne test is performed first, followed by Weber.

Rinne test

The tuning fork (512 Hz) is struck and placed first in front of the ear for a few seconds and then behind on the mastoid process. The patient is asked in which position the noise sounds loudest. Air is louder than bone conduction in a positive (normal) test.

Weber test

The tuning fork (512 Hz) is struck and then placed on the forehead in the midline. The patient is asked in which ear, if any, the noise sounds loudest (Fig 11.2). The sound will lateralize to the affected ear if the hearing loss is conductive, or to the opposite ear if it is sensorineural.

Pure tone audiometry

Pure tone audiometry is used to determine the pure tone hearing threshold within the speech range of frequencies (250–8000 Hz).

It detects the presence, severity, and nature of hearing loss as well as differentiating conductive, sensorineural, and mixed hearing loss. It detects the softest sound a subject can hear two out of three times that a pure tone is presented to the test ear.

- **Air conduction** tests the sensitivity to sound transmission through the outer, middle, and inner ear. The subject sits in a soundproof room. The sound is delivered via headphones, ear inserts or by sound-field (free-field) testing using external speakers. It is contraindicated if the external ear canal is blocked in some way, e.g. ear wax, foreign body, infection
- **Bone conduction** tests the sensitivity to sound transmission through the skull to the cochlea. An oscillator is placed on the mastoid process and transmits a signal via the bones to the cochlea, bypassing the outer and middle ears.

Impedance audiometry

Impedance audiometry is used to give an objective measure of middle ear function. The middle ear and mastoid air cells are a closed system from which air is constantly being absorbed. However, the Eustachian tube connects this system to the nasopharynx and when it opens the air pressure is equalized.

Sound transmission is best when there is no pressure difference across the tympanic membrane, i.e. middle ear pressure is equal to atmospheric pressure. Impedance is the resistance to the passage of sound through this system and is measured by tympanometry, acoustic reflex measurement or static compliance.

Evoked response audiometry

The basis of evoked response audiometry (electrical response audiometry) is that various parts of the auditory system produce electrical signals in response to a sound stimulus. Three different signals can be measured.

- **Electrocochleography** measures the signal produced by the cochlea and transmitted by the auditory nerve
- **Brainstem evoked response** measures the signal produced by the brainstem which is made up of a five-wave complex. Its use to detect acoustic neuroma has largely been superseded by MRI

- **Cortical electrical response** measures the signal produced by the cortex. It is not a primary signal but a secondary phenomenon to the sound stimulus and tests the whole auditory mechanism

Speech audiometry

Speech audiometry gives a qualitative assessment of a subject's perception of the spoken word.

The subject sits in a soundproof room with headphones on. Each ear is individually presented with standardized recordings of word lists. The contralateral ear is masked. The subject is asked to repeat the words back. This response is scored for accuracy and plotted on a graph.

Speech audiometry is also useful when investigating non-organic hearing loss or feigned hearing loss.

Otoacoustic emissions

Otoacoustic emissions (OAE) are outer hair cell vibrations detected in the external auditory meatus (EAM). They are classified as spontaneous, stimulus-frequency, transient evoked or distortion-product OAE.

Transient evoked OAE were initially used as a research tool to assess cochlear function objectively. However, as they are quick and easy to measure and have a high sensitivity and specificity for hearing loss, they now form part of the neonatal hearing assessment.

Tinnitus

Tinnitus is an auditory perception that can be described as the experience of sound, in the ear or in the head, that is not heard by anyone else. It affects up to 20% of the population, with 2–3% of cases being severe.

Tinnitus is often idiopathic although it can be associated with local conditions (middle or inner ear disorders and noise-induced hearing loss) or systemic conditions (hypertension, CCF, anaemia).

The underlying pathophysiology is uncertain. The neurophysiological model proposes that tinnitus results from abnormal processing of a signal generated in the auditory system.

Clinical assessment

History covers onset, timing, characteristics, and associated symptoms of the tinnitus. A full ENT and cardiovascular examination should be performed. Tuning fork tests, otoscopy, and facial nerve function are likely to be normal.

A pure tone audiogram is essential to document any hearing loss and an MRI excludes acoustic neuroma in cases of unilateral tinnitus or hearing loss.

Management

Several drugs can be used for the treatment of tinnitus, in particular tricyclic antidepressants. Other treatments include: acupuncture, hypnosis, tinnitus masking devices, and tinnitus retraining therapy.

Tinnitus retraining therapy is carried out over a variable number of sessions lasting up to 2 years. It includes education and counselling, with relaxation therapy and introduction of a white noise generator (masker) that produces a constant low-level noise which will help the auditory system to adapt to the tinnitus. This treatment has a 70% success rate.

Paediatric hearing assessment

Audiological testing in children includes distraction testing, visual reinforcement audiometry, play audiometry, toy testing, sound-field testing, and electrophysiological tests of hearing.

Screening tests

Screening tests are used to detect moderate or severe hearing loss at various points during a child's development.

- Neonatal (48 h)—OAEs +/- brainstem evoked response audiometry (BERA)
- 7 months—distraction testing
- 2–4 years—distraction testing or conditioned response audiometry
- 5 years—pure-tone audiometry

Subjective hearing tests

There are a number of subjective tests and they require experience to interpret the results.

- **Behavioural testing** (<6 months) assesses the change in a child's activity in response to a loud noise
- **Distraction testing** assesses whether a child turns to a distracting noise made behind or to the side of them whilst their attention is being sought by an assistant
- **Pure-tone audiometry** can be performed on cooperative children usually >5 years old

Objective hearing tests

- Auditory response cradle
- Otoacoustic emissions
- Evoked response audiometry

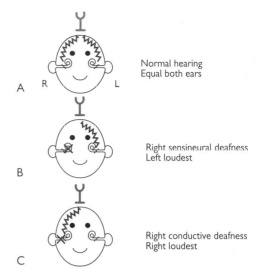

Fig 11.2 Weber test. **A** Normal result with equal detection in both ears. **B** Sensorineural deafness on right side means left side hears better. **C** Conductive deafness on the right side actually means right side hears best as bone conduction is not masked by background noise from air conduction.

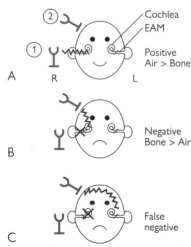

Fig 11.1 Rinne test of the right ear. **A** Positive (normal) test with air conduction better than bone conduction. **B** Negative test with bone conduction heard better than air owing to a conductive deafness. **C** False-negative occurs with an ipsilateral dead ear. Bone conduction is better than air conduction as it is being transmitted to the contralateral side. This can be overcome by masking the contralateral ear by making a rustling noise in front of it.

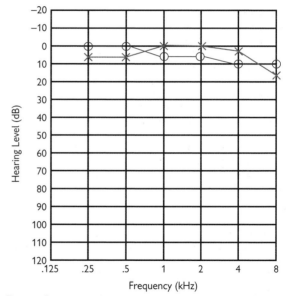

Fig 11.3 Pure-tone audiogram showing normal hearing. The red line represents the right ear, the blue line, the left ear. Sound intensity is measured in decibels (dB) and correlates with the perception of loudness. Sound frequency is measured in Hertz (Hz) and correlates with perception of pitch.

11.2 Hearing loss

Sudden hearing loss

Sudden hearing loss encompasses a spectrum of clinical presentations, from abrupt hearing loss through to progressive loss over a few days as well as distortions in sound and speech perception. Sudden hearing loss is almost always unilateral.

Aetiology

The causes can be divided into conductive or sensorineural.

Conductive

- Occlusion of EAM (foreign body, wax, middle ear effusion, infection)
- Trauma (temporal bone fracture, drum perforation, ossicular dislocation)

Sensorineural

- Idiopathic
- Infection—mumps, meningitis, syphilis
- Ototoxic drugs
- Trauma causing a perilymphatic fistula
- Vascular—CVA
- Tumour—acoustic neuroma
- Endocrine—diabetes mellitus, hypothyroidism

Pathophysiology

Conductive deafness occurs when there is impaired transmission of sound waves to the inner ear. Sensorineural deafness occurs when the sound waves reaching the inner ear are not converted to neuronal impulses or are not transmitted or interpreted by the brain in the correct way.

Clinical assessment

History

- Onset, timing, and associated symptoms (e.g. tinnitus and vertigo)
- Past medical history
- Drug history

Examination

- Head and neck examination
- Cranial nerve examination
- Otoscopy
- Tuning fork tests

Investigations

- Urinalysis
- Bloods—FBC, U+Es, glucose, CRP
- Autoimmune screen (ANA and ANCA)
- Syphilis serology
- Audiometry
- Vestibular function test only indicated if there is reasonable suspicion following clinical assessment
- CT or MRI if indicated to exclude an acoustic neuroma

Management

Management depends on the underlying aetiology. Patients with acute bilateral sensorineural hearing loss should be admitted for investigations. Patients with idiopathic unilateral sudden sensorineural hearing loss should be admitted for bed rest and given:

- oral steroids
- oral aciclovir if viral infection is suspected
- oral betahistine

- carbogen inhalation (mixture of 5% CO_2 and 95% O_2) for a minimum of 72 h or until hearing improves

Complications and prognosis

Spontaneous rates of recovery of hearing are good (60%). Poor prognostic factors include severe hearing loss, bilateral hearing loss, very young or old age, vestibular dysfunction, and raised inflammatory markers.

Otosclerosis

Otosclerosis is a rare autosomal dominant disease which causes areas of mature lamellar bone of the otic capsule to be replaced by woven bone. This leads to fixation of the stapedial footplate.

Patients present with hearing loss (>85% bilateral), tinnitus, and occasionally mild vertigo. Rinne test is negative (conductive hearing loss) in the affected ear and Weber lateralizes to the same ear. Pure tone audiometry shows a conductive hearing loss, which can progress to sensorineural hearing loss if the cochlea is involved.

Conservative management is with a hearing aid. Operative management is a stapedectomy. The stapes is removed and replaced with a prosthesis. Over 95% of patients see an improvement in their hearing postoperatively but there remains a 1–2% risk of a dead ear.

Presbyacusis

Presbyacusis is the deterioration of hearing acuity associated with advanced age. It affects both sexes equally and at least 20% of people >70 years of age will have a moderate hearing impairment (45 dB hearing level). The degeneration occurs both in the cochlea and neural pathways in the brain.

Patients find it difficult to follow conversations when there is significant background noise. Clinical examination is usually normal apart from the symmetrical bilateral sensorineural hearing loss on pure-tone audiometry (Fig 11.4).

Management aims to reduce the impact of the hearing loss on activities of daily life. The mainstay is hearing aids and auditory rehabilitation.

Ototoxicity

Ototoxicity is deafness caused by drug toxicity. Both the vestibulocochlear nerve (VIIIth CN) and cochlea can be affected. Drugs include:

- aminoglycosides (e.g. gentamicin) cause permanent degeneration of cochlea hair cells
- aspirin can cause reversible tinnitus
- furosemide causes reversible hearing loss
- phenytoin
- 5-HT antidepressants
- cisplatin
- quinine

Noise-induced hearing loss

Exposure to excessive noise levels can damage the cochlear mechanism. Occupational noise-induced hearing loss is a compensable disability, and health and safety legislation attempts to reduce the impact of noise in the work place.

Employees exposed to noise levels of 90 dB should be given hearing protection devices and entered into a hearing protection programme.

At first excessive noise leads to a temporary threshold shift (TTS) which is a reversible phenomenon. However, chronic exposure leads to permanent metabolic and mechanical damage to the outer hair cells and then the inner hair cells.

A careful history should be documented for medicolegal reasons. Patients with a TTS may complain of tinnitus but permanent threshold shift (PTS) is usually symptomatic. An audiogram might show a dip initially at 4–6 kHz in the early stages and then flattening with prolonged exposure (Fig 11.5).

Patients should be offered advice to prevent further noise damage and may benefit from hearing therapy to reduce the impact of tinnitus.

Non-organic hearing loss

Patients with non-organic hearing loss (NOHL) complain of a hearing loss when there is no detectable hearing deficit. The two main patient groups are adults who are pursuing a compensation claim and adolescents with psychological disturbance.

Diagnosis requires a high index of suspicion. Patients often give an inconsistent history, and initial investigations such as speech audiometry may be incompatible with their symptoms. Evoked cortical response audiometry and otoacoustic emissions help to establish the true auditory thresholds and confirm the NOHL.

Strong reassurance that the NOHL is only a transient problem is usually sufficient, especially in the younger age group. Occasionally a psychiatric referral may be warranted.

⊙ Auditory rehabilitation

Auditory rehabilitation uses hearing aids and other assistive devices. Surgical options include cochlear implantation, bone-anchored hearing aids (BAHA), and middle ear implants.

Conventional hearing aids

A hearing aid is an electroacoustic device used to amplify sounds. It is made up from a receiver (microphone or induction coil), a processor, a sound transmitter, and a power source.

Analogue systems are rapidly being replaced by digital systems that can better manipulate the signal to meet the needs of the patient. They are often smaller and have less energy demands.

There are different versions available, including behind-the-ear, in-the-ear, and body-worn aids.

Osseointegrated hearing aids

BAHA transmit mechanical vibrations directly to the bone of the mastoid bone via an implanted titanium screw. They are useful in patients in whom the external auditory canal cannot accept a conventional hearing aid as well as in patients with a unilateral total deafness to act as a cross-aid.

Cochlear implants

Cochlear implants are used in patients with severe or profound loss of hearing due to cochlear disease but who have normal auditory nerve and central processing.

There is an external component comprising the microphone, processor, and transmitter, and a surgically implanted internal component with a receiver and electrode array that stimulates the residual auditory nerve.

The outcome is variable and is partly dependent on whether the hearing loss was before or after developing language. Postlingual patients report improved lip reading and ability to identify environmental sounds.

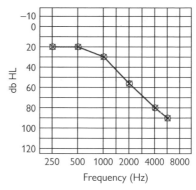

○ – Right ear   × – Left ear

Fig 11.4 Pure-tone audiogram showing a sloping high frequency loss seen in presbyacusis. Reproduced with kind permission from *The Oxford Handbook of Ear, Nose, and Throat.*

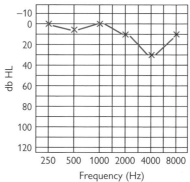

Fig 11.5 Pure-tone audiogram showing a 'notch' at 4 khz typical of noise-induced hearing loss. Reproduced with kind permission from *The Oxford Handbook of Ear, Nose, and Throat.*

The main peripheral causes of vertigo and associated symptoms are discussed below. When making a diagnosis do not forget that many other medical conditions present with similar symptoms.

Acute labyrinthitis

Acute labyrinthitis (vestibular neuronitis, acute vestibular failure) is inflammation of the labyrinth. The most common cause is viral infection, often following on from URTI, although it can be secondary to acute or chronic suppurative otitis media.

Clinical assessment

Patients present with a sudden onset of severe vertigo with nausea and vomiting but no hearing loss or tinnitus. Even the smallest head movement aggravates the vertigo so patients tend to lie still on their side in a darkened room.

On examination the ears are usually normal. Initially there is nystagmus which slowly improves with the clinical improvement. Any suggestion that the symptoms may be related to meningitis or a cerebellar abscess needs further investigation with an urgent CT or MRI. A swab of the ear is taken if there is evidence of infection.

Management

Bed rest, vestibular sedatives, and oral or intravenous fluids form the mainstay of therapy. Chronic cases occasionally progress to develop Ménière-like symptoms. Treatment is with prochlorperazine or an antihistamine for the acute attack of vertigo and vestibular rehabilitation in the longer term. Vestibular rehabilitation is the most successful conservative treatment. It promotes central compensation to improve symptoms of peripheral vestibular dysfunction. Vestibular rehabilitation is a combination of physical exercise (general fitness and Cawthorne–Cooksey exercises) and a psychological programme.

Benign paroxysmal positional vertigo

Vertigo is defined as the hallucination of movement in which there is sensory perception of movement without objective stimulus. Benign paroxysmal positional vertigo (BPPV) is thought to be caused by particles of calcium in the posterior semicircular canal making it more sensitive to movement.

Clinical assessment

There are many conditions that can cause dizziness or light-headedness and these must be differentiated from true vertigo. Patients with BPPV present with acute rotational vertigo when their head is in a certain position, usually tipped back and to one side or the other. They often wake with vertigo following re-positioning whilst sleeping. The symptoms are usually reproducible in clinic with the Dix–Hallpike manoeuvre and will fatigue with repetition.

The Dix–Hallpike manoeuvre is performed by moving the patient rapidly from a sitting to a supine position with the head turned 45° to the right. Rotatory nystagmus with latency and limited duration is pathognomonic of BPPV. The patient is returned to the sitting position and the manoeuvre is repeated with the head turned to the left.

Management

Various particle repositioning manoeuvres (e.g. Epley manoeuvre) can be performed as an outpatient. Vestibular sedatives have minimal success.

Ménière's disease

Ménière's disease is characterized by the triad of deafness, tinnitus, and episodic vertigo. The disease is bilateral in a third of cases. The underlying aetiology is unknown but there is a gradual increase in fluid in the endolymphatic compartment in the inner ear. This bursts out of the space and mixes with the perilymph which causes the acute symptoms.

Episodes often start with a feeling of fullness in the ear and may continue for up to a day. The deafness is usually transitory although may deteriorate over a long period of time. Interval audiograms may show a fluctuating sensorineural hearing loss.

Conservative management improves symptoms in 80% of patients. It includes lifestyle changes (reduced salt and fluid intake), diuretics, betahistines, and vestibular sedatives.

Operative management aims to decompress the endolymphatic sac. More radical surgery involves placing intratympanic gentamicin or intracranial sectioning of the vestibular nerve.

Vestibular function tests

Balance is maintained by the brain (brainstem, cerebellum, and cortex) processing sensory information from the eyes, vestibular apparatus, and peripheral proprioceptors. The two main tests used to assess the vestibular system are electronystagmography and caloric testing.

Caloric tests

The caloric tests consist of stimulation of the labyrinth by instilling warm (44°C) and cold (30°C) water or air into the ear canal and measuring the resulting nystagmus. This test assesses vestibular and cerebellar/brainstem pathology, with an abnormal response (canal paresis) seen on the affected side.

Electronystagmography

ENG is an electronic test used to evaluate the eye movements controlled by the visual system interacting with the vestibular and central nervous system (vestibulo-ocular reflex). This reflex maintains gaze stability and the analysis of this reflex helps to establish if the pathology is vestibular or in the brain. ENG measures saccades, smooth pursuit, and optokinetic nystagmus.

Rotation tests

Consists of stimulation of the vestibular system by rotating in a horizontal plane and recording the nystagmus response.

Posturography

Tests the vestibulospinal reflex, which maintains the relation between the vestibular and the proprioceptor systems connected by the vestibulospinal tracts. It is responsible for maintaining normal posture during head movement. The tests for vestibulospinal function can be static, by observing the postural sway on a fixed platform, or dynamic, by tilting the platform and/or removing visual clues.

Romberg's test

The patient stands feet together and arms by the side, with the eyes closed. It is useful to assess cerebellar and also vestibular function. The patient may fall towards the side of a non-compensated vestibular lesion.

Gait testing

Gait testing is useful to assess vestibular and central function. Patients with vestibular lesions will veer towards the affected side when walking. In those with central lesions the gait may be ataxic (cerebellar), Parkinsonian, or hemiplegic.

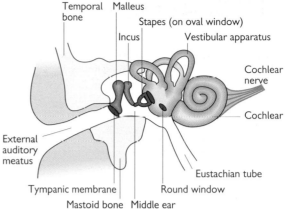

Fig 11.6 Diagram of the vestibular apparatus.

11.4 Otitis media

Acute suppurative otitis media

Acute suppurative otitis media (ASOM) is defined as acute infection (<3 weeks) of the middle ear mucosa with signs of inflammation and effusion. A condition lasting longer than this is classified as chronic. Peak incidence is in children 3–7 years old.

Aetiology

ASOM normally follows an acute viral upper respiratory tract infection (e.g. respiratory syncytial virus). Children are more susceptible as their Eustachian tubes are relatively narrow and short. Bacterial pathogens include *Streptococcus pneumoniae* (40%), *Haemophilus influenzae*, *Moraxella catarrhalis*, and *Streptococcus pyogenes*. Risk factors include prematurity, atopy, low socioeconomic class, and bottle feeding.

Pathophysiology

URTI causes obstruction of the Eustachian tube and stasis in the middle ear. Localized inflammation leads to exudate and pus formation. This increases the pressure on the tympanic membrane (TM) which causes pain and a conductive deafness. Localized necrosis of the TM may result in perforation, allowing the pus to drain and giving symptomatic relief.

Clinical assessment

History

- Upper respiratory tract symptoms (rhinitis, cough)
- Unilateral otalgia (deep and throbbing), pulling at ear
- Unilateral hearing loss

Examination

- Fever (>39°C) and malaise
- Otoscopy reveals a dull bulging tympanic membrane which progressively becomes red and inflamed. Following rupture there is mucopurulent fluid in the EAM

Investigations

- Swab of mucopurulent discharge for microbiology
- Audiometry is not routinely performed (conductive deafness)

Management

Conservative

Rest and analgesia is adequate in most cases. Systemic and topical decongestants are of no proven benefit.

Amoxicillin is the first line antibiotic although the common pathogenic bacteria in ASOM are becoming increasingly resistant.

Operative

Tympanocentesis may be considered for diagnostic purposes in immunocompromised and neonatal patients, or where medical treatment has failed. Tympanocentesis can be converted to a myringotomy by enlarging the hole in the TM.

Complications and prognosis

With treatment, clinical improvement should be seen within 48 h. Middle ear effusion will persist in 50% of cases at 1 month.

Extracranial

- Hearing loss
- Tympanic membrane perforation
- Chronic suppurative otitis media

- Mastoiditis with bone destruction should be suspected in patients with ASOM symptoms, erythema, and pain over the mastoid process. It should be treated early with intravenous broad spectrum antibiotics. Surgery in the form of cortical mastoidectomy is indicated if there is no improvement within 48 h
- Lower motor neuron facial nerve paralysis
- Labyrinthitis

Intracranial

- Meningitis
- Subdural empyema, epidural or cerebral abscess
- Lateral venous sinus thrombosis

Serous otitis media

Serous otitis media (glue ear) is the presence of thick sticky fluid in the middle ear. It has a bimodal distribution, with a peak at 2 and 5 years. It is more common in males.

Aetiology

The aetiology is unknown. Glue ear may precede an episode of ASOM. In children, the Eustachian tube is relatively easily blocked. The adenoids are relatively larger in the nasopharynx and are a ready source of bacteria. This can lead to occlusion of the Eustachian canal and inadequate ventilation of the middle ear.

Pathophysiology

Occlusion of the Eustachian canal causes a chronic negative pressure in the middle ear as a consequence of gas absorption. This change in environment leads to metaplasia of the cuboidal or flat epithelial lining to respiratory epithelium-containing globlet cells. These secrete a thick sticky mucus which accumulates in the middle ear. The fluid splints the eardrum and ossicles leading to a conductive deafness.

Clinical assessment

Hearing loss is the presenting complaint in 80% of cases and may be accompanied by delayed language skills and imbalance.

Otoscopy is very variable. Audiometry shows conductive hearing loss and a flat tympanogram (type B).

Speech and language therapy assessment may show a delay for their age.

Management

The majority of cases resolve spontaneously. Parents are reassured and the child followed up in clinic. Otoinflation using the Valsalva manoeuvre (expiration against a closed glottis) is recommended during the follow-up period.

Insertion of ventilation tubes (grommets) improves ventilation of the middle ear and is indicated if there is a persistent bilateral conductive hearing loss >30 dB on two assessments 3 months apart. Hearing aids are an alternative to grommets.

Complications and prognosis

The majority of cases resolve by age 10 years. Some children are left with a permanent hearing deficit and may require a hearing aid.

⊕ Insertion of grommets

Procedure
- General anaesthetic for children
- Patient supine with head ring for support
- Myringotomy incision in anteroinferior quadrant
- Middle ear effusion is aspirated
- Grommet is introduced through the incision with its waist in the tympanic membrane and a flange at either side of it
- Grommets are normally spontaneously extruded by the tympanic membrane after 7–9 months; 20% of children need repeat insertion

Complications
Infection (which responds well to antibiotic ear drops), continuing serous otitis media (20%), and residual tympanic membrane perforation (1%).

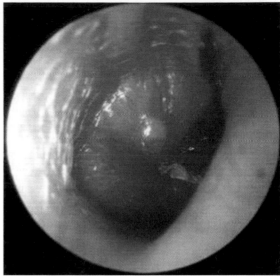

Fig 11.7 Left tympanic membrane of a 4-year-old boy with ASOM. The membrane is injected and bulging with visible pus.

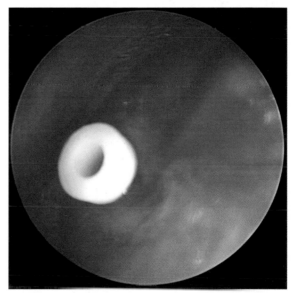

Fig 11.8 Serous otitis media showing a dull retracted tympanic membrane with a grommet in place.

11.5 Chronic suppurative otitis media

Chronic suppurative otitis media (CSOM) is a perforated tympanic membrane with persistent drainage from the middle ear. This chronic suppuration can occur with or without a cholesteatoma. In the past it was described as tubotympanic or tympanomastoid.

Aetiology

The underlying cause is likely to be migration of organisms from the EAM into the middle ear via a tympanic perforation. *Pseudomonas aeruginosa* is the most prevalent organism. Other organisms include *Staphylococcus aureus*, *Klebsiella* and *Proteus* species.

Pathophysiology

There is a degree of Eustachian tube dysfunction that predisposes to recurrent acute episodes of otitis media, causing perforation of the tympanic membrane which fails to heal owing to the continuation of the infection.

Recurrent attempts to heal the mucosal ulceration in the middle ear leads to granulation tissue and polyp formation and, eventually, destruction of surrounding bone.

Clinical assessment

History

- Hearing loss is common
- Chronic mucopurulent otorrhoea when disease is active
- Otalgia is uncommon

Examination

- Otorrhoea can be varied, from serous to purulent
- Otoscopy—TM perforation will be present through which the middle ear mucosa may be visible (oedematous, granulation tissue, polyp)
- Signs of complications—fever, vertigo, facial nerve palsy
- Tuning fork tests

Investigations

- Ear swab for microbiology
- Pure-tone audiometry will confirm conductive deafness
- CT scan of the temporal bones will identify a cholesteatoma
- Head CT and/or MRI to identify intracranial complications

Management

Conservative

- Topical rather than systemic therapy is usually successful in controlling CSOM
- Aural toilet
- Topical antibiotic–steroid preparation (short course)
- Oral antibiotics

Operative

Surgery is considered in patients with CSOM without cholesteatoma with a persistent perforation (>6 weeks), continuing discharge or conductive hearing loss. Tympanoplasty is performed to close the tympanic membrane perforation.

Cholesteatoma

Cholesteatoma is a benign keratinizing squamous cell cyst, with keratin in the centre, surrounded by several layers of squamous cells and inflammatory connective tissue. The cyst retracts and spreads into the middle ear and mastoid bone.

Cholesteatoma can be congenital or acquired (Eustachian tube dysfunction, trauma or iatrogenic).

Due to Eustachian tube dysfunction, the tympanic membrane develops a retraction pocket that grows into the middle ear and mastoid bone. Superadded infection causes a release of lytic enzymes which cause bone destruction and expansion of the cholesteatoma 'sac'.

Clinical assessment

Signs and symptoms are similar to CSOM without cholesteatoma. It tends to be painless and is characterized by a scant smelly discharge. A retraction pocket with cholesteatoma is visible in the tympanic membrane (usually in the pars flaccida). CT scan assesses the extent of disease.

Management

There is no role for conservative management; once the diagnosis is confirmed a mastoidectomy must be planned. The primary aim is to create a dry ear with complete removal of diseased tissue. A second stage procedure is used to reconstruct the ossicles and restore hearing.

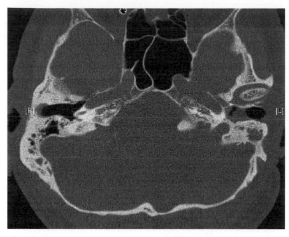

A

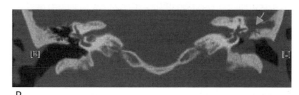

B

Fig 11.9 Left cholesteatoma. **A** Unenhanced CT scan (axial section); **B** coronal section demonstrating the same soft tissue and bony destruction.

11.6 External ear

Otitis externa

Otitis externa is inflammation of the skin and soft tissue of the EAM. Otitis externa is classified as acute (diffuse or localized) if present for <4 weeks or chronic beyond this point. Lifetime prevalence is 10%.

Aetiology

It is most commonly a bacterial infection. Various risk factors predispose to the condition.

Risk factors

- Prolonged exposure to water (swimming)
- Humid climate
- Skin disorders (eczema or psoriasis)
- Trauma (foreign body, hearing aid mould)
- Diabetes mellitus and immunosuppressive states

Pathophysiology

Acute diffuse otitis externa (swimmer's ear) causes generalized inflammation and oedema of the EAM. In acute localized otitis externa (furunculosis) a boil develops in a hair follicle in the hair-bearing outer third of the EAM.

Chronic otitis externa is caused by maceration of the stratified squamous epithelium lining the EAM. There is associated oedema and watery discharge. There may be a superimposed bacterial infection (Pseudomonas aeruginosa, Staphylococcus aureus) or, rarely, a fungal or yeast infection.

Clinical assessment

History

- Otalgia developing over a couple of days
- Hearing loss
- Itching, particularly in fungal infections
- Intermittent watery discharge
- Exposure to water (swimmers)
- Eczema or psoriasis

Examination

Acute

- Pain on gentle traction of the pinna
- Otoscopy reveals generalized oedema of the ear canal with debris or a boil occluding the EAM; often difficult to visualize TM
- Tuning fork tests show a conductive deafness

Chronic

- No pain on moving pinna
- Oedema of the external canal but not blocked
- Otoscopy also reveals debris in the EAM and oedema of the canal

Investigations

- Swab EAM for MC+S and fungal studies

Management

- Aural toilet ± insertion of an ear wick
- Diffuse otitis externa is initially treated with antibiotic–steroid drops. Oral antibiotics may be required if there is no response or evidence of cellulitis
- Furunculosis may require incision and drainage (use 21G needle) and/or insertion of a wick (ribbon gauze or Pope wick) soaked in either 10% glycerine and ichthammol solution or an antibiotic–steroid combination

Advice

- Keep the ear dry
- Stop swimming
- Do not use cotton buds or poke anything else in the ear

Complications and prognosis

With treatment, symptoms improve within 48–72 h. There is a small risk of chronic otitis externa becoming necrotizing otitis externa.

Necrotizing otitis externa

Necrotizing otitis externa (malignant otitis externa) is a very rare, progressive infection of the external ear canal that spreads beyond the canal, causing osteomyelitis of the skull base and multiple lower cranial nerve palsies. It has a high mortality rate.

The underlying bacterial infection is almost exclusively by Pseudomonas species and, rarely, Staphylococcus aureus. Risk factors include diabetes mellitus and immunosuppressive states.

Clinical assessment

Patients usually present with severe otalgia, often disproportionate to the clinical signs. Otoscopy shows evidence of otitis externa with granulations on the floor of the ear canal. There are progressive lower cranial nerve palsies: VII, IX, X, XI, and XII. Rare involvement of the petrous apex may result in VIth nerve palsy (Gradenigo's syndrome), and also Vth nerve palsy.

Investigations

- Swab EAM for microbiology
- Ear canal biopsy to exclude malignancy
- CT ± MRI scan of skull base and brain to assess skull base erosion and intracranial pathology
- Isotope bone scan helps to assess bone involvement

Management

Patients require admission and regular aural toilet. Systemic antipseudomonals and topical antibiotic–steroid drops are started pending microbiology results.

Surgical debridement is considered if there is no clinical improvement and to gain good microbiological and histological specimens.

Complications and prognosis

Complications include lateral and cavernous sinus thrombosis, meningitis, and death.

Pinna infection and inflammation

Cellulitis of the pinna occurs most commonly because of spread from an episode of otitis externa, or secondary to trauma such as ear piercing. Pathogens include Staphylococcus, Streptococcus, and Pseudomonas species.

Clinical assessment

- Current or incipient otitis externa
- Trauma to pinna (laceration, blunt trauma or piercing)
- Red, swollen, hot, and painful pinna
- Neck lymphadenopathy is uncommon
- Impetigo (caused by Staphylococcus) may also be present

Management

- Remove ear piercing and foreign bodies
- Microbiology swab
- Aural toilet if otitis externa present
- Systemic antibiotics (oral or intravenous)
- Abscess will need incision and drainage under LA or GA

Pinna trauma

Trauma to the external ear is common and is often associated with a head injury. It usually results in a laceration to the skin and the underlying cartilage. Depending on the mechanism, there may also be a haematoma (haematoma auris) which is a collection of blood between the perichondrium and cartilage. Poor management may result in pinna infection or a permanent 'cauliflower ear' deformity.

Clinical assessment

- Tetanus status
- Local assessment of external ear
- Otoscopy (perforated TM, blood/CSF otorrhoea, step in EAM)
- Tuning fork tests ± audiometry
- Cranial nerve examination (facial nerve palsy)

Management

Lacerations need debridement, irrigation, and closure under LA or GA. Skin edges should be well opposed and cartilage fully covered.

Pinna ring block—infiltrate LA + adrenaline 1 in 200 000 anterior and posterior to the pinna from the junction of the superior part of the helix and face; repeat from inferiorly from the junction of the earlobe and face.

A haematoma less than a third of the pinna can be aspirated. Larger ones require incision and drainage. In both cases, contoured packing of the pinna and a head bandage reduce re-accummulation.

Ear wax

The EAM (ear canal) is lined with superficial keratinized squamous epithelium. As it is a blind-ending lumen it has developed a self-cleaning mechanism involving epithelial migration. Ear wax is produced by modified pilosebaceous glands in the lateral portion of the canal. It mixes with the migrating squamous epithelium and other debris.

Clinical features include mass sensation, otalgia, and, if impacted, it can cause hearing loss. Irritation of the auricular branch of the vagus (Arnold's nerve) may cause coughing.

Management is with sodium bicarbonate ear drops or olive oil for 2–3 weeks before syringing to wash out the wax.

TM perforation and frequent otitis externa are contraindications to syringing. In these cases, microsuction under direct vision is more appropriate.

⊙ Otalgia

Primary otalgia arises directly from the pinna, EAM or middle ear, and is caused by ear pathology such as otitis externa or media.

Secondary (referred) otalgia is caused by local nerves and structures.

- Temporomandibular joint dysfunction and dental disease is related to trigeminal nerve (Vth CN) dysfunction
- Oropharyngeal and laryngeal pathology (including malignancy) related to glossopharyngeal (IXth CN) and vagus (Xth CN)
- Referred pain from C-spine through C2 and C3 spinal nerves

11.7 Epistaxis

Epistaxis is acute bleeding from the nostril, nasal cavity or nasopharynx. It is very common but only a tiny number of cases need specialist attention. There are two peaks in age distribution (2–10 years and 50–80 years) and there is an equal sex distribution.

Aetiology

Aetiology varies with age. Children tend to pick their nose and place foreign bodies up it. Adult epistaxis is more likely to be idiopathic or traumatic. Hypertension and neoplasia are more common in older people.

Local

- Idiopathic (80%)
- Trauma (nasal fracture, nose picking)
- Inflammatory/infective (rhinitis, sinusitis, vestibulitis)
- Iatrogenic
- Neoplasia (juvenile fibroangioma in young males)
- Desiccation (high altitude, air conditioning)

Systemic

- Drugs (e.g. warfarin)
- Hypertension
- Coagulopathy (e.g. haemophilia)
- Congenital—familial haemorrhagic telangiectasia (Osler–Rendu–Weber syndrome)

Pathophysiology

Most bleeds (90%) come from Little's area on the anterior nasal septum where there is a convergence of the anterior ethmoidal, superior labial, sphenopalatine, and greater palatine arteries (Kiesselbach's plexus). Posterior bleeding is more common in the elderly.

Clinical assessment

Initial approach follows ABC guidelines. If there has been significant bleeding, the patient may be shocked and require resuscitation.

History

- Onset, severity, laterality, frequency of bleeding
- Ask about methods used to control bleeding (often inadequate)
- Ask about risk factors (hypertension, drugs, liver disease)

Examination

- Wear gloves, apron and eye protection and have suction ready
- Anterior rhinoscopy
- Establish site of bleeding (anterior or posterior)
- Head and neck examination

Investigations

Blood tests are not routinely required. Patients with a significant bleed or underlying pathology require FBC, U+Es, LFTs, clotting, and G+S or cross-match.

Management

The aim is to identify and treat the cause of the bleeding. Patients with significant bleeding will require resuscitation. Packing the nose is unpleasant and often poorly tolerated. Calm reassurance is usually sufficient but occasionally sedation is required.

Conservative

After ABC, follow the outline below depending on where the source of the bleeding is and how persistent it is.

Simple measures

- Firm pressure of the nostrils between thumb and index finger for at least 10 min
- Ice pack on bridge of nose +/- sucking ice cube

Anterior nasal packing

- Remove blood clot with Luc's forceps or suctioning
- Spray mucosa with local anaesthetic
- Cauterize bleeding point with silver nitrate stick or electro-cautery. Do not cauterize both sides of septum as there is a risk of necrosis and septal perforation
- Use an inflatable nasal tampon to pack nose (e.g. Rapid Rhino®)
- Formal packing may be required if the tampon fails. Use bismuth iodoform paste-impregnated (BIPP) ribbon gauze
- Packing both sides increases the tamponade pressure
- Start broad spectrum antibiotics if packing for >48 h

Posterior nasal packing

- Insert a Foley catheter so that the balloon is in the posterior nasal space and inflate with 10 mL of air. To avoid airway obstruction, ensure the catheter is pulled forward and secured exteriorly
- Pack anterior nasal space and start broad spectrum antibiotics

Operative

In the rare instances that bleeding persists despite repeated packing, the patient needs examination under general anaesthesia.

- Submucosal resection of nasal septum (SMR) may be required to improve access for examination, cautery or packing of the nasal cavity
- General diathermy of nasal mucosa
- Arterial ligation is considered if EUA with diathermy and packing is unsuccessful. There are two main approaches:
- endoscopic endonasal ligation of the sphenopalatine artery
- external medial orbital incision to ligate the anterior ethmoidal artery
- Angiography and embolization is rarely used

Complications and prognosis

Complications of nasal packing include rhinosinusitis, Eustachian tube dysfunction, mucosal pressure necrosis, and toxic shock syndrome.

On discharge, give advice on epistaxis prevention and how to manage a recurrence. Arrange follow-up for patients following a severe bleed as they may require further investigation (CT/MRI head) to exclude neoplasia.

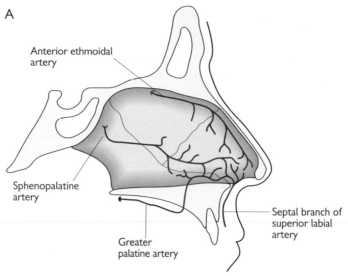

A

Anterior ethmoidal
artery

Sphenopalatine
artery

Greater
palatine artery

Septal branch of
superior labial
artery

Fig 11.10 Diagram of the arterial anatomy of the nose. Reproduced with kind permission from *The Oxford Handbook of Ear, Nose, and Throat.*

Allergic rhinitis

Allergic rhinitis is inflammation of the mucosal lining of the nose caused by an IgE-mediated, type 1 hypersensitivity reaction to an allergen. Common allergens include pollen and the house dust mite (*Dermatophagoides pteronyssinus*). Approximately 25% of the population suffers from allergic rhinitis.

Clinical assessment

In general, rhinitis can be diagnosed if two out of three of nasal congestion, rhinorrhoea, and sneezing are present for more than 1 hour every day for more than 2 weeks.

Patients may also complain of itching of the nasal cavity, mild facial pain, and hyposmia. Anterior rhinoscopy reveals inflamed nasal mucosa.

Investigations

- Skin prick tests or RAST—identify common airborne allergens (grass, pollen, house dust mite, cat and dog dander, feathers, and fungal spores)
- Bloods—FBC, ESR, U+Es, ANCA, RAST
- Sinus CT scan is indicated if there is coexisting sinus disease
- Saccharin clearance test or nasal biopsy to assess mucociliary dyskinesia

Management

Medical management includes allergen avoidance, saline nasal douches, and intranasal preparations: steroids, sodium chromoglycate, ipratropium bromide, and oral antihistamines.

Operative management includes inferior turbinate surgery and nasal septal or sinus surgery (if associated pathology).

Nasal polyps

Nasal polyps are benign, progressive inflammation and oedema of the mucosa of the nose and sinuses that eventually prolapse into the nasal cavity.

They are of unknown aetiology but associations include Samter's triad (nasal polyps, aspirin intolerance, and asthma) and ciliary immotility syndromes (cystic fibrosis, Kartagener's syndrome).

Clinical assessment

Patients present with nasal obstruction, rhinorrhoea, and/or postnasal drip, anosmia. On anterior rhinoscopy polyps appear as grey or yellowish masses in the nasal cavities. Gross polyposis can cause broadening of the nasal bridge.

Investigations

- See investigations for allergic rhinitis
- CT scan of paranasal sinuses if endoscopic sinus surgery or biopsy is planned
- Unilateral nasal polyps should be considered neoplastic until proven otherwise and should be biopsied

Management

Medical management is similar to that for allergic rhinitis and includes intranasal steroids and oral steroids for gross polyposis. Large nasal polyps or patients that fail medical treatment require endoscopic polypectomy. There is a high recurrence rate.

Nasal granulomas

This is an unusual condition caused by a variety of diseases that form granulomas, such as Wegener's granulomatosis, sarcoidosis, TB, and syphilis.

Clinical assessment

Anterior rhinoscopy reveals nasal crusting, granulations, ulceration, and septal perforation. There may also be systemic symptoms (cough, visual disturbance, weight loss, skin lesions), but this may take some time to develop after the sinonasal symptoms.

Investigations

- Biopsy of nasal granuloma
- Blood tests—FBC, ESR, U+Es, ANCA, ACE levels, TPA/VDRL
- Urinalysis ± renal biopsy
- Plain chest radiograph or chest CT scan
- Sinus CT scan to assess bone destruction

Management

Medical management is related to the long-term treatment of the underlying condition; this may include long-term systemic steroids and immunosuppressants (methotrexate or azathioprine).

Septal perforation

The causes of septal perforation include trauma (nose picking, surgery, cautery, and traumatic injury); chemicals (cocaine, chrome industry); granulomatous diseases; malignant neoplasia (SCC, BCC, T cell lymphoma).

Clinically they are asymptomatic or can cause epistaxis or whistling (if small perforation). Investigations are performed to exclude granulomatous disease and neoplasia with biopsy of the perforation edge.

Most asymptomatic septal perforations require no treatment. If symptomatic, use saline nasal douches or glucose in glycerine drops to prevent crusting, or close the perforation with a septal button or a formal surgical procedure.

Snoring and sleep apnoea

Snoring is a noise generated during sleep as a consequence of partial upper airway obstruction. It affects 25% of the male and 10% of the female population.

Apnoea is the cessation of airflow in the upper airway for at least 10 s and is a result of complete obstruction. Obstructive sleep apnoea (OSA) is present in ~6% of men.

Aetiology

- Nose and postnasal space—nasal polyps, deviated septum turbinate hypertrophy, adenoidal hypertrophy, choanal atresia, and nasal or nasopharyngeal tumours
- Mouth and oropharynx—tonsillar hypertrophy, long soft palate and uvula, oropharyngeal tumours, macroglossia or micrognathia
- Risk factors include—male sex, collar size >17, high BMI, family history, sedatives, smoking, alcohol intake, hypothyroidism, acromegaly, Marfan's, Down's syndrome, and muscular dystrophy

Pathophysiology

Narrowing of the airway causes acceleration of the airflow (Venturi effect), which will create negative pressure and a vacuum effect (Bernoulli), producing a vibration of the soft palate and pharyngeal wall, thus snoring. The worse the narrowing effect, the more severe the symptoms until reaching a critical point where there is collapse of the airway and apnoea.

Nasal obstruction increases inspiratory negative pressure and this compromises the airway.

Clinical assessment

Patients (and their partners) complain of day time somnolence and personality changes. Assessment includes full ENT and cardiovascular examinations. This includes nasopharyngoscopy to assess airway collapse (Müller manoeuvre).

Investigations

- Body mass index
- Epworth questionnaire (to assess daily somnolence at various activities and times of the day. Significant score 10/24)
- Bloods—FBC, TFT
- Plain chest radiograph and ECG to assess cor pulmonale in severe OSA
- Sleep study (polysomnography)
- OSA is diagnosed if there are more than 30 episodes of apnoea in 7 h of sleep or if the apnoea index (AI; number of periods of apnoea per hour) is greater than five
- If AI >20 the OSA is severe and needs treatment
- Imaging—CT, MRI, cephalometry (optional)

Management

Initial advice is to lose weight and avoid sedatives, smoking, and alcohol. Nasal obstruction needs to be addressed in individual cases (choanal atresia, polyps).

Mandibular advancement prosthesis can be helpful for significant tongue base narrowing for both simple snoring and OSA. Continuous positive airway pressure is the gold standard treatment for OSA.

Adenotonsillectomy is indicated in children with adenotonsillar hypertrophy.

There is a wide range of surgical procedures aimed to achieve stiffening or shortening of the soft palate to increase the airway (palatoplasty); however, the long-term results are discouraging.

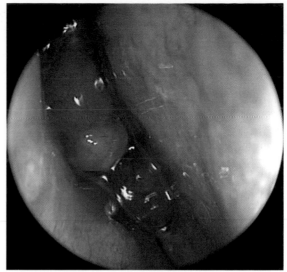

Fig 11.11 Endoscopic view of nasal polyps.

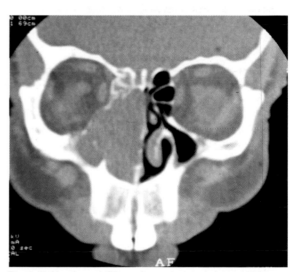

Fig 11.12 Unenhanced CT scan (coronal section) showing obliteration of the air space in the right nasal cavity and sinuses due to unilateral nasal polyps.

Laryngotracheobronchitis

Laryngotracheobronchitis (croup) is inflammation of the larynx, trachea, and bronchi. It is common in infants 3 months to 5 years old. It is most commonly caused by parainfluenza virus type 1; others include parainfluenza type 3, echovirus, and respiratory syncytial virus.

Clinical assessment

Viral infection causes local inflammation of the upper respiratory tract. With time, the subglottic area becomes oedematous and this causes stridor. It is crucial that acute epiglottitis is not missed (see below).

Management

Do not give sedatives or opiates as they will depress respiratory effort, and beware of bronchodilators and expectorants that might irritate the airway.

- Mild—paracetamol, humidified air
- Moderate—add nebulized budesonide 2 mg
- Severe—add systemic steroids and nebulized adrenaline. Child requires admission and, if there is severe respiratory distress with airways compromise, intubation and ITU may be required.

Table 11.1 Characteristics of croup and acute epiglottitis

Croup	Acute epiglottitis
History	
Onset over a couple of days	Rapid onset
Coryzal symptoms	Sore throat
Characteristic 'sea lion' barking cough	Dysarthria
Symptoms worse at night	Dysphagia (with drooling)
	Respiratory distress
Examination	
Fever	High fever
Stridor	Stridor
Respiratory distress	Drooling saliva

Acute epiglottitis

Epiglottitis is acute inflammation of the larynx, especially the epiglottis. It is uncommon and most prevalent in the winter. It is usually a bacterial infection caused by *Haemophilus influenzae* type B (HIB). The decreasing incidence may be related to the conjugated HIB vaccine given to 2-month-old infants.

Infection causes local inflammation of the epiglottis and supraglottis (aryepiglottic folds, false cords, and arytenoids). The associated oedema rapidly leads to obstruction of the airway and respiratory distress.

Clinical assessment

Initial approach is ABC. Emergency intubation is often required and should not be delayed by investigations. Do not place anything in the mouth to examine the throat or distress the child as this may precipitate complete airway obstruction. Investigations include throat swabs, bloods (FBC), and blood cultures.

Management

The first aim is to secure the airway. Keep the child sitting up in a quiet area with induction facilities. Emergency intubation by an experienced paediatric anaesthetist or rarely a tracheostomy may be indicated. Start IV antibiotics, fluid replacement, and systemic steroids.

There is usually a prompt response to treatment and the child is often extubated within 48 h of admission.

Laryngomalacia

Laryngomalacia is the commonest cause of stridor in neonates and early infancy. The epiglottis has a tubular (omega-shape) appearance and also the prominent mucosa of the arytenoid cartilages collapse into the airway during inspiration.

Clinically there is an intermittent and positional stridor from the age of 2–6 weeks, which is worse when supine, agitated, crying or feeding. Tracheal tug, costal recession, and failure to thrive can also be present. Investigations include flexible endoscopy or rigid microlaryngoscopy and bronchoscopy.

Mild cases improve in 6–9 months. Severe cases (respiratory distress and failure to thrive) will require aryepiglottoplasty (incision of aryepiglottic folds to allow a larger epiglottic inlet to the airway).

Vocal cord paralysis

Unilateral vocal cord paralysis can be congenital or acquired owing to birth trauma or cardiothoracic surgery (ligation of patent ductus arteriosus).

The stridor is biphasic and there is also a weak cry. Bilateral palsy is more severe and is associated with neurological abnormalities.

Subglottic stenosis

Narrowing of the airway in the subglottic region can be congenital or acquired following prolonged or repeated endotracheal intubation.

It presents with biphasic stridor, respiratory distress, and failure to thrive. Asthma is the main differential diagnosis although the stridor has no inspiratory phase, just an expiratory wheeze. Both can cause exercise-induced respiratory distress. Mild symptoms are treated conservatively. Severe stenosis requires surgical reconstruction.

Foreign bodies

A foreign body (FB) can be organic or inorganic. The upper respiratory tract is a common site (nose, pharynx, trachea, and bronchi).

Children often place objects into their ears or nose that they ought not to. Adults typically present complaining of having something stuck in their throat after swallowing a fish bone or large bolus of food which, if left, can cause local inflammation and infection.

Inhaled objects that occlude the larynx or trachea will cause airway obstruction. Those that pass the carina into a main bronchus (right>left) may cause respiratory symptoms.

Clinical assessment

- Nasal FB—unilateral smelly nasal discharge, bleeding, blocked nose
- Inhaled FB—cough, pain, and difficulty in breathing. Severity of respiratory symptoms will depend on level and degree of obstruction

- Swallowed FB—pain on deep palpation of the neck suggests FB. Indirect laryngoscopy can be used to visualize the pharynx
- Soft tissue neck radiograph will show a radio-opaque FB, e.g. watch battery
- Chest radiograph—complete occlusion of a main bronchus will cause ipsilateral lung collapse; partial obstruction may cause emphysema

Management

Conservative

- **Nose**—LA spray then use a right-angle hook, suction or forced exhalation
- **Pharynx**—if a FB is suspected but not detected, admission for observation and a soft diet. Buscopan and analgesia causes muscle relaxation and the object will often pass. If the dysphagia worsens, direct visualization and removal is required
- **Trachea**—prophylactic antibiotics for aspiration pneumonia

Operative

An oesophageal or bronchial FB identified on a plain radiograph needs urgent removal under GA.

◎ Stertor and stridor

Stertor is a noise caused by obstruction above the larynx. Causes include acute tonsillitis, OSA, choanal atresia, craniofacial abnormalities (Crouzon's, Treacher–Collins), macroglossia, and lingual thyroid.

Stridor is a noise during breathing caused by obstruction at the level of the larynx (supraglottis, glottis, or subglottis). Causes include laryngomalacia, epiglottitis, vocal cord pathology, subglottic stenosis, and laryngeal foreign body.

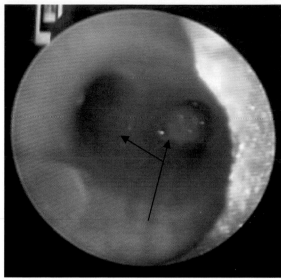

Fig 11.13 Paediatric bronchoscopy showing an inhaled foreign body (peanut) sitting in the right main bronchus. Foreign bodies tend to enter the right main bronchus in preference to the left as it divides from the trachea at less of an angle.

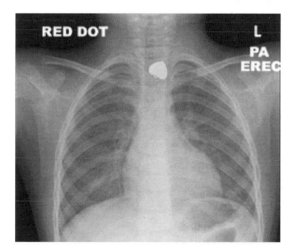

Fig 11.14 Plain chest radiograph showing a swallowed foreign body. The heart-shaped pendant is wider than the trachea which remains in its anatomical position and appears unobstructed. The lung fields are normal.

11.10 Adenoids and tonsils

The tonsilar tissue starts to develop in the 14th week of gestation. Mononuclear cells invade the mucosa of the tonsillar fossa, condense, and differentiate into five main areas of pharyngeal lymphoid tissue called Waldeyer's ring.

Tonsillitis

Tonsillitis is inflammation of the pharyngeal tonsils. It can be acute, recurrent acute, or chronic.

Aetiology

Inflammation of the tonsils is usually either viral or bacterial. β-Haemolytic streptococci and staphylococci are the most common bacteria. Viruses include rhinovirus, adenovirus, and Epstein–Barr.

Pathophysiology

There are two main types of acute tonsillitis which are both occasionally complicated by a peritonsillar abscess (quinsy). The first is parenchymatous, in which the whole tonsil is erythematous and swollen; the second is follicular, in which the tonsillar crypts are filled with infected fibrin and have a patchy appearance.

Clinical assessment

History

- Fever and malaise
- Sore throat
- Otalgia (earache)
- Odynophagia (pain on swallowing)
- Quinsy—severe pain, dysphagia and trismus (restricted jaw opening), and muffled voice

Examination

- Red, enlarged tonsils with pus
- Quinsy—unilateral peritonsillar swelling displacing the uvula to the contralateral side. Bilateral quinsies are very rare
- Neck lymphadenopathy

Investigations

- Swab each tonsil for MC+S
- Bloods—FBC (WCC ↑), CRP ↑
- Monospot test (Paul–Bunnell test) for infectious mononucleosis

Management

Initial management is conservative. Tonsillectomy is considered after the acute period if indicated (see box).

Conservative

- Oral or intravenous fluids
- Analgesia
- Soluble aspirin gargling (not in children—risk of Reye's syndrome)
- Penicillin V is the first line antibiotic. Ampicillin is avoided as those patients who actually have glandular fever have a risk of a hypersensitivity reaction causing a generalized maculopapular rash
- A quinsy should be incised and drained

Tonsillectomy

Absolute indications

- Airway obstruction (e.g. obstructive sleep apnoea syndrome)
- Suspected neoplasm

Relative indications

- Following peritonsillar abscess (quinsy)
- Recurrent tonsillitis (four or five episodes/year for at least 2 years) or chronic tonsillitis

Contraindications

- Tonsillitis or upper respiratory tract infection within 2 weeks of the operation date
- Coagulopathy
- Cleft palate is a contraindication to adenoidectomy

Complications and prognosis

During the acute phase of tonsillitis, complications include respiratory obstruction caused by severe swelling, abscess formation, and sepsis. Very rarely, rheumatic fever or glomerulonephritis develops following a streptococcal tonsillitis.

Adenoids

The adenoids are a condensation of lymphoid tissue in the posterior wall of the nasopharynx and form part of Waldeyer's ring, together with the palatine and lingual tonsils. The Eustachian tubes open immediately lateral to the adenoids, thus adenoid enlargement owing to repeated URTI may cause nasal obstruction as well as serous otitis media.

Clinical assessment

Enlarged adenoids can cause nasal and Eustachian tube obstruction with resultant hyponasal voice, mouth breathing, snoring, OSA, and hearing loss. Examination findings include:

- reduced or absent flow in nasal airway
- large adenoidal mass seen with mirror or endoscope
- otoscopic findings of serous otitis media

Investigations

Lateral neck soft tissue radiograph can help to assess the adenoidal shadow if difficult to visualize adenoids directly.

Management

Adenoidectomy (under GA) by curettage or suction diathermy.

Complications and prognosis

Haemorrhage is less common than in tonsillectomy. Palatal incompetence and nasal regurgitation and hypernasal speech. The operation is contraindicated in cleft or submucous cleft palate.

⊕ Drainage of pertionsillar abscess (quinsy)

This procedure can be performed under local anaesthetic by spraying the oropharynx with 1–2% xylocaine.

- The patient is in a sitting position with the mouth opened and instructed not to swallow the contents of the abscess
- The tongue is depressed and the abscess is incised with a No. 11 blade at the point of maximal fluctuation
- The incision is enlarged with an artery forceps or similar (nasal packing forceps) and a microbiology swab is taken. Recurrence is likely if the incision is not adequately enlarged as this will heal very quickly
- Alternatively, the quinsy can be aspirated with a syringe and 21G needle first and drained as above if it re-accumulates

→ **Extra**

National Prospective Tonsillectomy Audit

This audit collected information on tonsillectomies performed in England and Northern Ireland from July 2003 until September 2004. It aimed to investigate the occurrence of haemorrhage and other complications in the first 28 days following tonsillectomy.

Findings

- Adults had a higher haemorrhage rate than children and there was no sex bias
- Overall risk of haemorrhage was related to surgical technique
- A 'hot' technique for both dissection and haemostasis (diathermy or coblation) increased risk of haemorrhage threefold

Recommendations

- No advantage to using monopolar diathermy over other methods
- Trainees should become competent in using cold steel dissection and haemostasis using ties
- Care should be taken to ensure the correct settings when using diathermy machines
- Further research is required into the influence of diathermy and other hot techniques in wound healing and complications associated with the tonsillar bed

New tonsillectomy techniques

- Cold ablation (coblation) is a modified laser that generates lower tissue temperature than diathermy
- Laser (CO_2) used mainly for excision of malignant tonsillar tumours
- Harmonic scalpel is an ultrasonic dissection and haemostasis device

References

National Prospective Tonsillectomy Audit. Tonsillectomy technique as a risk factor for postoperative haemorrhage. *Lancet* 2004; **364:** 697–702

➕ **Adenotonsillectomy**

Procedure

- Laryngeal mask airway is usually used rather than endotracheal intubation
- Patient supine with roll under shoulders and neck extended
- Mouth gag placed
- Adenoidectomy is performed first by either 'cold' curettage or 'hot' suction diathermy. Then pack the posterior nasal space
- Blunt dissection with cold steel
- Incision made anterior pillar
- Tonsil shelled out
- Haemostasis with bipolar diathermy
- Occasional need for tonsillar ties
- Pack one side and then move to the other
- Remove the posterior nasal space, pack and suction any remaining blood clot to avoid any subsequent airway obstruction ('Coroner's clot')

Complications

Bleeding is the main complication of tonsillectomy (2%). It can be primary (intraoperative), reactive (<24 h) or secondary (5–10 days). Secondary haemorrhage is usually due to infection. Patients require admission and antibiotics and occasionally an emergency return to theatre.

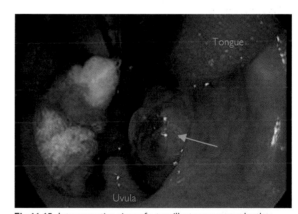

Fig 11.15 Intraoperative view of a tonsillectomy as seen by the operating surgeon. The left tonsil has been removed and the tonsillar fossa packed. The enlarged right tonsil (arrow) is next to be removed.

11.11 Paranasal sinuses

Acute sinusitis

Sinusitis is inflammation of the mucosal lining of the facial sinuses (acute <4 weeks, subacute 4–12 weeks, and chronic >12 weeks). Acute sinusitis is a common condition, with up to 5% of adults diagnosed with it annually.

Aetiology

A viral upper respiratory tract infection is usually the trigger for a superimposed bacterial infection. Around 0.5% of common colds are complicated by acute bacterial sinusitis.

Other predisposing factors include physical obstruction of the sinus ostia (polyps, tumours) and systemic disorders that reduce mucociliary clearance (cystic fibrosis, Kartagener syndrome).

Pathophysiology

The paranasal sinuses (frontal, maxillary, sphenoid, anterior, and posterior ethmoidal air cells) drain into the nasal cavity. They are lined with ciliated pseudostratified columnar epithelium interspersed with mucus-secreting goblet cells. The epithelium sweeps the mucus towards the sinus ostia (opening).

Viral infection and excess mucus secretion depresses their function. Obstruction of the sinus openings also leads to build up of mucus. The mucus becomes secondarily infected (*Streptococcus pneumoniae*, *Haemophilus influenzae*), leading to acute sinusitis. Maxillary sinus is most commonly affected.

Clinical assessment

History

- Upper respiratory tract symptoms
- Foul rhinorrhoea (nasal discharge)
- Hyposmia (reduced sense of smell)
- Headache and facial pain, and pressure worse when bending forward

Examination

- Malaise and mild fever
- Tenderness on palpation over the affected sinuses
- Anterior rhinoscopy may reveal red, oedematous nasal mucosa
- Nasal endoscopy will show congested middle meatus with or without mucopus

Investigations

- Sinus swab for microbiology. Nasal swab cultures do not correlate with sinus culture results
- Imaging is not required in the diagnosis and management of uncomplicated acute sinusitis

Management

The aim is to provide symptomatic relief, limit the course of the infection, and prevent complications. Conservative treatment is bed rest and analgesia. Nasal decongestants, antihistamines, and intranasal steroids are of unproven benefit. Antibiotics do not appear to shorten the disease course apart from bacteriologically confirmed acute sinusitis.

Functional endoscopic sinus surgery (FESS) is reserved for chronic disease or to manage complications.

Complications and prognosis

Over 60% of people have spontaneous resolution of symptoms without treatment. A small number go on to develop chronic sinusitis or a complication such as orbital cellulitis.

Chronic sinusitis

Chronic sinusitis is prolonged inflammation and/or infection of one or more of the facial sinuses lasting longer than 12 weeks. It is a common chronic condition.

Aetiology

Most cases follow on from acute sinusitis. However, it can have a much more insidious course and the bacterial species often differ from those seen in acute sinusitis (*Staphylococcus aureus* and mixed bacterial species). *Aspergillus fumigatus* is the commonest fungus involved in allergic fungal sinusitis.

Risk factors

- Recurrent upper respiratory tract infections
- Allergic rhinitis
- Nasal or sinus obstruction (e.g. nasal polyps and septal or uncinate process deviation)
- Immunosuppression (fungal infection)
- Primary ciliary dyskinesia
- Smoking and environmental pollution
- Gastrointestinal reflux disease

Pathophysiology

There is the same underlying process as acute sinusitis, although as time passes there may be permanent damage to the cilia.

Clinical assessment

Symptoms of chronic sinusitis are similar to acute sinusitis. They include postnasal drip, headache, and foul taste in the mouth. There is often percussion tenderness over the affected sinus.

Investigations

- Sinus swab for microbiology obtained at endoscopy
- Allergy testing if this is thought to be the underlying process
- Nasal endoscopy
- Plain radiographs have been superseded by screening CT
- CT scan of sinuses is used to assess chronic sinusitis not responding to medical therapy and to plan any operative procedure
- Sinus MRI is used in patients with fungal infection or with a suspected malignant tumour to assess intracranial or intraorbital extension

Management

Conservative

Initial approach is with prolonged broad spectrum antibiotics and intranasal steroids, along with treatment for any underlying cause, e.g. nasal polyps or allergic rhinitis.

Operative

Operative management is reserved for patients who have not responded to maximal medical therapy. Open sinus surgery has largely been superseded by FESS.

Complications and prognosis

Periorbital cellulitis and orbital abscess usually result from direct spread from the ethmoid sinuses. The eye may become displaced and proptosed. Tension on the optic nerve can lead to visual impairment. Osteomyelitis of the maxilla is rare.

Intracranial extension most commonly causes meningitis, but can also lead to encephalitis, intracranial abscess, and carvernous sinus thrombosis.

Mucocele is an accumulation of sterile pus and may occur if the sinus ostium becomes permanently blocked.

> ## ⊕ Functional endoscopic sinus surgery
>
> A preoperative CT scan is mandatory to show the anatomical landmarks. General anaesthesia is preferable, although can be done under local.
>
> *Indications*
> - Sinus disease (acute and chronic sinusitis)
> - Nasal polyps
> - Sphenopalatine ligation to control epistaxis
> - Orbital decompression
> - Dacryocystorhinotomy for nasolacrimal duct obstruction
>
> *Procedure*
> - Patient supine with head ring and head elevation
> - Nasal mucosa is prepared with topical anaesthetic and vasoconstrictor solution
> - Uncinate process of the ethmoid bone is excised. Care taken not to breach the medial orbital wall
> - Maxillary ostium widened (antrostomy)
> - Anterior and posterior ethmoidal cells are uncapped until healthy mucosa is reached
> - If disease extends to frontal and sphenoid sinuses, their drainage ostia are also widened
> - No packing needed if minimal oozing
> - Postoperative care includes saline nasal douches, intranasal steroids, systemic antibiotics, and regular nasal toilet
>
> *Complications*
>
> | *Intraoperative and early* | *Intermediate and late* |
> | --- | --- |
> | - Bleeding—epistaxis | - Intranasal adhesions |
> | - CSF leak | - Recurrent disease |
> | - Injury to orbit, internal carotid and optic nerve | - Intracranial infection |

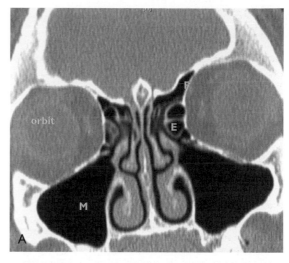

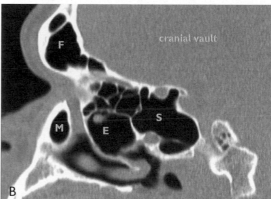

Fig 11.16 Sinus CT scan. A Coronal section; and A sagittal section showing normal sinus anatomy: maxillary (M), frontal (F), ethmoidal (E), sphenoidal (S).

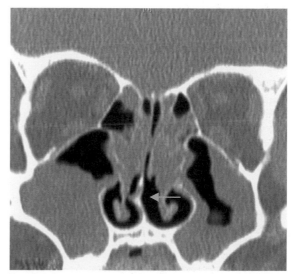

Fig 11.17 Sinus CT scan (coronal section) showing chronic sinusitis secondary to nasal polyps (compare with Fig. 11.12). There is moderately extensive mucosal thickening in the maxillary, ethmoid, and sphenoid sinuses bilaterally. The nasal septum is displaced to the right (arrow). Both osteomeatal complexes are occluded.

There are three main paired salivary glands (parotid, submandibular, and sublingual) and many hundreds of minor salivary glands scattered throughout the upper aerodigestive tract. The salivary glands have multiple functions, including production of saliva to lubricate the oral cavity and begin the enzymatic degradation of food. Salivary flow is primarily regulated by the parasympathetic nervous system.

The parotid is a serous gland contained within the parotid sheath. It has two lobes, superficial and deep in relation to the facial nerve and the retromandibular vein. The parotid duct drains in the buccal mucosa opposite the second upper molar tooth.

The submandibular gland is both serous and mucous. It also has superficial and deep parts divided by an anterior groove for mylohyoid muscle. The mandibular branch of the facial nerve is superficial to the gland, the hypoglossal and lingual nerves lie medial to the deep portion, and facial vessels groove the posterior aspect of the gland. The duct of the gland runs along the floor of the mouth and opens at the side of the frenulum of the tongue (one at either side).

The sublingual gland is mucus-secreting. It lies in the submental area and its duct opens into the submandibular gland duct.

Sialolithiasis

Sialolithiasis is the formation of calculi in a salivary gland or its duct system. Over 80% occurs in the submandibular gland and Wharton's duct.

Prolonged dehydration leads the secretions to settle out from the saliva, forming calculi. These then occlude the duct. The gland swells as the saliva accumulates behind the stone.

Clinical assessment

Patients often complain of pain and swelling which is worse whilst eating. On examination there is a painful swollen gland and often a palpable stone in the floor of the mouth. Ask the patient to suck on a lemon and the gland should increase in size as saliva accumulates.

Investigations include a plain radiograph of the floor of the mouth (calculi are made from calcium and magnesium salts and so are radio-opaque), CT scan or sialogram.

Management

If the stones are close to the opening of the duct they can be milked out or the duct cannulated and dilated to facilitate removal. Deep intraparenchymal stones or multiple stones require the whole gland to be surgically removed. Sialolithiasis can lead to sialoadenitis.

Sialoadenitis

Sialoadenitis is inflammation of a salivary gland. Acute sialoadenitis is usually due to viral or bacterial infection. The most common viral infection is mumps caused by paramyxovirus Other viral infections include Coxsackie, echovirus, and HIV. Acute bacterial infections usually occur in dehydrated patients, often with poor oral hygiene. The most common organism is *Staphylococcus aureus*; other organisms include *Streptococcus* spp., *Haemophilus influenzae*, and anaerobes.

Clinical assessment

The history should cover onset and duration of symptoms, recent dental work, and immunization history. The ductal opening of the gland should be inspected for pus and the gland palpated for stones.

Acute infection causes swelling, redness, and pain in the region of the affected gland. Mumps is characterized by bilateral parotid swelling, malaise, and trismus.

Management

Viral infection is usually self-limiting. Acute bacterial infections are managed with hydration and oral or IV antibiotics. Any pus should be bimanually milked from the gland and calculi can be managed as earlier described.

Chronic sialoadenitis can develop if there is a failure of salivary flow homeostasis. Treatment consists of massage and hydration. In refractory cases, the gland may have to be surgically removed.

Sialectasis

Sialectasis is dilatation of salivary duct systems. It is of unknown aetiology. The alveoli and parenchyma are progressively destroyed. There is duct stenosis and cyst formation. Occasionally calculi are found in the main ducts and patients give a history of gland swelling on eating.

Sialomegaly

Hyperplasia of the salivary glands can be caused by:
- drugs (thiouracil, OCP, coproxamol)
- metabolic (diabetes, myxoedema, gout, Cushing's, cirrhosis)

There are a number of conditions that may mimic a swollen parotid gland (pseudoparotomegaly). These include mandibular tumours, hypertrophic masseter, winged mandible, periauricular lymph node, dental cyst, lipoma, and sebaceous cyst.

Sjögren's syndrome

Sjögren's syndrome (Mikulicz disease) is an autoimmune disease characterized by periductal lymphocytes in multiple organs. Over 40% of patients have salivary gland involvement causing enlargement and reduced flow of saliva (dry mouth—xerostomia), and one in six patients will develop lymphoma. Clinically it can present with xerophthalmia, xerostomia, and a connective tissue disorder (SLE, scleroderma, polymyositis, primary biliary cirrhosis, etc.). Special blood tests include rheumatoid factor, antinuclear factor, electrophoresis, anti-Ro and La antibodies.

Salivary gland neoplasia

Salivary gland neoplasms constitute only 1% of all head and neck cancers. Eighty per cent of all tumours are in the parotid, 10% are in the submandibular gland, and 10% in the other minor glands. Eighty per cent of parotid tumours are benign and 80% of these are pleomorphic adenomas.

- Benign tumours of the glands include pleomorphic adenoma, Warthin's tumour (papillary cystadenoma lymphomatosum or adenolymphoma), and ductal papilloma

- Malignant tumours include adenoid cystic carcinoma (60% of minor salivary gland tumours), adenocarcinoma, SCC, mucoepidermoid carcinoma, and acinic cell carcinoma

Clinical assessment

- History of progression of mass
- Examine mass
- Oropharyngeal examination (assess deep lobe extension)
- Document facial nerve function. Pain or facial nerve paralysis suggests malignancy
- Head and neck examination (cervical lymphadenopathy)

Investigations

- FNAC is controversial as it often has a low sensitivity and specificity, especially in cystic lesions. There is no evidence that it causes seeding in parotid tumours
- MRI/CT scan is used to assess size and anatomical relations, e.g. facial nerve

Management

Parotidectomy is indicated for both benign and malignant tumours. Conservative parotidectomy aims to preserve the facial nerve with macroscopically normal tissue margins.

- Superficial parotidectomy (only the portion of the parotid lateral to VIIth nerve is removed)
- Total parotidectomy (includes gland and tumour deep to VIIth nerve)
- Radical parotidectomy involves sacrifice of the facial nerve

Adjuvant radiotherapy is given for malignant tumours if there is residual disease, adenoid cystic tumour, high grade or large (T3 and T4) tumours, and recurrence.

Complications and prognosis

Complications of parotidectomy include haemorrhage, facial nerve palsy (15% temporary, 1–2% permanent), salivary fistula, and Frey's syndrome (gustatory sweating). There is a low recurrence rate for pleomorphic adenomas. Malignant tumours have variable survival rate.

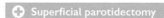

Superficial parotidectomy

Procedure

- Endotracheal intubation (with a short-acting muscle relaxant) with roll under the shoulders and head ring
- Facial nerve monitor is installed. Check patient is not paralysed
- 'Lazy S' cervicofacial incision starting in front of the tragus
- Subplatysmal flap elevated anteriorly until passed the anterior margin of the parotid lump (care with the VIIth branches as they become superficial anteriorly)
- Wide approach, exposing sternomastoid and posterior belly of digastric. Greater auricular nerve may have to be sacrificed if it restricts access
- Find VIIth nerve following the tragal pointer (1 cm anterior and inferior to it), the tympanomastoid groove, and/or the posterior belly of digastric and mastoid tip junction. If still not visible, a peripheral branch can be identified and tracked back to the main trunk of the nerve
- Once the nerve is identified, the part of the gland superficial is removed off the nerve until an adequate cuff of normal tissue surrounds the lump. Take care not incise the lump itself; this increases risk of recurrence
- Facial nerve is checked with stimulator before closure
- Haemostasis, drain, and closure in layers

Complications

Intraoperative and early	*Intermediate and late*
- Haemorrhage	- Frey's syndrome
- Facial nerve injury	- Great auricular nerve
- Salivary fistula	neuroma

Frey's syndrome occurs after 6 months. The main features are sweating and vasodilatation in the skin supplied by the auriculotemporal nerve. This is caused by misdirected re-innervation of the divided autonomic nerve fibres that previously supplied the parotid gland and skin.

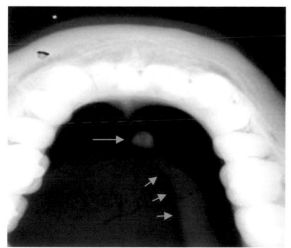

Fig 11.18 Intraoral occlusal radiograph after contrast into the submandibular duct (sialogram). There is a salivary calculus (arrow) obstructing Wharton's duct (small arrows).

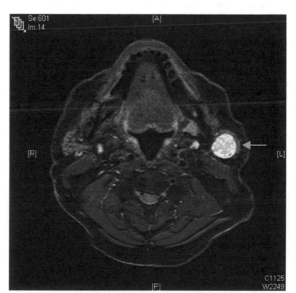

Fig 11.19 Left-sided parotid lump seen on STIR-MRI (short TI inversion recovery MRI scan) with gadolinium enhancement.

11.13 Neck lumps

Solitary lumps appearing in the neck are a common clinical problem. Their aetiology changes with age. The majority of lumps in children are benign and those in adults are malignant and frequently represent spread from ENT primary cancers, hence a full head and neck examination is essential.

Aetiology

Congenital
- Thyroglossal cyst
- Branchial cyst
- Cystic hygroma (lymphangioma)
- Dermoid cyst
- Thymic cyst
- Haemangioma (most have involuted in childhood)

Inflammatory
- Neck space infections and abscess
- Reactive lymphadenopathy
- Mycobacterial infection (TB and atypical)
- Sarcoidosis

Neoplastic
- Neoplastic lymphadenopathy (primary or secondary)
- Lipoma/liposarcoma
- Malignant neoplasia: lymphoma, rhabdomyosarcoma, medullary thyroid carcinoma, and salivary gland tumours

Vascular
- Carotid body tumour
- Carotid aneurysm

Endocrine
- Goitre or parathyroid lumps

Other
- Ranula
- Laryngocele

Clinical assessment

The neck can be anatomically divided into two main triangles (anterior and posterior) which can in turn be subdivided. The relative position of a lump will often give a clue to its aetiology.

History
- Lump—onset and duration, fluctuations in size, skin changes
- Associated symptoms—voice or speech changes, shortness of breath, stridor, cough, haemoptysis, dysphagia, and odynophagia
- Systemic symptoms—anorexia, weight loss, night sweats, fever, and malaise

Examination
- Full head and neck examination
- Examination of lump
- Systemic examinations guided by symptoms and differential diagnosis

Investigations
- Fine needle aspiration cytology and culture for TB
- Blood tests—FBC, CRP, infectious mononucleosis, ACE level, and toxoplasma serology
- MRI or CT scan of neck (MR angiogram or conventional angiography if vascular lump)
- Ultrasound for thyroid pathology
- Chest radiograph (exclude TB)
- Panendoscopy
- Excision biopsy

Thyroglossal cyst

In the fourth week of embryonic life a thickening develops at the base of the tongue (foramen caecum). This migrates down between the first and second branchial arches, divides, and becomes the thyroid gland.

In vivo lumps along this track are either thyroid tissue which failed to migrate fully (lingual thyroid) or a thyroglossal cyst. They are usually in the midline and at or below the level of the hyoid bone. They rise with tongue protrusion.

Cysts can become infected or form a sinus. In this instance they are best excised along with any remnants of the thyroglossal tract (Sistrunk's operation).

Branchial cysts and fistulae

These most commonly present in young adults. They present as a smooth swelling next to the anterior border of the sternocleidomastoid muscle at the junction of the upper and middle thirds. They commonly feel cystic but can be solid.

In adults the main differential diagnosis is metastatic squamous cell carcinoma, as both have squamous cells on FNAC. They must therefore be investigated and treated promptly, as described earlier with panendoscopy and excision biopsy.

Fistulae usually have an opening both in the pharynx just behind the tonsil and externally at the junction of the middle and lower of the sternocleidomastoid muscle.

They are cosmetically unattractive and are prone to infection so are normally excised.

Cystic hygroma

Cystic hygromas [G. moist tumour] are benign multiloculated cystic structures derived from lymphatics. Seventy-five per cent arise in the neck. They are usually large soft poorly circumscribed lesions and often present with stridor in the neonate or early infancy.

They can be extensive and MRI/CT is required to detail their relationship with other structures.

Surgical excision is usually required, although the use of sclerosing agents is an alternative. Recurrence rate is 10%.

Carotid body tumour

Carotid body tumours are also called paragangliomas or chemodectomas. They are rare tumours of the chemoreceptor cells in the carotid body. They present as a swelling at the bifurcation of the common carotid. A bruit may be heard over the lump. They are slow growing, but 10% can be bilateral, secretory of catecholamines, associated with phaeochromocytoma (in MEN syndrome), or even malignant.

Due to the risk of malignancy, they are usually resected.

⊕ Panendoscopy

Panendoscopy examines the whole upper aerodigestive tract.

Procedure

- Endotracheal intubation
- Patient supine with neck flexed and head extended to recreate the 'sniff the morning air position'. The upper teeth are protected with a gumshield to prevent damage
- The nasal cavity and postnasal space are visualized with a rigid nasendoscope after adequate decongestion
- The larynx, pharynx, and oesophagus are visualized using the relevant rigid endoscopes. If there is obvious laryngeal pathology, a suspension mechanism and a microscope can be used to obtain optimal biopsies
- When performing the oesophagoscopy the position of the neck may need changing to allow for an adequate and safe examination
- Finally, a rigid bronchoscope can be used to examine the tracheobronchial tree
- If the procedure is performed to investigate a suspected metastatic SCC in a neck node (on FNAC or clinical suspicion) and no obvious primary is found during the examination, then multiple 'blind' biopsies are taken from the nasopharynx, tonsil, tongue base and hypopharynx, as these are the most likely primary sites

Complications

Teeth damage, breathing difficulties (laryngeal spasm), and mucosal tear in pharynx or oesophagus which, if unrecognized or untreated, can lead to mediastinitis.

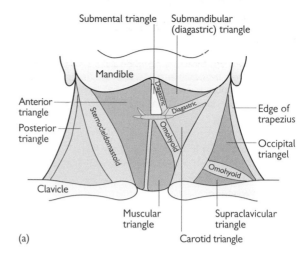

(a)

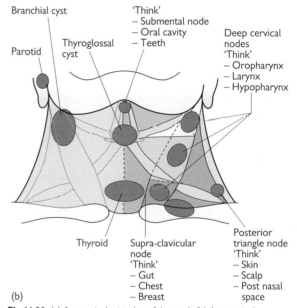

(b)

Fig 11.20 (a) Anatomical triangles of the neck (b) Anatomical positions of common neck lumps

Laryngeal cancer is the most common head and neck cancer after skin cancer. Incidence increases with age (peak 70+ years), and there is a male preponderance (M:F 5:1). It is most prevalent in areas with high rates of smoking (e.g. India and other developing countries).

Aetiology

Laryngeal carcinoma is almost exclusively found in smokers. Excess alcohol is an additional risk factor and appears to act synergistically with smoking.

Pathophysiology

The majority (70%) arise on the vocal cords (glottis), 20% in the supraglottis, and 10% in the subglottis. Tumour on the vocal cords quickly causes distortion of the voice and, as there is no lymphatic drainage, dissemination is slow. Squamous cell carcinomas account for 95% of all laryngeal neoplasms. Rare tumours include adenocarcinoma, adenoid cystic carcinoma, and lymphoma.

Clinical assessment

History

- Supraglottic—present late, with dysphagia, neck lump, otalgia, and muffled voice
- Glottic—present early with voice disturbance (hoarseness)
- Subglottic—rare, present with stridor
- General—weight loss and cachexia

Examination

- Head and neck examination (cervical lymphadenopathy)
- Flexible laryngoscopy to visualize the lesion and assess vocal cord function

Investigations

- FNAC of any cervical lymph neck nodes
- Direct laryngoscopy under GA to biopsy lesion and pandendoscopy
- Neck MRI or CT scan used for staging
- Plain chest radiograph—exclude primary bronchial carcinoma or metastatic disease. Chest CT scan may be indicated for further assessment

Staging

Clinical staging, particularly lymph node status, is the most reliable prognostic indicator, although there is still considerable variability. Supraglottic and subglottic tumours have good lymphatic drainage and often spread to local lymph nodes. The glottis has little drainage.

TNM classification of laryngeal cancer

Supraglottic tumour

T1	Limited to one site, normal vocal cord mobility
T2	Involving mucosa of more than one adjacent sub site of supraglottis or adjacent region outside the supraglottis, without fixation of the larynx
T3	Limited to larynx with fixed vocal cord or invades the postcricoid area, pre-epiglottic tissues or base of tongue
T4	Extension beyond the larynx

Glottic tumour

T1	T1a tumour limited to one cord T1b tumour involves both cords
T2	Extends to supraglottis and/or subglottis, or impaired cord mobility
T3	Limited to the larynx with fixed vocal cord
T4	Extends beyond the larynx

Subglottic tumour

T1	Limited to subglottis
T2	Extends to vocal cord(s), normal or impaired mobility
T3	Limited to the larynx with cord fixation
T4	Extends beyond the larynx

Regional lymph nodes

N1	Ipsilateral single node <3 cm
N2	Ipsilateral or bilateral nodes 3–6 cm
N2a	Single ipsilateral node 3–6 cm
N2b	Multiple ipsilateral nodes <6 cm
N2c	Bilateral or contralateral nodes <6 cm
N3	Any node >6 cm

Distant metastasis

MX	Cannot be assessed
M0	No distant metastasis
M1	Distant metastasis present

Management

Radiotherapy and/or surgical resection are the mainstay of therapy.

Glottic tumours

- T1/T2—radiotherapy or endoscopic resection
- T3—radiotherapy or laryngectomy depending on tumour volume. Patients with stridor need total laryngectomy. Adjuvant radiotherapy is indicated in high volume tumours
- T4—primary surgery (total laryngectomy) with radical neck dissection and adjuvant radiotherapy

Supraglottic and subglottic tumours

Small tumours are treated with radiotherapy or conservative resection. Larger tumours need laryngectomy and neck dissection.

Complications and prognosis

Complications include chondronecrosis (following chemotherapy and radiation therapy) and chronic aspiration following surgery. Prognosis of vocal cord tumours is good. Five-year survival is 95% for T1 and 40% for T4 tumours. Supraglottic tumours carry a slightly worse prognosis.

➕ Total laryngectomy

There are several types of laryngectomy, including partial, near total, and total. For large volume T3 and T4 glottic tumours the operation of choice is total laryngectomy. Neck dissection may also be carried out at the same time. Patients should have a preoperative speech therapy review and be made fully aware of their future with an end-tracheostomy with speech valve.

Procedure

- Endotracheal intubation
- Patient supine with roll under shoulders and head ring

- Skin infiltration and incision (Gluck–Sorenson 'U-shaped' flap)
- Elevation of subplatysmal flaps
- Exposure of the larynx which will be removed *en bloc* with strap muscles, hyoid bone, and one thyroid lobe (one should be preserved if possible)
- The larynx is mobilized by dissecting medial to sterno-mastoid. Identify and preserve the great vessels (carotid and jugular vein) and retract them laterally. The omohyoid muscle is divided (at the tendon), the middle thyroid vein is also divided to obtain access to the inferior thyroid pedicle; this is divided, and next is the superior thyroid pedicle (care in preserving the hypoglossal nerve)
- The same steps are performed on the opposite side, but preserving at least one thyroid pedicle (if possible both) and thyroid lobe
- The straps are divided inferiorly and superiorly. The muscular attachment above the hyoid bone and the bone is mobilized
- The trachea is exposed and divided (at the third ring), suturing the inferior margin of the stoma to the skin of the inferior aspect of the 'U-shaped' incision. A new endotracheal tube is inserted through the stoma
- The pharynx is then entered through the pre-epiglottic space (on the opposite side of the tumour). The larynx is released by dividing the constrictor muscles on the posterior border of the thyroid cartilage. The mucosa of the pharynx and postcricoid area are preserved to allow adequate reconstruction
- Once the larynx is removed, a cricopharyngeal myotomy is performed and a tracheo-oesophageal puncture (to accommodate a speaking valve) is carried out for post-laryngectomy voice rehabilitation
- The pharynx is then closed (without tension), a nasogastric tube is inserted and secured, haemostasis, drains inserted, superior skin flap is repositioned and sutured to the superior margin of the stoma

Postoperative care
- Antibiotic cover
- Nasogastric feeding commenced, with contrast swallow in 10 days to check for pharyngeal fistula
- Monitor serum calcium and thyroid function
- Speech rehabilitation

Complications

Intraoperative and early
- Haemorrhage
- Airway obstruction

Intermediate and late
- Wound infection
- Pharyngocutaneous fistula
- Stomal crusting
- Tumour recurrence

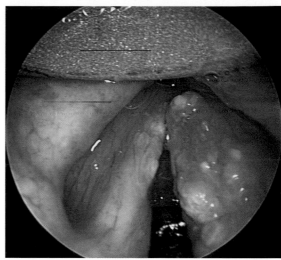
Fig 11.21 Endoscopic view of vocal cord squamous cell carcinoma.

11.15 Oropharyngeal, nasal, and nasopharyngeal cancer

Oropharyngeal neoplasia

Squamous cell carcinoma is the most common malignant tumour of the oropharynx. Adenocarcinomas and sarcomas are rare. Smoking and alcohol abuse are the main risk factors. SCC is most commonly found in the tonsil and tongue base, more rarely in the posterior pharyngeal wall, palate, and uvula.

Clinical assessment

Symptoms are variable and may include sore throat, mass sensation, dysphagia, otalgia, and bleeding. On examination there may be an obvious mass or ulceration in the oropharynx. The upper deep cervical lymph nodes are most commonly involved (jugulodigastric node).

Investigations

- Full ENT examination
- FNAC of neck nodes
- Panendoscopy and biopsy
- MRI or CT scan to assess local extension and metastatic disease

Management

T1 tumours may be treated with conservative surgery, i.e. tonsillectomy and radiotherapy or radiotherapy alone.

Larger tumours, especially T3–4, are treated with more radical surgery and chemoradiotherapy.

Commando operation involves dissection of the mandible, tongue, cheek, tonsil, and palate.

Five-year survival for tonsil tumours—stage 1, 90%; stage 4, 40%.

Nasopharyngeal neoplasia

Squamous cell carcinoma is a rare tumour in the western world, but of high incidence in South-East Asia and China. There are three factors involved in the development of nasopharyngeal carcinoma.

1. Genetic susceptibility (especially in the Cantonese)
2. Infection with Epstein–Barr virus
3. Environmental factor—diet rich in preserved salted fish (rich in nitrosamines)

Pathophysiology

The squamous epithelium of the nasopharynx undergoes metaplasia and malignant change. The tumour can be submucosal with deep invasion, causing pain in the side of the head (owing to invasion of the trigeminal nerve (Vth CN) at the foramen lacerum). Invasion of the Eustachian tube can cause unilateral conductive deafness and serous otitis media.

Clinical assessment

Symptoms include neck lump, epistaxis, nasal obstruction, and unilateral hearing loss. On examination there may be elevation of the ipsilateral soft palate, upper deep cervical lymphadenopathy, unilateral conductive deafness (serous otitis media), cranial nerve palsies, and a lump on direct vision with postnasal mirror or endoscope.

Investigations

- Nasopharyngoscopy
- Biopsy
- Epstein–Barr serology

- CT or MRI scan to assess local extension and metastatic disease

Management

- Radiotherapy or brachytherapy and chemotherapy
- Neck dissection for persistent lymphadenopathy
- 5-year survival is 35–60% with up to 80% with added chemotherapy

Nasal cavity neoplasia

Sinonasal tumours comprise approximately 10% of head and neck cancers. The commonest malignancies are SCC (70%), adenocarcinoma, and adenoid cystic carcinoma (10%). Others include lymphoma, anaplastic, olfactory neuroblastoma, and malignant melanomas. The common sites of origin are the ethmoid and maxillary sinuses and nasal cavity.

Risk factors include smoking, woodwork (hardwood dust for adenocarcinoma), work with nickel and chromium, and HPV infection.

Clinical assessment

Symptoms include nasal obstruction, epistaxis, facial pain, infraorbital anaesthesia, and visual disturbances. Trismus may occur with pterygopalatine fossa invasion. Signs include nasal mass, diplopia, and proptosis with orbital invasion.

Investigations

- Nasal endoscopy
- Biopsy of the mass
- FNAC of neck nodes
- CT or MRI scan to assess local extension and metastatic disease

Management

Management is usually a combination of surgery and radiotherapy. Surgical procedures include maxillectomy (partial or total), craniofacial resection, and orbital exenteration. Prognosis is poor.

⊕ Neck dissection

The lymphatic drainage of the upper aerodigestive tract is to the neck. It can be classified into seven levels (Fig 11.22).

Levels I–V are often involved in lymphatic regional spread of laryngeal and pharyngeal cancer. Levels VI and VII are mainly involved with thyroid cancer.

Radical neck dissection

Radical neck dissection consists of the excision of all lymphatic structures (levels I–V), as well as three non-lymphatic structures: spinal accessory nerve (XIth), sternomastoid muscle, and internal jugular vein.

Modified radical neck dissection

This comprises removal of all lymph node groups (I–V), with preservation of one or more non-lymphatic structures.
Type 1—accessory nerve preserved
Type 2—accessory nerve and jugular vein preserved
Type 3—accessory nerve and jugular vein and sternomastoid preserved

Selective neck dissection

One or more lymph node groups and all three non-lymphatic structures are preserved. It can be subdivided into:

- supraomohyoid: excision of all lymph nodes in levels I–III, the inferior limit being the superior belly of omohyoid muscle
- posterolateral: excision of levels II–V
- lateral: excision of levels II–IV

Extended radical neck dissection

As above plus excision of another lymph node group (levels VI and VII, retropharyngeal nodes, parotid nodes), or non-lymphatic structures (parotid, mandible, hypoglossal nerve, external carotid artery).

Procedure

- Endotracheal intubation with roll under shoulders, neck extended
- Skin incision from mastoid tip to chin two fingers below mandible (to prevent damage to mandibular branch of facial nerve) and inferiorly extended on a 'lazy S' shape (to prevent contracture) to the middle of clavicle
- Subplatysmal flaps are raised and accessory nerve is found at Erb's point (1 cm above the point where the great auricular nerve crosses the sternomastoid muscle on its way to the parotid gland)
- Sternomastoid muscle is then retracted and the deep investing fascia layer is dissected off the muscle in an anteroposterior direction
- The lymphatic group of the posterior triangle (level V) is now peeled off the cervical plexus, identifying the accessory nerve as it inserts into the trapezius muscle
- The dissection then continues anteriorly, dissecting the carotid sheath in the plane above the jugular vein and ligating the venous tributaries encountered during the dissection
- Lymph nodes in levels II, III, IV, and I are then removed. At level IV care must be taken to identify and either preserve or ligate the thoracic duct to prevent chylous leak
- Haemostasis, drains, and closure in layers

Complications

Intraoperative and early	Intermediate and late
• Haemorrhage	• Wound infection
• Airway obstruction	• Chylous fistula
• Facial oedema	• Seroma
• Raised ICP (ligation/ damage of one or both internal jugular veins)	• Carotid artery rupture
	• Fistula formation
• Pneumothorax	• Nerve damage
	• Tumour recurrence

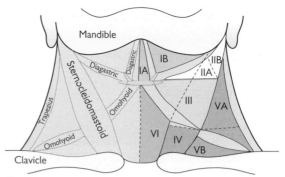

Fig 11.22 Head and neck lymphatic drainage.

- **I** Submental and submandibular
- **II** Upper jugular (above the level of carotid bifurca tion)
- **III** Middle jugular (from carotid bifurcation to upper part of cricoid)
- **IV** Lower jugular (from cricoid to clavicle)
- **V** Posterior triangle
- **VI** Anterior compartment (from hyoid to sternum, pretracheal and paratracheal)
- **VII** Upper anterior mediastinum

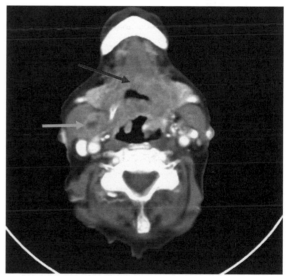

Fig 11.23 CT scan showing a base of tongue cancer (red arrow). There was circumferential soft tissue extending from the tongue base onto the lingual surface of the epiglottis and passing down the aryepiglottic folds, particularly on the right.

There are right-sided level 2/3 lymph nodes with central low attenuation suggestive of necrosis (green arrow).

11.16 Facial palsy

Facial palsy is the acute, unilateral paralysis of the muscles of facial expression. Lower motor neuron palsies affect the entire side of the face whereas upper motor neuron palsies spare the forehead muscles because of their bilateral innervation. This topic covers lower motor neuron facial palsy.

Aetiology

- Infection—ASOM, CSOM with cholesteatoma, Ramsay Hunt syndrome[2] (herpes zoster oticus)
- Trauma—base of skull fractures, facial injuries, barotraumas
- Iatrogenic—mastoid and parotid surgery
- Tumours—parotid tumours, acoustic neuroma
- Congenital—forceps delivery, Möbius syndrome (facial diplegia and other cranial nerve lesions)
- Systemic disease—diabetes mellitus, sarcoidosis, leukaemia, and multiple sclerosis

Pathophysiology

Initial nerve oedema is followed by ischaemia owing to compression against the bony canal that encases the nerve in the temporal bone. Bell's palsy is likely to be part of a viral polyneuropathy. Ramsay Hunt described a syndromic occurrence of facial paralysis, herpetiform vesicular eruptions, and vestibulocochlear dysfunction.

Clinical assessment

The aim is to identify the level of injury, underlying cause, and evaluate the severity.

History

- Recent infections (URTI)
- Associated symptoms
- Trauma or recent sugery
- History of previous palsy or family history of the condition

Examination

- Full head and neck examination, including otoscopy
- Full cranial nerve examination (check lacrimation, taste, and salivation)
- Examine muscles of facial expression; there are many different scales to grade the severity of motor weakness and associated symptoms. House–Brackmann is widely used
- Bell's phenomenon describes the incomplete closure of the upper eyelid, with the eyeball rolled up to protect the cornea
- Examine parotid gland for lumps

Investigations

- Audiometry to assess hearing loss
- MRI if suspected neoplasia of ear, parotid or acoustic neuroma
- CT scan of the head and skull base in trauma cases
- Electrophysiological studies to assess degree of injury and recovery

Management

Conservative

- Eye protection (eye pad) and ophthalmology review to assess and/or treat corneal ulceration
- Artificial tears; may require lateral tarsorrhaphy in the long term
- Facial massage and exercises

Specific management

- Bell's palsy and Ramsay Hunt syndrome require oral steroids (prednisolone 1 mg/kg, reducing over a period of 10–14 days) and oral antivirals (aciclovir 400–800 mg five times a day for 1 week)
- Infective cases can be treated medically with oral steroids and systemic antibiotics
- Chronic suppurative otitis media with or without cholesteatoma may require mastoidectomy and facial nerve decompression
- Immediate postoperative facial nerve palsy after otological surgery requires urgent re-exploration once the effect of local anaesthetic has been ruled out
- Delayed palsy can be due to pressure from an overtight mastoid packing following open mastoidectomy and the packing must be rapidly removed
- Temporal bone fracture causing immediate and total facial nerve palsy requires exploration and facial nerve decompression. If the palsy was not immediate or the diagnosis delayed, electrophysiological studies will be helpful to assess degeneration. If this is >90% within a week of onset, then surgical exploration is indicated.

Complications and prognosis

Facial palsy can cause considerable morbidity, as Bunnell reported:

'The eye cannot close and constantly weeps. The mouth dribbles, the speech is interfered with and mastication impaired. The delicate shades of continence are lost. Joy, happiness, sorrow, shock, surprise, all the emotions have for their common expression the same blank stare (Bunnell, 1927).'

Recovery is variable and can take up to 12 months, although in some cases it may be incomplete (10%). Reconstructive surgery such as cross face nerve graft and free muscle transfers aim to restore facial function in chronic cases.

> ### ➜ Extra
>
> #### Bell's palsy
>
> Sir Charles Bell [1774–1842, Scottish] was a surgeon, anatomist, and physiologist. In 1821 he described the trajectory of the facial nerve and a disease which led to the unilateral palsy of facial muscles[1] (Bell's palsy). He is also credited by some as the founder of modern neurology, as well as giving his name to other discoveries, including the long thoracic nerve of Bell.
>
> #### References
>
> 1. Bell C. On the nerves: giving an account of some experiments on their structure and function, which leads to a new arrangement of the systems. *Phil Trans Roy Soc (Biol)* 1821; **3:** 398–424
> 2. Hunt JR. On herpetiform inflammation of the geniculate ganglion: a new syndrome and its complications. *Nerve Ment Dis* 1907; **34:** 73

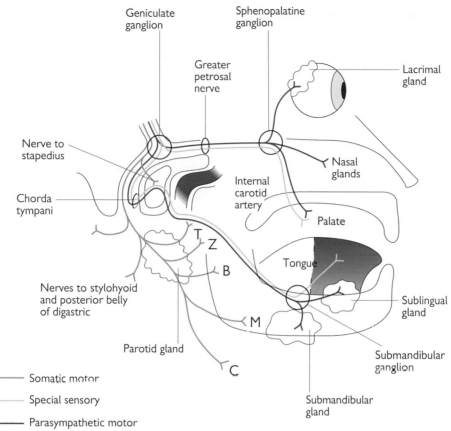

Fig 11.24 Diagram showing the anatomy of the facial nerve (CN VIII). The greater petrosal nerve, nerve to stapedius and chorda tympani branch inside the facial canal. The somatic motor branch emerges from the stylomastoid foramen and then branches to supply the muscles of facial expression (T – temporal, Z – zygomatic, B – buccal, M- mandibular, C – cervical).

11.17 Acute red eye

Acute red eye is a common presentation. It must be taken seriously as some conditions can lead to blindness.

Clinical assessment should include assessment of systemic causes of acute red eye. Check visual acuity and, whenever possible, use a slit lamp to examine the eye. Fluorescein staining and blue light is used if a corneal abrasion or ulcer is suspected.

Urgent referral to an ophthalmologist is needed if there is a history of trauma, pain, severe photophobia, pupil abnormality, ocular tenderness or evidence of raised intraocular pressure is found on examination.

Conjunctivitis

Conjunctivitis is inflammation of the conjunctiva. It is a very common eye condition that affects all age groups and both sexes equally.

Bacterial

Bacterial infection is a common cause of conjunctivitis. Common organisms include *Staphylococcus epidermidis, Staphylococcus aureus, Streptococcus pneumoniae,* and *Haemophilus influenzae.*

Patients present with acute redness, purulent sticky yellow discharge, burning, and gritty sensation. Papillary tarsal conjunctival changes may occur.

Initial treatment is with topical antibiotics such as chloramphenicol. Saline irrigation and artificial tears may also relieve symptoms. Conjunctivitis is contagious and so careful hand washing should be used to avoid transmission between eyes and to other people.

It is generally self-limiting and without long-term complications. However, *Neisseria gonorrhoea* infections can result in acute corneal perforations and therefore need systemic antibiotics in addition to topical therapy.

Viral

Viral conjunctivitis may be associated with a viral URTI. Adenovirus is frequently the culprit, with particular subtypes being epidemic keratoconjunctivitis and pharyngoconjunctival fever.

Typically there is a rapid onset of a watery, intense red eye with foreign body sensation. If the cornea is involved (keratoconjunctivitis), there is also soreness, photophobia, and blurred vision.

Management is usually conservative, with artificial tears and cool compresses, as the infection is self-limiting. Topical antibiotics are usually given to prevent secondary bacterial infection.

Allergic

Allergic conjunctivitis incorporates a variety of conditions, including seasonal allergic conjunctivitis, vernal keratoconjunctivitis, atopic keratoconjunctivitis, and giant papillary conjunctivitis.

Itching is the predominant complaint; however, chemosis (thickened conjunctiva), watery or mucoid discharge, and redness can occur.

Treatment is initially identifying and avoiding possible allergens. Artificial tears and topical mast cell stabilizers or antihistamines can be used if moderately symptomatic. A short course of topical steroids may be required in severe cases. Steroids carry the risk of raising intraocular pressure and so should be used with caution.

Chlamydial

Infection with *Chlamydia trachomatis* is almost always sexually transmitted, and is increasingly seen in young adults who may have an associated genital infection.

Features include mucopurulent discharge, lid oedema, lymphadenopathy, and peripheral corneal infiltrates.

Treatment is with topical antibiotics and systemic therapy using a tetracycline or erythromycin (in pregnant/breastfeeding women or in children).

Episcleritis and scleritis

Episcleritis is a mild inflammation of the fine episcleral tissue lying between the conjunctiva and sclera.

Patients present with acute onset of mild eye pain or photophobia. Redness is often confined to a sector of the conjunctiva, although it may be diffuse. In contrast to scleral vessels, inflamed episcleral vessels will blanch and move when examined with a cotton bud. Visual acuity is normal.

Patients should be reassured that episcleritis is self-limiting and there is unlikely to be any lasting eye damage. Symptomatic episodes may be treated with artificial tears and topical NSAIDs.

Patients with recurrent disease or a history suggestive of underlying disease (e.g. connective tissue diseases) should be referred for further investigations.

Scleritis is inflammation of the sclera in the anterior and/or posterior segments of the eye and is uncommon. Over 70% of episcleritis is idiopathic whereas over 50% of scleritis is caused by an underlying systemic condition such as rheumatoid arthritis, with 50% of cases being bilateral.

Patients present with a gradual increase in eye pain which may become severe with tenderness on palpation. There is diffuse or sectorial redness, increased watering, and photophobia. Nodules may be present, and scleral thinning and corneal ulceration and perforation can occur.

A full systems review should be carried out to exclude an underlying cause and urgent referral to an ophthalmologist is indicated.

Systemic immunosuppressants are commonly indicated, and scleral patching and corneal grafting may also be required.

Keratitis

Acute bacterial keratitis is an ophthalmic emergency and most commonly occurs in contact lens wearers. It presents with pain, foreign body sensation, diffuse or circumlimbal injection, photophobia, and tearing or discharge. A corneal ulcer (white area) is usually present, although this may be small and not visible without a slit-lamp in the early stages. *Staphylococcus aureus* and *epidermidis* are commonly isolated from corneal scrapes.

Patients should be referred urgently to an ophthalmologist where initial management is with intensive topical antibiotic use. Following this, topical corticosteroids may help the healing phase. Patients should be advised not to wear contact lenses.

Herpes simplex keratitis is a common condition that can also present with pain, redness, and blurred vision. A dendritic ulcer is commonly seen with fluorescein staining, and treatment is with topical aciclovir.

Corneal trauma

Trauma to the cornea is relatively common. Chemical injuries are particularly destructive. They require emergency irrigation to return to normal pH of 7, topical antibiotics and lubricants, and referral.

Most corneal foreign bodies are metallic. They present with pain, photophobia, injection, lacrimation, and blurred vision. Slit-lamp examination with fluorescein allows localization. Removal can be performed with topical anaesthetic instillation and use of a 25G needle. Topical antibiotics are given to reduce the risk of keratitis. Corneal abrasions are superficial injuries and should also be treated with topical antibiotics and cycloplegics for comfort.

Anterior uveitis

Anterior uveitis is inflammation of the anterior part of the uveal tract (iris and ciliary body). It accounts for over 75% of uveitis.

It is usually unilateral and presents with pain, photophobia, circumlimbal injection, and blurred vision.

Treatment is with frequent topical steroid titrated to the condition's progression. Anterior uveitis is associated with some systemic conditions, such as diabetes and sarcoidosis; these must be considered when assessing the patient.

Acute closed angle glaucoma

Acute closed angle glaucoma is an emergency and usually occurs in older patients. The outflow of aqueous fluid is acutely interrupted at the peripheral iris (iridocorneal angle), leading to an acute increase in intraocular pressure.

Systemic symptoms include abdominal pain, nausea, and vomiting. The eye is usually red, with a hazy cornea and mid-dilated, oval pupil. Visual acuity is usually decreased. Emergency referral to ophthalmology for reduction of intraocular pressure and YAG laser iridotomy is indicated.

Table 11.2 Diagnostic characteristics of common conditions causing a red eye

Characteristic	Conjunctivitis	Episcleritis	Scleritis	Acute glaucoma	Anterior uveitis	Keratitis
Redness	Diffuse Superficial	Localized sector	Diffuse Deep	Diffuse injection	Circumlimbal	Circumlimbal/diffuse
Discharge	Variable	Lacrimation	Lacrimation	None	Lacrimation	Variable
Pupil	Normal	Normal	Normal	Mid-dilated, oval	Small	Normal
Ocular pain	Mild/moderate	Mild	Severe	Severe	Moderate/Severe	Mild
Acuity	Usually normal	Normal	Usually Normal	Reduced	Often reduced	Often reduced

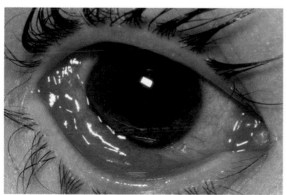

Fig 11.25 *Haemophilus* conjunctivitis showing characteristic conjunctival injection and mucopurulent discharge.

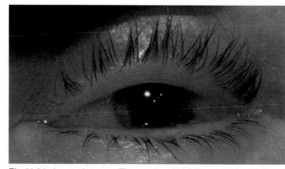

Fig 11.26 Acute glaucoma. The eye is red and the pupil is mid-dilated and fixed.

Case 1

A 61-year-old man is referred with epistaxis for an emergency ward review. He has had recurrent episodes over the last month and this morning has been unable to stop the bleeding. There is no other past medical history.

He walks in to the consultation room and sits down holding a bloodstained handkerchief to his nose. He is wearing braces to keep his trousers up over a large tight abdomen poking through his shirt.

- What is your initial approach?

He is talking and but feels slightly light-headed. His initial observations are HR 116, BP 150/88 mmHg, sats 97%. As you take a history you gain IV access, take bloods, and start fluids.

- What specific questions do you ask?
- What are you going to examine; why is an abdominal examination relevant?
- What blood tests do you request?

On rhinoscopy you identify a bleeding point in Little's area on the right-hand side. You cauterize it with a silver nitrate stick and then pack both sides with nasal tampons. You also find multiple bruises on his limbs and what feels like ascites.

Hb	10.5 g/dL	Na	136 mmol/L
WCC	6 x 10⁹/L	K	5.0 mmol/L
MCV	85 fl	Creat	150 µmol/L
Plts	155 x 10⁹/L	Urea	8 mmol/L
APTT	45 s	ALT	60 u/L
PT	2.3	ALP	110 u/L
		Bilirubin	17 µmol/L
		Albumin	17 g/L

- What is Little's area and which blood vessels are involved?
- What is your interpretation of his blood results?
- What is your differential diagnosis?

Discussion

The history from his wife was useful. She said that over 9 months he had become more short of breath, put on weight but had lost his appetite and started bruising easily.

He was urgently transferred to the physicians for further investigation and management of his bleeding diathesis. He was found to have metastatic disease in his liver.

Case 2

A 54-year-old woman is referred by her GP with a 2-month history of a lump in the right side of her neck.

- What key questions do you ask whilst taking a history?

She smokes 20 cigarettes and drinks 10 units a day and has done so for 30 years. On examination she has a well-defined, smooth rubbery lump 5 cm in diameter in the anterior border of the sternomastoid muscle, just lateral to the carotid pulse, with normal skin freely mobile over it.

- What investigations are indicated?
- What is your differential diagnosis?

The examination and investigations are consistent with a branchial cyst which she wants removed.

Six months later on the preoperative ward round you notice that the lump has got larger; it also feels firmer and the skin over it is quite indurated, and she has a peculiar anaerobic breath.

- What do you think has occurred?
- How should you have managed this situation in a better way?

Discussion

The details of risk factors and age are important so as to classify pathology into benign or malignant. A presumed clinical diagnosis of branchial cyst is a metastatic neck node until proven otherwise.

Even with a normal examination and FNAC (which may be undistinguishable from SCC metastases), a high index of suspicion should be maintained, and a formal panendoscopy with multiple biopsies should be performed sooner rather than later.

The most likely primary site is the tonsil, and a full tonsillectomy may also be indicated. Primary neck node SCC are rare, 5% or so of the head and neck SCC, and they are called primary if there is no other upper aerodigestive tract malignancy present for 5 years after initial diagnosis of the neck cancer. Thus, in this case the neck node metastases presented first and the primary in the tonsil later.

Case 3

A 62-year-old man has had a hoarse voice for 4 weeks following an URTI. He has also had episodes of coughing and choking, especially after drinking fluids, and has been missing the weekly choir practice. He is a well-controlled type II diabetic and hypertensive with no history of surgical operations. He smokes 1 oz of tobacco a week. On examination, he has an obvious dysphonia with a low phonation time and a poor cough.

- Describe a full head and neck examination.

The flexible laryngoscopy view of the vocal cords reveals a left cord paralysed in abduction, with a poor glottic closure during phonation and coughing, thus an incompetent larynx.

- What investigations would you request?
- The GP arranged a chest X-ray before the consultation which reveals a mediastinal mass
- What is your differential diagnosis before and after this result?
- What is the management of your working diagnosis?
- What can be done to prevent the episodes of aspiration?

Discussion

The rule of thumb of aetiology of vocal cord palsy is: one-third idiopathic, one-third postoperative, and one-third neoplastic.

The left recurrent laryngeal nerve descends into the chest, where it hooks around the arch of the aorta before returning to the neck. Compression from a mediastinal/lung mass will cause palsy. The position of the paralysed cord is irrelevant to the type of pathology. Vocal cords in abduction predispose to aspiration pneumonia. Early diagnosis and speech and language therapy assessment is important.

In the long term, a medialization procedure can be attempted to prevent aspiration and improve the quality of the voice. Initially the management of the lung carcinoma takes priority.

Chapter 12

Plastic and reconstructive surgery

◎ Clinical skills

- Cutaneous scarring
- Flap monitoring
- Estimation of burn depth
- Estimation of total burn surface area
- The 7Rs of major burn care

➕ Technical skills and procedures

- Wound debridement
- Split thickness skin grafting
- Nail bed repair
- Zone II flexor tendon repair
- Dupuytren's disease surgery
- Open carpal tunnel decompression
- Excision of a skin lesion

12.1 Acute inflammation

Acute inflammation is the response of living tissues to injury. It usually lasts as long as the stimulus remains. Although it has a protective function, disorders of inflammation can lead to serious illness and death.

Aetiology
Tissue injury may be endogenous or exogenous.

Endogenous
- Hypersensitivity reactions
- Autoimmune conditions (e.g. rheumatoid arthritis)

Exogenous
- Infection
- Mechanical (e.g. sprained ankle)
- Physical (e.g. ionizing radiation)
- Chemical (e.g. acid burn)
- Tissue necrosis (e.g. ischaemic infarction)

Pathophysiology
Local changes seen in acute inflammation are mediated by changes in the microcirculation and leucocyte activity. They act to dilute the inflammatory stimulus, deliver oxygen and nutrients, and stimulate an immune response.

A systemic acute phase response is caused by release of proinflammatory cytokines, such as IL-1, IL-6, and IL-8. These stimulate the liver to produce acute phase proteins.

Microcirculation
Following injury there is transitory vasoconstriction followed by prolonged vasodilatation of arterioles and venules, leading to increased capillary blood flow. There is also an increase in vascular permeability. The combination of these factors leads to an inflammatory exudate.

Plasma-derived components
In addition to the changes in microcirculation, there are plasma-derived mediators.
- Clotting cascade results in platelet aggregation and clot formation
- Fibrinolytic system (fibrin-related peptides and plasmin) keeps the clotting in check and results in the release of other inflammatory mediators
- Kinin system (kallikrein and bradykinin) results in vasodilatation and increased vascular permeability
- Complement cascade mediates the early inflammatory response, helps with chemotaxis (C5a), and aids phagocytosis by opsinization (C3b)

Cellular components
Initially, neutrophils migrate from the circulation to the site of injury along a chemotaxic gradient. An early peak of neutrophils is followed by migration of mononuclear phagocytes (macrophages).

Emigration of neutrophils into the interstitium follows a number of steps (Fig 12.2): margination and rolling along the periphery of the blood vessel, adhesion to the endothelium, and transmigration between the endothelial cells into the tissues.

Once in the tissues, a process of chemotaxis directs the neutrophils towards the site of injury. They must be able to understand and act on these signals (reception and transduction).

They then act as either phagocytes ingesting micro-organisms and debris or release enzyme containing lysosome granules (degranulation). There are also various inflammatory mediators derived from these cells (Fig 12.1)

Clinical assessment
Inflammation can have both local and systemic features.

Local
Celsus, the Roman patrician, originally described four cardinal signs of inflammation. Others include excessive secretion (fluor) and loss of function (functio laesa).
1. Heat (calor) is a result of increased local blood flow
2. Pain (dolor) is caused by stretching and distortion of the tissues. Some of the inflammatory mediators, such as bradykinin, induce pain
3. Redness (rubor) is a result of capillary dilatation
4. Swelling (tumour) is caused by localized collection of excess interstitial fluid (oedema)

Systemic
Systemic symptoms are a result of an acute phase response. Features include fever, malaise, and anorexia. In severe cases this may develop into a systemic inflammatory response syndrome.
- Pyrexia is caused by endogenous pyrogens released by polymorphs and macrophages. These act on the thermoregulatory mechanism in the hypothalamus
- Reactive hyperplasia of the reticuloendothelial system

Investigations
No investigations are usually needed. Serum C-reactive protein (CRP) is a non-specific marker of inflammation. It has a half-life of 6 h and so can be used to track the progression of inflammation.

Outcome
Resolution
Resolution is complete restoration of the tissues to their normal state. This is most likely to occur if there is minimal cell death, rapid destruction of the causative agent (e.g. bacteria), and rapid removal of fluid and debris by a good vascular system.

Suppuration
Suppuration is the formation of pus. This can lead to a localized collection (abscess) or empyema if it is in a body cavity. *Staphylococcus aureus* is a common pus-forming organism.

Organization
Organization is the replacement of the inflammatory exudate with granulation tissue. It is likely to occur if a large amount of fibrin is formed but not cleared. Capillaries grow into the inflammatory exudate and fibroblast proliferation results in fibrosis.

Chronic inflammation
Acute inflammation can progress to chronic inflammation if the causative agent is not removed. However, chronic inflammation is often a primary event and is not preceded by acute inflammation.

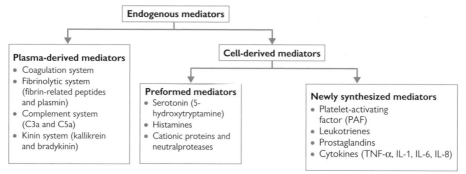

Fig 12.1 Classification of endogenous mediators of acute inflammation. Exogenous mediators include formylated peptides produced by micro-organisms.

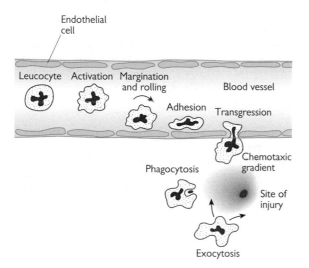

Fig 12.2 Leucocyte activity in acute inflammation.

1. Margination and rolling

2. Adhesion

3. Transmigration

4. Chemotaxis

5. Phagocytosis

6. Killing.

12.2 Cutaneous wound healing

Cutaneous wound healing is the body's response to a breach of the skin and underlying tissues, and almost always results in scar formation. It is likely that this imperfect regeneration was an evolutionary trade-off for rapid wound healing under the pressure of natural selection. Wound healing has two main aims:

1. epithelial regeneration
2. connective tissue repair to restore the tensile strength of the underlying tissues

Definitions

- Primary intention describes the direct apposition of cleanly incised wound edges. This is usually achieved by suturing the wound
- Delayed primary intention describes delayed surgical closure of a wound. This may allow time to ensure that wound debridement has been adequate before closure
- Secondary intention describes the healing that occurs when direct apposition is not possible owing to the size of the skin defect. Wound contraction and granulation tissue combine to achieve wound closure

Pathophysiology

Wound healing by primary intention is a complex process of coordinated events which can be divided in to four overlapping phases.

1. Coagulation (fibrin–fibronectin clot formation)

A wound invariably causes blood vessel injury and bleeding. This stimulates vasoconstriction and haemostasis (□ Topic 7.1). Platelets release cytokines and growth factors, which stimulate inflammation. The resulting clot protects the wound as well as providing a matrix through which the inflammatory cells can migrate.

2. Inflammatory cell recruitment

Neutrophils and monocytes are rapidly recruited to the wound by chemotactic signals, including complement factors, TNF-α, IL-1, PDGF, TGF-α, and TGF–β. Neutrophils remove bacteria and provide further pro-inflammatory cytokines.

3. Proliferation

This phase can be summarized as fibroplasia, matrix deposition, angiogenesis, and re-epithelialization. It begins within hours of injury and continues until the wound is fully covered.

4. Remodelling

Remodelling results in wound contracture and a gradual increase in tensile strength. Some fibroblasts become myofibroblasts which pull the opposing dermis and adipose tissue together.

Mature scar fibroblasts increase the amount of types I and III collagen. The maximum tensile strength only returns to 70% of the original tissue because of the haphazard arrangement of the collagen fibres.

Wound healing by second intention

Wounds in which the edges are not apposed follow a similar sequence to wound healing by primary intention, but there are some distinguishing features.

- Wound contraction is a major feature of healing by secondary intention. This is mediated by myofibroblasts and helps to reduce the size of the wound
- Granulation tissue fills the space before spontaneous epithelial migration covers the wound. The excess of granulation tissue leads to more scar formation

Clinical assessment

History

- Mechanism of injury and progression of wound
- Nutritional status
- Immune status
- Systemic conditions affecting healing e.g. diabetes mellitus

Examination

The wound needs to be described in detail.

- Location and size
- Wound edges and surrounding skin
- Wound base and exudate
- Evidence of infection

Investigations

Investigations are not routinely indicated during wound healing unless there is a delay or suspected infection.

Management

The main aim is to optimize the wound healing environment. Local factors include removing devitalized tissue and foreign bodies, maintaining a moist environment, and reducing any pressure or tension.

Systemic factors include optimizing nutritional status, medical co-morbidities, and drugs that may affect wound healing.

Delayed wound healing

Delayed wound healing takes longer than anticipated given the type of wound and use of appropriate therapy.

Pathophysiology

There are both local and systemic factors that may cause a delay in wound healing, often by prolonging an abnormal inflammatory response.

- Local factors include ischaemia or poor venous drainage, infection, poor apposition, foreign bodies, and high skin tension or excess local mobility
- Systemic factors include advanced age, malnutrition, vitamin deficiency (zinc, vitamins A and C), immunosupression, diabetes mellitus, chemotherapy/radiotherapy, and malignancy

Clinical assessment

- Persistent pain or discomfort
- Increased fragility or change in appearance of granulation tissue
- Necrotic tissue in wound bed with excess exudate or slough
- Extending margin or surrounding erythema
- Local swelling/oedema
- Recurrent wound breakdown

Investigations

- Microbiology specimens: tissue (preferable) or wound swabs
- Bloods—FBC (anaemia, leucocytosis), U+Es, CRP, albumin (low protein delays healing), glucose, micronutrients (zinc, magnesium, copper, iron)
- Special bloods—autoimmune screen (connective tissue disorders), cryoglobulins (haematological disorders), haemoglobinopathy screen (sickle cell anaemia and thalassaemia), clotting factors (vascular thrombosis), serum electrophoresis (myeloma), viral screen (HIV)

Management

- Regular debridement of non-viable tissue and early treatment of wound infection
- Address underlying cause, e.g. reduce pressure
- Optimize systemic co-morbidities
- Appropriate wound dressings to optimize the wound healing environment (📖 Topic 12.3)

➕ Wound debridement

The aim of wound debridement [Fr. desbrider; unbridle] is to improve the wound healing environment by removing devitalized tissue and foreign material.

Devitalized tissue acts as a medium for bacterial growth, elicits an excessive inflammatory response, and delays the natural progression of wound healing.

It should be performed by an experienced surgeon at an appropriate time, i.e. not in the middle of the night.

Surgical debridement

- Surgical debridement is performed in theatre and enables proper assessment of the wound and definitive debridement
- Tissue samples are sent to microbiology. If there is a subsequent wound infection, then the original wound isolates guide antimicrobial therapy
- Sharp debridement uses a scalpel but is performed on the ward or in clinic

Other techniques

- Autolytic therapy encourages debridement using the body's own enzymes. Occlusive or semi-occlusive dressings as well as hydrocolloids and hydrogels encourage autolytic debridement by keeping wound fluid in contact with necrotic tissue
- Larvae therapy (*Lucilia sericata*) selectively digests dead tissue and debris back to healthy viable tissue
- Mechanical debridement occurs when dressings are removed that are stuck to the wound material. It is cheap but not very selective
- Enzymatic debridement rapidly breaks down necrotic tissue. It is not routinely used

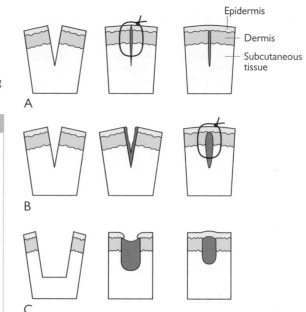

Fig 12.4 (A) Primary wound healing – the tissues are well apposed and heal with minimal scarring. (B) Delayed primary wound healing – often following debridement of a contaminated wound. (C) Secondary wound healing – wound is left to heal by itself with no closure. There is a higher risk of poor scarring.

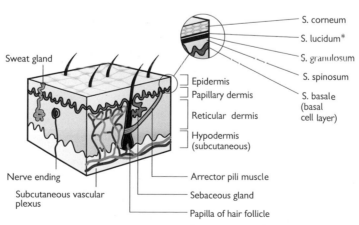

*S. lucidum only present in thick skin of the palm and soles of the feet

Fig 12.3 Anatomy of the skin. The epidermis acts as a renewable outer barrier. The dermis gives the skin strength and flexibility, and contains the adnexal structures (sebaceous glands, sweat glands, hair follicles) and neurovascular structures.
The main blood supply to the skin is derived from direct perforators (cutaneous and septocutaenous) and indirect perforators (e.g. musculocutaneous) which are less important to its survival. Confluence of adjacent vascular networks derived from these perforators occurs at multiple levels in the skin.

The reconstructive ladder describes the hierarchy of options available for closing a wound. It ranges from simple wound dressings through to complex free tissue transfer.

Step 1: dressings

Dressings allow the wound to heal by secondary intention. The aim is to maintain a moist environment without excess exudate. Many wound dressings need secondary dressings to soak up exudate, keep them secure, and provide bulk and protection.

Low adherence dressings

These dressings maintain a moist wound bed and allow exudate to pass through into a second dressing such as gauze. They are generally easier and less painful to remove although they can still get stuck to the wound. They come as tulles which are open weave cloth soaked in paraffin (Jelonet, Paranet, Urgotul); textiles (Mepilex, Mepitel, Tegapore) or plastic films.

Semi-permeable films

Semi-permeable films consist of a polyurethane sheet coated with hypoallergenic acrylic adhesive (Bioclusive, Tegaderm). They are permeable to air and water vapours but impermeable to fluids and organisms. They are transparent and are very flexible, enabling dressing of difficult areas.

Foam dressings

The foam is either polyurethane or silicon and is manufactured as a sheet (Allevyn). It is highly absorbent and usually comes with a hydrophobic backing to prevent strikethrough.

Hydrocolloids and hydrogels

Hydrocolloids come as sheets, foam or paste, and consist of sodium carboxymethylcellulose, gelatin, pectin, and elastomers. The dressings are virtually impermeable. They form a gel at the wound interface which helps to rehydrate dry necrotic wounds and promote autolytic debridement. Hydrogels come as a viscous gel and consist of a matrix of insoluble polymers with a high water content.

Alginates

Alginates are derived from calcium and sodium salts of alginic acid found in brown seaweed. They are very absorbent and should only be used on wounds with a high exudate.

Antimicrobial dressings

These dressings aim to reduce microbiological load in colonized or infected wounds. Silver is the most commonly used agent (Aquacel Ag, Acticoat), although iodine-based products are also effective (Inadine).

Vacuum-assisted closure (VAC)

Vacuum-assisted closure creates a controlled sub-atmospheric pressure environment. The negative pressure is thought to draw excess exudate away from the wound, promoting tissue oxygenation, angiogenesis, and formation of granulation tissue.

A piece of open cell foam is cut to fit the wound. This is then covered and secured to the surrounding skin with polyethylene adhesive film. The sealed wound environment is then connected to a vacuum pump with a rubber tube. An intermittent vacuum force of up to 125 mmHg is applied to the wound. A lower continuous pressure (75 mmHg) may be used to secure a skin graft.

Step 2: primary or delayed closure

Primary closure aims to appose and then secure incised wound edges. This can be achieved using sutures, adhesive strips, staples, and tissue adhesive. Traumatic wounds may need debridement followed by delayed primary closure.

Principles of suturing skin wounds

Interrupted sutures

Simple sutures

- Simple interrupted cutaneous sutures allow accurate placement and fine adjustment of each stitch. They can be placed alone in tension-free wounds.
- Buried absorbable intradermal sutures can be used to eliminate dead space and to close wounds which are under tension. This reduces stretching when the cutaneous sutures are removed
- Length of time, wound tension, body region, and suture material all contribute to the likelihood of developing suture marks and a poor scar

Mattress sutures

- Vertical and horizontal mattress sutures are double stitches. They are strong and less likely to cut out
- They improve wound eversion and closure of subcutaneous dead space (Fig 12.5)

Continuous

- Continuous over-and-over sutures (locked or unlocked) are fast to place and are haemostatic so are are often used for closure of scalp wounds. Mattress sutures can also be continuous
- Continuous subcuticular (intradermal) sutures avoid suture marks and are excellent in tension-free wounds

Optimal scar placement

A skin incision will leave a scar. Various methods have been described to achieve the best aesthetic and functional result.

Scars should follow relaxed skin tension lines (wrinkles) which lie parallel to dermal collagen bundles and perpendicular to muscle contraction. Langer's lines are a similar concept but are based on the direction of the ellipses seen when a circular punch is made in cadaveric skin. Natural junction lines and concealed areas are also good areas for scar placement.

Z-plasty

Z-plasty is a technique used to treat and prevent scar contractures or to change the direction or length of a scar, especially on the face.

A single Z-plasty involves the transposition of two interdigitating triangular flaps (Fig 12.6). Multiple Z-plasties can be joined together in a row or used in more complex geometric formations.

Cutaneous scarring

Scarring is a common clinical problem and is often associated with problems such as poor cosmesis, loss of function, and an adverse psychological outcome.

Pathophysiology

Most scars take over a year to mature fully. Wound healing resulting in problematic scarring is more common in younger people.

- **Atrophic** scarring leaves a pale depressed scar (e.g. acne scarring)
- **Stretched** scars occur early in wound healing when the edges are under tension. They are usually flat and pale and look unattractive but are otherwise asymptomatic
- **Hypertrophic** scars have a higher incidence in younger people. They generally occur early in wound healing and are limited to the boundary of the original wound. They spontaneously regress but not back to 'normal' and are more likely to form scar contractures. Wound tension and delayed healing increase risk
- **Keloid** scars have a higher incidence in younger age groups and pigmented skin types. There is often a familial tendency. They extend beyond the boundary of the original wound and occur later in wound healing (>3 months). They do not regress and usually recur following excision. Unrelated to wound tension, they may be autoimmune phenomenon.

Clinical assessment

History

- Details of original injury and risk factors for poor wound healing
- Symptoms: discomfort, pain, itching, loss of function
- Psychological impact

Examination

- Anatomical location (sternum and deltoid region particularly prone to bad scarring)
- Scar characteristics: extent, width, raised/depressed, evidence of hypertrophic or keloid scarring. Scoring system such as the Vancouver scar scale can be used

Management

The initial approach is usually watchful waiting as scars can take over a year to remodel and mature.

Conservative approaches include scar massage, compression therapy with pressure garments, topical silicon pads, and creams. Invasive approaches include local steroid injections and surgical revision.

- Hypertrophic or stretched scars can be excised and re-sutured
- Keloid scars have a very high recurrence rate following excision (>50%). Intralesional excision combined with steroid injection or radiotherapy may reduce recurrence
- Scar contractures can be released (see Z-plasty). Resurfacing with skin grafting or flap reconstruction may be indicated in severe cases

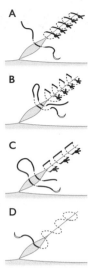

Fig 12.5 Suture techniques. A Simple interrupted; B vertical and C horizontal mattress sutures; D continuous subcuticular suture.

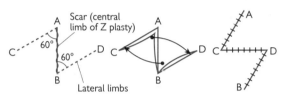

Fig 12.6 Z-plasty. There is lengthening in the direction of the common limb which also changes direction. The length of the limbs should all be the same. The angles can be varied and determine the increase in length.

Angle	Lengthening
30°	25%
45°	50%
60°	75% (usual design)
75%	100%
90°	125%

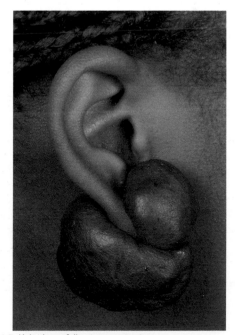

Fig 12.7 Keloid scar following ear piercing.

Step 3: skin grafting

Skin grafts are either split-thickness (epidermis and variable depth of dermis) or full-thickness (epidermis and full thickness of dermis).

The survival of the graft relies on both the graft and the graft bed. Generally, more vascular beds give a better take. Muscle and fascia accept grafts; bare cortical bone and exposed tendons do not.

Stages of graft take

1. **Adherence** (<8 h): fibrin bonds develop between the graft and its bed. They are easily disrupted by shear forces
2. **Plasmic imbibition** (<day 2): breakdown of intracellular proteoglycans in graft cells leads to osmosis and swelling of the graft with oedema
3. **Inosculation** (days 2–5): ingrowth of blood vessels occurs and there is restoration of lymphatic circulation
4. **Remodelling** (>1 week): the graft may become pigmented, re-innervated, and there may be regeneration of skin appendages

Split-thickness skin graft (Tiersch graft)

Split-thickness skin grafts (SSG) are very versatile. A large surface area can be harvested, leaving a donor area that will heal spontaneously. To increase its surface area, the harvested skin can be meshed.

The choice of donor site depends on the amount of skin required, cosmetic outcome, and convenience of dressings. Commonly used sites include the thigh and upper arm. SSG usually take easily but do not have volume and often develop patchy pigmentation.

Full-thickness skin graft (Wolfe graft)

Full-thickness skin grafts (FTSG) are limited in size because they leave a defect with no healing potential. The defect needs either direct closure or SSG.

Donor skin needs to be chosen carefully to obtain a good colour and texture match. Common sites include postauricular, supraclavicular, upper eyelid, and flexural skin (groin and antecubital fossa).

FTSG do not take as well as SSG because the relatively thick dermis acts as a barrier to the 'take' process and they gain most of their blood supply from the margins rather than the base. However, they do retain their volume and pigmentation.

Step 4: tissue expansion

Tissue expansion increases the surface area of locally available skin. An expander implant is placed in a subcutaneous pocket. An injection port enables serial inflation with saline over a period of weeks or months.

The expander is then removed and the skin advanced to cover the defect. This technique is particularly useful for scalp and breast reconstruction.

Step 5: flaps

A flap is a unit of tissue transferred from one place (donor site) to another (recipient site) whilst maintaining its own blood supply. The classification and nomenclature is often confusing but essentially flaps can be described in terms of their blood supply, donor site, and tissue components.

Blood supply

- **Random pattern flaps** are not based on a named blood vessel but rely on the random pattern of cutaneous vessels. This usually limits them to a length to breadth ratio of 1:1
- **Axial pattern flaps** are based on a named arteriovenous system running the length of the flap. Axial flap dimensions are limited by length rather than breadth

Improved understanding of the anatomy and physiology of the skin has led to the use of custom-made flap designs based on specific perforating vessels (**perforator flaps**)

Location of donor site

- **Local** flaps have their donor site next to the recipient site. They are either pivotal (rotation, transposition, interpolation) or advancement (single pedicle, bi-pedicle or V–Y)
- **Distant** flaps have their donor site at a distant site from their recipient site. They are either pedicled or free. Free flaps refer to tissue moved from one area of the body to another with disconnection and then re-anastomosis of their blood supply. Almost any tissue can be used, including skin, fascia, muscle, bone, and intestine.

Tissue components

Any tissue with an intrinsic arterial and venous network of vessels can be used as a flap. Flaps are composed of single or multiple types of tissue (composite flap).

Cutaneous and fasciocutaneous flaps

Inclusion of the underlying fascia with a cutaneous flap (fasciocutaneous flap) improves the blood supply and reliability of the flap.

Muscle and myocutaneous flaps

Muscle flaps can be classified based on their blood supply (Fig 12.9). Muscle flaps with a single dominant pedicle are most reliable. If possible, function is preserved at the donor site by leaving a portion of muscle with its anatomical attachments intact.

Myocutaneous (musculocutaneous) flaps have a skin paddle as well. This is generally supplied by the terminal branches of the myocutaneous perforators although it may get some direct branches.

➕ Split-thickness skin graft

The recipient bed should be prepared and its surface area estimated.

Procedure

- Select donor area and position the patient appropriately
- Infiltrate with local anaesthetic or use topical EMLA™
- Skin usually harvested with powered dermatome or Watson knife. Check the width of the blade and thickness setting
- Once harvested the skin should be placed in a damp swab and the donor site dressed
- Donor site usually dressed with a haemostatic layer (e.g. kaltostat) and then jelonet/gauze/crepe
- The skin is meshed or fenestrated and placed on the bed and secured (suture, staples or tissue glue) before being dressed to reduce the risk of shear and haematoma formation
- Tie over dressings are often used to secure the graft in place and a splint may be needed to help immobilize grafts near joints
- Grafted site checked at 48 h to 5 days depending on site and concern about take. The donor site is left intact for 2 weeks.

Complications

Loss of graft is usually related to shear, haematoma, infection or grafting on to an inappropriate (avascular) bed.

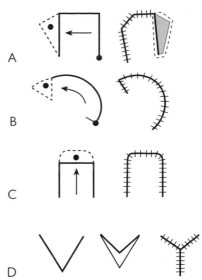

Fig 12.8 Local flap designs. Pivotal flaps include transposition flaps (A) and rotation flaps (B). They are often used to cover primary defects that are not amenable to skin grafting. The secondary defect (shaded area) is either directly closed or may require a skin graft. Examples of advancement flaps include single pedicle (C) and V–Y flaps (D).

⊙ Flap monitoring

Postoperative monitoring of flaps is crucial, as early detection of failure can enable emergency re-exploration and potential salvage.

There are many other methods used in free flap monitoring but they are often unreliable, and experienced clinical assessment remains the criterion standard.

The table below gives a simple overview of clinical findings in a failing flap. In reality, signs are often more subtle and depend on the type of flap being monitored.

	Arterial insufficiency	Venous insufficiency
Colour	Pale	Dusky purple
Temperature	Cool	Cool
Turgor	Reduced	Increased
Capillary return	Delayed	Brisk
Post-puncture dermal bleeding	Slow	Brisk dark bleeding

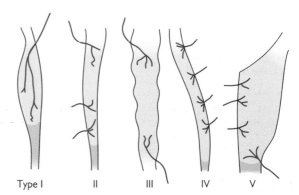

Fig 12.9 Mathes and Nahai classification of muscle flaps.
 I One vascular pedicle (e.g. gastrocnemius)
 II Dominant pedicle and minor pedicle (e.g. gracilis)
 III Two dominant pedicles (e.g. gluteus maximus)
 IV Multiple Segmental pedicles (e.g. sartorius)
 V One dominant pedicle and secondary segmental pedicles (e.g. latissimus dorsi).

12.5 Congenital conditions

This topic gives an overview of the congenital conditions that plastic surgeons often manage. Congenital urological and breast conditions are discussed elsewhere.

Hand

Upper limb anomalies are seen in 1 in 600 live births; ~5% are associated with a clinical syndrome. Polydactyly, camptodactyly, and syndactyly are the most common anomalies.

Upper limb embryology

Limb development occurs between the third and eighth week of gestation. The limb buds (apical ectodermal ridges) are condensations of mesenchyme covered with ectoderm that appear on the ventrolateral aspect of the embryo. The mesoderm gradually elongates and differentiates into cartilage and muscle. By day 33 there is a visible hand paddle and at 50 days there is digital separation and a full skeletal structure.

Swanson classification of congenital hand anomalies

I Failure of formation

Arrest of development can occur at any level from the shoulder to phalanges. Central longitudinal arrest leads to clefts of the hand.

II Failure of differentiation

Failure of differentiation can occur in both the skeleton and soft tissues.

- Syndactyly [Gr. *syn*, with; *dactyly*, finger] is partial or complete fusion of two or more digits. Simple cases just involve the soft tissues; complex cases also have bony fusion. Middle–ring finger fusion is most common
- Camptodactyly [Gr. *campto*, bent] is a finger flexion deformity in the anteroposterior plane
- Clinodactyly [Gr. *clino*, deviated] is finger deviation in a radial or ulnar direction. It is often bilateral and commonly affects the little fingers

III Duplication

In extreme cases this may apply to the whole limb. Polydactyly [Gr. *poly*, many] is the most common abnormality. The extra digits may be preaxial (radial), central or postaxial (ulnar), which is most common.

IV Overgrowth

Overgrowth is rare and includes macrodactyly.

V Undergrowth

Conditions include radial hypoplasia, brachysyndactyly, and brachydactyly.

VI Constriction band syndrome

This syndrome is a result of annular bands of chorionic tissue encircling the limb or digit. Proximal anatomy is normal but the distal anatomy is abnormal or even amputated in extreme cases.

VII Generalized anomalies and syndromes

This category covers all other anomalies.

Cleft lip and palate

Cleft lip and palate are the commonest congenital craniofacial conditions seen in the UK.

Craniofacial embryology

- During the first trimester of pregnancy, the face and jaw is formed by five facial elements coming together (frontonasal, two lateral maxillary, two mandibular)
- The primary palate is a triangular area of hard palate anterior to the incisive foramen and includes the four incisor teeth. It forms during the fourth to seventh week of gestation. It is the palatal component of the intermaxillary segment
- The secondary palate forms the rest of the hard palate and the whole of the soft palate. It develops during the sixth to ninth weeks of gestation

Aetiology and pathophysiology

The aetiology is multifactorial and involves both genetic and environmental factors (phenytoin, alcohol, diabetes).

- Cleft lip and palate (60%) can be unilateral or bilateral, and can range from incomplete clefts of the lip, alveolus and palate through to complete clefts of the lip, alveolus and palate
- Cleft palate (40%) ranges from partial clefts of the soft palate (velum) through to complete clefts of the soft and hard palates. Up to 50% are syndromic

Clinical assessment

There are a number of problems associated with cleft lip and palate. The degree of functional and aesthetic deficit is related to the type and severity of the cleft.

- **Speech** is affected by both the altered anatomy of the soft palate and lip as well as dysfunction of the palatal muscles
- **Hearing** may be affected as the abnormal soft palate interferes with Eustachian tube function
- **Feeding** is affected if there is a communication between the oral and nasal cavities. There is nasal regurgitation and the baby is unable to suck during breastfeeding
- **Dentition** is abnormal if the alveolus is involved
- **Appearance** is altered in cleft lip and hypoplastic growth of the midface
- **Psychological** disturbance often affects social interaction

Management

Management in the UK is provided by dedicated cleft lip and palate centres. The multidisciplinary team includes surgeons (plastic and ENT), orthodontists, specialist nurses, speech therapists, psychologists, geneticists, and paediatricians.

Management aims to restore form and function, including speech, dentition, appearance, and social integration.

Timeline

The approximate timeline for management of a child with cleft lip and palate is outlined below.

Age	Event
3 months	Repair of cleft lip, nose, and anterior palate
6 months	Repair of remaining soft and hard palate +/- grommets
3 years	Speech assessment. Re-exploration of the palate and pharyngoplasty may be required
8 years	Orthodontic treatment ready for bone grafting in those with clefts involving the alveolus
7–9 years	Alveolar bone grafting
10+ years	Definitive orthodontic treatment
17+ years	Maxillary advancement +/- rhinoplasty in patients with maxillary retrusion and cleft lip

Craniofacial

Craniofacial clefts

Craniofacial clefts are a result of failure to fuse of the ectomesenchymal tissues.

- **Craniofacial clefts** are very rare and have a complex pathogenesis. The Tessier classification numbers them from 0 to 14. The lower numbers (0–7) represent facial clefts and the higher numbers (8–14) their cranial extension
- **Orbital hypertelorism** is defined as an increased interorbital distance measured between the medial walls of each orbit. Hypertelorism is a physical finding in many congenital conditions

Craniofacial microsomia

Craniofacial microsomia (hemifacial microsomia) encompasses a wide spectrum of clinical deformities resulting from morphogenetic anomalies of the second and third branchial arches.

It results in asymmetrical hypoplasia of the face, most commonly affecting the external ear, vertical ramus of the mandible, and temporomandibular joint.

Management to restore the facial contour may involve both lengthening of the skeletal structures and soft tissue augmentation.

Craniosynostosis

Craniosynostosis is the rare premature fusion of one or more of the sutures in the cranial vault or cranial base. Non-syndromic sporadic cases tend to involve just one suture, whereas syndromic cases are inherited and tend to have multiple congenital abnormalities.

- **Apert's syndrome** is characterized by multiple craniosynostoses, exorbitism, midface hypoplasia, and symmetrical syndactyly of both the hands and feet
- **Crouzon's syndrome** has similar facial features to Apert's syndrome but no associated digital anomalies

Miscellaneous

Accessory auricles

The external ear arises from the first and second branchial arches; the external auditory meatus arises from the first branchial groove between them.

Abnormal development may leave accessory tissue which usually sits anterior to the tragus. It ranges from a simple skin tag to a lesion containing a deep root of cartilage. Management is complete excision, including the cartilage root if present.

Prominent ears

Prominent ears ('bat ears') are caused by excessive protrusion of the external ear from the temporal scalp (>25°). The main features are: (1) underdeveloped or absent antihelical fold; (2) deep concha; and (3) increased conchoscaphal angle.

Many different operations have been described to correct the deformities mentioned. Surgical correction (otoplasty) is usually performed after the child is 3 years old and before they go to school. By this time the ear is almost full size.

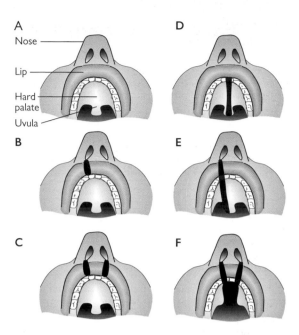

Fig 12.10 Diagram showing an overview of cleft lip and palate. A Normal; B unilateral cleft lip; C bilateral cleft palate; D isolated cleft palate; E unilateral cleft lip and palate; F bilateral cleft lip and palate.

Burns are common and affect 1% of the UK population per year. Approximately 10% need hospital admission and 1% of these will be life-threatening.

Burns affect people of all ages, but are particularly prevalent in young children and the elderly.

Burn prevention

At least 90% of burns are avoidable. The main public health strategies to reduce the incidence of burns are education and legislation.

- **Education** attempts to change people's behaviour. Successful campaigns have included installing smoke alarms in the home and not using deep fat fryers
- **Legislation** attempts to prevent burns by altering the environment in which people live and work (e.g. Health and Safety at Work, etc., Act, 1974). Examples include sprinkler systems in public and commercial buildings

Aetiology

Most burns occur at home, with the kitchen and bathroom being the most dangerous places. The aetiology changes with age. Children are most likely to suffer scalds whereas in adults flame burns are more common.

Thermal

Wet thermal injuries such as scalds are common in young and old patients. They are often caused by spilling hot liquid and are usually superficial partial-thickness.

Flame burns are the most common burn injury in adults and are often associated with inhalational injuries. Flash burns are usually due to sudden ignition of a volatile substance and are usually deep partial-thickness or full-thickness.

Contact burns can be caused by prolonged contact with moderately hot objects (e.g. elderly person falling and becoming trapped next to a radiator) or brief contact with a very hot object. The depth is dependent on the length of contact; they are usually deep partial-thickness or full-thickness.

Chemical

Chemical burns are rare and tend to cause deep partial-thickness or full-thickness burns. Although household products can cause chemical burns, they are most commonly caused by accidents involving industrial chemicals.

Alkaline substances (e.g. cement) penetrate deeper than acids (e.g. hydrochloric acid) as they cause liquefaction necrosis rather than coagulative necrosis. Certain chemicals have specific treatments. For instance, the fluoride ions in hydrofluoric acid rapidly penetrate through the skin and chelate calcium ions, potentially leading to hypocalcaemia. Following irrigation, calcium gluconate should be applied to chelate the fluoride ions.

Electrical

Electrical burns constitute <5% of burns admissions. The degree of tissue damage is related to the amount of heat generated ($0.24 \times (voltage)^2 \times resistance$).

High voltage injuries (>1000 V) are either true electrocutions in which current passes through the body between an entry and exit point, or flash injuries where a person is near an arc of current from a high-tension source. They cause extensive tissue damage and, occasionally, loss of limbs.

Domestic electricity is a low voltage (240 V) alternating current which causes local deep burns at the entry and exit sites. Electrical injuries can cause cardiac arrhythmias and so patients require an ECG and then monitoring if there are abnormalities. If everything is normal they can go home.

Pathophysiology

Burns cause tissue injury which initiates an inflammatory response. There are both local and systemic effects.

Local response

Normal capillary function is disrupted and this leads to loss of fluid and protein into the interstitial space and oedema. Jackson described the local zones of injury seen in a burn (Fig 12.11).

Systemic response

Burns involving >25% of the total body surface area often lead to a systemic inflammatory response with the following consequences:

- hypovolaemia and hypoperfusion owing to increased capillary permeability
- decreased myocardial perfusion
- increased basal metabolic rate
- hypoperfusion of the gut and bacterial translocation
- acute lung injury leading to ARDS
- immunosuppression

First aid

First aid is usually administered in the community.

1. **Stop the burning process** by extinguishing the source of the burn and removing the victim to a safe environment. Clothing should be removed except adherent nylon. Rescuers should avoid burning themselves

2. **Cool the burn** with tepid water (15°C). This helps to stop the burning process, reduce pain, minimize oedema, and cleanse the wound. Ideally this should be done within 20 min and continued for up to 20 min with thermal burns and longer with chemical burns. Avoid ice cold water as it causes excessive cooling and intense vasoconstriction which can lead to burn progression. Hypothermia is also a risk

3. **Cover the burn** with polyvinyl chloride (clingfilm). It is clean, pliable, non-adherent, impermeable, and allows inspection. Lay the clingfilm on loosely to avoid constriction of limbs. Hands can be put in a plastic bag

Emergency assessment

Burns may be associated with other immediately life-threatening injuries. Rapid assessment following ATLS and Emergency Management of Severe Burns (EMSB®) guidelines saves lives (📖 Topic 8.1).

- Primary (ABCDEF) and secondary survey. First estimation of burn depth and total burn surface area (TBSA) is done during 'exposure'. This guides early fluid resuscitation
- Burn and AMPLE history: timing, type, and duration of burn
- First aid—was it immediate? Were clothes removed? Type of cooling and length of application
- Associated injuries, e.g. inhalational injury and head injury
- Assess risk of non-accidental injury, especially in children
- Co-morbidities and tetanus status
- Routine investigations needed in larger burns include FBC, U+Es, glucose, clotting, and G+S/cross-match
- Other investigations to consider include ABG, ECG, chest radiograph, therapeutic drug levels (e.g. antiepileptics), and carboxyhaemoglobin

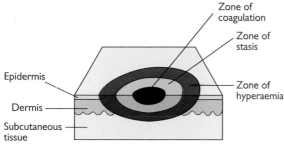

Fig 12.11 Jackson's burn wound model. This model divides the local tissue response to a burn into three-dimensional zones.

1. Zone of coagulation is at the maximum point of injury. The tissue is irreversibly damaged due to denaturation of proteins
2. Zone of stasis surrounds the zone of coagulation and is hypoperfused. The tissue is reversibly damaged and so potentially salvageable with adequate resuscitation and proper wound care
3. Zone of hyperaemia is the outer zone and has hyperperfusion. This tissue usually survives

Estimation of burn depth

There are a number of ways of describing burn depth. Clinically, burns often have varying depths and the area of each of these should be estimated. The depth of a burn gives some indication of its healing potential.

Superficial burns involving just the epidermis are not included in estimation of total burn surface area. They cause erythema as a result of local hyperaemia. Healing is rapid and without scarring.

All other burns involve the dermis to some degree and can be divided into partial- (superficial or deep) and full-thickness.

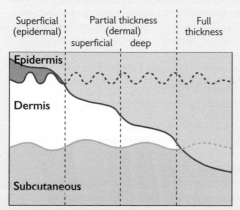

Fig 12.12 Diagram showing depth of burns.

Table 12.1 Clinical assessment of burn depth

Depth	Superficial (epidermal)	Partial-thickness (dermal)		Full-thickness
		Superficial	Deep	
Sensation	Painful	Painful	Less painful	Insensate
Appearance	Pink, dry, no blisters	Pink, wet, fine blisters	Bright red, thick blisters	Dry, leathery no hair
Blanching	Brisk	Brisk	None, fixed staining	None
Bleeding	Brisk	Brisk	Delayed	Fixed

Estimation of total burn surface area

Assessing burn area and depth can be difficult. Where possible, the burns should be cleaned and blisters de-roofed before carrying out an assessment. In major burns this is not appropriate and an initial estimate will need to be reviewed following resuscitation.

- **Wallace rule of nines** is quick and easy to estimate total burn surface area for medium or large burns, but is inaccurate for small burns and in children (use paediatric rule of tens)
- **Lund and Browder chart** is most commonly used in clinical practice as it takes account of variation in body shape with age
- **Palmar surface** can be used to estimate small (<15%) or large (>85%) burns. The patient's palm, including fingers, is thought to be about 1% of total body surface area. Rough estimate: patient's hand = 1% although this varies by sex

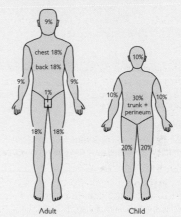

Fig 12.13 Wallace rule of nines and paediatric rule of tens.

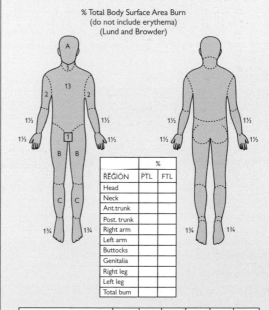

Fig 12.14 Lund and Browder chart. Reproduced from Longmore et al, (2007) Oxford *Handbook of Clinical Medicine*, 7e, with permission from Oxford University Press.

Emergency assessment will usually occur at the nearest hospital. There are now clear guidelines for referral to a regional burns unit where further expert multidisciplinary care can be provided.

Referral

The British Burns Association National Burn Injury Referral Guidelines are based on overall complexity rather than just TBSA. Complex burns need referral to a burns centre and non-complex burns to a local plastic surgery unit.

Complex

- TBSA (full-thickness or deep dermal) paediatric >5%, adult 10%
- Age <5 years or >60 years
- Chemical or acid burns
- Inhalation injury
- Burn to special areas (hands, face, perineum, flexural surfaces) or circumferential burns to limbs or chest
- Burn in a multiply injured patient
- Burn in a patient with co-morbidities

Non-complex

- Paediatric: 2–5% deep dermal and any full-thickness
- Adult: 5–10% deep dermal and smaller if full-thickness

Complex burns

Burn wound

Partial thickness burns can be managed with biologically compatible dressings such as mepitel, biobrane, opsite or duoderm. Deep dermal and full thickness wounds can be dressed daily with topical antimicrobials such as silver sulphadiazine, especially if there was a delay in transfer. The burn wound should undergo regular assessment over the first few days to check it has not deepened.

Deep partial and full thickness

Deep partial-thickness burns will invariably heal with conservative management. However, this is associated with delayed wound healing, hypertrophic scarring, and a poor aesthetic functional outcome. Surgical debridement and skin grafting is preferable.

Full thickness burns will not heal unless they are very small. Patients with large full thickness burns require surgical excision of the burn wound. This can be achieved using serial excisions, although more recently early total burn excision has been shown to reduce mortality rates and wound healing time.

Following excision, the wound needs to be closed. Sheet or narrowly meshed autologous SSG is preferable although temporary skin substitutes or allograft can be used whilst waiting for donor sites to heal and be available for repeated harvest.

Escharotomy

Circumferential full-thickness burns of the chest can restrict chest wall excursion and impair ventilation. In limbs or digits they can cause distal ischaemia. All circumferential full thickness burns require escharotomies. These can be performed either at the bedside or in theatre. Fasciotomy is usually unnecessary, except in patients with very deep burns in the extremities and burns from electrical injuries.

Inhalational injuries

Smoke inhalation is a serious complication of burn injury. Smoke contains numerous noxious chemicals, including soot and carbon monoxide.

Supraglottic injuries

- Supraglottic injuries are usually thermal. They result in rapid upper airway obstruction due to oedema
- Assessment: facial burns with swelling, burnt nasal hairs, soot in the nose or mouth, intraoral swelling, oedema on laryngoscopy, hoarseness of voice, and stridor
- Spontaneous resolution is expected, but patients may need intubation and ventilation in the short term

Subglottic injuries

- Subglottic injuries are usually chemical. The tracheobronchial mucociliary apparatus is damaged. Necrotic cellular debris, mucus, and exudate obstruct bronchi, causing atelectasis which predisposes to secondary infection
- Risk of subglottic injury is increased by fires in an enclosed space. In addition to the findings in supraglottic injuries, there may be reduced consciousness, anxiety, impaired gas exchange, and carbonaceous sputum
- ABG and chest radiograph are often normal. Carboxyhaemoglobin levels are helpful but normal levels do not exclude smoke inhalation injury. Bronchoscopy is the most useful investigation and has characteristic appearances

Management of inhalation injuries

- Chest physiotherapy
- Drug therapy: nebulized heparin (fibrinolytic), salbutamol (bronchodilator), and acetylcysteine (mucolytic)
- Therapeutic bronchoscopy removes plugs and secretions
- Mechanical ventilation with lung-protecting strategies. Early tracheostomy is indicated in patients with extensive head and neck burns and severe smoke inhalation injury

Fluid resuscitation

Vital and prompt. Give early. Following burn injury, loss of capillary integrity results in leakage of fluid and proteins from the intravascular to the interstitial space. The aim is to restore circulating volume and maintain tissue perfusion to stop the burn deepening beyond the zone of stasis. Burns >15% of total body surface area in adults and >10% in children require formal fluid resuscitation.

The Parkland formula is commonly used and calculates the volume of Hartmann's required over the first 24 h; half is given over the first 8 h and the second half is given over the next 16 h. Children are also given maintenance fluids (0.45% saline, 5% dextrose). Resuscitation is a dynamic process and patients may require additional fluids to make up for increased insensible losses (e.g. inhalation injury, pyrexia). Beware of hyponatraemia.

Total fluid in first 24 h = 4 ml x (%TBSA x body weight (kg))

The starting point is the time of injury, not the time of admission. Any fluids already given by paramedics should be subtracted from the volume required in the first 8 h. The endpoint is a urine output of 0.5–1.0 ml/kg/h for adults and 1.0–1.5 ml/kg/h in children.

Nutrition

The hypermetabolic response to a burn injury is greater than that seen with any other injury or disease state. This response can be modulated by environmental, nutritional, and hormonal manipulation.

Ambient temperature should be increased to abolish shivering and reduce evaporative heat loss. Enteral feeding (via nasoentric tube) is started as soon as possible. This preserves the integrity of gut mucosa, which reduces bacterial translocation and prevents stress ulceration.

Energy requirements should follow standard formulas, with the majority of calories coming from carbohydrates, high protein, and low fat feed. Additional vitamins and trace elements should also be given.

Infection

The burn wound is rapidly colonized and is at high risk of infection. Topical antimicrobials are used to reduce bacterial colonization. Products containing silver are particularly effective against common burn wound organisms, including *Staphylococcus aureus*, *Pseudomonas aeruginosa*, and *Candida albicans*.

Sepsis can be more difficult to diagnose in the burns patient as usual indicators are usually abnormal. Quantitative microbiological surveillance is important and invasive infection ($\geq 10^5$ organisms per gram) should be treated with appropriate antibiotics.

Non-complex (minor) burns

Non-complex and minor burns are washed with soapy water and debrided following first aid. They can then be fully assessed and dressed. Some cases will need admission for pain relief and close monitoring of the burn wound, but most can be followed-up in outpatients.

Superficial partial-thickness

Superficial partial-thickness burns should spontaneously re-epithelialize. Good analgesia allows the wounds to be properly cleaned including removal of loose epidermis and blisters. An appropriate choice of dressings then helps to maximize the speed of healing by promotion of a moist healing environment and prevention of infection. Minimizing the number of dressing changes is important for patient comfort and infection control.

Small burns (<5% TBSA) are dressed with low adherence dressings. Topical antimicrobials (e.g. Flamazine) can be added to reduce bacterial colonization. Larger burns may benefit from application of a semi-biological dressing such as Biobrane®.

Rehabilitation

This is integral to burn care and starts as early as possible, and should involve all members of the multidisciplinary team. The aims are to preserve function, improve aesthetic outcome, through scar management, and offer psychological support. The overall goal is to return the patient to independent living and their pre-injury activities.

In general burns, reconstruction can be divided into release of contractures, resurfacing of unstable or unsightly scars, and reconstruction of missing parts. Many techniques are available; however, simplicity is often a virtue.

Morbidity and mortality rates have progressively improved, with advances in early closure of the burn wound, fluid resuscitation regimes, nutrition, and antimicrobials. The delivery of burn care by specialist multidisciplinary teams in burns centres has also contributed. A child with a 95% full-thickness burn will have a 50% chance of survival in some specialist units. Morbidity is mainly associated with delay in wound healing and scarring, aesthetic outcome, and psychological well-being.

> **⊙ The 7Rs of major burn care**
>
> 1. **Rescue** the person from the burn situation and give first aid
> 2. **Resuscitate** the patient on admission to hospital
> 3. **Retrieve** the patient to a specialist burns unit if required
> 4. **Resurface** the patient's skin—dressing or grafting
> 5. **Rehabilitate** the patient to their pre-injury state
> 6. **Reconstruct** function
> 7. **Review** regularly to identify problems with patient's care

> **➲ Extra**
>
> 1. British Burns Association (britishburnsassociation.co.uk)
> 2. Burns Surgery (burnsurgery.org)
> 3. Burns prevention (firekills.gov.uk)

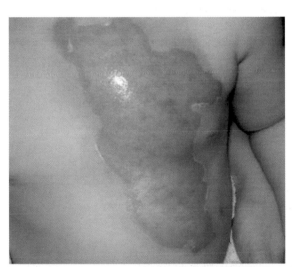

Fig 12.15 Superficial partial-thickness scald on the chest of a toddler sustained when they pulled a cup of hot tea off a table.

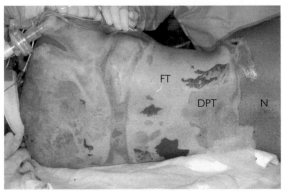

Fig 12.16 Mixed depth flame burns sustained by a black patient. Full-thickness (FT), deep partial-thickness (DPT), and normal skin (N).

12.8 Emergency hand surgery

Hand injuries are very common. They require a careful history and examination to assess both the severity of injury and risk of infection. Most injuries, whether managed conservatively or operatively, benefit from hand therapy to improve the functional outcome and reduce the risk of long-term disability.

Nail bed and finger tip injuries

Subungal haematoma

A subungal haematoma accumulates beneath the nail plate. Haematomas <25% of the nail can be drained by trephining the nail with a hot needle. Haematomas >25% of the nail require removal of the nail and repair of the nail bed.

Nail bed injury

Peak incidence is in children and young adults. The injury is usually a simple laceration, although 50% are associated with an underlying open distal phalanx fracture. If the fracture is unstable and displaced, it requires reduction and stabilization with a Kirschner wire (K-wire).

Finger tip amputation

There are many management options for amputation. These are guided by the presence of the amputated tip and its quality and whether there is exposed bone. Options include dressings, replantation, composite graft of the tip, closure with flaps (e.g. V–Y) or grafts or revision amputation. Complications include cold intolerance and hypersensitivity.

Skin and soft tissue

Loss of skin and soft tissue is commonly associated with injuries to the hand. The reconstructive ladder should be used to guide management. The aims of dorsal and volar soft tissue cover are different. Dorsal skin should be thin and elastic, whereas volar skin should be thicker but loose enough to maintain function and sensibility.

Replantation

Replantation refers to the reattachment and revascularization of an amputated part. Revascularization refers to restoration of the circulation in a devascularized part which has not been fully amputated.

Following an amputation the part should be wrapped in a piece of damp sterile gauze and placed in a bag. This bag is then placed in a further bag containing ice and water (~4°C).

Clinical assessment

- ATLS protocol—treat life-threatening injuries first. Establish tetanus status. Give broad spectrum antibiotics
- History—mechanism of injury (crush or avulsion), ischaemia time, contamination, co-morbidities, hand dominance, occupation, and treatment of amputated parts
- Plain radiographs are indicated to identify associated fractures and confirm level of amputation

Management

Initial management follows ATLS guidelines. Try and keep ischaemic time to a minimum. The aim is to restore function and cosmesis. A functionally poor outcome with good cosmesis may still be worse than an amputation if the replanted part gets in the way.

Infections of the hand

Paronychia

Paronychia is infection of the perionychium or eponychium. Acute infection is very common and is mainly caused by *Staphylococcus aureus*. Chronic infection is usually caused by *Candida albicans*. The hyponychium is most resistant to infection. Early infection can be managed with oral antibiotics and warm soaks. A pointing abscess should be incised and drained. Complete removal of the nail may be needed for adequate decompression.

Felon

A felon is a subcutaneous infection of the distal pulp space of a digit. It presents as a tense swelling of the finger distal to the distal interphalangeal joint associated with throbbing pain. Initially, it can be managed conservatively with antibiotics. Surgical incision and drainage is indicated if there is fluctulance in the pulp.

Flexor sheath infection

Infection of the flexor tendon sheath is usually caused by a penetrating injury to the volar surface of the finger. Purulent infection can rapidly destroy the gliding mechanism, cause adhesions, and lead to necrosis of the tendon.

Four cardinal signs of acute flexor sheath infection:

1. semi-flexed position of the finger
2. fusiform swelling of finger (like a sausage)
3. excessive tenderness limited to the course of the flexor tendon
4. severe pain along the flexor tendon on passive extension of the finger

Early infections (<12 h) can initially be treated with IV antibiotics; however, there should be a low threshold for surgical decompression and washout.

Deep space infections

The palm has three potential spaces (thenar, midpalmar, and hypothenar). Abscess formation is usually caused by a penetrating injury. Hand radiographs are used to exclude a foreign body. Management is with broad spectrum IV antibiotics and early surgical incision and drainage.

Animal and human bites

The majority of animal bites are from dogs. Any bites from outside the UK must be assumed to be at risk of rabies and post-exposure prophylaxis must be given. Cat bites have a higher rate of bacterial infection, commonly with *Pasteurella multocida*.

Human bites often occur during fights when a closed fist makes contact with teeth. Tendons and joints are at risk of injury, and inoculation with oral bacteria (e.g. *Eikenella corrodens*) can lead to wound infections.

All types of bite wound should undergo thorough wound toilet and are left to heal by secondary intention or delayed primary intention. The use of prophylactic antibiotics is controversial, but many units give 48 h of broad spectrum intravenous antibiotics followed by a course of co-amoxiclav.

> ### ✚ Nail bed repair
>
> Isolated nail bed lacerations should be repaired early under a digital nerve block and finger tourniquet.
>
> #### Procedure
>
> - Patient supine with hand out on hand table
> - Digital nerve block
> - Prep and drape hand then apply a finger tourniquet
> - Remove the nail, irrigate the underlying nail bed, and debride any non-viable tissue
> - Repair the nail bed and nail fold (6/0 absorbable suture)
> - Splint the nail fold open by replacing the nail or using a substitute
> - Release the tourniquet
>
> #### Complications
>
> Patients should be warned of the potential for abnormal or absent nail growth. Infection is also a risk.

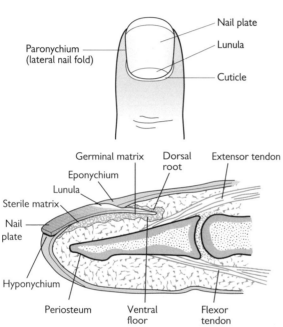

Fig 12.17 Anatomy of the finger nail.

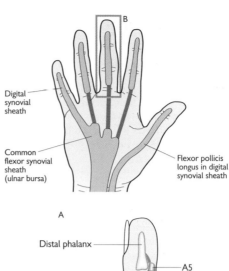

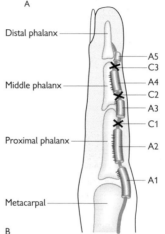

Fig 12.18 (A) Anterior view of flexor synovial sheaths. (B) Lateral view of fibro-osseous digital sheath showing the annular and cruciate pulleys. The pulleys prevent bowstringing of the tendons during flexion (especially A2 and A4).

12.9 Tendon injuries

Flexor tendon injuries

Flexor anatomy

- Flexor digitorum profundus (FDP) flexes the DIPJ of the index, middle, ring, and little fingers
- Flexor digitorum superficialis (FDS) flexes the proximal interphalangeal joint (PIPJ) of the index, middle, ring, and little fingers
- Flexor pollicis longus flexes the thumb

The flexors enter the hand through the carpal tunnel. They cross the palm and then enter their respective fibro-osseous digital sheaths. Their nutrient supply comes from both the vincula system of small blood vessels and diffusion from the synovial fluid within the sheath.

Clinical assessment

Preserved movement with increased pain or weakness suggests a partial tendon injury.

- Position and extent of soft tissue injury
- Neurovascular status of the hand
- FDP injury: unable to flex DIPJ of affected digit actively whilst its PIPJ is kept extended along with all the uninvolved digits
- FDS injury: unable to flex metacarpophalangeal joint (MCPJ) of affected digit actively whilst all uninvolved digits are kept extended
- Plain radiographs of the affected digit if a fracture is likely

Management

Complete division and partial tendon lacerations >50% of the cross-sectional area are usually repaired.

Zone I

Avulsion of FDP from its insertion into the distal phalanx may or may not take a fragment of bone. The tendon is reattached to the bone. If attached to a large fragment, this can be K-wired or screwed back in place.

Laceration leaving a stump of FDP <1 cm allows direct advancement of the FDP and primary repair to the bone. If the stump is >1 cm, a primary tendon repair is performed.

Zone II

Zone II injuries can usually be primarily repaired. The proximal tendon will often have to be retrieved from the palm (see box).

Zones III, IV, and V

These are approached in a similar way to more distal injuries. Lacerations frequently injure multiple tendons and also involve neurovascular structures (e.g. median or ulnar nerves, and radial or ulnar arteries). There is less risk of adhesions causing impaired function.

Extensor tendon injuries

Extensor anatomy

The extensor tendon divides at the proximal half of the proximal phalanx into three slips, one central and two lateral. Wing tendons form interossei on the ulnar side and interossei and lumbricals on the radial side.

- Wrist extensors are extensor carpi radialis longus (ECRL) and brevis (ECRB), and extensor carpi ulnaris (ECU)

- Thumb extensors are abductor pollicis longus (APL), extensor pollicis brevis (EPB), and extensor pollicis longus (EPL)
- Finger extensors are extensor indicis proprius (EIP), extensor digitorum communis (EDC), and extensor digiti minimi (EDM)

The fascia surrounding the extensors condenses at the wrist to form the extensor retinaculum. The space below is divided in to six compartments.

Extensor compartments (radial to ulnar)

1. APL, EPB
2. ECRL, ECRB through floor of anatomical snuff box
3. EPL bends around Lister's tubercle which separates it from the second compartment
4. EDC, EIP
5. EDM
6. ECU

Clinical assessment

The skin on the dorsum of the hand is thin and has little subcutaneous fat. The extensor tendons are therefore superficial and prone to injury. Examine each finger in turn. Check for passive and active movement and extensor lag.

Management

Management depends on the zone of injury and clinical findings. Distal injuries with active but weak movement with no lag can often be managed conservatively.

Open repair of distal injuries is with a simple running mattress suture. It is often possible to place a core suture in zone V and more proximal injuries.

Zone I—mallet finger

Mallet finger is a characteristic flexion deformity of the DIPJ owing to disruption of the terminal slip and the loss of extension. The injury is usually a result of forced flexion of the extended finger tip. There may be an associated avulsion fracture of the distal phalanx. Management is usually conservative, with immobilization of the DIPJ in extension using a splint for 6 weeks. Open repair is considered if there is skin loss or a displaced distal phalanx fracture.

A mallet finger can develop into a swan neck deformity if left (hyperextension of PIPJ with flexion of DIPJ).

Zone III—Boutonnière deformity

A Boutonnière deformity occurs if the central slip is divided over the PIPJ before it inserts into the base of the middle phalanx. This lets the lateral bands slip to the volar side of the PIPJ where they act to flex the joint. With time they also cause hyperextension of the DIPJ. Acute closed Boutonnière injuries are usually splinted with the PIPJ in extension. Open injuries with an extensor lag need surgical repair.

Zone V

Zone V injuries over the MCPJ are often the result of a 'fight bite.' The closed fist makes contact with the opponent's mouth, causing a laceration that may involve the joint. However, the wound often looks superficial and inocuous when the finger is extended. Antibiotics, wound exploration +/- delayed repair, and closure is needed (📖 Topic 12.7).

➕ Zone II flexor tendon repair

There have been a number of different techniques described. A modified Kessler technique is the most commonly taught core suture technique. Tendon injuries associated with neurovascular injury are an emergency; otherwise they are best repaired within 3 weeks.

Procedure

- Patient supine with arm out on hand table. High brachial tourniquet (250 mmHg)
- Wound extended proximally and distally to allow adequate exposure
- Retrieve the proximal tendon end and secure ready for repair. A small incision at the distal palmar crease may be needed for access and the A4 pulley may have to be dilated
- Place two continuous modified Kessler core sutures (four-strand technique) using 3/0 or 4/0 non-absorbable suture. Strength of repair is related to the number of strands crossing the gap. The transverse parts should be approximately 1 cm from the ends being repaired
- Placing a running peripheral (epitendinous) suture makes a major contribution to strength, reduces gapping, and smooths the edges of the repair. Use a 6/0 Prolene suture. Then close the skin
- Hand therapy referral

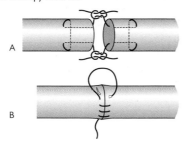

Fig 12.19 A Modified Kessler core suture; **B** Running epitendinous suture.

Complications

Intraoperative and early	Intermediate and late
• Nerve injury	• Adhesions between FDP/FDS
• Re-rupture (~POD 10)	• Contracture PIPJ ± DIPJ

Hand therapy

Postoperative regimes will be specific to the tendon repaired and the zone of injury. Early referral for hand therapy is essential, and exercises following zone II flexor tendon injuries should ideally commence within 48 h of repair.

The regime will usually include controlled active exercises or specific passive exercises to minimize tendon adhesions through protected tendon movement, with the ultimate aim of achieving maximum function. The hand therapist will need to know exactly which structures have been repaired. Details of the injury or repair that may compromise tendon healing are also helpful in guiding the choice of regime and any modifications to it (e.g. segmental injury or repair under tension). The plaster of Paris backslab applied in theatre is usually replaced by a custom-made thermoplastic splint which remains on the hand at all times for up to 6 weeks, depending on the level and site of the tendon injury. The tendon may take up to 3 months to heal to full strength, and therapy may continue for longer.

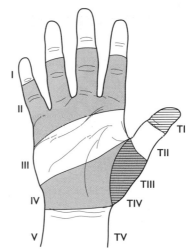

Fig 12.20 A Flexor tendon zones. I, insertion of FDP; II, from FDS insertion to the A1 pulley (distal palmar crease); III, between distal palmar crease and distal extent of carpal tunnel; IV, carpal tunnel; V, proximal to carpal tunnel.

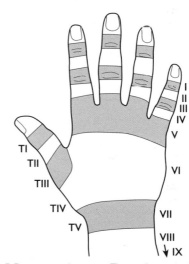

Fig 12.21 B. Extensor tendon zones. The tendons cross 8 zones (zone IX added for forearm musculature). The thumb has 6 zones although zones V and VI are shared with the digital extensor tendons. Digital zones: I – DIPJ (mallet injury), II – over middle phalanx (central slip going to DP), III – PIPJ, IV – over proximal phalanx, V – MCPJ, VI – dorsum of hand (metacarpals), VII – dorsal retinaculum, VIII – distal forearm.

Peripheral nerve injuries are common. They are frequently associated with vascular injuries and fractures owing to their anatomical relations.

Aetiology
Traumatic injuries can stretch, compress or lacerate nerves. Stretch and compressive injuries tend to be closed and continuity is retained. Lacerations are more likely to cause complete transection.

Classification and pathophysiology
Seddon classified nerve injury into three categories; Sunderland later expanded them to five.

1. **Neuropraxia** is a temporary physiological block to nerve conduction with focal demyelination. There is mild local demyelination at most and so recovery is quick without the need for true regeneration
2. **Axontmesis** is disruption of the axon while the sheath remains in continuity. Axontmesis and neurotmesis lead to axonal (Wallerian) degeneration of the distal axon. The axon is degraded and removed by local macrophages and Schwann cells, leaving only a sheath. This then guides the axon as it regenerates at 1 mm/day in adults
3. **Neurotmesis** is complete transection of the nerve axon and sheath. Neurotmesis also leads to axonal degeneration but because of the lack of continuity has a lower potential for useful regeneration

Clinical assessment
Clinical signs of nerve injury include alteration or loss of sensation and motor function.

Investigations
Plain radiographs may be indicated following acute injury if an associated fracture is suspected. Electrodiagnostic studies are not performed acutely, but are done after at least 3 weeks and then again at 2 months.

- Electromyography is performed >3 weeks following injury. When a needle is inserted, normal muscle shows a brief burst of activity whereas fibrillations or no electrical activity is detected in denervated muscle. When activated, normal muscle shows a full interference pattern of motor unit potentials (MUP). Innervated muscle following a nerve injury shows reduced activation and recruitment of MUPs
- Nerve conduction studies (NCS) assess the large myelinated fibres of motor and sensory neurons carrying vibration and light touch but not pain or temperature. Recorded parameters include duration, amplitude, latency, and conduction velocity

Management
Conservative
Closed injuries can be observed. Electrodiagnostic studies are performed at 3 weeks and again at 2 months. If there is no sign of recovery at 6 months, surgical exploration is considered.

- Splints and other supports help to protect and offload joints
- Physiotherapy at an early stage helps to maintain a good passive range of movement and strength in unaffected muscles

Operative
- Open lacerations should be explored and a primary repair performed if the gap is <2.5 cm
- Nerve graft is considered when the gap is >2.5 cm to give a tension-free repair

Complications and prognosis
Outcome from neuropraxia is usually excellent, with full recovery within 6 weeks. Prognosis is poor for axontmesis and neurotmesis.

Upper limb

Brachial plexus (C5–T1)
Injuries are either traumatic (high energy RTC) or obstetric (forceps delivery).

- Upper plexus lesions (Erb–Duchenne palsy) are caused by excessive traction or rupture of C5 and C6 nerve roots. Weakness of rotators of the shoulder, arm flexors, and hand extensors leaves the upper limb held in a 'waiter's tip' position with medial rotation of the arm and pronation of the forearm and flexion of the wrist
- Lower plexus lesions (Klumpke's palsy) are much rarer, and are caused by excessive traction on C8 and T1 nerve roots during extension of the upper limb. A clawed hand develops due to paralysis of the intrinsic hand muscles and weakness of the ulnar flexors

Long thoracic nerve of Bell (C5,6,7)
Traumatic injury results in paralysis of serratus anterior and winging of the scapula.

Median nerve (medial and lateral cords C5–8, T1)
Anatomy

- Motor: PT, FCR, FDP (radial half), FDS, PL, FPL, PQ; 'LOAF' (1st and 2nd **l**umbricals, **O**P, **A**PB, **F**PB).
- Sensory: palmar cutaneous branch (radial half of the palm and the palmar surface of the radial three and a half fingers as well as the nail beds)

Injury at elbow or above

- Arm held supine
- Weak wrist flexion with wrist held adducted (FCU, FDP, FCR paralysed)
- Index and middle fingers stay extended when making a fist (long flexors paralysed except for part of FDP supplied by ulnar)
- Thumb is laterally rotated and adducted owing to paralysis of the thenar eminence which wastes over time
- Sensory changes in the median distribution

Injury at the wrist

- Paralysis of the thenar eminence and sensory changes in the median nerve distribution

Radial nerve (posterior cord C5–C7)
Anatomy

- Motor: triceps (long, medial, and lateral heads), anconeus, brachialis (lateral part), brachioradialis (small part), ECRL, ECRB, supinator, ED, EDM, FCU, APL, EPL, EPB, EI
- Sensory: posterior cutaneous nerve of arm, lower lateral cutaneous nerve of arm, posterior cutaneous nerve of forearm, superficial branch of radial nerve (radial side of dorsum of hand and radial three and a half fingers)

Axilla injury

- Loss of elbow, wrist, and finger extension (wrist drop caused by unopposed flexors of the wrist)
- Loss of grip strength due to wrist held flexed.
- Supination preserved by biceps brachii
- Variable sensory loss down posterior arm and forearm

Mid-humerus (spiral groove injury)

- Preserved elbow extension
- Wrist drop
- Sensory loss

At or below elbow forearm injury

- Forearm injury (posterior interosseous branch) means
  - Supinator and ECRL preserved
  - No wrist drop owing to ECRL action
  - No sensory loss

Ulnar nerve (medial cord C8, T1)

Anatomy

- Motor: FCU, FDP (ulnar half), ADM, FDM, ODM, AP, third and fourth lumbricals, seven interossei, PB
- Sensory: joints (elbow, wrist, hand), palmar cutaneous branch (ulnar side of dorsum of hand and ulnar one and a half fingers), posterior cutaneous branch

Injury at the elbow

- Claw hand due to hyperextension of the MCPJ and flexion of the IPJ
- Loss of adduction and abduction of the fingers (intrinsic hand muscles except 'LOAF' paralysed)
- Froment's sign—flexion of terminal phalanx and contraction of flexor pollicis longus used to grip a piece of paper between thumb and index finger, indicating weak AP

- Wrist abducts when flexed (paralysis of ulnar flexors)
- Wasting of the ulnar border of the forearm, hypothenar eminence, and between the metacarpal bones
- Sensory change ulnar one and a half fingers

Injury at the wrist

- The FDP and FCU are spared, which results in a worse claw hand (ulnar paradox). The wasting of the hypothenar eminence and intrinsic hand muscles remain, as does the sensory loss

Lower limb

Sciatic nerve (L4,5, S12)

The sciatic nerve is derived from the lumbosacral plexus. It innervates the hamstrings, all muscles below the knee, and sensation below the knee.

Injury at the hip joint causes loss of knee flexion and movement in the ankle and foot. There is altered sensation over the foot, posterolateral calf, and posterior thigh.

Injuries following trauma often resolve spontaneously. Deficit following surgery needs re-exploration.

Common peroneal nerve (L4,5)

The common peroneal nerve is a terminal branch of the sciatic nerve. It innervates the anterior and lateral compartments of the leg and sensation to the dorsum of the foot and the dorsal surface of the first web space.

It is typically injured at the neck of the fibula. This results in a dropped foot and altered sensation over the dorsum of the foot and lateral aspect of the leg. If there is no recovery, a tendon transfer can be use to improve the foot drop.

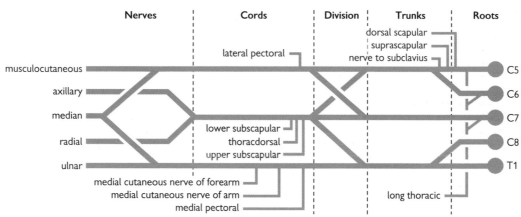

Fig 12.22 Diagram of the brachial plexus (C5, 6, 7, 8, T1).

Dupuytren's disease

Dupuytren's disease (DD) is a progressive fibroproliferative disorder characterized by benign thickening and contracture of the palmar and digital fascia, leading to permanent contracture of the digits. It usually involves both hands. It most commonly affects men over 50 years old (M:F 5:1). There is an increased incidence in northern Europe (Celtic origin).

Aetiology

Aetiology is unknown but it is associated with other fibroproliferative conditions, including Garrod's pads of the knuckles; penile fibrous plaques (Peyronie's disease) and plantar fibromatosis (Lederhose disease).

Risk factors

- Family history (30% have a first degree relative with DD)
- Diabetes mellitus
- Chronic alcohol abuse
- Anticonvulsant therapy in epileptics
- Hand trauma

Pathophysiology

DD is a progressive disease. During the early stages fibroblasts predominate. These are replaced by myofibroblasts as the contractures develop. Clinically, its development can be divided into three phases.

1. Thickening and nodularity develops adjacent to the distal palmar crease
2. Contracture begins with palpable cords proximal to the nodules
3. Significant contracture with tendinous cords but no nodules

Clinical assessment

The cardinal features are a nodule in the palm, cords running up to the digits, and flexion contracture at the MCPJ and PIPJ in the affected digits. The range of movement in the fingers should be documented.

Management

Management depends on how disabling the patient finds the disease. Conservative options include splinting and steroid injections, but these are rarely successful.

Surgery will not completely remove or prevent disease but can reduce deformity and improve function (see box).

Indications for surgery

- Painful palmar nodules
- MCPJ flexion >30°
- PIPJ contracture
- Thumb deformity

Complications and prognosis

The disease is incurable. Recurrence rates vary and may be lower following dermofasciectomy.

> ### ➔ Extra
>
> #### Dupuytren's disease
> The disease process seen in Dupuytren's disease was first described by Sir Astley Cooper [1768–1841, English surgeon] and then by Baron Guillaume Dupuytren [1777–1835, French surgeon] in 1831.

Carpal tunnel syndrome

Carpal tunnel syndrome (CTS) describes the features associated with compression of the median nerve in the carpal tunnel. It is often bilateral.

Most patients are over 40 years old, and there is a female preponderance (F:M 6:1).

Aetiology and pathophysiology

Most cases are idiopathic. Risk factors include female sex, pregnancy, diabetes mellitus, rheumatoid arthritis, obesity, alcoholism, and hypothyroidism.

Compression causes ischaemia of the nerve and subsequent fibrosis and degeneration.

Clinical assessment

History

- Pain, numbness, and tingling in radial two and a half fingers
- Weakness or clumsiness of the hand
- Worse at night. Relieved by exercising the hand and dangling the arm out of bed

Examination

- Paraesthesia or numbness in median distribution. Wasting of thenar eminence and weakness of thumb abduction (APB) occur late
- Tinel's sign—the course of a nerve is lightly percussed from distal to proximal. At the point of nerve regeneration (i.e. carpal tunnel), a positive test elicits tingling in the nerve's distribution
- Phalen's test is positive if pressure of the carpal tunnel with flexion of the wrist reproduces the symptoms felt by the patient

Investigations

Electrodiagnostic tests (NCS and EMG) help to confirm the clinical diagnosis of CTS. NCS show prolonged sensory and motor latencies in the median nerve, with decreased amplitude. Normal latency does not exclude CTS. EMG is usually normal until late in the disease process. These studies may also help to exclude more proximal compression caused by cervical disc disease and other neuropathies.

Management

Night timing splinting with the wrist held in neutral, local steroid injection, and NSAIDs are all possible modes of conservative therapy. Relief of symptoms following steroid injection is a good prognostic indicator for success following surgical decompression.

Operative

Carpal tunnel decompression is recommended if conservative therapy fails. The open approach (see box) is often favoured, although minimally invasive and one or two port endoscopic techniques are used with success.

Minimal and endoscopic techniques reduce the scar but increase the risk of nerve injury and incomplete release.

Complications and prognosis

Carpel tunnel decompression is successful in most cases. Recurrence may be caused by incomplete division of the transverse carpal ligament, compression by scar tissue or flexor tenosynovitis. Re-exploration is warranted if Phalen's and NCS remain positive after 3–6 months.

Ganglion cysts

Ganglion cysts are the most common soft tissue tumour of the hand. The highest incidence is in middle-aged women. They contain mucin and are usually attached to an adjacent joint capsule, tendon or tendon sheath. They are usually solitary and can be associated with almost every joint in the hand, although they are usually found in specific locations such as the dorsum of the wrist. A **mucous cyst** is a ganglion of the DIPJ.

Patients present for a variety of reasons, including poor cosmesis, pain, weakness, and concern regarding malignant potential. Conservative management includes injection of sclerosing agents (hyaluronic acid) and aspiration. Excision using an open or arthroscopic technique is used if conservative management fails. The main complication is recurrence, which is usually caused by incomplete excision.

⊕ Dupuytren's disease surgery

The key aim of surgery is to reduce the contracture and restore hand function. There are three challenges. (1) the skin, which may be of poor quality; (2) the fascial disease; and (3) joint contractures. Warn the patient about the high risk of recurrence.

Procedure

- GA or brachial plexus block
- Hand supine on hand table with arm tourniquet
- Many skin incisions have been described. They should take account of the planned procedure, i.e. fasciectomy or dermofasciectomy
- The fasciectomy is described in terms of how radical it is. A very limited approach aims to remove enough fascia to release the contracture. Limited removes all of the diseased fascia, and a radical approach removes uninvolved fascia in an attempt to reduce recurrence
- PIPJ contracture poses more of a problem than the MCPJ and its release remains controversial
- Loose wound closure is important. Dermofasciectomy is closed with a full-thickness skin graft taken from the forearm or groin.

Complications

Intraoperative and early	Late
● Digital nerve injury	● Recurrence
● Digital artery injury	● Loswss of finger flexion
● Haematoma	● CRPS
● Infection	
● Skin flap necrosis	

⊕ Open carpel tunnel decompression

Document preoperative examination of the upper limb and pain distribution.

Procedure

- LA or regional anaesthesia
- Hand supine on hand table with arm tourniquet
- 3 cm skin incision parallel and ulnar to the thenar crease. Avoid the palmar cutaneous branch in the distal part of the incision
- Under direct vision, divide the transverse carpal ligament from distal to proximal on the ulnar side of the nerve to avoid the motor branch. Push the scalpel down in slow controlled movements on to an instrument to protect the median nerve
- Direct skin closure and local anaesthetic to the wound if not already used
- Hand therapy can start on day 2 or 3. Night-time splinting should continue for a couple of weeks

Complications

Intraoperative and early	Intermediate and late
● Haematoma	● Recurrence
● Nerve injury (recurrent motor branch of median)	
● Incomplete division of ligament	

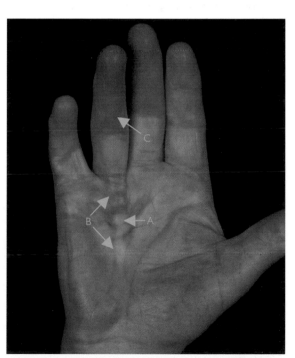

Fig 12.23 Dupuytren's disease of the fourth ray of the right hand. Classic signs include: (A) palmar nodule; (B) palpable cords; and (C) fixed flexion contracture of ring finger

Cutaneous malignant melanoma (MM) is a tumour of epidermal melanocytes. It accounts for ~4% of skin cancers but >75% of all skin cancer-related deaths. Its incidence in the UK has doubled over the past 10 years and it is now the most common cancer in 20–40-year-olds, with an incidence of 10 per 100 000 per annum in the UK.

The peak age is 50–60 years. It is slightly more common in women (F:M 1.3:1) and most common in fair-skinned people (very rare in blacks).

Prevention
Preventative measures are targeted at the general population to try and reduce the risk of melanoma. Countries such as Australia have run very successful public health campaigns such as 'slip, slop, slap' (slip on a t-shirt, slop on some sun cream, slap on a hat).

- Use clothing to protect against sun exposure
- Avoid sunbeds
- Broad spectrum sunscreens (sun protection factor of 30+)
- Avoid direct exposure to intense sunshine (i.e. midday sun)
- Children and people with fair complexion need to take particular care

Aetiology
The aetiology is multifactorial, involving both genetic and environmental factors. Ultraviolet light exposure (UVB in sunlight) is the most important risk factor for developing MM.

Risk factors
- Increased numbers of dysplastic naevi or a giant congenital melanocytic hairy naevus (>5% total body surface area)
- Unusually high sun exposure, especially during childhood
- Blistering sun burns
- Previous malignant melanoma
- Skin type (fair or red hair and pale complexion)
- Family history (first degree relative with MM)
- Immunosuppressed state, e.g. transplant patients

Pathophysiology
Melanocytes are derived from neural crest cells. Only ~10% of melanomas arise in a pre-existing naevus. In <5% of cases there is no primary tumour identified and MM presents with lymph node disease or distant metastasis (lung, liver, and brain). There are four main cutaneous histological subtypes.

1. Superficial spreading melanoma (65%)
2. Nodular melanoma (20%)
3. Lentigo maligna melanoma (Hutchinson's melanotic freckle) is the invasive from of lentigo maligna (LM; melanoma *in situ*). Up to 50% of LM will become invasive
4. Acral lentiginous melanoma is found on the palms, soles, subungual, and myocutaneous junctions. It is the most common MM in dark-skinned populations

Clinical assessment
Diagnostic accuracy has been improved by using the ABCDE system to assess pigmented lesions. Nodular and amelanotic melanoma may not exhibit these features and require a high index of suspicion. Local lymph nodes should also be examined.

ABCDE system
A   Asymmetry in two axes
B   Border irregularity (ragged, notched, or blurred)
C   Colour variegation: non-uniform shades of brown and black; white, red, or blue discoloration is of concern
D   Diameter >6 mm
E   Evolving: changes in the lesion over time are characteristic; ulceration and bleeding

Investigations
Suspicious lesions should be fast-tracked for excision biopsy. Non-excisional biopsy may lead to inadequate histology and should be avoided. Essential features of a melanoma pathology report include:

- Breslow thickness
- Clark level (if Breslow thickness <1 mm)
- ulceration
- growth phase
- regression
- lymphovascular invasion and microscopic satellites
- microscopic margins (mm)

Histological prognostic indicators
- Breslow thickness is the single most important prognostic indicator. It is measured from the stratum granulosum to the deepest part of the tumour: superficial <1 mm; intermediate 1–4 mm; deep >4 mm
- Clark level defines the depth of invasion by anatomical level and is a strong prognostic indicator in tumours with a Breslow thickness <1 mm

Clark levels
I   Confined to epidermis
II   Invasion into papillary dermis
III   Filling of papillary dermis
IV   Filling of papillary dermis
V   Invasion into subcutaneous fat

- Growth phase correlates strongly with prognosis. Vertical growth conveys a worse prognosis than radial growth
- Epidermal ulceration is a prognostic indicator
- Regression
- Lymphovascular invasion
- Histiogenic type and melanoma cell type do not appear to influence prognosis

Further investigations
Imaging techniques, such as chest radiography, ultrasound and CT scan, and blood tests have been shown to be unhelpful in assessing the extent of disease and likelihood of metastasis. However, they are used to stage advanced disease and their use in follow-up of asymptomatic patients is debated.

Staging
TNM classification of melanoma
Primary tumour
T1   ≤1 mm*
T2   1.01–2 mm
T3   2.01–4 mm
T4   >4 mm

Regional lymph nodes

N1	1 node
N2	2–3 nodes
N3	≥4 nodes

Distant metastasis

M1	Distant skin, subcutaneous or nodal metastasis
M2	Lung metastasis
M3	All other visceral metastasis, any distant metastasis

*Breslow thickness

Overall stage grouping and survival

Stage	TNM category	Breslow	5-year survival
0	Tis, N0, M0	≤1 mm	97%
IA	T1a, N0, M0	≤1 mm	95%
IB	T1b or T2a, N0, M0	1.01–2 mm	90%
IIA	T2b or T3a, N0, M0	2.01–4 mm	85%
IIB	T3b or T4a, N0, M0	>4mm	75%
IIC	T4b, N0, M0	>4 mm	50%
III	any T, N1–3, M0	>4 mm	45%
IV	any T, any N, any M	>4mm	10%

Management

Excision biopsy is usually diagnostic. Following this, definitive treatment is achieved by wide local excision (WLE). The margin used is determined by Breslow thickness (see table).

Recommended WLE surgical excision margins

TNM	Breslow	Margin
pTis	*In situ*	2–5 mm
pT1	< 1 mm	1 cm
pT2	1–2 mm	1–2 cm
pT3	2.1–4 mm	2 cm
pT4	>4 mm	2 cm

Regional lymph nodes

Nodal metastasis is the most significant predictor of outcome in MM. The risk increases with tumour depth (60% in tumours >4 mm thick).

Palpable lymph nodes should undergo FNAC. Confirmation of metastatic deposits is an indication for radical dissection of that lymph node basin.

Impalpable nodes can undergo sentinel node biopsy. This provides a method of earlier detection of nodal metastases before they become clinically apparent. It identifies the first node in the local lymph node basin that would drain the lesion and thus is at the greatest risk of metastatic disease. There is not yet definitive evidence of improved survival using this technique.

Isolated limb perfusion

This technique allows the localized delivery of high dose chemotherapy to recurrent disease in an isolated lower limb below the knee. More recently, isolated infusion using percutaneous interventional radiology has reduced complications.

Stage II and III disease

Adjuvant therapy in stage II and III disease is mainly experimental. Radiotherapy following lymph node dissection is not indicated and other options such as immunotherapy are being trialled.

Stage IV disease

Survival in patients with stage IV disease is limited (6–9 months). Surgery to remove metastatic deposits may prolong survival and prevent complications such as ulceration.

There is little evidence that chemotherapy or chemoimmunotherapy is beneficial although dacarbazine is often given.

MM is relatively radioresistant, although radiotherapy is often helpful in symptom control of bone metastases.

Complications and prognosis

Recurrence is the main complication. Wound complications associated with any excision are minimal. The main one to avoid is incomplete excision that will require a further procedure. Lymphoedema of the upper or lower limbs may complicate axillary or groin lymph node dissections.

All invasive melanomas need follow-up, which should be prolonged in those with stage III disease. The annual risk of recurrence for tumours <1.5 mm thick is <6 % in the first 5 years and then 1% thereafter. *In situ* melanoma does not need follow-up.

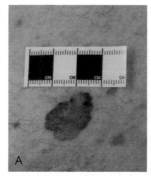
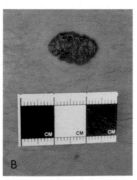

Fig 12.24 (A)Superficial spreading melanoma; (B) Nodular malignant melanoma.

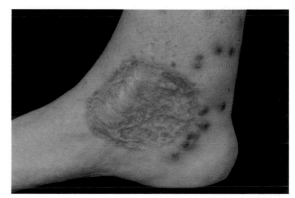

Fig 12.25 MM nodules next to a skin graft used to resurface the defect left by the primary resection.

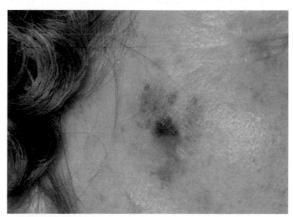

Fig 12.26 Lentigo MM.

Basal cell carcinoma

Basal cell carcinoma (BCC; basal cell epithelioma, rodent ulcer) is a malignant neoplasm derived from the basal cell layer of the skin. BCC is the commonest malignant skin neoplasm in Caucasians but is rare in non-Caucasians. Incidence is 5 per 1000 population per year. It is most common in later life (>50 years) with a male preponderance (M:F 3:2).

Aetiology

The main causes are chronic exposure to sunlight (ultraviolet radiation) and ionizing radiation. Pale skin, tendency to freckle, and high sun exposure are risk factors. Rarely, BCC may be inherited (e.g. Gorlin syndrome).

Pathophysiology

BCC arise from pluripotential cells of the basal layer of the epithelium or pilosebaceous follicles. There are five main clinical and histological subtypes. It is important clinically to try and differentiate between them as some are more aggressive (micronodular, infiltrating, and morpheaform tumours).

1. Nodular BCC are the most common subtype. They are often found on the face. If the contents can be expressed, they are termed cystic
2. Superficial BCC are pink/brown scaly papules with a low risk of local infiltration but they bleed easily
3. Micronodular BCC are aggressive. They have a well defined edge and rarely ulcerate
4. Infiltrating and morpheaform BCC look sclerotic and ill defined and have the appearance of scar tissue. They rarely ulcerate or bleed

Clinical assessment

Over 90% are on sun-exposed sites (face, scalp, and dorsum of hands). Patients present with a slow-growing skin lesion (often multiple lesions). They classically appear as a pink or pearly translucent mass with telangiectasia and a well defined rolled border. They may have an area of central ulceration. There is unlikely to be regional lymphadenopathy as BCC rarely metastasize. Diagnosis is confirmed histologically from a biopsy specimen.

Management

Small superficial BCC can be managed with topical drugs or immune modulating agents. More aggressive subtypes need excision.

- Surgical excision should be with margins of 3–5 mm for well defined primary tumours
- Topical 5-fluorouracil (5-FU) and external beam radiotherapy can be used as adjuvant therapy
- Mohs micrographic surgery giving frozen section margin control has the lowest recurrence rates and is used in high risk areas such as the face
- Cautery, and curettage and cryotherapy are useful on superficial non-aggressive lesions
- Imiquimod 5% cream modifies the cell-mediated immune response and induces apoptosis in the tumour cells. The length and intensity of treatment is tailored to the patient but is usually over a period of 6 weeks. It can be used on early, small superficial BCC

Complications and prognosis

Patients require follow-up and are advised on self-examination to detect recurrence. Management of incompletely excised tumours varies, ranging from further excision to watchful waiting. Two-thirds of recurrences occur in the first 3 years. Patients rarely die from BCC.

Squamous cell carcinoma

Squamous cell carcinoma (SCC; squamous epithelioma) is derived from keratinocytes of the epidermis or its appendages. It is the second most common skin cancer. Incidence is 1 per 1000 per year and increases with age (>70 years). It is most common in men (M:F 2:1) and Caucasians.

Aetiology

The main cause is chronic exposure to ultraviolet and ionizing radiation. Risk factors include fair skin, advanced age, severe sun burns, immunosuppression (transplant, leukaemia, lymphoma), and human papilloma virus infection.

Pathophysiology

Histology shows dermal invasion of atypical Malpighian cells. Well differentiated neoplasms exhibit parakeratosis and keratin pearls. Actinic keratoses can go on to SCC *in situ* (Bowen's disease) and they can also form in burns scars (Marjolin's ulcer).

SCC have a low metastasis rate via lymphatic spread and, rarely, haematogenously. High-risk factors include location (lip and ear), diameter (>2 cm), depth (>4 mm), and histological differentiation.

Clinical assessment

They present as painless slow-growing skin lesions commonly found on sun-exposed areas. They have a variable morphology but are often indurated nodular keratinizing tumours with central ulceration. They may present as an ulcer without keratinization. Metastatic spread is usually a late feature. Diagnosis is made histologically from a biopsy specimen.

Management

There are three main factors that influence treatment.

1. Aim to excise or treat the primary SCC completely
2. Possibility of local 'in transit' metastases
3. Likelihood of lymphatic spread to lymph nodes

Operative

- Surgical excision is the treatment of choice for the majority of cutaneous SCC. For well defined tumours <2 cm in diameter the margins should be over 5 mm. High-risk tumours require margins over 1 cm
- Curettage and electrosurgery or cryosurgery for small well defined low-risk tumours
- Mohs micrographic surgery for high-risk and recurrent tumours

Complications and prognosis

Patients require follow-up and are advised on self-examination to detect recurrence. They must also protect their skin from the sun.

⊕ Excision of a skin lesion

The aim is to excise the lesion completely and send it for histological examination.

Procedure

1. **Mark**—use pen to mark the extent of the lesion, the required margin, and method of closure depending on location and skin availability
2. **Infiltrate** area with local anaesthetic slowly and avoid entering lesion. Use LA with adrenaline if no end arteries
3. **Prep** the area with cleaning agent
4. **Drape** the area to create a sterile field
5. **Excise** skin lesion, taking cuff of fat or down to fascia. The margins of clinically normal-looking skin depend on the type of lesion
6. **Marker** suture in superior pole of specimen (not through lesion) and send for histology
7. **Close** the wound with appropriate choice of suture
8. **Dress** the wound
9. **Follow-up** the patient by arranging removal of sutures, wound check, and outpatient appointment for histology report

Complications

Intraoperative and early	**Intermediate and late**
• Haemorrhage	• Abnormal scarring
• Haematoma	• Incomplete removal
• Wound infection	• Recurrence
• Wound dehiscence	

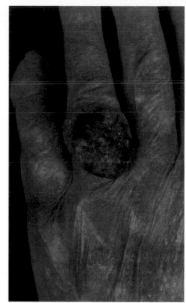

Fig 12.29 Squamous cell carcinoma at the base of the left ring finger.

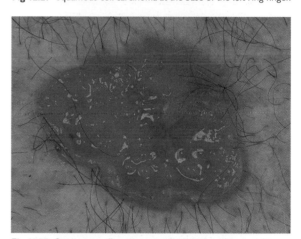

Fig 12.30 Squamous cell carcinoma.

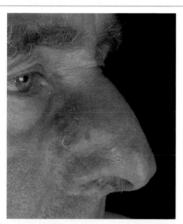

Fig 12.27 Morphoeic BCC.

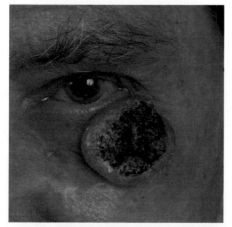

Fig 12.28 Nodular BCC. Differential diagnosis would include keratoacanthoma (📖 Topic 12.15)

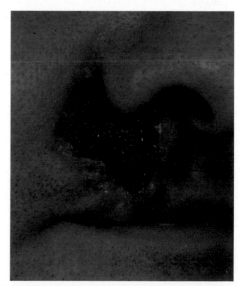

Fig 12.31 Squamous cell carcinoma of the upper lip with central ulceration.

Naevi

Melanocytic naevi (mole, pigmented naevi) are common benign skin lesions. They are caused by a proliferation of melanocytes. They vary in colour (pink flesh tones to dark brown or black) and the number depends on genetic factors and sun exposure.

Moles may darken following sun exposure or during pregnancy. During adulthood, they often lose their pigmentation, and they may even disappear in old age. Mole mapping is useful when there are multiple lesions. Suspicious lesions should be excised.

Congenital naevi

Congenital naevi are present at birth and tend to enlarge with the child's growth. They are caused by disturbed migration of melanoblasts, resulting in an ectopic population of cells.

These are usually uniformly pigmented and may darken and become hairy with age. They are classified by diameter as small (<1.5 cm), medium (up to 10 cm), large (up to 20 cm), and giant (>20 cm).

Giant congenital naevi have a lifetime risk of malignant transformation of ~5%.

Most congenital naevi do not need any intervention. Cosmetically unattractive naevi and those at high risk of malignant transformation or with suspicious characteristics are excised.

Acquired naevi

- Non-hairy moles are usually uniformly pigmented and <1 cm in diameter. Early naevus cells form nests on the junction between the epidermis and the dermis (junctional naevi). With maturity, nests of naevus cells can also form in the dermis (compound naevi). Cells confined to the dermis (intradermal naevi) are often thickened and protrude from the skin surface
- Hairy naevi are always intradermal
- Freckles (ephilides) are small benign flat brown lesions usually found in sun-exposed areas. They are caused by accumulation of melanin in keratinocytes derived from local melanocytes. They fade in the winter as the melanocytes are less active. These are different from solar lentigines (age spot, liver spot) which are benign flat brown spots arising in later life as a result of sun damage
- Dysplastic or atypical (Clarke's) naevi often have a 'fried egg' appearance, with a central papule and surrounding pigmented macule with varying pigmentation
- Blue naevi have heavy brown–black pigmentation and, because of an optical effect, take on a blue appearance
- Halo naevi are caused by the loss of colour in the skin surrounding the naevus which appears as a white ring. Both the naevus and ring usually disappear with time
- Spitz naevi often appear as a pink papule and are difficult to distinguish from acquired naevi
- Mongolian spots are blue/black patches usually found over the lower back or buttocks. They are very common in Asians and blacks but are rare in whites. They usually regress in childhood

Seborrhoeic keratosis

Seborrhoeic keratoses (senile wart, basal cell papilloma) are common benign skin tumours of late middle age. There is a familial predisposition.

The aetiology is unknown. They can occur in all areas of the body irrespective of previous sun exposure.

The macroscopic appearance is often of a 'stuck on' brown thickened lesion with a rough surface. The lesions are usually asymptomatic although patients present with concerns about cosmesis and malignancy.

An eruption of multiple seborrhoeic keratoses is a very rare manifestation of an underlying gastrointestinal malignancy (Leser–Trelat sign).

Management

Seborrhoeic keratoses do not need to be removed if the clinical diagnosis is certain. Patients often ask for them to be removed owing to cosmetic appearance, discomfort or snagging on clothes. If the diagnosis is in doubt they should be removed for histological examination.

- Cryotherapy, cautery, and curettage remove the lesion but do not allow histological examination
- Shave biopsy or excision biopsy, allowing histological examination, is indicated if a malignant lesion is suspected

Actinic keratosis

Actinic keratoses (solar keratoses) are usually multiple, scaly, erythematous patches on sun-exposed areas presenting in later life. They are precancerous and may give rise to SCC.

The hyperplastic form is commonly found on the hands and may become a skin horn. The spreading pigmented form is usually found on the face.

Microscopically, there is focal parakeratosis with loss of underlying granular layer. There is loss of orderly arrangement of the epidermis, with large atypical keratinocytes.

Management

It is not possible to remove all actinic keratoses on extensively sun-damaged skin.

- Cryotherapy with liquid nitrogen is effective. It causes blistering and shedding of the affected skin, and may leave a pale scar
- Curettage and cautery is preferred with thicker keratoses, or early SSC
- 5-FU cream (Efudix) is used to treat multiple facial keratoses. The cream is applied onto facial skin once or twice daily for 2–4 weeks. Skin healing follows completion of the therapy
- Imiquimod 5% cream
- Diclofenac cream
- Photodynamic therapy involves applying a photosensitizer (a porphyrin chemical) to the affected area. Exposure to strong visible light causes a burn which subsequently heals
- Complete surgical excision offers the highest cure rate but is often impractical given the number of lesions and their anatomical location

Cysts

A cyst is a benign, sac-like growth in the deeper layers of the skin. They form from the lining of a hair follicle that becomes blocked. Common types include:

- **Acne comedone**—whitehead
- **Acne cyst**—large uninflamed acne lumps
- **Dermoid cyst**—a developmental inclusion cyst

- **Milia**—tiny surface white balls often found on the cheeks after sun exposure or following an injury. Milia can easily be squeezed out
- **Epidermoid cyst**—often incorrectly termed sebaceous cyst. The sac is filled with a soft, whitish brown material that sometimes oozes out onto the skin's surface. This material, which is keratinous debris (dead skin cells), smells like rotten cheese
- **Trichilemmal cyst**—scalp cyst, often multiple and familial, arising from hair root sheath
- **Pilar cyst**—firm white content
- **Labial mucous cyst**—cyst in the lip
- **Apocrine hidrocystoma**—clear jelly-like cyst of eyelid

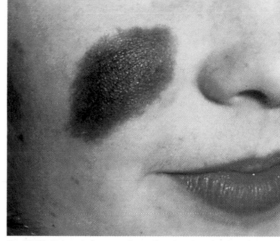

Fig 12.33 Congenital naevus. Reproduced with permission from Warrell et al. (2005). *The Oxford Textbook of Medicine*, 4e, with permission from Oxford University Press.

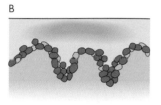

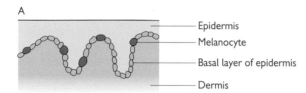

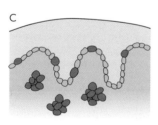

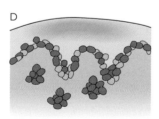

A — Epidermis, Melanocyte, Basal layer of epidermis, Dermis

Fig 12.32 Patterns of naevus cell distribution in melanocytic naevi. (A) normal skin – melanocytes are scattered along the basal layer of the epidermis. (B) junctional naevus – naevus cells are clustered along the junction between epidermis and dermis. The lesion is pigmented. (C) Intradermal naevus – naevus cells in dermis only. The lesion is raised but not pigmented. (D) Compound naevus – mixture of junctional and intradermal naevus cells. The lesion tends to be both pigmented and raised.

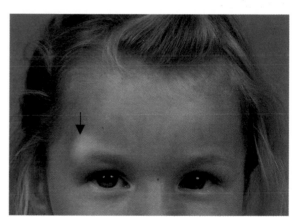

Fig 12.34 Dermoid cyst.

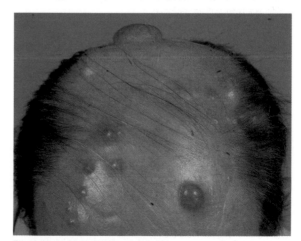

Fig 12.35 Multiple trichilemmel cysts.

Benign fibroepithelial papilloma

Benign fibroepithelial papillomas (skin tag, acrochordon, soft fibroma) are very common soft harmless lesions that appear to hang off the skin.

Macroscopically, they may be pedunculated or filiform. They are skin-coloured or darker, and range in size from 1 mm to 5 cm. They are most often found in the skin folds (neck, armpits, and groin). They tend to be more numerous in obese persons and in those with type 2 diabetes mellitus.

Microscopically, they are made up of loosely arranged collagen fibres and blood vessels surrounded epidermis.

Skin tags can be removed for cosmetic reasons by cryotherapy, surgical excision, electrosurgery or ligation.

Warts

A wart (verruca vulgaris) is caused by infection with one of the many strains of human papilloma virus (HPV).

It presents as a hard, rough surfaced papule 0.2–2 cm (solitary or multiple). Microscopically, there is an exophytic, symmetric, papillomatous lesion with large keratohyaline granules and characteristic in-turning of the rete ridges.

The majority of warts disappear without treatment. Topical salicylic acid liquid or pads and regular removal of dead warty skin with pumice stone is effective but takes time.

Cryotherapy or electric needle can be used to burn off warts. CO_2 laser is not recommended as the smoke contains viable virus particles. Multiple treatments are often needed.

Keratoacanthoma

Keratoacanthoma (adenoma sebaceum, molluscum sebaceum) is a benign cutaneous tumour that presents predominantly in sun-exposed skin of elderly patients. Men are more affected than women.

The lesion grows rapidly in size over a few weeks and then resolves spontaneously, leaving an atrophic scar.

They appear as a solitary nodule with a central keratin plug. Microscopically, it is an exoendophytic, symmetrical lesion characterized by deep bulbous lobules of keratinizing well differentiated squamous epithelium with a central keratin-filled crater. Management is excision and histological examination.

Fibromatosis

Fibromas are fibrous overgrowths of dermal or subcutaneous connective tissue. Superficial (fascial) fibromatoses include Dupuytren's disease and dermatofibroma. Deep (musculoaponeurotic) fibromatoses include desmoid tumours.

Dermatofibroma

Dermatofibroma (fibrous histiocytoma) is a common benign fibrous skin lesion of unknown aetiology. It often develops following minor trauma.

They are most common in young to middle-aged women and often occur on the legs and arms. They usually persist for years.

Macroscopically, they are a firm-feeling nodule, often yellow–brown in colour, sometimes quite dark, especially in dark-coloured skin. Microscopically, there is proliferation of dermal fibroblasts with normal overlying epidermis. Treatment is surgical excision.

Neurofibroma

Neurofibromatosis (NF) is a genetic disorder that affects the bone, soft tissue, skin, and nervous system. It is classified into neurofibromatosis 1 (von Recklinghausen disease) and neurofibromatosis 2 (bilateral acoustic neurofibromatosis), which is much rarer.

NF1 is characterized by the presence of:

- six or more café-au-lait spots
- multiple neurofibromas
- freckling (under the armpits and areas of skin folds)
- Lisch nodules (tiny tumours on the iris of the eye)

NF2 is characterized by multiple tumours and lesions on the brain and spinal cord. Patients usually present with hearing loss due to tumours growing on the auditory nerves.

Most tumours in both NF1 and NF2 are benign but are symptomatic because of local pressure effects.

There is no cure for NF. The main goal of treatment is to monitor its development. Neurofibromas that become large and painful can be excised to reduce the risk of malignancy and other complications. Genetic counselling and education about NF is important.

Pyogenic granuloma

Pyogenic granuloma (granuloma telangiectaticum) is a relatively common benign skin lesion. The aetiology is unknown, although trauma, infection, and underlying microscopic blood vessel malformations may play a role in its development.

Macroscopically, the surface has a raspberry-like or raw minced meat appearance. The condition usually first appears as a small pinhead-sized red, brownish–red or blue–black spot that grows rapidly over a period of a few weeks. They bleed easily and may ulcerate and form crusted sores. Treatment is excision with cautery to the base.

Rhinophyma

Rhinophyma [Gr. *rhis*, nose; *phyma*, growth] is marked skin thickening owing to hypertrophy and hyperplasia of the sebaceous glands of the nose. It affects white men >40 years old, and is often associated with longstanding acne rosacea but not excessive alcohol consumption.

The nose has a thick bulbous appearance, with yellow skin. Management is partial thickness excision using cryosurgery, chemical peel, dermabrasion, electrosurgery, laser or surgical excision.

Xanthelesma

Xanthelesma is the accumulation of fat in skin macrophages, presenting as soft, yellow plaques. Xanthelesma palpebrum is the most common form, with plaques on the upper and lower eyelids.

The condition may be associated with hyperlipidaemia, which needs to be excluded. The aim of management is to treat the underlying condition, which often leads to resolution of the xanthomas. Those that do not regress can be treated with topical trichloroacetic acid, electrodissection or excision.

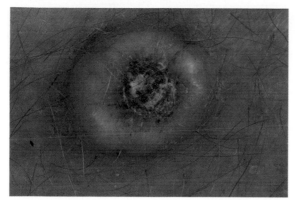

Fig 12.36 Keratoacanthoma.

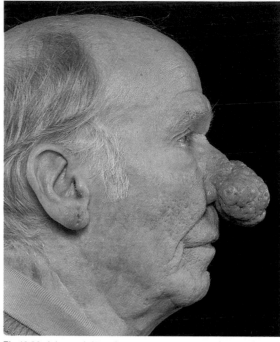

Fig 12.38 Advanced rhinophyma.

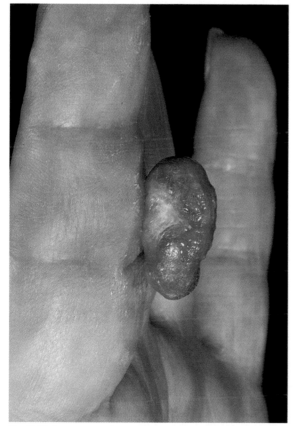

Fig 12.37 Pyogenic granuloma over the middle phalanx of the left index finger which developed following trauma to the skin.

Case 1

A 3-year-old child is referred with a scald estimated as 7% TBSA, having knocked a fresh cup of tea down her front.

- What key questions will you ask in your history?
- What is your initial approach? Is fluid resuscitation indicated?

She is given opioid analgesia and has the burn cleaned and debrided. You review her (Fig 12.15).

- Describe the burn and estimate the TBSA
- Describe the different dressings that could be used to dress the wound

Case 2

A 40-year-old man is referred by his GP with a pigmented lesion on his left thigh. His wife has been nagging him for some time to see a doctor. She feels that it has increased in size and become darker in colour.

- What are the risk factors for malignant melanoma?
- How would you assess the lesion? What suspicious characteristics would you look for?

On examination there is a pigmented lesion with irregular borders and a maximum diameter of 7 mm. There is no ulceration or bleeding and no local lymphadenopathy.

- Discuss the different types of biopsy. Which would you use in this case?

He undergoes an urgent biopsy. The histological report confirms that it is a superficial spreading malignant melanoma. The Breslow thickness is 1.6 mm.

- What features should be contained in the report?
- What is a Breslow thickness and Clark level?
- How would you manage him?

He undergoes a wide local excision and subsequent follow-up. At his 6month follow-up you discover groin lymphadenopathy. The scar from his previous excision is well healed and there is no sign of local recurrence.

- What is your approach to his further assessment and management?

Discussion

The patient presented with a pigmented lesion which had suspicious features as assessed by the ABCDE system. Excision biopsy is the gold standard for gaining a histological diagnosis in a suspected malignant melanoma.

The tumour was of intermediate Breslow thickness and required wide local excision of the excision biopsy scar.

Tumours of >1.5 mm have a high risk of recurrence. The discovery of groin lymphadenopathy immediately makes the tumour stage III.

Case 3

A 40-year-old man presents with a rapidly growing fungating lesion on his back which has grown to 4 cm in diameter in 1 month. It has rolled edges with a central area of ulceration. It is itchy and occasionally bleeds.

- What is your initial approach to this lesion?
- What is the differential diagnosis?

An urgent biopsy shows squamous cell carcinoma (SCC) and he is listed for urgent excision.

- What is the aetiology and pathogenesis of non-melanoma skin cancer?
- Describe how you would excise the lesion and the margins you would use
- What options do you have for wound closure with reference to the reconstructive ladder?

The lesion is excised and closed, with a skin graft taken from his thigh. The histology shows complete excision with adequate margins.

- Describe the different types of skin graft
- What are the stages of skin graft take?

Unfortunately the SCC recurs and requires re-excision.

- Does he require any further investigations?
- Is there a role for adjuvant therapy?

Case 4

You review a 23-year-old man in clinic who has been referred with possible Dupuytren's disease of his right hand. His father developed the disease at an early age and had a number of operations.

- What other points will you cover in your history?
- What signs do you look for on examination?

He has classic Dupuytren's disease, affecting the palm and ring finger of his right hand. The ring PIPJ is held in 100° flexion. There appears to be early disease in the palm.

- What are the management options?
- When counselling him about the disease and management, what key points do you cover?

Chapter 13

Paediatric surgery

⊕ Technical skills and procedures

- Open pyloromyotomy
- Air-reduction enema
- Circumcision
- Scrotal exploration
- Paediatric inguinal herniotomy
- Orchidopexy

⊘ Clinical skills

- Paediatric appendicitis versus mesenteric adenitis
- Neonatal bowel obstruction
- The vomiting infant

343

The first two decades of life are spent, among other things, reaching physiological and anatomical maturity. It is important to be aware of these differences when assessing and managing children. They are not small adults.

The terminology used to describe different age ranges is often poorly defined and varies between societies. However, important age definitions are neonate (<44 weeks post-conceptual age) and infant (1 month–1 year). Beyond this, the broad divisions are child and adolescent.

Size and weight

Paediatric patients are not just small; they also have different body proportions. The head is relatively large compared with the rest of the body, which contributes to the high body surface area:volume ratio. This ratio has implications for thermoregulation and fluid balance, as discussed below.

Thermoregulation

Thermoregulation in neonates is underdeveloped and poorly sustained. To maintain a stable temperature they need a higher ambient temperature with limited variation. Despite the contribution of brown adipose fat to non-shivering thermogenesis, neonates are susceptible to labile body temperature owing to:

- high body surface area:volume ratio, which increases loss or gain of heat
- reduced subcutaneous fat for insulation
- poor peripheral vasomotor control
- inability to shiver or sweat
- inability to control their environment voluntarily

Cardiovascular system

The cardiovascular system undergoes significant changes at birth (📖 Topic 3.3).

Heart rate and rhythm

The neonatal heartbeat is rapid and reaches a peak at 1 month, before declining to adult levels following puberty (Table 13.2). Marked beat-to-beat variation and sinus arrhythmia are common.

Oxygen carriage

In the first few months of life, oxygen carriage is impaired by the high percentage of circulating fetal haemoglobin. This causes a left shift of the oxygen–haemoglobin dissociation curve and associated decrease in oxygen release in the peripheral tissues. To counteract this, there is a higher haemoglobin concentration, blood volume, and cardiac output.

Myocardial contractility

The myocardium is relatively stiff and non-compliant. Left ventricular filling is unable to increase cardiac output by increasing stroke volume. This is achieved by an increase in heart rate instead.

Respiratory system

Following delivery, the lungs adapt rapidly to extrauterine life. There are a number of differences between the paediatric and the adult airway and respiratory system which may complicate airway management (Fig 13.1).

Airway

- Large occiput tends to flex head, causing obstruction
- Narrow nares (neonates are obligate nasal breathers)
- Large tongue with a small mandible
- Large floppy U-shaped epiglottis
- Short trachea
- Narrowest point is the cricoid ring, not the vocal cords
- Airway diameters are small and easily blocked by secretions

Respiratory system

- Neonates tend to increase respiratory rate rather than tidal volume in response to increased oxygen demand
- Respiratory muscles are immature and fatigable
- There is a mechanical disadvantage as the chest wall is very compliant and ribs are positioned horizontally

Renal system and fluids

The neonatal kidney has a lower glomerular filtration rate and concentrating ability than the adult kidney. Creatinine measurement during the first days of life is uninformative, as it reflects maternal and not neonatal renal function.

- High solute loads require an obligatory urine volume which can lead to dehydration and hyponatraemia owing to the reduced ability to conserve sodium
- The water content of a neonate is very high, at 80% of body weight. Of this, 40% is held as extracellular fluid, compared to 20% in adults. As a consequence, there is a high turnover of fluid which can be rapidly lost, leading to dehydration
- Fluid balance needs to be carefully calculated in relation to weight and ongoing fluid losses

Calculation of paediatric maintenance fluids

Neonatal and infant fluid requirements vary with respect to age, and prescription of fluid type and volume requires a detailed understanding of neonatal physiology. Standard fluid requirements for newborns are usually 60, 90, 120, and then 150 mL/kg/24 h for days 1, 2, 3, and 4 onwards.

Prescribing fluids for children >10 kg is less complicated. An easy method for estimating hourly maintenance fluid requirements is shown in Table 13.1.

Half normal saline (0.45%) with 5% dextrose is a standard crystalloid used for paediatric maintenance fluids. Fluid resuscitation is routinely performed using 0.9% normal saline, but in some settings colloids are preferred.

Liver and nutrition

The liver is immature and many of the enzyme systems are not at full capacity. This has implications for the metabolism of drugs and toxins, placing the neonate at an increased risk of drug toxicity.

Table 13.1 Estimation of maintenance fluid requirements

Body weight	Per hour	Per 24 h
First 10 kg	4 mL/kg	100 mL/kg
Second 10 kg	2 mL/kg	50 mL/kg
Subsequent kg	1 mL/kg	20 mL/kg
e.g. for a 35-kg child: (4 x 10) + (2 x 10) + (15 x 1) = 75 mL/h.		

Table 13.2 Normal physiological parameters by age				
	Neonate	**Infant**	**5 years**	**Adult**
Heart rate (beats/min)	130 (110–160)	120 (95–140)	90 (80–120)	77 (60–100)
Systolic BP (mmHg)	65	70	95	120
Blood volume (mL/kg)	85	80	75	70
Haemoglobin (g/dL)	17	11	12	14
Respiratory rate (breaths/min)	30–40	20–30	15–20	12–16
O_2 consumption (mL/kg/min)	6	5	4	3

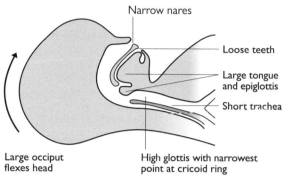

Narrow nares

Loose teeth

Large tongue and epiglottis

Short trachea

High glottis with narrowest point at cricoid ring

Large occiput flexes head

Fig 13.1 Diagram showing unique features of the paediatric airway.

13.2 Paediatric abdominal pain

Abdominal pain in children is very common. It is important to differentiate new onset acute abdominal pain, needing surgery, from recurrent pain.

Aetiology

Some conditions should be considered in all age groups (see below); others peak at certain ages. Do not forget extra-abdominal causes of abdominal pain.

- Non-specific abdominal pain (60%) is the commonest diagnosis in children with acute abdominal pain but is a diagnosis of exclusion. There are usually no focal signs and investigations are normal
- Appendicitis (30%) is commonly mimicked by mesenteric adenitis (see box). 📖 Topic 8.13
- Urinary tract infection (2%)
- Others: gastroenteritis, pneumonia, constipation, sickle cell crisis

Less common causes by age

- Neonates and infants: midgut malrotation with volvulus, intussusception, irreducible or incarcerated inguinal hernia
- Children: pancreatitis, Meckel's diverticulum
- Adolescents: testicular or ovarian torsion, ruptured ovarian cyst, pelvic inflammatory disease (PID), pancreatitis, cholecystitis

Pathophysiology

The characteristics and location of abdominal pain are related to the structures involved and their embryological origin. Abdominal pain is generally divided into visceral, parietal or referred pain.

Clinical assessment

Young children and those with learning difficulties are unable to give a reliable history and may prove difficult to examine.

Perform the assessment in a quiet, warm, safe environment. Distraction of the child by a parent, nurse or toys is helpful. 📖 Topic 8.12 for assessment of the acute abdomen in adults.

History

- Detailed history of the onset and progression of pain
- Associated symptoms such as nausea, vomiting, change in bowel habit, and non-GI symptoms
- Level of activity and eating/drinking habits
- Gynaecological history: menstrual history, sexual activity
- Exclude child abuse and non-accidental injury

Examination

- Well or unwell? Children are usually active
- Peritonism is often subtle. Abdominal distension may be the most prominent sign of intra-abdominal sepsis. A child able to hop on one leg is not peritonitic
- Board-like rigidity is unusual. Whilst children do demonstrate guarding, it seldom equates to the 'board-like rigidity' typically seen in adults. Distraction will often help to discern involuntary from voluntary contractions
- Formal testing for rebound tenderness is unacceptable. Percussion tenderness is a more reliable gentle method of revealing peritonism. Deep palpation often causes discomfort regardless of underlying pathology
- Full systems examination, including chest and ENT. (URTI may precede mesenteric adenitis)
- DRE and PV are not routine and should be considered an investigation only to be performed if the result would influence management
- Repeated clinical examination over a number of hours will often help the surgeon make a diagnosis

Investigations

- Urinalysis (exclude UTI and pregnancy)
- Bloods—FBC (raised WCC in infection, anaemia), U+Es (if vomiting or dehydrated), CRP, amylase
- Other bloods, if indicated: βHCG following consent to exclude pregnancy in girls who have started to menstruate; sickle cell screen
- Plain abdominal radiograph to detect intestinal obstruction, and erect chest radiograph if perforation or pneumonia is suspected
- Abdominal ultrasound may be indicated to assess intra-abdominal masses, and the renal tract, biliary tract, adnexae, and scrotum

Management

- Intravenous fluid resuscitation if dehydrated
- Analgesia and antiemetic. Do not withhold analgesia
- NBM
- For further management, see individual conditions

Recurrent abdominal pain

Recurrent abdominal pain (RAP) is characterized by more than two similar episodes of abdominal pain within a 3 month period.

Prevalence in school-aged children is approximately 15%. Whilst children with RAP may be assessed by paediatric surgeons, the vast majority benefit from non-surgical multidisciplinary management (e.g. pain team and paediatric gastroenterologist).

Causes include:

- functional gastrointestinal disorders: functional dyspepsia, IBS, abdominal migraine
- gastrointestinal conditions: IBD, peptic ulcer disease
- gynaecological: ovulatory or perimenstrual pain
- neoplasia, especially if associated unexplained weight loss, anorexia, mass

⊚ Paediatric appendicitis versus mesenteric adenitis

Mesenteric adenitis (MA) is the commonest mimic of acute appendicitis (📖 Topic 8.13) in children. Its peak incidence is in pre-pubertal children and is uncommon after 15 years of age.

Mesenteric adenitis is caused by viral or, less commonly, bacterial infection of mesenteric lymph nodes. Lymph node biopsies show non-specific reactive hyperplasia.

Clinical assessment

- Preceding viral URTI with high fever, malaise, headache, sore throat, and cough is commonly seen in mesenteric adenitis. Appendicitis usually has a fairly rapid onset with progressive deterioration
- Abdominal pain in mesenteric adenitis is diffuse, central, and colicky. Appendicitis may initially present in this way but tends to deteriorate and localize to the RIF with signs of peritonism
- Anorexia is a feature of both. Appendicitis is more commonly associated with nausea and vomiting
- Temperature is generally higher in mesenteric adenitis (>39°C)
- ENT examination in mesenteric adenitis may reveal cervical lymphadenopathy, ± erythematous upper respiratory tract. Usually normal in appendicitis

Management

- A confident diagnosis of mesenteric adenitis can be managed at home with simple analgesia and oral fluids
- If early acute appendicitis is suspected, the child should be admitted for active observation for signs of sepsis and peritonism
- Some children will have the diagnosis of mesenteric adenitis confirmed during diagnostic laparoscopy or negative appendicectomy for presumed appendicitis. Typical findings include free, serous fluid together with numerous, enlarged mesenteric lymph nodes and oedematous associated mesentery
- Mesenteric adenitis usually settles uneventfully within 48 h; acute appendicitis continues to deteriorate and needs an operation

There are two main types of congenital abdominal wall defect (CAWD).

1. Gastroschisis: organs herniate through an open abdominal wall defect and are not contained within a sac
2. Exomphalos: organs herniate through an abnormal umbilical ring and are contained within a sac

General principles

Embryology of the anterior abdominal wall

The abdominal wall is formed by lateral and craniocaudal folding of the trilaminar embryo. Folding occurs during weeks 3 and 4 of gestation and is caused by disproportionately vigorous growth of embryonic disc and amnion compared with the yolk sac.

Lateral folding culminates with ventral midline fusion of the endoderm, mesoderm, and ectoderm to derive a primary gut tube (endoderm) bounded ventrally by the anterior abdominal wall (mesoderm and ectoderm).

Fusion occurs first at the cranial and caudal extents of the embryo, progressing in 'zipper'-like fashion towards the umbilicus. The protruding vitelline duct and connecting stalk prevent fusion at the umbilicus. Expansion of the amnion to enclose these protruding structures defines the umbilical ring. The open umbilical ring permits physiological herniation (weeks 6–7) and retraction (weeks 10–11) of the midgut, with accompanying midgut rotation. Normally, umbilical ring closure follows retraction of the midgut.

Concurrent with folding, anterior abdominal wall muscles differentiate in segmental fashion from somitic mesoderm and migrate anterolaterally towards the ventral midline.

Antenatal diagnosis

The primary diagnosis is typically made at the 20 week anomaly USS when the presence or absence of a covering membrane is usually detectable.

Maternal serum alpha-fetoprotein (αFP) is elevated in over 90% of cases owing to enhanced passage of fetal αFP into the amniotic fluid followed by the maternal circulation. The levels are highest in gastroschisis (2.5× maternal median) as the bowel is directly exposed to amniotic fluid. Other fetal disorders that raise maternal serum αFP include neural tube defects and trisomy 21 (Down's syndrome).

Following the diagnosis, further detailed USS scans and karyotype examinations are performed to confirm or exclude associated organ and chromosomal anomalies. In the presence of associated lethal chromosomal anomalies, antenatal counselling should discuss the option of termination.

Antenatal management

Premature spontaneous delivery is common. Beyond 32 weeks gestation the mother has a weekly USS to check for fetal or bowel compromise (thickening or reduced mesenteric blood flow). Planned preterm delivery for such complications improves outcome.

The delivery should take place in a centre with both neonatal surgical and intensive care units. Mothers are encouraged to have a spontaneous normal vaginal delivery. This is not associated with increased sepsis or intestinal trauma. Delivery is optimal at 37 weeks, and elective Caesarean section may be considered to ensure delivery when the surgical and neonatal units are maximally staffed. Absolute indications for Caesarean section are maternal or fetal distress.

Exomphalos (omphalocele)

Exomphalos minor (hernia of the umbilical cord) and major are on a spectrum of the same abdominal wall defect. They are uncommon, with an incidence of 1 per 7000 live births and have a male preponderance.

Aetiology

Genetic anomalies are associated with over 50% of cases, and include Beckwith–Wiedemann syndrome (exomphalos, macroglossia, and gigantism) and Pentalogy of Cantrell (exomphalos, ectopia cordis, and defects of distal sternum, anterior diaphragm, and diaphragmatic pericardium).

Pathophysiology

The protruding structures are covered by a trilaminar sac comprising amnion, Whartons jelly, and peritoneum. Exomphalos is subdivided into minor and major.

- Exomphalos minor has a small abdominal defect (<4 cm). The umbilical cord inserts to the left of the hernial sac rather than the apex
- Exomphalos major has a large abdominal wall defect (>4 cm) and the umbilical cord inserts into the apex of the sac. It may contain liver, stomach, colon, and spleen in addition to midgut (Fig 13.2)

Management

Immediate

- Wide bore nasogastric tube for decompression
- Intravenous maintenance fluids and urinary catheter
- Monitor serum glucose (hypoglycaemia is common)
- Intravenous broad spectrum antibiotics
- Warm environment
- Protected the hernia to prevent torsion of vascular pedicles supplying structures within the sac
- Wrapping exposed bowel in clingfilm minimizes insensible fluid losses and allows monitoring of bowel viability
- Assess for associated anomalies. In severe cases, palliative care may be appropriate rather than surgery

Operative

Primary reduction of the protruding abdominal organs may not be possible and so a staged reduction can be required.

Gradual reduction is achieved by suspension of the sac or organs (if the sac is excised). Overzealous reduction may result in abdominal compartment syndrome.

- Primary closure of the abdominal wall defect is well suited to infants with a small defect and an abdominal cavity of sufficient capacity to hold the reduced contents
- Delayed closure ± prosthetic patch is used for infants with large defects and/or paucity of abdominal wall musculature and skin
- Escharotic therapy is often used to close 'giant' defects or in those with severe associated anomalies which preclude surgical closure

Complications and prognosis

Exomphalos major has the worst prognosis of the CAWDs. Prognosis is determined largely by co-morbid anomalies. Over 60% of cases with chromosomal anomalies die *in utero*. Other factors carrying a poor prognosis are large defects, prematurity, and sac rupture.

Abdominal compartment syndrome

Overzealous reduction of sac contents (especially liver) may cause excessive intra-abdominal pressure. Increased intra-abdominal pressure impedes venous return with resultant decreased cardiac output, and splints the diaphragm, impairing ventilation. Multiorgan failure ensues owing to visceral hypoperfusion and escalating intracerebral pressures. Indicators of excessive intra-abdominal pressure include ventilatory pressures >35 cmH$_2$O and type II respiratory failure.

Gastroschisis

Gastroschisis is more common than exomphalos, with an incidence of 1 per 3000 live births which has risen threefold in the last 25 years. It also has a male preponderance.

Aetiology

In contrast to exomphalos, associated genetic anomalies are rare. Environmental factors are implicated in many cases. Prevalence is highest amongst teenage mothers who smoke and use recreational drugs during early pregnancy.

Pathophysiology

Exposed midgut protrudes through a small open abdominal defect. The defect is typically to the right of a normally sited umbilicus, from which it is separated by a narrow skin bridge. The intestines are often oedematous owing to exposure to amnion and fetal urine *in utero* (Fig 13.3). Intestinal atresia or stenosis occurs in 15% of cases following strangulation at the neck of the defect.

Management

Immediate management is similar to exomphalos, albeit lack of a hernial sac increases risks of sepsis and insensible losses.

Operative

Primary reduction of protruding abdominal organs and closure of the defect is possible in 80% of cases. Excessive intra-abdominal pressure is an indication for staged reduction within a silo and then delayed closure. Preformed silos (e.g. Medicina silo) are gaining in popularity. To minimize sepsis risks, surgeons aim to achieve reduction within 7–10 following surgery.

Neonates often require prolonged TPN owing to ileus of the inflamed bowel. Survival rates exceed 85%.

Other abdominal wall defects

Prune belly syndrome

Prune belly syndrome (abdominal wall dysplasia) is failure of development of the anterior abdominal wall musculature; it is associated with dilatation of the urinary tract and testicular maldescent. It is rare and 95% of cases occur in males. The abdominal wall is thin, flaccid, and wrinkled. Surgery is used to correct each of the anomalies.

Bladder exstrophy

Bladder exstrophy results in bladder protruding from the lower abdominal wall. It is often associated with anomalies of the external genitalia, e.g. epispadias. Operative management aims to close the defect and restore continence.

Table 13.3 **Exomphalos versus gastroschisis**		
	Exomphalos	**Gastroschisis**
Location of defect	Umbilical ring	Right of umbilicus
Sac	Present	Absent
Cord	On to sac	Normal
Liver herniation	Yes	No
Non-rotation	Yes	Yes
Gut appearance	Normal	Matted, thickened
Gut function	Normal	Dysmotile
Atresia	Rare	Common
Other anomalies	Common	Rare

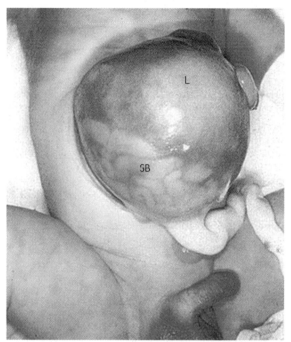

Fig 13.2 Exomphalos major. Liver (L), and small bowel (SB) are seen within the sac. Reproduced with permission from *The Oxford Textbook of Surgery*.

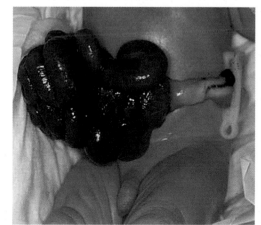

Fig 13.3 Gastroschisis with defect right of umbilicus. The loops of bowel are not contained within a sac and are oedematous with venous congestion.

13.4 Anorectal malformations

Congenital anorectal malformations (ARMs) incorporate a spectrum of conditions affecting the rectum, distal anus, urinary tract, and genital tract, with an incidence of 1 per 5000 live births. There is a male preponderance. (M:F 4:1).

Embryology of the anus

The cloacal membrane is an ectodermal membrane which spans the common outlet for the intestinal and urogenital tracts (cloaca) during early fetal development.

During the fourth and fifth weeks of gestation, transformation of the cloaca by approximation of the cloacal membrane and urorectal septum defines an anterior urogenital sinus and posterior hindgut. The cloacal membrane becomes the urogenital and anal membranes, which rupture at 10 weeks gestation to produce patent urogenital and rectal tracts.

Aetiology

ARMs are of unknown aetiology. The high incidence of associated anomalies affecting multiple organ systems suggests many ARMs result from global insults to fetal development. Experimental models implicate anomalies or absence of the cloacal membrane in the aetiology of ARMs.

Rectal atresia

Rectal atresia is a rare form of ARM, the aetiology of which differs from other ARMs. Akin to proximal small intestinal atresia, rectal atresia is most likely the result of intrauterine vascular accident and resultant ischaemia.

Pathophysiology

Bowel fistulae in ARMs are histologically and physiologically ectopic anal canals.

- Histology: normal anal epithelium including transitional zone, anal glands
- Physiology: internal anal sphincter muscle encircles the ectopically sited bowel fistula

To maximize continence, surgical reconstruction aims to retain internal anal sphincter with associated distal bowel.

The external anal sphincter is normally sited, indicating that its development is at least partly separate to that of the ectopic anus and internal anal sphincter. The external sphincter is, however, universally hypoplastic. The severity of such hypoplasia is proportional to: (1) the distance between rectal pouch and perineum; and (2) severity of associated sacral anomalies.

Associated syndromes

- VACTERL: vertebral, anorectal, cardiac, tracheo-oesophageal, renal, limb
- CHARGE: colobomata, heart disease, atresia choanae, retarded growth, genital anomalies (males), ear anomalies
- Currarino triad: anorectal malformation, presacral mass, and sacral bony defect

Clinical assessment

Primary diagnosis of ARMS usually occurs at the routine screening examination post-delivery. Subsequent assessment aims to establish the underlying anatomy of the ARM and diagnose any associated anomalies.

Examination

Characterization of the ARM, including any associated fistulous bowel openings, will include assessment of:

- anus: present or absent, position, calibre, and tone of anomalous anus noted
- fistula opening sites may be difficult to identify. Suggestive signs are: 1) bead of meconium, 2) dark green/black subcutaneous tracking of meconium within fistula (Fig 13.4).
- gentle probing of perineal fistulae sites may reveal position of the rectum
- anomaly screen, including: low birth weight, syndromic facies, heart murmur, abnormal genitalia in males, and limb malformations

Investigations

- Urinalysis showing meconium (dark green) suggests a rectourogenital fistula
- Plain chest/abdominal radiograph to show distal bowel obstruction, and abnormal vertebrae/ribs/sacrum
- Cross-table lateral supine plain radiograph ('invertogram') with buttocks raised shows a terminal gas shadow outlining the distal rectal pouch, allowing measurement of distance to perineum
- Ultrasound measures the distance from distal rectal pouch to perineum. Renal USS shows renal anomaly in 40%. Spinal USS may demonstrate tethering or anomalies of the spinal cord, conal anomalies, or a presacral mass
- MRI measures distance from distal rectal pouch to perineum and assesses sphincter muscle or perisacral pathology
- Distal loopogram (i.e. via colostomy) shows anatomy of distal bowel and *anterograde* delineation of perineal fistula
- MCUG (micturating cystourethrogram) for *retrograde* delineation of rectourogenital fistula, i.e. which communicates with urinary tract

Classification

Krickenbeck International Classification (2005) classifies ARMs by fistula type into major clinical groups as well as rare or regional variants (not shown). The major clinical groups are:

- perineal (cutaneous) fistula
- rectourethral fistula
- prostatic
- bulbar fistula
- rectovesical fistula
- vestibular fistula
- cloaca
- no fistula
- anal stenosis

Alberto Pena, a world leader in ARMs, has described an alternative classification in which ARMs are defined as either low (with a perineal fistula or <1 cm on plain radiograph between bowel and skin) or high (without a fistula or >1 cm between bowel and skin).

Management

Immediate

Associated anomalies are the predominant cause of preoperative morbidity. Wide bore NGT ensures upper GI decompression, allowing safe deferral of surgery for 24 (or more) h, whilst ancillary investigations are performed.

Neonatal colostomy

Neonatal colostomy decompresses the bowel, enables further investigation with a distal colostogram, and reduces the risk of wound complications following definitive repair.

Divided, sigmoid colostomies are preferred and are typically reversed 3–6 months later, following definitive repair. Select patient groups may not require colostomy, and are suitable for primary definitive repair.

Definitive repair

Definitive reconstruction aims for a continent neo-anus, and restoration of the relationships between bowel, internal anal, and external anal sphincters.

Optimal surgical approach varies according to ARM and fistula anatomy.

- Reconstructive approaches may be perineal, anterior sagittal, sacroperineal, as well as the posterior sagittal anorectoplasty (PSARP) developed by Alberto Pena
- Pull-through approaches include abdominosacroperineal, abdominoperineal, and, more recently, laparoscopic-assisted surgery

Postoperative care

Some surgeons advocate serial anal dilatation, for example starting 2 weeks after surgery, to prevent anal stenosis. Good perineal skin care and bowel management are also needed to prevent wound breakdown, constipation, and soiling.

Complications and prognosis

Operative complications include damage to nerve plexuses innervating bowel and bladder, peritonitis, retraction/dehiscence of pull-through, recurrence of fistula, anal stenosis, mucosal prolapse, constipation and overflow incontinence, and sphincter incompetence.

Function outcome is assessed according to voluntary bowel movements, constipation (20–60%), and soiling. Factors predictive of good functional outcome include:

- favourable ARM type (e.g. perineal, rectal atresia)
- limited external anal sphincter hypoplasia
- normal sacrum

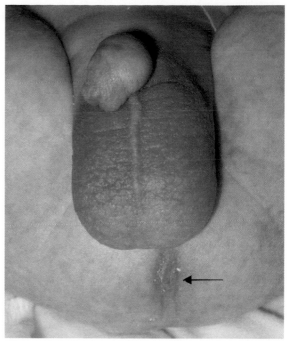

Fig 13.4 Example of an imperforate anus with perineal fistula (arrow). The external genitalia appear normal.

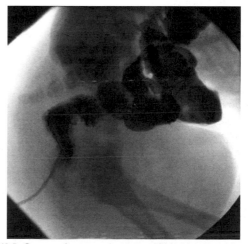

Fig 13.5 Gastrografin enema showing an ARM with perineal fistula. The distal rectal pouch is ~1 cm from the perineum. Note also hypoplastic sacrum and passage of feeding tube, used to instil the contrast, outlining the perineal fistula.

Neonatal bowel obstruction

Bowel obstruction is the commonest surgical emergency in neonates, and occurs in 1 in 2000 live births. Excluding meconium plug syndrome, the commonest causes are bowel atresia or stenosis (30%), meconium ileus (20%), Hirschsprung disease (15–20%), and midgut volvulus.

Congenital bowel obstruction may present antenatally, with polyhydramnios or bowel dilatation on ultrasound. Postnatal presenting features will vary according to level of bowel obstruction, and include bile-stained vomiting, abdominal distension (see box), together with failure to pass meconium within the first 24 h of life. Distal bowel obstruction usually causes distension; a non-distended (scaphoid) abdomen suggests proximal obstruction.

Duodenal atresia or stenosis

The duodenum is the commonest site for congenital atresia or stenosis, with an incidence of up to 1 in 5000 live births. Fifty per cent present prenatally with maternal polyhydramnios and 30% are associated with Down's syndrome.

Bile-stained vomiting is the typical postnatal presentation, but this is absent if the atresia is proximal to the ampulla of Vater. A 'double bubble' on ultrasound or plain abdominal radiograph is pathognomonic, reflecting dilated stomach and obstructed duodenum (Fig 13.7).

Jejunoileal and other intestinal atresias

Jejunal and ileal atresia result from intrauterine vascular accidents, which may be idiopathic but can also arise as a result of volvulus, intussusception, gastroschisis, and exomphalos. Multiple atretic segments are uncommon. Colonic atresia is less common, and may be associated with cloacal extrophy.

Meconium plug syndrome

Meconium plug syndrome occurs in 1 in 500 live births and is the commonest cause of bowel obstruction in neonates. Its aetiology is unknown, but a plug of thick and dry (inspissated) meconium typically obstructs the distal colon. Contrast enema is both diagnostic and therapeutic by causing passage of the plug and bowel decompression. The majority of neonates go on to have normal bowel function with no complications; however, there is an infrequent association with both cystic fibrois and Hirschsprung disease (see below).

Meconium ileus

Meconium ileus occurs in up to 1 in 5000 live births. Although over 90% of patients have cystic fibrosis, meconium ileus occurs in only 15% of neonates with cystic fibrosis. Failure of pancreatic enzyme secretion causes inspissated meconium which obstructs the bowel lumen. The colon is small and unused (microcolon) and meconium is not passed. The proximal bowel dilates, with subsequent abdominal distension and bile-stained vomiting on the first day of life. 'Complicated' meconium ileus is seen in up to 50%, with associated intrauterine volvulus, atresia, perforation, and/or meconium peritonitis.

Hirschsprung disease

Hirschsprung disease occurs in 1 in 5000 live births. A variable length of distal gut extending proximally from the anus is aganglionic. The development of the enteric nervous system is abnormal as a result of failure of migration of neural crest cells. Various gene mutations (e.g. *RET*) have been implicated. There is delayed passage of meconium >24 h, with resultant distension and vomiting. Diagnosis is made by rectal biopsy (usually suction). Aganglionic bowel is hypertonic, resulting in obstruction or severe constipation.

Treatment is resection of the aganglionic segment with or without primary colostomy. The most serious complication is enterocolitis, which can also occur following corrective surgery.

Malrotation with midgut volvulus

Malrotation with midgut volvulus (volvulus neonatorum) occurs in 1 in 6000 live births. Malrotation is caused by failure of normal midgut rotation and mesenteric fixation. This diagnosis must be considered in all newborns with bilious vomiting (even a single vomit), as an unrecognized midgut volvulus will be fatal.

Embryology

Between weeks 5 and 10 of gestation the midgut rotates anti-clockwise through 270° in association with physiological midgut herniation and subsequent reduction.

Midgut rotation is followed by elongation of the ascending colon and descent of the caecum into the RIF. Both changes contribute to the formation of a broad-based small bowel mesentery between the ligament of Treitz and the RIF. Malrotation gives rise to a spectrum of disorders, the most pathological of which is a narrow-based small bowel mesentery predisposed to volvulus with resultant bowel strangulation.

Clinical assessment

- Identify and treat hypovolaemia and sepsis
- Upper GI contrast study is the criterion standard. Colour Doppler ultrasound may also aid assessment

Management

Initial management is fluid resuscitation, antibiotics, and a wide-bore nasogastric tube (8Ch) before emergency surgery (Ladd procedure). Midgut infarction is catastrophic (Fig 13.8), and resection of necrotic bowel may result in short gut syndrome. The mortality rate is 65%, with 75% for small bowel length necrosis.

Congenital diaphragmatic hernia

Congenital diaphragmatic hernia (CDH) occurs in 1 in 2500 births. Its aetiology is unknown, but it results from failure of formation or fusion of one of the parts of the diaphragm during gestational weeks 7–8. The posterolateral (Bochdalek) defect is more common than the anterior (Morgagni) defect, and is more frequently left-sided. Stomach, bowel, and other organs herniate into the thoracic cavity. Associated lung hypoplasia was previously considered to be secondary to external compression by the CDH contents, but may actually be the primary problem, with resultant failure to push bowel caudally at the time of diaphragmatic development.

Clinical assessment

Diagnosis is most often antenatal, prompting specialist investigation to characterize the hernia and associated anomalies. Postnatal presentation with respiratory compromise is confirmed by plain chest radiograph.

Management

Emergent management is cardiorespiratory support and nasogastric tube decompression of the herniated bowel. The mortality rate is >60%. Surgical repair is not urgent, and is usually only undertaken following complete stabilization and improvement of the associated pulmonary hypertension.

Oesophageal atresia and tracheo-oesophageal fistula

Oesophageal atresia (OA) with tracheo-oesophageal fistula (TOF) occurs in 1 in 3000–5000 live births. Five anatomical variants are described (Fig 13.6). OA with TOF is often associated with other anomalies, including the VACTERL and CHARGE syndromes.

Clinical assessment

Presentation may be antenatal with polyhydramnios or postnatal with frothy oral secretions and feeding difficulties. Aspiration of saliva or feed (or gastric contents via TOF) causes respiratory distress with pneumonitis and sepsis. Inability to pass a nasogastric tube into stomach confirmed on plain radiograph is diagnostic. TOF variant may be surmised from the presence or absence of stomach gas. Further investigations to confirm or exclude common associated anomalies should be obtained prior to surgical intervention.

Management

The goals of preoperative management are prevention of aspiration by continuous suctioning of proximal pouch with a specialized nasogastric tube (Replogle), sepsis treatment, and respiratory and nutritional support. Early definitive surgical correction is very successful in the absence of other congenital anomalies, with survival approaching 100%.

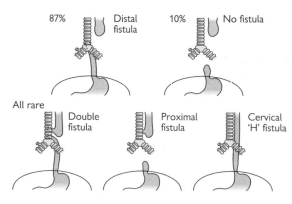

Fig 13.6 Diagram of classification of tracheo-oesophageal fistulae.

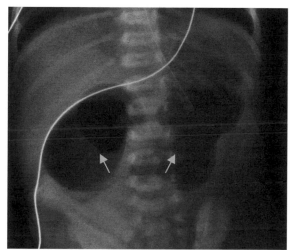

Fig 13.7 Plain abdominal radiograph showing the double bubble appearance of duodenal atresia (arrows).

⊙ Neonatal bowel obstruction

Bowel obstruction without bile-stained vomiting
- Duodenal atresia (proximal to ampulla of Vater, 20%)
- Duodenal stenosis
- Rare: pyloric atresia, pyloric stenosis, annular pancreas

Bowel obstruction with bile-stained vomiting
- Duodenal atresia (distal to ampulla of Vater, 80%)
- Malrotation with midgut volvulus
- Jejunal atresia

Bowel obstruction with marked abdominal distension
- Meconium plug
- Meconium ileus
- Hirschsprung disease
- Anorectal malformation
- Uncommon: ileal atresia
- Rare: small left colon syndrome, colonic atresia

Necrotizing enterocolitis

Nectrotizing enterocolitis (NEC) or other systemic sepsis may cause ileus, and so present with bile-stained vomiting and abdominal distension, mimicking bowel obstruction. NEC is common in pre-term infants and is due to bowel ischaemia and infection, resulting in intestinal necrosis. Plain radiographs show intramural gas (pneumatosis coli). Indications for surgery include refractory sepsis and bowel perforation.

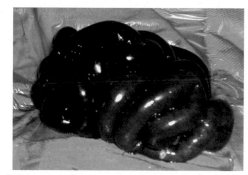

Fig 13.8 Intraoperative appearance of midgut volvulus resulting in catastrophic bowel infarction.

Infantile hypertrophic pyloric stenosis (IHPS) is narrowing of the pyloric canal caused by thickening of the smooth muscle wall. IHPS is the commonest cause of intestinal obstruction and vomiting in the first 2 months of life. Incidence is 2–5 per 1000 live births, with a peak at 2–8 weeks. There is a male preponderance (M:F 4:1).

Aetiology

IHPS is a multifactorial genetic disorder. Familial clustering indicates a polygenic trait.

Genetic

Familial incidence does not follow Mendelian inheritance. First-born infants are most commonly affected (30%). Predominance in children of affected parents approaches 10%. However, similar concordance in monozygotic compared with dizygotic twins (or non-twin siblings) suggests that environmental factors are also important.

Environmental

- Nitric oxide (NO) synthase deficiency: NO is a myenteric plexus neurotransmitter responsible for smooth muscle relaxation
- Abnormal myenteric plexus: abnormal nerve terminal distribution, immature neurons, and ganglia
- Hypergastrinaemia: hyperacidity causes repeated pyloric contraction, resulting in overwork hypertrophy
- Antibiotics: prenatal exposure to non-erythromycin macrolides

Pathophysiology

IHPS is typified by hypertrophy and hyperplasia of circular and longitudinal muscle layers of the pylorus, leading to thickening and elongation of the pyloric canal.

The thickening, along with pyloric spasm and mucosal oedema, causes a functional gastric outlet obstruction. Marked stomach dilatation occurs in advanced cases.

Clinical assessment

History

- Onset of vomiting at 2–8 weeks. Rare before 10 days or after 3 months
- Postprandial vomiting is initially mild, then forceful, and eventually projectile
- Vomiting is strictly non-bile-stained, and, once established, occurs after every feed
- Exclude sepsis, e.g. fever, offensive urine, diarrhoea

Examination

- Early: active and hungry but losing weight
- Late: weak and lethargic, indicative of dehydration
- Visible peristalsis: left to right across epigastrium during a test feed
- Examine for an 'olive'-shaped pyloric mass in the RUQ. Start from infant's left, palpating with the left hand. A well performed test feed may assist mass palpation by relaxing the baby and distending the stomach

Investigations

- Bloods—FBC (increased HCT), U+Es, including chloride
- Capillary blood gas—repeated vomiting typically results in hypochloraemic, hypokalaemic metabolic alkalosis through loss of electrolyte-rich acidic vomitus. Compensatory renal retention of H^+ in favour of K^+ exacerbates hypokalaemia
- Abdominal USS is diagnostic. The classic appearance in the transverse plane is a 'doughnut': echogenic centre of mucosa with circumferential thickened echopenic pyloric muscle (Fig 13.9)
  Diagnostic measurements vary between institutions. Typical values are muscle wall thickness >4 mm, canal length >16 mm
- Contrast studies of the upper gastrointestinal tract are rarely used. They may show gastro-oesophageal reflux, malrotation or other causes of proximal obstruction

Management

IHPS itself is not a surgical emergency. It is the accompanying dehydration and acid–base disturbance that needs to be addressed urgently.

Immediate

- Rehydrate and correct electrolyte imbalance using 0.45% NaCl over 24–48 h
- Wide-bore nasogastric tube (8Ch). The viscosity of gastric secretions in children is no different to adults, and narrow lumen nasogastric tubes are of no benefit. Ongoing nasogastric losses must also be replaced
- Nil by mouth

Pyloromyotomy

Operative management is pyloromyotomy (see box). Ramstedt first described an open pyloromyotomy via a RUQ incision in 1911. Modifications commonly used in the UK include open pyloromyotomy via a periumbilical incision, and laparoscopic techniques.

Endoscopic balloon dilatation and local injection (e.g. atropine sulphate) of the stenosed pylorus are not clinically proven.

Complications and prognosis

Following adequate resuscitation, complications are infrequent and death extremely rare.

Failure to correct the dehydration and acid–base disturbance prior to surgery may result in refractory hypotension and an inability to extubate the infant, as the physiological response to uncorrected metabolic alkalosis is hypoventilation.

➕ Open pyloromyotomy

Procedure
- Skin incision in RUQ (Ramstedt) or periumbilical
- Incise rectus sheath, peritoneum, and deliver stomach/pyloric mass
- Serosal incision made from pyloroduodenal junction to antrum. Muscle split is achieved using curved mosquito forceps (or Denis–Browne pyloric spreader) with care to avoid mucosal perforation (Fig 13.10)
- The risk of perforation, commonest at the pyloro-duodenal junction, is reduced by Whiting's manoeuvre (invaginating the duodenal mucosa)
- Air leak test may be used to detect mucosal perforation. About 40 mL of air is instilled into the stomach via a nasogastric tube. Appearance of air bubbles suggests a perforation that requires closure
- In the event of a perforation, a nasogastric tube is kept in place and feeds delayed for 48 h

Postoperative care
- Feeds are recommenced 6–12 h postoperatively. Hydration is maintained intravenously until feeds are re-established

Complications
Complications are rare but include inadequate myotomy, haemorrhage, and wound infection. This is commonest in malnourished infants, and may be further complicated by dehiscence and incisional hernia.

⊙ The vomiting infant

Vomiting is common in neonates and infants. It is most frequently related to feeding or medical problems. The characteristics that are concerning include:

- persistency
- projectile
- bile-stained
- blood-stained
- failure to gain weight or weight loss

- Surgical diagnoses
- Pyloric stenosis
- Gastro-oesophageal reflux
- Strangulated inguinal hernia
- Malrotation and volvulus

Medical diagnoses
- Overfeeding
- Gastroenteritis
- UTI
- Meningitis
- Septicaemia
- Rare: raised intracranial pressure, congenital adrenal hyperplasia, or other inborn errors of metabolism

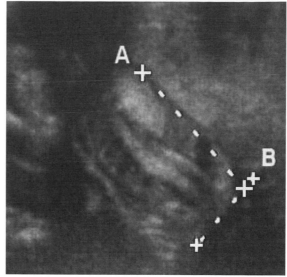

Fig 13.9 Abdominal ultrasound showing a thickened and lengthened pyloric canal in a case of IHPS.

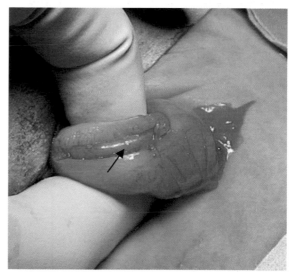

Fig 13.10 Open pyloromyotomy. Serosa and muscle have been longitudinally incised, allowing the underlying mucosa (arrow) to bulge outward, overcoming the stenosis.

Intussusception is the invagination of one bowel segment (intussusceptum) inside the lumen of the adjacent distal segment (intussuscipiens). Intussusception is the commonest cause of intestinal obstruction in infants, with an incidence of 1–4 per 1000 live births. It has a peak at 3–7 months, with over 90% of cases presenting before 3 years of age (M:F 3:2).

Aetiology

Over 90% of cases are labelled idiopathic as no abnormality is detected. It is suggested the lead point might be lymphoid tissues from Peyer's patches in the terminal ileum. This explains the relationship to preceding respiratory or GI tract infection and the increased incidence after administration of early versions of the rotavirus vaccine.

Mechanical lead points are typically seen in older children and include Meckel's diverticulum (75%), polyp, and lymphoma. Intussusception may complicate Henoch–Schönlein purpura and cystic fibrosis.

Pathophysiology

Antegrade peristalsis carries the intussusceptum apex ('lead point') and associated mesentery into the distal bowel (Fig 13.11)

Intussusception causes compression of the intussusceptum mesenteric vessels and obstruction of intussuscipiens lumen. This in turn causes venous and lymphatic congestion, leading to intestinal ischaemia and later perforation which may present with 'redcurrant jelly' stools and peritonism.

The most common type of intussusception is ileocolic (75% are ileocaecal), i.e. a portion of terminal ileum intussuscepts through the ileocaecal valve into the colon and sometimes extends all the way around to the rectum. Rarer types of intussusception are ileo–ileocolic, ileal–ileal and colo–colic.

Clinical assessment

The condition can progress rapidly over 24 h, with the infant becoming dehydrated and septic. Initial assessment and management should follow APLS guidelines if the infant is unwell. The classic triad of colicky abdominal pain, vomiting, and redcurrant jelly stool is seen in a minority of cases.

History

- Prodromal febrile illness often with diarrhoea
- Early: paroxysms of colicky abdominal pain lasting a few minutes. Infant screams and draws-up knees (>80%)
- Vomiting becomes bilious and more frequent as intestinal obstruction develops
- Late: mucoid, bloody 'redcurrant jelly' stools suggest intestinal ischaemia

Examination

- Pale and lethargic or irritable in between episodes of pain
- Palpable abdominal mass, often described as 'sausage-shaped' (Dance's sign), is typically found in the RUQ
- Abdominal distension and tenderness increase as the obstruction develops
- DRE is sensitive for blood (>80%). A palpable rectal mass or transanal prolapse is uncommon

Differential diagnosis

- Colicky abdominal pain: wind colic, milk intolerance, acute appendicitis
- Intestinal obstruction: strangulated inguinal hernia, adhesive/Meckel's band, volvulus
- Bloody stools—gastroenteritis, Meckel's diverticulum

Investigations

- Bloods—FBC (raised WCC), U+Es (dehydration)
- Plain abdominal radiograph is often normal or may show a non-specific abnormality early on. Small bowel obstruction causes fluid-filled loops of bowel with paucity of right-sided bowel gas. Pneumoperitoneum is an indication for urgent laparotomy
- Abdominal USS is the gold standard investigation. The intussusception can be recognized because of interposition of hyperechoic intussusceptum mesenteric fat between hypoechoic and oedematous intussuscipiens bowel wall, which is classically described as the target sign (transverse, Fig 13.12), sandwich sign (longitudinal) or pseudokidney (oblique), according to orientation

Management

All infants require aggressive fluid resuscitation to replace third space losses prior to reduction of the intussusception. Peritonitis, perforation, and shock refractory to fluid resuscitation are absolute indications for emergency operative reduction.

Immediate

- Intravenous fluid resuscitation
- Intravenous broad spectrum antibiotics
- Wide-bore nasogastric tube on free drainage
- Analgesia
- Nil by mouth

Non-operative

Air reduction enema under fluoroscopic guidance is the criterion standard for non-operative treatment of intussusception. Saline reduction under ultrasound guidance may also be used, but hydrostatic reduction using water-souble contrast or barium is no longer in wide-spread use.

Laparotomy

Site of intussusception and viability of involved bowel is assessed. Frankly ischaemic bowel is excised without attempt to reduce the intussusceptum–intussuscipiens complex to prevent systemic circulation of toxins on re-perfusion. Where reduction is appropriate, non-viable bowel is excised with either stoma formation or primary anastomosis. More recently, laparoscopy has been used to manage irreducible intussusception.

Complications and prognosis

Prompt diagnosis and management leads to a low complication rate and excellent prognosis. Untreated intussusception leads to sepsis and death. Complications include:

- intestinal haemorrhage
- bowel wall necrosis, intestinal perforation, sepsis
- recurrence (5–10%) usually occurs within first 24 h and is more common following air-reduction enema
- intestinal stricture, which is caused by marginal ischaemia of reduced bowel and subsequent fibrosis

➕ Air reduction enema

Air reduction enema is successful in 80–85% of cases. Failure after three attempts is an indication for laparotomy. Delayed re-attempts may succeed, but the patient's condition takes precedence. It can be performed under fluoroscopic (Fig 13.13) or ultrasound guidance.

Procedure
- Intubate rectum with Foley catheter
- Tape buttocks to secure position and promote seal which may be aided by judicious catheter balloon inflation
- Scout plain film excludes pneumoperitoneum
- Instil air whilst recording the pressure with manometry, keeping the pressure below 120 mmHg
- Imaging is used to monitor the retrograde movement of the intussusceptum by the column of distal air
- Successful reduction is confirmed by the sudden appearance of air throughout the small bowel

Complications
- Failure of reduction is more common at extremes of age (<3 months or >5 years) and if symptoms have lasted longer than 48 h
- Perforation (<2%) occurs in normal bowel owing to excessive enema pressure at sites of transmural necrosis
- Perforation during air reduction causes a tension pneumoperitoneum. Emergency decompression by low midline wide-bore needle stab is followed by a laparotomy

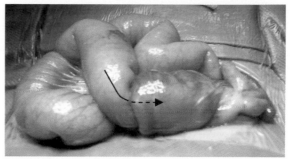

Fig 13.11 Intraoperative photograph showing an ileo–ileal intussusception (arrow denotes path of intussusceptum).

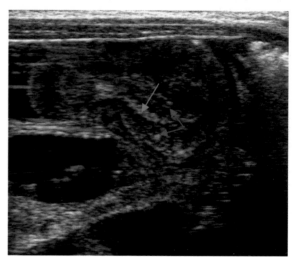

Fig 13.12 Abdominal ultrasound showing characteristic target sign with hyperechoic mesenteric fat (green arrow) interposed between intussuscipiens bowel wall (red arrows).

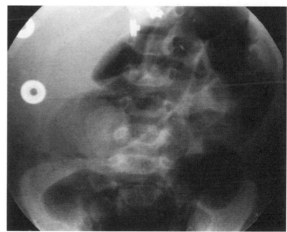

Fig 13.13 Air reduction enema, showing the distal colon distended by insufflated air and a filling defect (intussusceptum) in the proximal transverse colon close to the hepatic flexure.

Phimosis

Phimosis is the inability to retract the foreskin proximally over the glans penis.

Aetiology

Phimosis is usually a normal physiological phenomenon, with retraction prevented by a narrow preputial orifice and fusion of the inner foreskin and glans epithelia. The prevalence decreases with age (96% in neonates; 10–15% at 4 years; 1% at 18 years).

Pathological phimosis (preputial stenosis) is caused by scarring of the foreskin orifice as a result of balanitis xerotica obliterans (BXO), recurrent balanoposthitis, or trauma, including paraphimosis. Pathological phimosis occurs in all age groups, with a prevalence of 4–10%.

Pathophysiology

Resolution of physiological phimosis occurs with maturation of the developing foreskin. The foreskin separates from the glans, with keratinization of opposing epithelia. The foreskin orifice also widens, allowing retraction.

Clinical assessment

History

- Ballooning (or inflation) of foreskin during micturition occurs when the foreskin is partially or completely separated but remains non-retractile. Ballooning in the context of physiological phimosis is normal
- White, cheesy discharge (smegma)
- History suggestive of pathological phimosis: recurrent inflammation of the foreskin ± shaft of penis, dysuria, or difficulty passing urine, worsening phimosis, which may completely occlude the foreskin orifice

Examination

Examination must distinguish between physiological and pathological phimosis.

- Physiological phimosis: non-inflamed healthy foreskin, which is free from scarring, pliable, and 'pouts' during attempts to gently retract over the glans (Fig 13.14)
- Pathological phimosis: acute and/or chronically inflamed foreskin, with scarring of the foreskin orifice preventing retraction (Fig 13.15)

Management

Physiological phimosis

Management options for physiological phimosis vary with age but are based around reassurance, daily retraction, and topical steroids in adolescents. Delayed physiological phimosis which is refractory to non-operative management warrants consideration for preputioplasty (widening of the distal foreskin) or circumcision.

Pathological phimosis

Conservative options (topical steroids or preputioplasty) are rarely effective and circumcision is usually performed.

Complications and prognosis

Physiological phimosis generally resolves spontaneously, with fewer than 10% needing surgery. Pathological phimosis caused by BXO can lead to meatal stenosis with or without a urethral stricture.

Balanitis xerotica obliterans

BXO is a chronic, progressive, sclerosing dermatosis of unknown aetiology. It is similar to lichen sclerosis seen in females.

Initially it affects the foreskin, leading to phimosis, but may progress to affect the glans, urethral meatus, and urethra, with complications including meatal stenosis and urethral stricture.

BXO may be a premalignant condition, and is the only absolute indication for circumcision (see box). Some paediatric urologists consider a role for corticosteroid ointments in early disease.

Paraphimosis

Paraphimosis is the inability to reduce a retracted foreskin back over the glans penis into its normal position.

Constriction, typically at the coronal sulcus, results in increasingly painful oedema with venous engorgement. If untreated, ischaemia and necrosis of glans and foreskin ensue.

Emergency reduction is achieved under local or general anaesthesia. Typically, the resulting foreskin is more easily retractile. Foreskin scarring may predispose to recurrence, needing a preputioplasty or circumcision.

Balanitis

Balanitis is inflammation of the glans penis. Balanoposthitis is balanitis that also involves foreskin and prepuce in uncircumcised patients. It is a common condition and affects men of all ages, but is particularly common in infants and toddlers.

It results from infection (bacterial>viral) or dermatitis. Candidal species are most common in diabetics. In adult men, obesity and poor personal hygiene are risk factors.

Clinical assessment

Symptoms include penile discharge, tenderness, and itching. It is a common cause of phimosis (see below).

On examination, the glans penis and foreskin may be inflamed and oedematous.

Investigations

- Routine bloods not normally indicated
- Send swab for MCS

Management

The majority of cases are self-limiting or resolve without sequelae following antibiotic treatment.

Twenty per cent develop recurrent episodes, and may progress to foreskin scarring and pathological phimosis. Circumcision is an effective treatment for pathological phimosis owing to recurrent balanoposthitis, but balanoposthitis may also occur in circumcised males.

✚ Circumcision

The only absolute indication for circumcision is BXO. Relative indications include recurrent balanoposthitis, paraphimosis, and delayed physiological phimosis.

Circumcisions are also performed for non-medical indications, i.e. religious, cultural or social reasons.

It is contraindicated in congenital penile conditions (e.g. hypospadias) as the foreskin may be needed for future reconstruction.

Procedure
- GA or LA
- Skin incisions are made using either a scalpel or scissors. Inner preputial incision should run circumferentially approximately 5 mm proximal to the corona, and outer incison circumferentially at level of corona. Sleeve of skin between incisions is then removed
- Place interrupted or running suture along cut edges
- Particular care around frenulum (bleeding and underlying urethra)

Complications

Intraoperative and early
- Asymmetrical skin excision
- Injury to glans or urethra
- Haemorrhage (1%)
- Infection

Intermediate and late
- Meatal stenosis
- Urethral fistula
- Painful erection

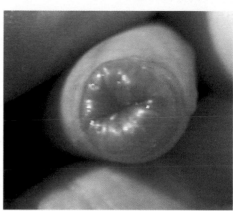

Fig 13.14 Physiological phimosis. The foreskin is healthy and not inflamed and without scarring. It 'pouts' during attempts at gentle retraction.

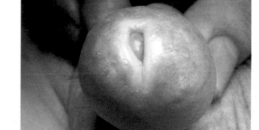

Fig 13.15 Balanitis xerotica obliterans. The foreskin is scarred and cannot be retracted over the glans of the penis. There is circumferential white scarring, plaques, and a narrowed foreskin meatus.

13.9 Testicular torsion

Testicular torsion or, more correctly, torsion of the spermatic cord, is an emergency. It is the commonest cause of an acute scrotum in pubescent boys and young men.

The incidence is 1 per 4000 males under 25 years old, with a bimodal (neonatal and puberty) age distribution. It peaks in winter months and at northern latitudes, possibly being caused by cremaster contraction in response to cooler ambient temperatures.

Aetiology

Intravaginal torsion (95%, Fig 13.16)

This usually develops in older boys. Attachment of the tunica vaginalis is abnormally high, allowing testis to hang free (bell clapper anomaly) within the tunica vaginalis.

Extravaginal torsion (5%)

This presents during the neonatal period, but usually develops prenatally (in utero), either before completion of testicular descent or owing to failure of normal fusion. The torsion occurs proximal to the tunica vaginalis and so is extravaginal.

Pathophysiology

Torsion of the spermatic cord and vessels causes venous congestion, and oedema, haemorrhage, and, finally, arterial occlusion resulting in testicular ischaemia, infarction, and necrosis (Fig 13.17). Most torsions are medial (70%) and typically rotate 180–720°. Left is more common than right; less than 5% are bilateral.

Clinical assessment

History

- Acute onset of unilateral severe testicular pain
- Recent episodes of pain may be intermittent torsions
- Abdominal pain, nausea, and vomiting are possible
- No urinary symptoms

Examination

- Distressed child with wide-based gait
- Firm and diffusely tender testis lying in a high transverse position in the scrotum ('bell clapper'). Note that the right testis usually lies higher in the scrotum than the left
- Erythematous and oedematous hemiscrotum
- Reactive hydrocele may be present, especially if the presentation is delayed
- Cremasteric reflex is typically absent, but presence does not exclude torsion
- Spermatic cord may be thickened and tender owing to congestion of vessels

Investigations

Investigations should not delay surgery once the clinical diagnosis is made. Testicular colour Doppler USS demonstrating no arterial flow to testis in acute torsion is yet to be adopted into routine practice owing to concerns regarding its specificity and sensitivity. Urinalysis helps to exclude UTI and epididymitis.

Management

A high suspicion of testicular torsion is an indication for emergency exploration of the scrotum irrespective of fasting status (see box). If emergency surgery is delayed, manual de-torsion should be attempted as a temporary manoeuvre. Its success rate approaches 70%.

Complications and prognosis

The rate of testicular salvage and subsequent morbidity is related to the duration of torsion (<6 h leads to >95% salvaged; >24 h, <5% salvaged).

Testicular atrophy develops in 30–50% of salvaged testis and subfertility in up to 30–40%. Subfertility may be related to ischaemia, anti-testicular antibodies, and secondarily reduced microcirculation affecting contralateral testis.

Patients requiring orchidectomy are offered a testicular prosthesis. This is carried out at least 6 months after the initial surgery and inserted via an inguinal incision.

Torsion of testicular appendages

Torsion of a testicular appendage is the commonest cause of an acute scrotum in pre-pubertal children (peak 7–11 years). Testicular appendages are present on 85–90% of testes. Only a minority will develop a torsion.

Aetiology

Of the four types of testicular appendage, the commonest is the appendix testis, a remnant of the paramesonephric (Mullerian) duct. The rest are remnants of the mesonephric (Wollfian) duct.

- Appendix testis (hydatid cyst of Morgagni)
- Appendix epididymis
- Paradidymus (organ of Giraldes)
- Ductulus aberrans (vas aberrans of Haller)

Pathophysiology

Testicular appendages are often pedunculated and so prone to torsion. Localized acute inflammation of the tunica vaginalis and/or epididymis is responsible for symptoms of localized scrotal pain.

Clinical assessment

Compared with testicular torsion, the testicular pain has a slower onset and is less severe. Most cases present after 6 h.

- Hemiscrotum is usually normal, but may be inflamed with a reactive hydrocele present, especially with a delayed presentation. Cremasteric reflex is typically present
- Testicular orientation and palpation is normal. Tenderness is localized to the upper pole
- Necrotic testicular appendage is occasionally visible through scrotal skin as the 'blue dot' sign
- Exclude intra-abdominal sepsis and inguinal herniae

Management

If the diagnosis is certain, the patient can be managed conservatively with analgesia. If there is any doubt the scrotum must be explored.

Complications and prognosis

Non-operative management may occasionally be associated with ongoing discomfort (>48 h), and delayed exploration to remove the appendage may be required.

The necrotic, torted appendage atrophies, and is absorbed without sequelae.

✚ Scrotal exploration

The symptomatic side should be marked preoperatively and the parent warned about the possibility of orchidectomy.

Procedure

- Skin incision is transverse scrotal or midline raphae
- Scrotal layers (skin, dartos fascia, tunica vaginalis)
- Incision of tunica vaginalis heralded by evacuation of secondary hydrocele and deliver testis by incision and eversion of tunica vaginalis
- Inspect for torsion of the spermatic cord, noting the direction and degree of torsion (typically medial to lateral, 360–720°)
- Assess testis for viability
- Infarcted or necrotic testis should be removed (orchidectomy) before de-torting as there is a theoretical risk of releasing antitesticular antibodies, which may cause subfertility in the contralateral testis
- Ischaemic but salvageable testis should be de-torted and placed in warm damp swabs. De-torsion is guided by orientation of the lateral sulcus between epididymis and testis, with care to avoid partial de-torsion if >360°
- Orchidopexy of the contralateral testis is indicated if there is testicular torsion confirmed, as the predisposing 'bell clapper' anatomy is bilateral in 40% of cases. The midline raphae incision allows both procedures to be performed via a single incision
- If no torsion is identified, any pedunculated testicular appendage is removed but contralateral orchidopexy is contraindicated
- Close scrotum in two layers or *en masse* using interrupted sutures

Complications

Intraoperative and early	Late
• Infection	• Testicular atrophy
• Haematoma	• Subfertility
• Incomplete de-torsion	

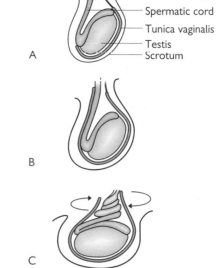

Fig 13.16 (A) Normal testis with posterolateral attachment of the tunica vaginalis. (B) 'Bell clapper' testis with abnormally high attachment of the tunica vaginalis. (C) Intravaginal torsion of a 'bell clapper' testis. The torted testis is lying transverse in a raised position.

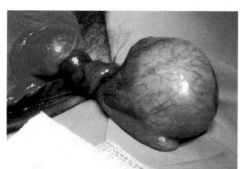

Fig 13.17 Ischaemic torted testis and spermatic cord found at scrotal exploration. The appearance of this testis improved after de-torsion, and orchidectomy was avoided.

Epididymitis is inflammation of the epididymis. Orchitis is inflammation of the testis. Epididymitis most commonly occurs on its own although it is often referred to as epididymo-orchitis. It is as common as testicular torsion in pre-pubertal males. There is a bimodal age distribution, with peaks at puberty > infancy. It affects both sides equally.

Aetiology

Epididymitis

- Most commonly a bacterial infection (*Escherichia coli*, *Proteus mirabilis*)
- Non-infective causes such as Henoch–Schönlein purpura (HSP), drugs (amiodarone), and trauma are rare
- Renal tract anomalies predispose children to urinary tract infection, which can cause epididymitis by retrograde ascent along the vas deferens

Orchitis

- Viral infection (mumps orchitis) is most common. It occurs via haematogenous spread and so is independent of renal tract. Bacterial and atypical infections are rare

Pathophysiology

Infection typically begins in the tail of the epididymis, spreading towards the body and head, causing concomitant orchitis in 20–40% of cases.

It is thought that retrograde passage of infected urine from the prostatic urethra reaches the epididymis via the vas deferens. Urethra–vasal reflux does not normally occur and so patients should undergo screening for urinary tract anomalies.

Clinical assessment

Testicular pain has a more insidious onset and is less severe than torsion of the spermatic cord. There may be accompanying dysuria, lower abdominal pain, and fever.

Examination

- Epididymitis: tenderness and oedema start in the tail, then body and spermatic cord
- Prehn's manoeuvre (elevation of scrotum above pubis symphysis) leads to the relief of epididymitis pain but exacerbation of testicular torsion pain
- Hemiscrotum may be inflamed and the cremasteric reflex is typically present. Testicular orientation is normal
- Orchitis: testis is enlarged and tender. There may be a reactive hydrocele. The epididymis is non-tender

Investigations

- Urinalysis and MCS if a urinary tract infection is suspected
- Bloods not routine. FBC shows raised WCC
- Colour Doppler USS: thickened, hyperaemic epididymis +/- testis and scrotal skin
- Renal USS +/- MCUG performed during outpatient follow-up to exclude underlying renal tract anomalies

Management

If testicular torsion cannot be excluded, the scrotum must be explored. If the diagnosis is certain, the patient can be managed conservatively. Admission and intravenous antibiotics are given if the patient is systemically unwell.

- Rest and scrotal support
- Analgesia and ice
- Antibiotics

Complications and prognosis

Complications of bacterial epididymo-orchitis include abscess, pyocele, gangrene, and infarction. Late complications include testicular atrophy, chronic pain, and subfertility.

Idiopathic scrotal oedema

Idiopathic scrotal oedema is uncommon and tends to be pre-pubertal, with a peak incidence at 5–7 years. Over 50% of cases are bilateral.

The aetiology is unknown, although it is likely to be viral or allergic. The scrotal swelling and light erythema develop over 2–4 h. On examination there is marked scrotal oedema, often extending to inguinal and perineal regions (Fig 13.19). The testes are normal and non-tender.

The condition is occasionally tender and can lead to diagnostic uncertainty in the early stages. In this situation, the testis can be manoeuvred into the groin for examination to confirm the absence of testicular signs.

No investigations are required. The condition is self-limiting and resolves over 48–72 h but often recurs.

Table 13.4 Differential diagnosis of acute scrotum

Diagnosis	Age	Onset	Tenderness	Urinalysis	Treatment
Testicular torsion	Pubertal (>12 years) (or neonatal)	Acute	Testis and cord	Negative	Emergent exploration
Torsion of appendage	Pre-pubertal (<12 years)	Subacute	Upper pole testis +/- over 'blue dot'	Negative	Analgesia +/- exploration for pain
Epididymo-orchitis	Pubertal (or neonatal)	Subacute	Epididymis +/- testis	Positive (or negative)	Antibiotics
Idiopathic scrotal oedema	Pre-pubertal	Acute	Skin may be tender, testis non-tender	Negative	Reassure

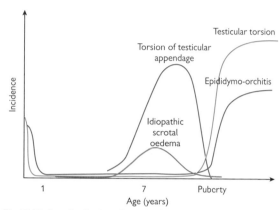

Fig 13.18 Age distribution of causes of acute scrotum.

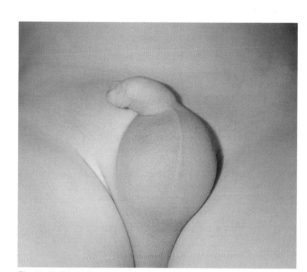

Fig 13.19 Idiopathic scrotal oedema. There is marked scrotal erythema and swelling, extending both into the groin and perineum.

13.11 Infantile inguinal hernia and hydrocele

Inguinal hernia is the commonest condition requiring surgery during childhood. It occurs in 2 per 100 live births (including 30 per 100 live premature births). Its peak incidence is in infancy and there is a male preponderance (M:F 6:1). Most are right-sided (60%), some occur on the left (30%), and bilateral is uncommon.

Inguinoscrotal embryology

Indeterminant phase (weeks < 8)
The urogenital ridge and development of the male and female gonads is morphologically identical up to 7–8 weeks of gestation. Over the following weeks the male testis descends to the scrotum in two sequential phases.

Transabdominal phase (weeks 8–15)
This phase is controlled by Müllerian-inhibiting substance (MIS) secreted by the Sertoli cells. It causes regression of the cranial suspensory ligament of the testis and swelling enlargement of the gubernaculum (caudal suspensory ligament). The gubernaculum anchors the testis near the internal inguinal ring. Somatic fetal growth results in net migration of the testis from just below the kidneys to the level of the internal inguinal ring.

Processus vaginalis (weeks 20–25)
The processus vaginalis (PV) is a peritoneal diverticulum attached to the lower pole of the testis which elongates with the gubernaculum. The PV extends further, with caudal gubernacular growth towards the base of scrotum 'hollowing' out the inguinal canal.

Inguinoscrotal phase (weeks 28–35)
Under the guidance of the gubernaculum, the testis descends with the PV along the inguinal canal and into the scrotum. Descent is controlled primarily by testosterone and calcitonin gene-related peptide (CGRP). CGRP is released by the genitofemoral nerve in response to androgen. It causes rhythmic contraction and shortening of the gubernaculum. Once descent is complete, the patent PV is obliterated and the gubernaculum becomes secondarily attached to the scrotum.

Aetiology
Indirect inguinal hernia and congenital hydrocele are both caused by a patent PV. The width of the PV channel determines which occurs: the PV is wide in indirect inguinal herniae, and narrow in the case of congenital hydrocele.

Risk factors for indirect inguinal herniae
- Prematurity and low birth weight
- Chronic respiratory disease of prematurity
- Increased peritoneal fluid, e.g. VP shunt, ascites, CAPD
- Genital anomalies: testicular maldescent, hypospadias
- Congenital abdominal wall defects
- Connective tissue disorders

Direct inguinal herniae
Direct inguinal herniae are very rare in childhood.

Non-communicating hydroceles
Non-communicating hydroceles are less common than congenital (i.e. communicating) hydroceles in childhood. Examples include reactive hydroceles due to trauma, tumour or infection, hydrocele of cord and rare varieties such as hydrocele of the canal of Nuck (female cord hydrocele equivalent) and abdominoscrotal hydrocele.

Pathophysiology
The clinical significance of inguinal herniae is their predilection (~50%) to incarceration. Occlusion of the gonadal and mesenteric vessels at the level of the internal ring and inguinal canal results in venous and lymphatic congestion followed by ischaemia of the gonad and/or bowel.

Clinical assessment
The aim is to exclude a condition that requires emergency surgery such as a strangulated hernia, intestinal obstruction or intra-abdominal sepsis.

History
- Painless groin or scrotal swelling is the most common presentation
- Ask about the onset, variation in size, and intermittent reducibility
- Colicky abdominal pain, vomiting or absolute constipation suggests bowel obstruction owing to incarceration or strangulation of a hernia

Examination
Examine both groins and the abdomen.
- Groin swelling (Fig 13.20) extends from internal inguinal ring towards scrotum/labia, cannot 'get above', tender; +/- reducible, inflamed overlying soft tissue, ovary within sac (female), undescended testis (male)
- Abdomen—distended, peritonism
- If no groin swelling is evident, increased abdominal pressure (palpation, cough, and laugh) may evoke hernia. If not, features suggesting a reduced inguinal hernia include: thickened spermatic cord and 'silk sign' (movement of hernial sac over cord structures)

Investigations
- Urinalysis (UTI)
- Plain abdominal radiograph if obstruction is suspected

Management
Owing to a greater than 50% risk of incarceration/complications, all cases of inguinal herniae must undergo surgical repair. Decision between elective, urgent or emergent repair is based on age of child and reducibility together with clinical status.

Manual reduction of inguinal hernia
Manual reduction of an incarcerated hernia should be attempted to minimize the risk of bowel and gonadal ischaemia. Contraindications include intra-abdominal or systemic sepsis, indicative of strangulation.

The fingers of one hand support the neck of the hernia and guide reduction towards the external ring. The other hand applies firm, continuous pressure upward from the base, slowly reducing the hernia. If initially unsuccessful, judicious sedation may facilitate manual reduction.

Herniotomy (see box)
Children with strangulated hernia, intra-abdominal sepsis, or a failed manual reduction need fluid resuscitation and emergency surgery. When manual reduction is successful, urgent inguinal herniotomy may be deferred for 24–72 h to allow inflammation to settle, as oedematous tissues increase the risk of complications.

Congenital hydrocele

Congenital hydroceles spontaneously resolve by age 2 years in over 90% of cases, and so surgery should be deferred until early childhood. Open or laparoscopic surgery to ligate the patent PV is similar to that performed for an indirect inguinal hernia (see box).

Simple aspiration (or injection of sclerosing agents) is not performed owing to the risk of recurrence, intra-abdominal sepsis, and bowel injury in an undiagnosed inguinal hernia.

Complications and prognosis

The main complication of untreated inguinal herniae is incarceration (30–70%), which can lead to bowel ischaemia, perforation, sepsis, and, rarely, death.

Complications of congenital hydroceles are uncommon. They include concomitant inguinal hernia, testicular atrophy with resultant subfertility, infection.

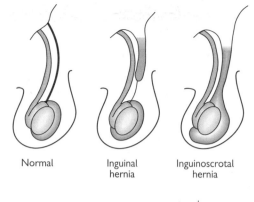

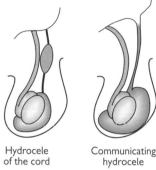

Fig 13.20 Diagram showing the different conditions arising from a patent processus vaginalis depending on its size and extent.

⊕ Paediatric inguinal herniotomy

A reliable parental history of an intermittent inguinal swelling is enough to prompt elective surgery, even in the presence of equivocal examination findings.

Procedure (open)

- Transverse lower abdominal skin crease incision
- Divide fat, Scarpa's fascia, and external oblique aponeurosis to expose patent spermatic cord complex
- PPV dissected free from the spermatic cord. Mosquito forceps placed across sac only, which is divided distally; proximal sac dissected to deep internal ring
- To minimize risk of injury, never grasp vas or vessels and avoid the use of diathermy
- Transfixion and division of PPV +/- reduction of sac contents: proximal sac may be opened to exclude sliding component, inspect for ischaemic bowel and/or ovary prior to transfixion and division
- Close in layers. In males, scrotal position of testis is confirmed
- Postoperative care: day cases require simple analgesia for 48 h, and abstinence from contact sports for 2 weeks.

Contralateral groin exploration

Surgical exploration of the contralateral groin to identify and treat contralateral PPV/inguinal hernia remains controversial. Growing consensus is that contralateral exploration is not indicated in the absence of clinical evidence except in uncomplicated female cases in which injury to the vas/gonadal vessels is not a consideration.

Laparoscopic inguinal herniotomy

Laparoscopic inguinal herniotomy is now routinely used in many UK paediatric surgical centres. Possible benefits include direct assessment and targeted treatment of contralateral PPV, reduced risk of injury to vas deferens, and easier examination of adnexal structures.

Complications

Intraoperative and early	Intermediate and late
• Injury of vas deferens	• Recurrence (6%)
• Injury of spermatic vessels	• Testicular atrophy (1–10%)
• Failure to identify ischaemic bowel	• Testicular ascent (1%)
• Wound infection (2%)	

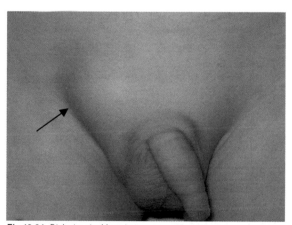

Fig 13.21 Right inguinal hernia.

13.12 Testicular maldescent

Testicular maldescent (also termed cryptorchidism) is the failure of a testis to descend and rest in the normal position in the scrotum. Incidence is approximately 1 in 20 male live births, with diagnosis made post-delivery or at the 6-week screening. Eighty per cent are unilateral (right > left); the rest are bilateral.

Classification

Maldescended testes are classified according to their position relative to path of normal descent.

- Undescended testes (UDT) are the most common (90%), and are found along the path of normal descent. They may be palpable (inguinal, 65%; emergent, 25%) or impalpable (intra-abdominal, 10%)
- Ectopic testes (10%) are found outside the path of normal descent. Ectopic sites are: pre-penile, femoral, perineal, and transverse ectopia (ectopic descent along the contralateral inguinal canal)

Retractile testes

Retractile testes are normally descended, and often wrongly grouped together with maldescended testes. Unlike an UDT, retractile testes may be brought to the base of the scrotum without undue tension on the cord structures, and do not require corrective surgery.

Aetiology

Congenital

The testis descends via two sequential phases (transabdominal and inguinoscrotal), as outlined in Topic 13.11. Failure of hormonal or anatomical (i.e. mechanical) mechanisms during each phase may arrest descent at that level.

Acquired or 'ascending testis'

Childhood growth increases the distance between the base of the scrotum and the external inguinal ring. The spermatic cord needs to lengthen to keep the testis in the scrotum.

An ascending testis is caused by failure of the cord to lengthen. Causes include cremasteric muscle spasticity (e.g. cerebral palsy), fibrous processus vaginalis remnant or complication of inguinal surgery.

Pathophysiology

Testicular descent brings the testes down into the cool environment of the scrotum which is kept at 2–3°C lower than core body temperature. Three anatomical features promote scrotal heat loss.

1. Scrotal skin rugae (increased surface area)
2. Lack of subcutaneous fat
3. Countercurrent heat exchange mechanism between the testicular pampiniform venous plexus and arterial vessels

Tubular dysplasia occurs in testes that reside outside the scrotum by 6–12 months of age, progressing to testicular atrophy in childhood, and this may explain increased risks of neoplasia in maldescended testes.

Temperature-induced germ cell degeneration results in irreversible azoospermia with increased rates of subfertility unless the testis is placed back in the scrotum before puberty.

Clinical assessment

The aims are to exclude a retractile testis, establish the diagnosis of undescended or ectopic testis and whether it is palpable or impalpable, and to exclude an intersex infant with bilateral impalpable UDT.

History

- Maternal hormone environment (*in utero* exposure to oestrogens and anti-androgens)
- Gestational age and weight at birth
- Family history of testicular maldescent, intersex, or congenital adrenal hyperplasia

Examination

Examine in a warm, relaxed environment.

- Inspect external genitalia for abnormalities (e.g. hypospadias) and the scrotum for asymmetry
- Check the cremasteric reflex which should make the testis retract but stay in the scrotum
- Palpate both hemiscrotums for testes. Compensatory hypertrophy of the descended, contralateral testis may occur if UDT is non-functional or absent
- Palpate for the UDT along the path of normal descent, starting lateral to internal inguinal ring and 'milking' contents of inguinal canal towards scrotum
- Gentle traction on the UDT and spermatic cord will show if testis can be brought into scrotum, and exclude normal but retractile testis or testicular masses
- If no UDT is palpable in the path of normal descent, examine ectopic sites (e.g. femoral and perineal areas)

Investigations

Routine investigations are not indicated in UDT unless bilateral or associated with hypospadias.

- Diagnostic laparoscopy is the best method for detecting impalpable testes, and is usually combined with definitive surgery
- Patients with hypospadias need further genetic and metabolic screening to exclude intersex disorders

Management

Over 95% of UDT descend in the first 3–6 months of life. Only 1% of infants have a persistent UDT at 1 year. Descent is unlikely after this age and so examination under anaesthetic and orchidopexy or orchidectomy (see box) is usually performed before 2 years of age.

Intravenous human chorionic gonadotropin and intranasal luteinizing hormone have been used to promote descent but these techniques are not clinically proven.

Complications and prognosis

Prognosis of UDT is good. Parents must be counselled about the increased risk of subfertility and cancer.

- Subfertility: occurs in 5% of men with maldescended testes, and is attributed to temperature-induced germ cell degeneration. Recent reports suggest early (≤2 years) orchidopexy reduces the risk of subfertility
- Testicular cancer: seminomas are most common in patients with UDTs, and NSGCT in testis following orchidopexy. It must be made clear that orchidopexy may not reduce the risk of cancer, but may assist in detection by self-examination

✚ Orchidopexy

Orchidopexy aims to place the testis in the scrotum to prevent torsion, improve fertility and cosmesis, and enable easy self-examination for testicular cancer. Orchidopexy for a palpable UDT has a success rate of 95%.

Examination under anaesthesia

- Palpable testes that are normal undergo orchidopexy; abnormal or atrophic testes need orchidectomy
- Impalpable testes need laparoscopy. This may identify the testis in the abdomen or show the cord entering the internal inguinal ring. If this is the case, groin exploration is needed. The procedure then follows the indications above
- Contralateral testicular fixation may be performed in infants requiring orchidectomy

Single stage procedure

- A scrotal, subinguinal, inguinal, suprainguinal or laparoscopic approach is used depending on the location of the testis
- Identify UDT within its tunica vaginalis
- Divide gubernaculum to allow mobilization of testis
- Ligate the PPV to obtain maximal length
- Deliver testis by incising and everting the tunica vaginalis
- Inspect the testis and excise any appendix testis
- Place testis into a sub-dartos pouch in scrotum. Fixation is achieved by adhesions forming between the testis and raw dartos pouch surfaces
- Testicular sutures are discouraged owing to risk of trauma to the testis and immunological consequences of breaching tunica albicans (anti-testis antibodies)

Two stage procedure (Fowler–Stephens)

When the length of the gonadal vessels is insufficient to bring testis into scrotum (e.g. intra abdominal testis), a staged procedure is employed (open or laparoscopic).

- First stage is division of gonadal vessels, leaving the testis to form a collateral circulation with the cremasteric and vasal vessels
- Second stage is performed 6 months later. A healthy testis indicates adequate collateral blood supply. It is moved down into the scrotum with its vascular pedicle and fixed. Atrophic or abnormal testes are excised

Complications

Intraoperative and early	Late
• Bleeding and haematoma	• Testicular ascent (<5%)
• Injury to vas deferens (1%)	• Testicular atrophy (1–5%)
• Epididymo-orchitis	
• Hydrocele	

Case 1

A 6-week-old infant is referred by the GP with an 8-day history of persistent vomiting. She has started to lose weight and has not wet her nappy for the past 12 h.

- What features of the vomiting would you ask about?

The infant is unsettled but consolable. She is both tachycardic and tachypnoeic. Abdominal examination is made difficult by the infant's movements and crying, but you suspect fullness in the RUQ.

- How would you assess her hydration status?
- What are the typical examination findings of a pyloric mass?
- What is a 'test feed' and how might it help the diagnosis?

Urinalysis is normal. Her blood results are below:

Venous bloods		Arterial blood gas	
Na$^+$	131 mmol/L	pH	7.50
K$^+$	3.0 mmol/L	HCO$_3^-$	37.4 mmol/L
Cl$^-$	84 umol/L	BE	14.6

- Discuss the blood results
- What imaging study would you arrange and what might it show?

Discussion

She has pyloric stenosis, complicated by hypochloraemic hypokalaemic metabolic alkalosis.

- Discuss immediate management. Does she need to go to theatre as an emergency?
- What are the options for managing pyloric stenosis?

Case 2

A 6 month-old infant is brought by his parents to the paediatric emergency department. The child has been non-specifically unwell for a week, and for the past 12 h has been periodically very upset with what appear to be colicky spasms. Despite being too sleepy to show any interest in his last two feeds he has just had a large vomit.

- What is the pathophysiology of colicky abdominal pain?
- Discuss the presentation and causes of bowel obstruction in infancy. What is the most likely diagnosis in this child?

On examination he is quiet and lethargic. He looks dehydrated. There is mild abdominal distension with a tender fullness in the RIF. Hernial orifices, external genitalia, and rectal examination are all normal. A spasm of colicky pain interrupts your examination, making cardiorespiratory examination impossible.

No urine sample is obtainable for urinalysis. A plain supine abdominal radiograph shows bowel obstruction.

- What would your approach be to managing this infant?
- What additional imaging study will confirm a clinical impression of intussusception and what are the findings?

Discussion

This infant has acute bowel obstruction due to intussusception. He is dehydrated and requires fluid resuscitation.

- Describe the pathophysiology of intussusception?
- What additional immediate management would you institute to treat and prevent the sequelae of intussusception?
- What are the indications for surgical intervention?

Case 3

A 3-year-old boy is referred to the outpatient clinic for assessment for circumcision. His parents are anxious that he has a 'tight foreskin'. The foreskin balloons notably as he passes urine, and he tends to spray everywhere. The GP has told them that a circumcision is indicated.

- What is phimosis and paraphimosis?
- What symptoms are suggestive of pathological phimosis?

You examine the genitalia (Fig 13.14). The remainder of the examination is unremarkable.

- What signs are sought to identify pathological phimosis?
- Are any further investigations required in this case?

Discussion

You reassure the parents that their child has a normal foreskin with physiological phimosis. His parents remain very concerned about the tightness of the foreskin. His cousin had a tight foreskin which needed surgery after he pulled it back and it got stuck.

- What is your management plan for this young boy?
- What advice will you give regarding retraction of the foreskin?
- Discuss, with reference to indications for treatment, whether this child warrants circumcision.

Case 4

A 12-year-old girl is referred by the out-of-hours GP service for assessment of lower abdominal pain. It started as diffuse abdominal discomfort 2 days ago and has been getting gradually worse, particularly over the past 12 h.

- Describe the history you will take
- What signs will you look for on examination?
- What is your differential diagnosis?

The girl appears flushed and walks stooped towards the examination couch. She declines your request to hop or jump. ENT and cardiorespiratory examination is unremarkable. Tenderness is prominent in the lower abdomen and maximal in the RIF. Rectal exam is not performed.

The observation chart shows temperature is 37.8°C, HR 121 and RR 28.

- What is peritonism and how might the presentation differ between children and adults?
- Are any investigations necessary?

Discussion

This girl has localized peritonism, with a clinical diagnosis of acute appendicitis. Urinary βHCG is negative. You recommend appendicectomy and gain consent from her mother.

- What must you cover during the consent process?
- Can the girl refuse consent for the operation?

Chapter 14

Transplant surgery

Basic principles

Knowledge

◎ Clinical skills

- HLA tissue typing
- Brainstem death
- Patient assessment for transplantation

✚ Technical skills and procedures

- Renal transplant biopsy
- Multiple organ retrieval
- Renal transplantation (deceased donor)
- Liver transplantation
- Heart transplantation

14.1 Immunology

An individual's immune system consists of cells and cell products that protect against potentially harmful substances. It is divided into innate and acquired systems. Each has cellular and non-cellular (humoral) components.

Innate immunity

This is an inherited and evolutionary primitive system. Its components form an immediately available first line of defence but are unable to adapt or remember previously encountered pathogens.

Acquired immunity

Acquired immunity is a complex system mediated by cells (lymphocytes) and antibodies. It is able to recognize what is foreign, i.e. distinguish between self and non-self.

Although slower to respond, it mounts a very specific response to the foreign material. It acquires a memory and so the second encounter of a pathogen elicits a faster and greater response.

Table 14.1 Immune system

	Innate	Acquired
Cellular	Neutrophils Macrophages Natural killer cells Dendritic cells	Blymphocytes Tlymphocytes
Humoral	Complement Cytokines Antibacterial agents Lactoferrin	Antibodies Cytokines

Immune components

Antigens

Antigens are substances that provoke an immune response and the production of antibodies. They are either foreign (non-self) or native to the host (self). The immune response they elicit depends on the similarity to the host, size, and chemical composition.

Autologous antigens are usually recognized as 'self' and do not elicit an immune response. However, a breakdown in this process is the cause of autoimmune diseases.

Major histocompatibility complex

The group of genes responsible for the cell surface molecules that present antigens are termed the major histocompatibility complex (MHC) and are found on the short arm of chromosome 6. As these molecules were first discovered on human leucocytes they are known as human leucocyte antigens (HLA). In the human MHC there are two major groups, termed class I and class II.

- Class I HLA (HLA-A, HLA-B, and HLA-C) are expressed on the surface of almost all nucleated cells in the body
- Class II HLA (HLA-DP, HLA-DQ, and HLA-DR) are usually found on immune related cells

T cells

T cells are lymphocytes that mature in the thymus. On their cell surface they have T cell receptors and various co-receptors (e.g. CD3, CD4, and CD8) which aid the recognition of antigens presented to them by antigen-presenting cells.

T cells are divided into helper T cells (CD4+) or cytotoxic T cells (CD8+). Helper T cells are subdivided in to proinflammatory cells (Th1) and B helper cells (Th2).

Antibodies

Antibodies (immunoglobulins) are glycoproteins secreted by terminally differentiated B lymphocytes called plasma cells or are found on their cell surface.

The basic structure of an antibody is 'Y' shaped (Fig. 14.1), and comprises two identical heavy chains joined to two light chains. The amino acid sequence in the variable region determines the single antigen to which it can bind.

Antibodies are grouped into five isotopes (classes): IgG, IgA, IgM, IgD, and IgE. These groups are determined by the constant region of the heavy chain.

Antibodies work in a number of different ways.

- Binding and neutralization of bacterial toxins
- Agglutination and lysis of bacteria
- Activation of the 'classical' complement system, leading to opsonization and phagocytosis
- Antibody-dependent cell-mediated cell death

Histocompatibility typing

Before transplantation can take place, the compatibility of the donor and recipient immune systems has to be assessed.

The degree of tissue matching performed depends on the organ being transplanted. Renal transplants undergo the most detailed matching; corneal grafts require none. Tests performed include:

1. ABO blood group determines whether the graft will be a target of preformed anti-ABO antibodies in the recipient. Incompatible blood groups cause hyperacute rejection
2. HLA tissue typing (see box)
3. Cytotoxic cross-match involves a small amount of the recipient's serum being mixed with donor white cells. It is used to detect any potential recipient anti-HLA class I antibodies against the donor. A graft transplanted into a host with a positive cross-match would lead to hyper-acute rejection
4. Antibody screening—the host has their blood tested against a bank of control specimens. This gives an indication of how much antibody to HLA phenotypes is present (percentage antibody is called the panel reactive antibody)

HLA-specific antibodies are formed in response to pregnancy, blood transfusion or previous transplants. They can change and so require repeated monitoring.

⊙ HLA tissue typing

Tissue typing is usually limited to looking for six HLA antigens, one inherited from each parent at the HLA-A, HLA-B, and HLA-DR loci. Each locus has a high number of possible alleles. An example tissue typing is presented below.

	A	A	B	B	DR	DR
Donor	1	2	7	8	15	17
Recipient	1	9	8	37	15	17

A mismatch is used to describe the difference in HLA phenotype between individuals and is recorded in the form A-B-DR. A perfectly matched donor–recipient pair will have a 0-0-0 mismatch. A donor–recipient pair with no common HLA phenotype will have a mismatch of 2-2-2. The example above has a mismatch of 1-2-0. HLA-DR is the most important match, as a mismatch here is associated with a higher incidence of rejection.

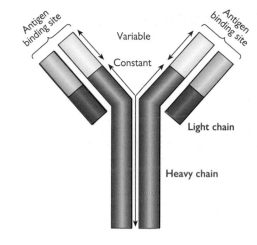

Fig 14.1 Antibody structure.

Early allograft transplants failed because of the inability to control the host immune response. The development of immunosuppressive agents in the 1980s (e.g. ciclosporin) dramatically improved graft survival and fostered a new age of transplant surgery.

Types of transplant

The immune response of the host is dependent on the type of transplant.

- **Autograft:** transplantation from one site to another in the same individual. It does not provoke an immune response
- **Isograft:** transplantation to a genetically identical individual (i.e. identical twin). It carries a very small risk of an immune response
- **Allograft:** transplantation to another individual of the same species. It provokes an immune response
- **Xenograft:** transplantation from one species to another. It provokes an immune response

Rejection

Rejection is an acquired immune response mediated by cellular (T cells) and humoral (antibody) mechanisms.

Donor-specific antigens recognized by recipient antigen-presenting cells (macrophages, B cells, dendritic cells) generate a cascade which ultimately leads to tissue attack by activated T cells, NK cells, and dendritic cells either directly or via antibody binding. This rejection process will lead to loss of graft function and, if untreated, graft loss.

Hyperacute rejection

Hyperacute rejection occurs within minutes to hours following transplantation. Preformed allospecific recipient IgG antibodies react against class I HLA in the transplanted tissue. There is rapid loss of the graft owing to antibody deposition, complement activation, and vascular destruction. The graft must be removed. This is now a rare event owing to preoperative ABO matching and histocompatibility testing.

Acute rejection

Acute rejection can occur at any time following transplantation but most frequently occurs in the first 6 months. It is mediated by T cells, which infiltrate the graft, undergo clonal expansion, and cause tissue destruction.

Immunosuppressive drugs are usually effective in preventing this type of rejection. Thirty per cent of renal transplant patients experience at least one episode of acute rejection.

First line treatment is with a short course of intravenous methylprednisolone followed by antibody therapy if unsuccessful. Plasmaphoresis is considered if antibody-mediated rejection is confirmed and the initial therapy has failed.

Chronic rejection

Chronic rejection is the term used when allograft function slowly deteriorates and there is histological evidence of intimal hypertrophy of small to medium-sized arteries leading to interstitial fibrosis, atrophy, and eventual failure of the organ. Its aetiology is unknown and in renal transplantation it has been re-termed chronic allograft nephropathy to reflect both immunological and non-immunological aetiologies.

Although chronic rejection is most likely to occur late in the post-transplantation course, it may develop as early as 6–12 months after transplantation. There is no standard treatment for chronic rejection and it may require a new graft.

Graft versus host disease (GVHD)

Donor T cells are transferred to the host in the graft tissue. These cells then undergo monoclonal expansion and attack the host. Bone marrow transplantations are particularly prone but this process can also occur with solid organ transplants. Acute GVHD can be treated in the same way as acute rejection.

Immunosuppression

The two possible strategies for modulating the host immune response to prevent rejection are immunosuppression and induction of a tolerant state.

Evidence of a tolerant state is seen in a very small number of transplant patients who stop their immunosuppressant medications but do not go on to reject the graft. Research is under way to understand this phenomenon and develop drugs that one day will achieve this for all patients.

Immunosuppressant regimens

The choice of immunosuppressant regimen is dependent on the type of graft and patient factors along with drug side effect profiles and risk assessment.

Table 14.2 Typical immunosuppressant regimens

	Induction	Maintenance
Low-risk patient	Corticosteroid Azathioprine Ciclosporin	Corticosteroid Azathioprine Ciclosporin
High-risk patient	Antibody therapy Corticosteroid Mycophenolate mofetil (MMF) Tacrolimus	Corticosteroid MMF Tacrolimus

Complications

The acquired immunosuppressed state leaves patients at an increased risk of infection and neoplasia. Other side effects include dyslipidaemia, hyperglycaemia, hypertension, peptic ulcer disease, and nephrotoxicity.

Infection

Immediately infection is suspected, specimens should be sent for microscopy, culture, and sensitivity. Empirical antibiotics are used in the first instance, followed by carefully targeted therapy guided by sensitivity results. All types of infection are seen, especially opportunistic organisms.

The immunosuppressive therapy may need to be reduced or stopped, despite placing the organ at risk of rejecting.

Neoplasia

Transplant recipients are at a 100-fold increase compared with the general population of developing a cancer. The most common cancers are skin cancers, lymphoproliferative disorders, and solid tumours associated with viral infections (e.g. Kaposi's sarcoma and cervical carcinoma).

⊚ Immuunosuppressant drugs

Antimetabolites—azathioprine

Azathioprine is a purine analogue that acts as an antimetabolite to decrease RNA and DNA synthesis. It is used for maintenance immunosuppression.

Corticosteroid—prednisolone

Prednisolone inhibits T cell activation as well as interleukin production by macrophages (IL-1, IL-6). Corticosteroids are used for induction and maintenance immunosuppression as well as to treat acute graft rejection. Side effects include weight gain, Cushing's syndrome, glucose intolerance, and osteoporosis.

Calcineurin inhibitors—ciclosporin/tacrolimus

These prevent T helper cells (Th2) from secreting IL-2. Ciclosporin is used for induction and maintenance immunosuppression.

Ciclosporin has many potential side effects, including nephrotoxicity, cosmetic changes (hypertrichosis, hirsutism), and has multiple drug interactions (particularly agents affecting the cytochrome P450 system).

Tacrolimus is another calcineurin inhibitor that is active against T helper cells. It is used as maintenance therapy and produces fewer cosmetic changes than ciclosporin.

mTOR inhibitors—sirolimus/everolimus

Sirolimus inhibits cell division and is used as maintenance therapy as well as treatment of chronic rejection.

Mycophenolate mofetil (MMF)

MMF impairs B and T cell proliferation by inhibiting inosine monophosphate dehydrogenase. It is used as maintenance therapy as well as treatment of chronic rejection. Its principal side effects are on the gut.

Antibody therapy

Polyclonal antibodies induce the complement lysis of lymphocytes. Commonly used agents include horse antithymocyte globulin (Atgam) and rabbit antithymocyte globulin (Thymoglobulin).

Monoclonal antibodies are also used to deplete T cells and are often used as induction agents and to treat acute rejection. Muromonab-CD3 (OKT3) has been largely superseded by the CD25 monoclonal antibodies basiliximab and daclizumab as induction agents.

⊕ Renal transplant biopsy

Renal transplant biopsy is commonly used to investigate impaired graft function. It is performed under ultrasound guidance. The tissue is immediately analysed to confirm the presence, type, and severity of rejection.

Procedure

- Aseptic technique
- Duplex ultrasound is used to exclude hydronephrosis as a cause of renal dysfunction and to guide the biopsy needle
- Infiltrate local anaesthetic
- Advance biopsy needle into renal cortex and fire gun under direct vision. Deposit sample in storage medium (formalin buffer)
- Repeat at least once to minimize sampling error

Complications

Complications include bleeding, infection, arteriovenous fistula formation, and graft loss (1 in 3000).

14.3 Organ donation

In the UK the annual demand for organ transplants continues to outstrip supply. Ever increasing numbers of patients are waiting and dying whilst on the UK Transplant National Transplant Database.

UK Transplant

United Kingdom Transplant (UKT) is the organization that has a nationwide remit to ensure that donated organs are matched and allocated in a fair and unbiased way.

It administers the NHS Organ Donor Register. So far over 13 million people have registered and carry a donor card which specifies which organs they wish to donate.

Potential donor audit

In 2003, UKT started a Potential Donor Audit as part of a drive to improve organ donation. It records details on every intensive care unit death (7% of ICU patients are potential donors). From this data it identifies the reasons why potential donors do not go on to become actual solid organ donors

Reasons for relatives refusing consent

- Patient stated a wish not to be an organ donor
- Unsure or divided over their decision
- Felt patient had suffered enough
- Did not want the body to undergo surgery

Consent

Current system ('opt in')

The Human Tissue Act 2004 (England, Wales, and Northern Ireland) states that if a person has, while alive and competent, given consent for organ donation following his or her death (by joining the NHS Organ Donor Register or by other means) then that consent is sufficient to go ahead.

Once consent is established, relatives or other relevant people should be advised of the fact and encouraged to respect the deceased's wishes. They will be treated with the utmost sensitivity but advised that they have no legal right to veto or overrule the deceased.

If there is no record of the deceased's wishes, the medical staff will approach the relatives or other relevant people to establish any known wishes of the deceased. Consent to donate can be given by a person nominated by the deceased to deal with the use of their body after death or by someone in a 'qualifying relationship' immediately before their death.

Alternative ('opt-out')

Two other systems of organ donation are used around the world—'opting out' and 'required request'. Both aim to increase levels of donation.

Opting out/presumed consent

Under a system of 'opting out' or 'presumed consent,' every person living in that country is deemed to have given their consent to organ donation unless they had specifically 'opted out' by recording in writing their unwillingness to give organs.

There are two main concerns with this policy. First, it risks causing major distress to a close relative or partner and creating ill-will which would outweigh any advantages in the longer term. Second, if an individual does not register an objection, this silence may indicate a lack of understanding rather than an agreement with the policy.

Required request

The USA operates a policy of required request or referral. Required referral is defined 'that it shall be illegal, as well as irresponsible and immoral, to disconnect a ventilator from an individual who is declared dead following brainstem testing without first making proper enquiry as to the possibility of that individual's tissues and organs being used for the purposes of transplantation.' The policy means opportunities for donation are less likely to be overlooked. Although the introduction of this scheme saw an initial increase in the availability of organs, over time the numbers have declined.

Types of donor

Deceased donor

The deceased (formerly cadaveric) form the majority of donors and are either brain-dead or after cardiac death donors.

Brainstem-dead donors still have a beating heart. Although their organs remain perfused there are still detrimental physiological changes. They are usually suitable for multiorgan donation.

Donation after cardiac death (formerly non-heart beating donors) is progressively expanding the donor pool. Death rarely occurs in a controlled environment and so the physiological quality of the organs is poor.

Living donor

Living donors remain alive and donate organs and tissues that can be regenerated or compensated for by remaining tissue (e.g. single kidney, partial liver).

Most donors are friends or relatives of the recipient. Two other mechanisms now exist.

Altruistic non-directed donation allows an individual to donate a kidney to a stranger.

Paired/pooled donation pairs an incompatible donor/recipient couple anonymously with another couple in the same situation to exchange matched organs.

The main benefits of living donation are the short cold ischaemia time and avoidance of donor brainstem death.

Organ allocation

All patients waiting for an organ transplant are registered on the UKT National Transplant Database. The system of allocation varies according to the type of organ. Each has guidelines and a computer program is used to identify the best matched patient or transplant unit for each organ.

Patients waiting for a heart or liver who are classified as urgent are given priority because of limited life expectancy.

If there are no urgent patients on the waiting list, the organ is offered to patients on the non-urgent list who are nearest in age, tissue type, and blood group to the donor (tissue type is not a consideration for cardiac or liver transplantation). The location of donor and recipient is also considered to minimize the delay between retrieving and transplanting organs.

Children are given priority for kidneys because they tend not to thrive on dialysis and may suffer growth impairment. Organs donated by children generally go to child patients to ensure the best match in size.

There is a reciprocal agreement for organ donation in the European Union. Occasionally, if there are no suitable patients in the UK for an organ it will be sent abroad.

Brainsteam death

Before organs can be retrieved from a deceased donor the diagnosis of brainstem death must be confirmed.

Pre-conditions

1. Diagnosis compatible with brainstem death

2. Presence of irreversible structural brain damage

3. Presence of apnoeic coma

The following must be excluded before carrying out the tests:

- therapeutic drug effects (sedatives, hypnotics, muscle relaxants)
- hypothermia (core body temperature <35°C)
- metabolic abnormalities
- endocrine abnormalities
- alcohol intoxication

Clinical tests

The clinical tests are carried out by two experienced practitioners, one of whom must be a consultant separate to the transplant team. The tests are undertaken on two separate occasions, although there is no prescribed time interval between them.

They are used to confirm the absence of brainstem reflexes and presence of a persistent apnoea.

Absent brainstem reflexes

- No pupillary response to light
- No corneal reflex
- No motor response within cranial nerve distribution
- No gag reflex
- No cough reflex
- No vestibulo-ocular reflex

Test for confirmation of persistent apnoea

- Pre-oxygenation with 100% oxygen for 10 min
- Allow $PaCO_2$ to rise above 5.0 kPa before test
- Disconnect from ventilator
- Maintain adequate oxygenation
- Allow $PaCO_2$ to climb above 6.65 kPa
- Confirm no spontaneous respiration
- Reconnect ventilator

Inclusions to organ donation

- Brainstem death confirmed
- Consent obtained
- No exclusion criteria are met

Exclusions to organ donation

- Active malignancy
- Toxicity/poisons
- Sepsis
- HIV and other communicable infections

Multiple organ retrieval

Multiple organ retrieval is facilitated by a donor transplant coordinator and often involves multiple surgical teams.

Following the confirmation of brainstem death, the donor is taken to theatre ventilated and with circulatory support if necessary.

The abdominal dissection is performed first but the organs are left *in situ*. The thoracic dissection is then performed and heart and lungs removed. The abdominal organs can then be removed in sequence—liver, pancreas then kidneys.

Organ preservation and transfer

Organ preservation is a vital element of the transplantation process. Currently the liver and pancreas can be preserved for a maximum of 18 h and kidneys for 2 days by flushing the organs with UW (University of Wisconsin) solution and storing at hypothermia (0–5°C). This solution prevents cellular swelling during cold ischaemic storage and helps stimulate recovery of normal metabolism upon reperfusion.

Despite this, 20–30% of kidneys do not function well following transplantation and there is growing evidence that continuous perfusion of organs may reduce preservation-related injury. The golden rule is to transplant organs as quickly as is safely possible to minimize the cold ischaemia time.

Ischaemic preconditioning of grafts is another strategy aimed at improving graft outcome. The theory is that by exposure of potential transplant organs to a more minor ischaemic insult will upregulate protective proteins that will protect them during the subsequent prolonged ischaemia.

14.4 Renal transplantation

Renal transplantation is the gold standard for treating end-stage renal failure (ESRF).

The first successful renal transplant was between identical twins in 1954. Since the 1960s the success of the procedure has improved in parallel with advances in immunosuppressant therapy.

Renal replacement therapy

The aims of treating ESRF are to slow progression, treat complications, such as hypertension and anaemia, and plan appropriate renal replacement therapy.

The options for replacement therapy are haemodialysis, continuous ambulatory peritoneal dialysis, and renal transplantation.

Renal transplantation is the most successful form of renal replacement therapy in patients with ESRF. When compared to dialysis it offers improved quality of life, longer life expectancy, and is cheaper.

Indications for renal transplantation

ESRF is the main indication and is caused by one of the following conditions.

- Diabetic nephropathy (30%)
- Chronic glomerulonephritis (30%)
- Hypertensive nephrosclerosis (10%)
- Polycystic kidney disease (5%)
- Other causes: IgA nephropathy, chronic pyelonephritis, drug toxicity, obstructive uropathy, Alport syndrome

Contraindications

Physiological age rather than actual age is considered. There is no absolute age limit. Standard contraindications to transplants include active infection or malignancy, cardiopulmonary insufficiency, morbid obesity, and smoking. Vascular disease is particularly important in renal transplantation and, if severe, is also a contraindication.

Organ donation

Deceased donor

The majority of donated kidneys are from brainstem-dead donors. These are matched to recipients via the National Transplant Database.

Living donor

Living donation forms around 30% of kidney transplants in the UK. The wellbeing of the living donor is of paramount importance. They must be fully informed and volunteer their kidney without coercion. At least one member of donor team should have no connection with the recipient's care.

Laparoscopic live donation is the gold standard and is currently practised in a number of centres in the UK and widely in the USA. The procedure is more appealing to donors and this has a positive effect on increasing the donor pool.

The donor nephrectomy is performed either via an open or laparoscopic approach. The left kidney is usually removed as it has a longer renal vein. The recipient operation can either follow the donor or occur synchronously.

Transplant assessment

Generally, the clinical assessment for transplantation runs in parallel with renal replacement therapy (see box). Some fortunate patients receive an organ before becoming dialysis-dependent. On average, 60% of patients will receive a kidney within 2 years of being on the waiting list, with a median time of 490 days in the UK.

Perioperative transplant care

On the day of transplantation the patient is admitted and undergoes a final health check. Repeat investigations include urinalysis, bloods, ECG, and chest radiograph. Dialysis is required if they are hyperkalaemic or fluid-overloaded.

Immunosuppression regimen

The induction and maintenance regimen depends on the patient's risk of rejection (Table 14.2). A typical prophylactic drug regimen is outlined below. The regimen is started pre-operatively.

- Aspirin to reduce risk of renal vascular thrombosis
- Antihypertensive agents depending on blood pressure
- Nystatin prophylaxis for oral candidiasis
- Antiviral prophylaxis (e.g. valganciclovir) for CMV-positive donors to CMV-negative recipients
- Co-trimoxazole prophylaxis for *Pneumocytis jiroveci*

Complications and prognosis

There have been significant improvements in surgical technique and immunosuppressive drugs over the past 20 years which have led to reduced early complications.

Unfortunately, longer term complications such as the increased risk of cancer and infection still pose a challenge, and transplant patients require long-term outpatient follow-up.

Prognosis is best in recipients of living donor kidneys (85% 5-year survival) compared with recipients of deceased donor organs (73% 5-year survival).

Renal and pancreas transplantation

The main indication for combined kidney and pancreas transplantation is patients with ESRF due to type 1 diabetes mellitus.

The operation usually involves placing the kidney extraperitoneally in the left iliac fossa and the pancreatic graft intraperitoneally in the right iliac fossa with its exocrine pancreatic secretions draining into a loop of small bowel.

◎ Patient assessment for transplantation

The potential recipient undergoes a full assessment before being placed on the transplant waiting list. The aim is to identify any medical conditions requiring optimization and contraindications to transplantation.

The history and examination assesses the patient's general state of health and guides further investigations. A psychosocial review is also carried out to assess their social support structure and predict future compliance with treatment.

Bloods
- FBC (anaemia)
- Clotting
- U+Es (hyperkalaemia, uraemia, high creatinine)
- LFTs, bone profile (hypermagnesaemia, hypocalcaemia)

Cardiorespiratory screening

Full cardiac screening is reserved for those candidates with known IHD or those at high risk (e.g. diabetics).
- ECG
- Chest radiograph
- Exercise tolerance test
- Lung function tests
- Echocardiography
- Coronary angiography

Infectious disease screening
- Urinalysis
- Tuberculosis
- Hepatitis B and C serology
- Cytomegalovirus (CMV) serology
- Epstein–Barr virus (EBV) serology
- Varicella-zoster virus serology
- Syphilis (rapid plasma reagin test)
- HIV

Immunological screening

Renal transplant patients undergo the most rigorous immune screening.
1. ABO blood group
2. HLA tissue typing
3. Cytotoxic cross-match
4. Screening for antibody to HLA phenotypes

Other investigations

Symptoms or signs discovered during the evaluation may require further investigation. For instance, patients with biliary colic require an abdominal USS followed by cholecystectomy if gallstones are found. Acute cholecystitis in transplant patients carries an increased mortality.

⊕ Renal transplantation (deceased donor)

Before the operation begins the patient is started on immunosuppressants and aspirin. They have a urinary catheter placed in theatre.

Graft

In theatre, 'back table' surgery prepares the organ for implantation. An all clear allows the transplantation to go ahead.
- General appearance and evidence of macroscopic disease
- Inspection of blood vessels and repair of any damage
- Inspection of ureter to ensure adequate length
- Renal artery perfused and confirmation of perfusate from vein ensures flow through organ

Transplant procedure
- 'Hockey stick' skin incision in either iliac fossa
- Dissect down through the layers of the abdominal wall to expose the retroperitoneal iliac vessels
- Iliac vessels clamped whilst avoiding entering peritoneum
- Renal vein to common iliac vein (end-to-side anastomosis)
- Renal artery to common iliac artery (end-to-side anastomosis)
- The clamps are released (arterial then venous) following administration of intravenous mannitol and furosemide
- Ureteric anastomosis to bladder wall following clamping of urethral catheter and back filling. Optional ureteric stent and drain placed

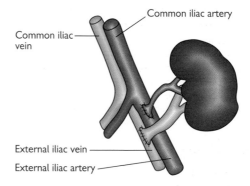

Fig 14.2 A right-sided renal transplant. The heterotopic graft lies extraperitoneal in the pelvis.

Post-transplant
- Maintain SaO_2 >95%, stable blood pressure, and good urine output (>50 mL/h)
- Daily blood tests (FBC, U+Es, LFTs, bone profile)
- Urinary catheter remains *in situ* for 5 days
- Monitor for signs of sepsis or rejection
- Abdominal USS to assess graft blood flow, resistive index, and presence or absence of hydronephrosis

Complications

Intraoperative and early
- Bleeding
- Renal vein thrombosis
- Arterial thrombosis or stenosis
- Ureteric obstruction/stricture
- Urinary fistulae
- Urinary leak
- Hyperacute rejection
- Acute rejection

Late
- Hypertension
- Hyperlipidaemia
- Metabolic bone disease
- Chronic allograft nephropathy
- Retained ureteric stent
- Lymphocele
- Chronic rejection
- GVHD

Liver

Liver transplantation was first pioneered by Thomas Starzl [American b. 1926] in the 1960s. The procedure remained experimental until the introduction of ciclosporin by Sir Roy Calne [British b. 1930]. In the 1980s it was finally recognized as a treatment for acute and chronic end-stage liver failure. Over 6000 liver transplants are carried out annually in the USA and Europe.

Indications for liver transplantation

There is no effective 'liver replacement' therapy and so liver transplantation should be considered in almost all patients with advanced hepatic failure for which the underlying aetiologies are outlined below.

In addition, an increasing number of patients are undergoing retransplantation following technical complications or non-function of their primary graft.

Acute hepatocellular failure

- Viral hepatitis (hepatitis C is the most common indication)
- Drug reactions and poisoning (e.g. paracetamol)

Chronic hepatocellular failure

- Alcoholic cirrhosis
- Chronic active hepatitis
- Primary hepatoma (<5 cm diameter or <3 tumours)
- Postviral cirrhosis
- Autoimmune hepatitis

Cholestatic disease

- Biliary atresia (especially children)
- Primary biliary cirrhosis
- Sclerosing cholangitis

Inborn errors of metabolism

- Glycogen storage disease
- α_1-antitrypsin deficiency
- Wilson's disease

Contraindications for liver transplantation

General contraindications are similar to those in renal transplantation. Active drug or alcohol addiction is a definite contraindication as post-transplantation compliance is poor.

Organ donation

The liver is often relatively unaffected by systemic diseases (e.g. hypertension), and so age and medical co-morbidities are often not contraindications to donation. Absolute contraindications include HIV infection, malignancy (apart from primary brain and non-melanoma skin cancers), and hepatitis B surface antigen-positive.

The liver is usually from a deceased donor and is transplanted whole. It is important to try and match the size. This can be difficult when using adult donors for children.

Split-liver transplantation is possible in some cases. The donor liver is divided into two and the parts transplanted into two recipients. An adult usually receives the larger right lobe and a child or small adult the smaller left lobe. Approximately 10% of liver transplant recipients in the UK receive split livers.

Living-related liver donation involves similar pre-donation assessments to those described for renal transplantation. The use of extended donors and reduced size, split, and living-related liver transplants continues to expand the organ donor pool

Transplant assessment

Potential recipients undergo similar pre-transplant assessment to those having a kidney transplant. Bloods are taken for liver tumour markers and for the model for end-stage liver disease (MELD) scoring system.

This assesses the severity of disease and helps rank patients on the basis of clinical priority. It is based on serum bilirubin, serum creatinine, and INR.

Patients are entered into the UK Transplant Database. Those with acute liver failure are placed on a super-urgent waiting list. Patients waiting for transplantation often require treatment for complications of end-stage liver failure such as pruritis, ascites, spontaneous bacterial peritonitis, encephalopathy, and oesophageal varices.

Complications and prognosis

Graft and patient survival rates continue to improve with better patient selection, technical skill, and immunosuppressive regimens, giving a 5-year graft survival of 66%.

Heart

In 1967 the first successful human heart transplant was performed by Christiaan Barnard [South African, 1922–2001] at Groote Schuur Hospital in Cape Town. Since then over 3000 heart transplants have been performed worldwide.

The majority of candidates have end-stage congestive cardiac failure (NYHA class III or IV) that is refractory to medical or surgical therapy, leaving them with a life expectancy of 12–18 months.

- Dilated cardiomyopathy (54%)
- Ischaemic cardiomyopathy (45%)
- Congenital heart disease (children)
- Valvular heart disease

Clinical assessment

Candidates initially undergo a detailed outpatient assessment and, if suitable, are admitted for the standard transplant investigations and psychosocial assessment. In addition, most candidates routinely undergo coronary angiography and lung function tests.

Complications and prognosis

There is a 30-day mortality rate of ~4% and 5-year survival of ~70%.

Heart and lung

Combined heart and lung transplantation is rarely performed, as organ blocks tend to be divided up for more successful individual transplantations. The most common indications are congenital heart disease with secondary pulmonary hypertension or Eisenmenger's syndrome followed by primary pulmonary hypertension.

The greatest postoperative challenge is managing the ventilation to minimize barotrauma and volume overload. Five-year survival is 50%.

✚ Liver transplantation

The donor hepatectomy is usually part of a multiple organ retrieval. Following removal, the portal vein and hepatic artery are flushed through, and then immersed in UW preservation solution for cold storage. At the time of retrieval the liver is inspected to ensure it is macroscpically disease-free.

Liver transplantation is orthotopic, which means that the recipient liver is excised and the donor liver placed in the same anatomical position. In heterotopic transplantation, the diseased organ is left *in situ* and the donor organ placed in another position, e.g. renal transplantation.

Procedure

- Bilateral subcostal incision with vertical extension to the xiphoid
- Recipient hepatectomy followed by meticulous haemostasis
- Gallbladder removed
- The donor liver is sited in an orthotopic position
- The end-to-end suprahepatic vena cava, infrahepatic vena cava, and portal vein anastomoses are performed first to allow early reperfusion of the graft
- Arterial reconstruction is to the recipient hepatic artery or, more typically, to the common hepatic artery
- Biliary drainage is achieved with an end-to-end choledo-chocholedochostomy in adults with a normal common bile duct (+/- T-tube placement)
- In the presence of an inadequate recipient bile duct or sclerosing cholangitis, a Roux-en-Y choledochojejunostomy is required

Complications

Intraoperative and early	Late
• Hepatic artery thrombosis	• Bile duct stricture
• Bile leak	• Chronic rejection
• Primary non-function	
• Acute rejection	

✚ Heart transplantation

The viability of a cold perfused heart is approximately 6 h. This means there is not normally time for tissue typing and cross-matching. This is only carried out if the potential recipient is at high risk for rejection. Geographical location of the recipient relative to the donor is also of great importance owing to transportation time.

Procedure

- Median sternotomy
- Recipient placed on cardiopulmonary bypass with systemic cooling to 28°C and aorta cross-clamped
- Donor heart inspected before starting recipient cardiectomy
- Donor heart brought into operative field. Anastomoses performed between donor and recipient left atria, right atria, pulmonary artery, and aorta (bicaval anastomosis technique). The classical technique preserves both the recipient and donor atria
- The heart is de-aired and the aortic cross-clamp removed, followed by discontinuation of the cardiopulmonary bypass
- Optional pacing wires placed
- Sternum closed

Postoperative course

The donor heart is denervated and so maintains an intrinsic rate. Initially, it requires inotropic support and well maintained circulating calcium ions. The graft undergoes regular endomyocardial biopsies to assess for rejection.

Induction immunosuppression is antithymocyte globulin (ATG) and intravenous high-dose corticosteroids followed by a maintenance regimen of oral corticosteroids (tapering over 6–12 months), azathioprine (or MMF) and cyclosporin (or tacrolimus).

In addition, antiobiotic prophylaxis is given for 48 h as well as nystatin therapy for 6 weeks to prevent oral candidiasis.

Complications

Intraoperative and early	Late
• Bleeding	• Graft vessel arteriosclerosis
• Acute rejection	• Chronic rejection
• Non-function	
• Pneumothorax	
• Haemothorax	
• Cardiac tamponade	
• Sepsis	
• Pneumonia	
• Wound infection	

379

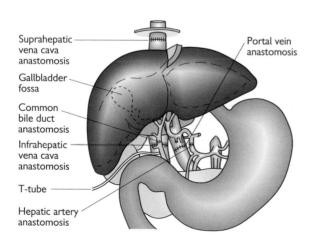

Suprahepatic vena cava anastomosis

Gallbladder fossa

Common bile duct anastomosis

Infrahepatic vena cava anastomosis

T-tube

Hepatic artery anastomosis

Portal vein anastomosis

Fig 14.3 Liver transplant. There are five anastomoses. The biliary reconstruction is decompressed and stented with a T-tube.

Case 1

A 27-year-old man sustains severe head injuries during an RTC. His GCS is 6/15 on arrival and he is intubated. A CT scan confirms massive cerebral contusion and oedema. The patient is admitted to neurological ICU and an intracerebral pressure monitoring device is inserted.

On ICU he remains cardiovascularly stable with artificial support. Four days later he still has a GCS of 3/15 and there is no sign of any respiratory effort.

- At what point should brain death be considered?
- What other factors must be excluded prior to proceeding with testing?
- How do you confirm brainstem death?

An organ donor card was found in his wallet. The family have been at his bedside throughout and are unaware of his wish to donate. They do not understand how the patient can appear alive and yet be brainstem-dead.

- Is the patient a potential organ donor?
- Is the organ donor card sufficient for consent?
- Is consent from the family required and, if so, who should you discuss this with?
- Who should be contacted as this decision is being made?

Discussion

Brainstem death is confirmed and the patient is a potential donor. The fact that the family is unaware of his wish is a potential problem. By law, they are unable to withhold consent, but it is prudent to gain their consent before proceeding.

- What conditions must be excluded to allow organ donation to proceed?
- What information about the potential donor will the transplant coordinator require to find a suitable recipient?

Case 2

A 53-year-old mother-of-three with type 1 diabetes has previously had a renal transplant for end-stage renal failure secondary to diabetic nephropathy.

The graft has chronic allograft nephropathy and she is back on haemodialysis three times a week (Monday, Wednesday, and Friday).

She is a candidate for a second graft and has undergone full outpatient assessment. She is called by the transplant co-ordinator on a Sunday night with news that a kidney is available.

- Outline the assessment of a potential transplant patient.
- When admitted before transplant, what further investigations are performed?

On admission, she is found to be 5 kg above her 'dry weight' with a serum potassium of 5.9 mmol/L.
Explain these findings and how you would manage them?
The HLA tissue typing result is below.

	A	A	B	B	DR	DR
Donor	1	8	10	2	7	11
Recipient	1	8	2	10	7	11

- Describe the mismatch.
- What other immune tests are required for renal transplantation?

No contraindication is identified and the transplant goes ahead.

- What are the main complications of renal transplantation?
- What immunosuppression regimen should be started?

The operation is successful and the first 5 days are uneventful. The drain and urinary catheter have been removed, the patient has been free from dialysis, and serum urea and creatinine have declined to near normal levels.

However, on postoperative day 6 the blood tests show a sharp increase in her creatinine.

- What is your differential diagnosis?
- How would you investigate this further?

Despite adequate hydration and a normal USS of the graft, the creatinine is slightly worse when checked later that day.

- What investigation would you arrange?
- What is the first line anti-rejection therapy?

Discussion

On admission, the patient's blood tests were abnormal as she was due for haemodialysis the following day. Owing to her previous rejection, she required the high risk regimen of immunosuppressant drugs.

Following the operation she had an episode of acute rejection which was confirmed on renal biopsy. This was treated with IV steroids and antibody therapy. She made a good recovery was discharged home a few days later.

Chapter 15

Core surgical skills and knowledge

Clinical skills
- Surgery in hepatitis and HIV carriers
- Surgical thromboprophylaxis
- Hypoglycaemia
- Hyperglycaemia
- Hyperkalaemia (K^+ >6.5 mmol/L)
- Alcohol
- Sickle cell crisis

Technical skills and procedures
- Insertion of central venous catheter
- Renal replacement therapy in ARF

Perioperative management
- Preoperative fasting and medications
- Respiratory tract infection
- Asthma
- COPD
- Cardiac risk in non-cardiac surgery
- Heart failure
- Arrhythmias
- Hypertension
- Diabetes mellitus
- Stroke
- Acute confusion
- Haematological conditions

Normal body fluid distribution

In the normal 70 kg adult man, body water accounts for 60% of the total body weight (45 L); this is slightly less in women as, proportionally, they have more body fat.

The body water is distributed across the intracellular and extracellular compartments. The extracellular compartment is subdivided into intravascular, interstitial, and transcellular (e.g. CSF and synovial fluid).

Intracellular compartment

The intracellular and extracellular compartments are separated by the cell membrane which is highly permeable to water but has a low permeability to electrolytes. It also has sodium pumps (Na^+–K^+ ATPase) which pump sodium out of the cell. This means that the distribution of water between the two compartments is largely determined by the osmotic effect of electrolytes in the extracellular fluid (e.g. Na^+ and its associated anions—Cl^-, HCO_3^-) and the proteins within the cell.

Extracellular compartment

The capillary membrane divides the intravascular and interstitial spaces and is permeable to water and electrolytes but relatively impermeable to protein. Therefore the distribution of fluid between these spaces is largely determined by the balance of hydrostatic and colloid (protein) osmotic pressure across the membrane. This relationship is described by the Starling hypothesis (Fig 15.1).

Osmosis and osmotic pressure

- Osmosis is the net diffusion of water across a selectively permeable membrane (i.e. capillary membrane) from a high water concentration to a low water concentration
- Osmotic pressure is the pressure required to prevent osmosis and is directly proportional to the concentration of osmotically active particles in the solution
- Osmole (osm) is the number of osmotically active particles in a solution; it is the standard unit of osmotic pressure
- Osmolality is the number of osmoles of solute per kilogram of solvent. Osmolarity is the number of osmoles of solute per litre of solution

  Plasma osmolarity (mOsmol/L) = $2(Na^+ + K^+)$ + urea + glucose = ~290 mosmol/L
- Tonicity is the effective osmolality of a solution in relation to a particular membrane (i.e. osmolality less any solutes ineffective at exerting an osmotic force across the membrane)

Fluid homeostasis

Water balance and osmoregulation

Body water is controlled by the thirst–ADH axis and mediated by highly sensitive osmoreceptors found in the anterior hypothalamus. They respond to changes in plasma tonicity which is usually directly related to the ECF sodium concentration.

The thirst centre is located in the lateral hypothalamus. It is stimulated by hypertonicity, hypovolaemia, hypotension, and angiotensin II. It controls the input of water into the body (i.e. drinking) whilst ADH and the kidney act to regulate water excretion.

Volume regulation

High pressure arterial baroreceptors (carotid, juxtaglomerular apparatus) predominate over low pressure arterial baroreceptors (right atria and great veins) in their response to changes in intravascular volume. They are less sensitive than osmoreceptors.

Significant hypovolaemia (~10% volume loss) is a more potent stimulus for ADH release than hypertonicity detected by osmoreceptors. Intravascular volume is therefore preserved at the expense of tonicity.

Water and sodium imbalance

Sodium and its associated anions (mainly chloride) account for the majority of osmotically active particles in the ECF. Plasma sodium concentration therefore gives an indication of ECF osmolarity.

Hyponatraemia

Hyponatraemia is common. Assessment of the ECF volume and plasma osmolarity is crucial for diagnosis.

- Reduced ECF—dehydrated patient with urinary sodium >20 mmol/L suggests renal loss of sodium (e.g. Addison's, renal failure, diuretics). Sodium <20 mmol/L suggests losses elsewhere (sweating, GI tract)
- Normal ECF—syndrome of inappropriate ADH secretion or hypothyroidism
- Increased ECF—excessive water administration, heart failure, renal failure

Hypernatraemia

- Excessive water loss from the ECF is the most common cause. This occurs following increased loss (e.g. sweating) or reduced intake (e.g. fasting). A rarer cause is inappropriate urinary excretion of water seen in diabetes insipidus (pituitary or renal)
- Excessive sodium load (e.g. parenteral nutrition, hypertonic saline)

Imbalance of other electrolytes

Potassium

- Hypokalaemia is caused by infusion of fluids without potassium and increased renal excretion owing to diuretic therapy. It is usually asymptomatic, although severe depletion may cause muscle weakness and arrhythmias. Treat the underlying cause and consider slow release oral potassium or in severe cases IV potassium (cardiac and regular serum K^+ monitoring needed if faster than 20 mmol/L per hour)
- Hyperkalaemia (K^+ >6.5 mmol/L) is an emergency (Also see Topic 15.18)

Magnesium

Magnesium is absorbed in the small intestine and excreted by the kidneys. It is an important intracellular cation and is needed for normal neuromuscular function. Hypomagnesaemia is caused by reduced intake or GI absorption or increased renal or GI loss. Hypermagnesaemia occurs in chronic renal failure.

Table 15.1 Daily fluid balance in 70-kg adult man	
Input	**mL/day**
Oral fluid	1500
Water from food	750
Water from metabolism	250
Total	2500
Output	**mL/day**
Insensible-skin	400
Insensible-lungs	400
Sweat	100
Urine	1400
Faeces	100
Total	2500

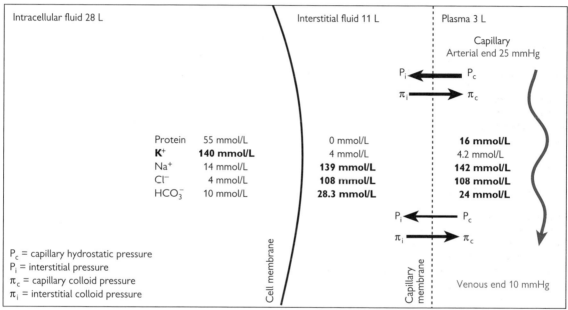

Fig 15.1 Body fluid compartments and their ionic composition (transcellular compartment not shown). Blood contains both ECF (plasma) and intracellular fluid within the circulating cells. The effective circulating volume is the volume of ECF in the arterial circulation and is usually directly related to ECF volume.

Starling hypothesis

Starling's hypothesis states that the fluid movement due to filtration across the wall of a capillary is dependent on the balance between the hydrostatic pressure gradient and the oncotic pressure gradient across the capillary.

Net filtration pressure = $(P_c - P_i) - (\pi_c - \pi_i)$

P_c = Capillary hydrostatic pressure (arteriolar 25 mmHg, venous 10 mmHg)
P_i = Interstitial hydrostatic pressure (−6 mmHg)
π_c = Capillary oncotic pressure (25 mmHg)
π_I = Interstitial oncotic pressure (5 mmHg)

Fluid management in the surgical patient requires an understanding of the distribution of across-the-body fluid compartments, the type of losses, and the fluid balance problems that can occur during the perioperative period.

Clinical assessment of fluid and electrolyte status

History
- Obvious fluid loss—bleeding, vomiting, diarrhoea
- Potential 'third space' losses (e.g. pancreatitis)
- Recent surgery
- Co-morbid conditions altering fluid status
- Drug history

Examination
- Clinical indices (Table 15.2)
- Observation charts (heart rate, lying/standing BP)
- Fluid balance charts (input and output)
- Daily weights
- Central venous pressure (JVP or invasive measurement)

Investigations
- Bloods—FBC (haemoconcentration), U+Es (raised urea may represent dehydration, electrolyte balance)

Types of fluid therapy
Fluids are generally divided into crystalloids and colloids. They have different properties and indications for their use.

Crystalloids
A crystalloid solution contains a water-soluble crystalline substance capable of diffusion across a semi-permeable membrane. Crystalloid solutions are inexpensive and non-allergenic.

- **0.9% sodium chloride** (normal saline) is 'isotonic' but provides a slightly higher sodium and chloride load than is found in normal plasma. The high chloride content can cause hyperchloraemic metabolic acidosis if overused.
- **Compound sodium lactate** (Hartmann's solution) is an isotonic balanced salt solution. It does not cause hyperchloraemic metabolic acidosis.
- **5% glucose** (dextrose) contains 50 g/L of glucose and no electrolytes. The glucose is metabolized to leave free water which equilibrates across all body fluid compartments. It is used to replace whole body water loss but is ineffective at resuscitating the intravascular space. Dextrose–saline (4% dextrose, 0.18% saline) reduces the risk of sodium overload but can cause water overload

Colloids
A colloid is not a solution but a suspension of finely divided particles in a continuous medium. There are different types of colloid solutions but all contain a base constituent solution which is usually 0.9% sodium chloride.

- **Gelatins** (e.g. Gelafusin®, Haemaccel®, Volplex®) contain modified gelatin with a molecular weight of 30–35 kDa. The effective half-life within the circulation is approximately 3 hours. They have the highest potential for anaphylactic reactions
- **Starches** (e.g. Voluven®, HAES-steril®) consist of starch with various numbers of additional hydroxyethyl groups and contain a wide variety of particles, ranging from 10 to 450 kDa
- **Dextrans** contain polysaccharides and are classified according to their molecular weight. They have less allergenic potential than the gelatins but have been associated with renal impairment, clotting abnormalities, and can interfere with the cross-matching of blood
- **Blood** and albumin are natural colloids (📖 Topic 8.5)

Fluid prescription
Three main factors should be considered when deciding on a fluid and electrolyte prescription.
1. Current deficit
2. Continuing losses
3. Maintenance requirements

Resuscitation fluids
Resuscitation fluids aim to expand the intravascular compartment urgently in response to a significant deficit. Colloids and blood are most effective as they contain osmotically active particles that do not easily cross the capillary membrane. Normal saline and Hartmann's equalize across the whole ECF compartment and so only a third of their volume remains in the intravascular space.

Replacement fluids
The fluid prescription should replace like with like. Most fluid losses are of a similar composition to ECF (e.g. blood, vomit, diarrhoea, 'third space') and should be replaced with 0.9% saline with added potassium. Increased insensible losses are mainly water and are replaced with 5% dextrose.

Maintenance fluids
The normal 24 h fluid and electrolyte requirements for a 70-kg adult man are 40 mL/kg of water, 2 mmol/kg of Na^+, and 0.5–1 mmol/kg of K^+. A regimen for 24 h is:
- 1 L of normal saline + 20 mmoL K^+ over 8 h
- 2 L of 5% dextrose + 40 mmoL K^+ over 16 h

Postoperative fluids
The physiological stress response to surgery increases ADH secretion and so water is retained. Potassium may also be raised owing to reduced renal excretion, cell lysis, and increased efflux of potassium from cells.

Route of administration
Ideally, fluids are delivered orally or enterally if the gut mucosa is intact and functioning. Intravenous delivery is used in emergencies or if the oral route is contraindicated.

Monitoring of fluid status

Non-invasive
- Regular clinical assessment and observations (Table 15.2)
- Suprasternal transcutaneous Doppler ultrasound estimates cardiac output

Invasive
- A central venous catheter can be used to estimate volume status and gives access for blood sampling and administration of drugs. Use of pulmonary artery catheters (Swan–Ganz) is rare other than in cardiac surgery owing to their associated morbidity and mortality rates
- Arterial catheters allow continuous blood pressure monitoring as well as access for repeat ABGs
- Transoesophageal Doppler is a minimally invasive technique to estimate cardiac output and is increasingly used intraoperatively and in the ITU setting

⊕ Insertion of central venous catheter

Central venous catheter (CVC) insertion is used for haemodynamic monitoring, administration of drugs, renal replacement and nutrition, and endoluminal interventions.

Pre-procedure

Identify and gather all of the equipment needed and, if possible, obtain skilled assistance. Choose an appropriate anatomical site for central venous cannulation considering the following factors: indication for insertion, skill of practitioner, anatomical landmarks, and any risk factors individual to the patient.

Seldinger technique for insertion of internal jugular line

The procedure should be performed in a clean environment with space, light, and monitoring equipment. Communicate with the conscious patient at all times.

- Ultrasound guidance should be used to identify anatomical landmarks in most clinical situations
- Position patient with head down and neck turned towards the contralateral side
- Strict aseptic technique (hat, mask, gown, and gloves)
- Administer local anaesthetic
- Check the equipment and flush all of the lumens of the catheter to ensure patency
- Cannulate the central vein, removing the needle, and leaving the plastic cannula *in situ*
- Ensure that there is appropriate flow of venous blood. Pass the J-wire through the cannula, taking care not to insert the wire too far and watching for ectopic atrial activity or arrhythmias on ECG monitoring
- Remove the cannula, leaving the wire in the vein and pass the dilator over the wire, nicking the skin at the entry point with the scalpel blade
- Remove the dilator, the wire remaining in the vein and pass the catheter over the wire, ensuring that the end of the wire is visible at all times. Usually, insert to a maximum of the 15 cm mark on the catheter at the skin
- Aspirate blood from all of the lumens of the catheter and flush with normal saline solution
- Suture the catheter in position, ensuring it is securely fixed, and cover with a sterile translucent dressing
- Request and review a chest radiograph to check the position
- Other markers that confirm correct placement include a central venous pressure trace, an appropriate transduced pressure (0–15 cmH₂O), and a venous blood sample on blood gas analysis

Complications

Intraprocedure and early	Late
• Failure to cannulate vein	• Infection, both local and catheter-related bloodstream infection
• Misplacement of catheter	
• Arterial puncture or placement	• Thrombosis
• Haematoma, haemothorax	
• Pneumothorax	
• Cardiac tamponade	
• Arrhythmia	
• Thoracic duct damage and chylothorax (with left subclavian lines)	
• Nerve injury	
• Air embolism	

Table 15.2 Dehydration in a 70-kg adult

Level of dehydration	Clinical indicators
Minimal >4%**, >2500 mL*	• Thirst • Reduced skin turgor • Dry tongue
Mild >6%, >4200 mL	Plus: • Orthostatic hypotension • Oliguria • Nausea • Low CVP • Apathy • Haemoconcentration
Moderate >8%, >5600 mL	Plus: • Cool peripheries • Thready pulse • Hypotension
Severe 10–15%, 7000–10 500 mL	Plus: • Hypovolaemic shock • Coma • Death

**Percentage body weight lost as water; *volume of fluid loss.

Table 15.3 Constituents of crystalloid solutions

	0.9 % NaCl	CSL	4% dextrose/ 0.18% NaCl	5% dextrose
Osmolarity (mO5m/L)	308	280	202	278
Na⁺ (mmol/L)	154	131	30	0
K⁺ (mmol/L)	0	5	0	0
Cl⁻ (mmol/L)	154	111	30	0
HCO₃⁻ (mmol/L)	0	29*	0	0
Ca²⁺ (mmol/L)	0	2	0	0
Glucose (g)	0	0	40	50

*As lactate.

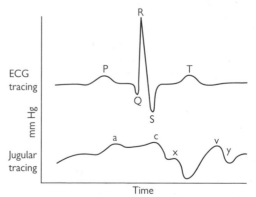

Fig 15.2 Central venous pressure wave (jugular) with an ECG to compare the timings of the different waves. A 'normal' CVP is approximately 3–8 mmH₂O but the trend is more useful than absolute values.

- a wave = increased right pressure caused by atrial contraction
- c wave = early ventricular contraction pushes the closed tricuspid valve into the atrium slightly, leading to an increase in pressure
- x descent = continuing ventricular contraction moves the ventricle down and reduces atrial pressure
- v wave = blood filling the atrium increases the pressure
- y descent = tricuspid valve opens, allowing blood to flow into the ventricle

15.3 Healthcare-associated infection

Healthcare-associated infections are a common, and largely preventable, cause of surgical morbidity and mortality.

Infections in surgical patients may be surgical site infections (SSI), or elsewhere such as the respiratory tract and urinary tract.

Risk factors

- Advanced age
- Immunosuppression
- Diabetes mellitus
- Poor nutritional status
- Emergency operation
- Increased duration and complexity of operation
- Surgical site and level of contamination
- Increased length of hospital admission

Pathophysiology

Definitions

- Contamination is the transient presence of microorganisms without injury or invasion
- Colonization is the continuing presence of microorganisms, again without injury or invasion
- Infection is the active invasion of microorganisms causing tissue injury

Stages of infection

1. Acquisition of organism by the host by direct contact, inhalation, ingestion, or inoculation
2. Colonization is the survival and multiplication of the organism so that it persists
3. Invasion leads to infection and is dependent on the organism being able to evade and survive the host's innate and specific immune systems
4. Spread through the local tissue and beyond establishes the ongoing infection
5. Injury to the host may be mediated by toxins, altered host function, and response to infection (i.e. overwhelming inflammatory response)
6. Resolution occurs if the host's immune response overcomes and destroys the invading organism. The acute inflammatory response usually resolves but can become chronic

Virulence and immunity

Virulence is related to characteristics of the organism and how it interacts with the immunity of the host. Immunosuppression leaves the host particularly susceptible to infection.

Clinical assessment

Nosocomial infections develop 48 h after hospital admission or in patients with a recent documented admission or operation. Infection may present with localized or systemic signs of inflammation (📖 Topic 12.1).

A full history and examination may be accompanied by investigations to assess the severity of infection, and the type and sensitivity of the microorganisms involved.

Investigations

- Microbiology—tissue, pus, and fluid should be sent for microscopy, culture, and sensitivities. Serological tests and PCR are used for organisms that cannot be cultured
- Bloods—raised WCC and CRP
- Imaging (e.g. CT scan or ultrasound) is often used to localize infection and/or guide drainage of abscesses
- Interventional techniques—laparoscopy, guided biopsy

Management

Once a diagnosis is made, treatment aims to eradicate the causative organism. This may include antibiotic therapy (📖 Topic 15.4), drainage, and washout of an abscess or infected cavity, and excision of infected tissue and removal of infected prosthetic material.

Prevention of infection

Definitions

- Asepsis is the exclusion of microorganisms from tissues
- Antisepsis is the prevention of multiplication of microorganisms that cause infection in living tissue

Hand hygiene

This is the single most important factor in preventing nosocomial infection. Plain soap has little antimicrobial action but facilitates mechanical removal of microorganisms. Antimicrobial soaps are effective but alcohol-based products are usually used as they have a rapid action, do not need towels, and are highly effective.

Disinfection and sterilization

- Cleaning removes visible contamination and should precede all attempts at disinfection and sterilization
- Disinfection reduces microorganisms to a very low level, but may leave active viruses and spores. Disinfection methods include low pressure steam, boiling water, and a variety of chemical methods
- Sterilization is the complete destruction of all viable organisms on inanimate objects; it cannot be achieved in living tissues. Methods include irradiation, filtration, chemicals, and heat
- Re-usable surgical instruments are usually autoclaved using high pressure saturated steam or dry heat if they are sensitive to moisture. Ethylene oxide and irradiation are used industrially to sterilize large batches of products, including disposable instruments

Operating environment

- Clean environment with regular disinfectant in between cases.
- Limit personnel in the theatre and movement in and out
- Positive pressure air changes or ultra-clean using laminar air flow. These measures reduce the airborne spread of bacteria
- Gloves, gowns, masks, and impermeable gowns protect the surgeon from the patient but may play a limited role in prevention of infection in many operations

Surgical technique

- Use appropriate antibiotic prophylaxis
- Avoid shaving operative site as it mobilizes deep skin flora and increases the bacterial count. If it has to be done, keep to a minimum and perform at start of operation
- Antiseptic preparation with povidone iodine (Betadine®) or 4% chlorhexidine (Hibiscrub®); 70% alcohol is effective but rarely used owing to skin irritation and fire risk

- Sterile drapes to create operating field
- Good surgical technique: reduce theatre time, minimal tissue handling, remove all devitalized tissue, avoid dead space, good haemostasis, use appropriate suture material, and use closed drain systems away from the wound
- Maintain postoperative glucose control to avoid hyperglycaemia
- Maintain normothermia perioperatively

Table 15.4 Classification of surgical wounds

Class	Definition
Clean	No inflammation No entry of respiratory, GI or GU tracts Aseptic technique maintained
Clean-contaminated	Respiratory, GI or GU tracts entered but no significant spillage
Contaminated	Acute inflammation Visible contamination Open injuries <4 h old
Dirty	Presence of pus Perforated viscus Open injuries >4 h old

⊙ Surgery in hepatitis and HIV carriers

Bloodborne viruses

Hepatitis B and C are bloodborne viruses. They can both cause hepatitis that in some becomes chronic and results in liver failure and an increased risk of hepatocellular cancer. All healthcare professionals involved in patient care must be immune to hepatitis B.

Human immunodeficiency virus (HIV) is increasingly prevalent. High-risk groups include homosexuals and intravenous drug users; however, there is an increasing incidence amongst heterosexuals and other population groups.

HIV infection is asymptomatic in the early stages. The immune deficiency eventually leads to opportunistic infections and tumours, some of which define the acquired immune deficiency syndrome (AIDS).

Needlestick injury

Injury with a sharp that is contaminated with patient fluids carries the risk of viral inoculation. Particular risk factors for transmission include large bore needle, puncture of a blood vessel with visible blood, and patient with known viral infection. Hepatitis B and C have a much higher viral load than HIV and so are more likely to be transmitted. The advent of post-exposure prophylaxis has reduced the transmission rates (<1 in 1000).

Needlestick protocol

The management of a needlestick injury should follow local guidelines. These usually involve contacting the occupational health department during working hours or the emergency department out of hours.

- Immediately wash area with soap and running water and encourage bleeding
- Early risk assessment of the patient. If indicated, post-exposure prophylaxis should be started early (<1 h)
- Antibiotics and hepatitis immunization may also be indicated
- Blood samples for virology tests (HIV, hepatitis B and C) are needed from both the patient and injured worker. The consent process should be approached sensitively

Prevention

- Standard precautions—every patient should be assumed to be a carrier. Apron, gloves, and eye protection should be worn during exposure-prone procedures
- Easy access to sharps disposal boxes and immediate disposal of used sharps
- Do not re-sheath needles (implicated in 40% of injuries)
- Do not pass sharp instruments between people, use a tray instead

15.4 Microorganisms and antimicrobials

Microorganisms

Only 10% of the estimated 10^{14} cells in a human body are actually of human origin; the majority are microbial flora. Few are pathogenic; many are actually beneficial.

Bacteria

Bacteria are simple unicellular structures that lack a cell nucleus. They are generally classified by shape or their ability to retain crystal violet–iodine dye when treated with acetone or alcohol (Gram stain).

The human commensal flora is mainly bacterial. The majority is harmless and often play important roles, such as competitive exclusion of pathogenic bacteria.

Viruses

Viruses are acellular parasites that rely on the host cell for replication. They are the commonest cause of human infection. They are generally classified according to their host, possession of an envelope, and the type of nucleic acid in their structure.

Antibiotics

Antibiotic action is either bacteristatic or bactericidal. Bacteristatic agents depend on the body's immune system to kill and remove the damaged bacteria.

Antibiotic mechanisms of action

- Cell wall inhibitors are bactericidal as they block the synthesis of cell wall peptidoglycans, causing cell lysis
- Protein synthesis inhibitors are bacteristatic. Once the antibiotic levels decrease, the protein synthesis restarts
- Nucleic acid synthesis inhibitors are limited in number as all cells synthesize nucleic acids. They target a few pathways or enzymes that are specific to bacteria

Antibiotic prescribing

1. Consider the patient: renal or hepatic impairment, history of allergy, other medications, pregnancy, breastfeeding
2. Consider the likely organism and its sensitivities. Local hospital antibiotic prescribing policy should always be followed as they take account of the local flora and resistant strains
3. Take specimens for culture and sensitivity testing. Empirical antibiotic therapy should be changed following sensitivity results
4. Dose is determined by the age, weight, renal function, hepatic function, and severity of infection. Combination therapy should be considered
5. Duration is determined by the type of infection and response to treatment. Stopping a course early can result in a relapse and antibiotic resistance. Deep infections and those associated with prosthetic implants often need prolonged therapy for a number of weeks
6. Route of administration is determined by the severity of infection and bioavailability of the antibiotic. Life-threatening infections need intravenous therapy
7. Monitoring of serum levels is needed for some antibiotics with narrow therapeutic indexes and significant toxicity (e.g. gentamicin, vancomycin). This is important in patients with renal or hepatic dysfunction

Antibiotic prophylaxis

Antibiotic prophylaxis aims to reduce surgical site infections. It is used when the benefits outweigh the risks (e.g. hypersensitivity reactions, antibiotic resistance, colitis).

Elective surgery

- Prophylactic antibiotic must cover the majority of common pathogens expected at that surgical site
- A single dose of intravenous antibiotic is usually administered just before or at induction of anaesthesia
- A further dose may be given during the operation if there is greater than 1500 mL blood loss or significant haemodilution
- Prophylactic antibiotics may be continued for 24 h and then stopped

Emergency surgery

Clean and clean-contaminated procedures follow the guidelines for elective surgery. Emergency procedures with contaminated or dirty wounds need a course of antibiotic therapy rather than just prophylaxis.

Antibiotic hypersensitivity

Adverse drug reactions occur in approximately 10% of patients prescribed beta-lactam antibiotics.

- Associated symptoms in increasing severity are rash, urticaria, and anaphylaxis
- Cross-sensitivity may occur with penicillin derivatives, cephalosporins, and carbapenems
- Patients should not be prescribed beta-lactams if there is a history of hypersensitivity
- A rash or problem occurring more than 72 h after giving penicillin is unlikely to be an allergy

Antibiotic resistance

Antibiotic resistance is increasing owing to extensive agricultural use, overprescribing, and use of broad spectrum drugs. Mechanisms include loss of permeability to the antibiotic, enzymatic destruction of the drug (e.g. beta-lactamases), loss of the target site, and development of alternative biosynthetic pathways. Bacteria acquire resistance through single point mutations and transfer of genetic material between microorganisms.

Meticillin-resistant Staphylococcus aureus (MRSA)

Staphylococcus aureus is a common pathogen which can display resistance to a number of antibiotics, with the increased prevalence of meticillin-resistant strains (MRSA), including meticillin, penicillin, tetracycline, and erythromycin. Vancomycin became the antibiotic of choice, although vancomycin-resistant *S. aureus* has also been reported. Linezolid has similar efficacy to vancomycin and there is little resistance to it.

Vancomycin-resistant enterococcus (VRE)

This is most commonly a nosocomial infection and is usually only a problem in immunocompromised patients. It is classified on the sequence of the resistance gene.

Multi-drug resistant Acinetobacter baumannii (MRAB)

A. baumannii is an opportunistic pathogen that can cause serious infections usually in immunocompromised patients. They are difficult to treat and can have a high mortality rate. If the strain is susceptible, imipenem is the first line antibiotic, along with strict infection control measures.

Table 15.5 Surgically important bacteria

Gram-positive cocci (stain blue/purple)	Gram-negative cocci (stain pink/red) and coccobacilli
Staphylococci Grow in clusters and classified by coagulase production • *S. aureus* (coagulase-positive) is a common virulent primary pathogen and skin commensal that causes infections in different tissues and through different mechanisms (toxins, enzymes) • *S. epidermidis* (coagulase-negative) is a normal skin commensal and opportunistic pathogen. It has a particular affinity for prosthetic material such as catheters and orthopaedic implants *Streptococci* Grow in chains and classified by ability to haemolyse blood. Most are facultative anaerobes. Enterococci are now classified separately and include *E. faecalis* • *S. pneumoniae* (alpha-haemolytic) and *S. pyogenes* (beta-haemolytic) are virulent primary pathogens that are often found in the upper respiratory tract. *S. pneumoniae* is an important cause of pneumonia, meningitis, and septicaemia • *S. pyogenes* causes throat infections and wound infections	*Neisseria* spp. Grow in pairs (diplococci) • *N. meningitides* is the most important cause of meningitis • *N. gonorrhoea* causes gonorrhoea *Haemophilus* spp. *H. influenzae* is a coccobacillus and non-encapsulated forms are normal flora in the respiratory tract although they can cause local infection. Encapsulated forms are more virulent and can cause meningitis *Acinetobacter* spp. These coccobacilli can be carried as normal flora. They are opportunist pathogens and are becoming increasingly important hospital-acquired infections (ventilator-associated pneumonia)
Gram-positive bacilli	**Gram-negative bacilli**
Clostridia These are spore-forming aerobic bacteria • *C. difficile* is the most important in the surgical patient. It can develop when the normal gut flora is removed following antibiotic use • *C. perfringens* is a cause of gas gangrene, *C. tetani* causes tetanus, and *C. botulinum* causes food poisoning (botulism) *Bacillus* spp. *Bacillus* spp. are spore-forming aerobes (facultative anaerobes). *B. anthracis* and *B. cereus* are human pathogens; the rest are opportunistic. They are usually from a soil or animal reservoir *Corynebacteria* *Corynebacteria* aerobes (facultative anaerobes) are benign commensals; *C. diphtheriae* is the exception to this rule and causes diphtheria	*Enterobacteriaceae* ('coliforms') These are all aerobic (facultative anaerobic) bacilli, mainly derived from the GI and urogenital tracts. Most are opportunist pathogens and can cause intra-abdominal, urinary, and wound infections • *Escherichia coli* is a normal commensal of the bowel but certain strains are pathogenic • Other members include *Proteus*, *Enterobacter* spp., *Klebsiella* spp., *Salmonella* spp., and *Shigella* *Pseudomonas* spp. These are strict aerobes which are widely distributed in the environment. They are generally opportunistic and can be antibiotic-resistant. They often cause infection in the immunocompromised, e.g. burns patients (*P. aeruginosa*) *Helicobacter pylori* This is a curved microaerophilic bacteria that causes gastritis and peptic ulcer disease

Table 15.6 Commonly prescribed antimicrobial drugs

Class	Examples	Details
Beta-lactams	Penicillins	Beta-lactam antibiotics inhibit bacterial cell wall synthesis and are bactericidal Narrow spectrum: benzylpenicilliin, penicillin V Broader spectrum: ampicillin and amoxicillin Antistaphylococcal: flucloxacillin Antipseudomonal: piperacillin Penicillin/beta-lactamase inhibitor combinations such as amoxicillin–clavulanate (co-amoxiclav) and piperacillin–tazobactam extend the spectrum of the antibiotics
	Cephalosporins	Broad spectrum antibiotics used to treat septicaemia, pneumonia, meningitis, biliary tract infections, peritonitis, and urinary tract infections First generation (e.g. cefradine) have generally been replaced by newer cephalosporins Second generation (e.g. cefuroxime) have better Gram-negative activity and are often used in severe infection. Less susceptible to beta-lactamases Third generation (e.g. ceftazidime) have even better Gram-negative activity and some are antipseudomonal
	Carbapenems	Carbapenems (e.g. imipenem, meropenem) have very broad spectrum and good CSF penetration. Used in severe infections and sepsis
Macrolides	Erythromycin Clarithromycin	Inhibit ribosomal function and protein synthesis Similar spectrum to penicillin and so often used in penicillin-sensitive patients
Aminoglycosides	Gentamicin Amikacin	Inhibit ribosomal function and protein synthesis, bactericidal Good Gram-negative activity. Poor GI absorption so given by injection
Quinolones	Ciprofloxacin Ofloxacin	Inhibit DNA gyrase and hence DNA synthesis Used in uncomplicated UTI. Ciprofloxacin is the only oral antipseudomonal available
Tetracyclines	Oxytetracycline Doxycycline	Inhibit ribosomal function and protein synthesis Coverage against Gram-positive and -negative organisms. Limited use now due to resistance
Sulphonamides + trimethoprim		Inhibit bacterial folic acid synthesis and hence purine and thymidine synthesis Combined therapy co-trimoxazole used in UTI. Increasing resistance
Miscellaneous		Rifampicin and fusidic acid are used in combination to treat MRSA. Fusidic acid has good bone penetration Vancomycin and teicoplanin are glycopeptide antibiotics active against Gram-positive bacteria. No Gram-negative activity Metronidazole is active against anaerobic bacteria (e.g. *Bacteroides fragilis*) and protozoa. It is used to treat colonic sepsis and antibiotic-associated colitis Linezolid, clindamycin, and daptomycin are predominantly active against Gram-positive bacteria and are used to treat complicated infections of skin, soft tissue, bone, and joint (e.g. MRSA). Clindamycin was the first drug recognized to cause antibiotic-associated colitis

Patients undergoing surgery need preoperative assessment to identify and arrange investigation of any potential problems that may lead to an adverse outcome. It also allows them to be fully informed of their risks and prognosis during the consenting process (📖 Topic 1.7).

Surgical risk

Cardiac risk

Coronary artery disease is very prevalent and poses the greatest proportion of operative risk. It is discussed in more detail later in the chapter (📖 Topic 15.13).

Non-cardiac risk

- Smoking inhibits clearance of pulmonary secretions, suppresses the immune system, and causes wound hypoxia. Ideally a smoker should stop for 2 months preoperatively. However, there is an advantage in stopping even for 12 h before surgery as the blood carboxyhaemoglobin level falls and ciliary function improves
- Alcohol dependence is associated with hepatic dysfunction, malnutrition, and haematological dysfunction
- Malnutrition and obesity both convey increased risk
- Endocrine disorders, particularly poorly controlled diabetes mellitus

Grading systems

Both the patient and the planned surgery is graded to help predict outcome and to guide further investigations.

Patient

The American Society of Anesthesiologists (ASA) grading system (Table 15.7) subjectively classifies patients by their preoperative physical fitness. The peroperative system for the surgical enumeration of mortality (POSSUM) is another scoring system often used.

Functional capacity of a patient can be expressed in terms of metabolic equivalents (METs). Patients unable to reach four METs have an increased risk (Table 15.8).

Surgery

The type of surgery is graded by the degree of stress it will cause. Each type of surgery carries its own risks and often needs different levels of preoperative assessment (e.g. cardiothoracic surgery and neurosurgery).

Clinical assessment

History

- Details of surgical condition and procedure
- Details of previous anaesthetic
- Respiratory—smoking, control of asthma, and COPD
- Cardiovascular—angina, recent MI, exercise tolerance
- Renal—renal impairment
- Gastrointestinal—gastro-oesophageal reflux, hiatus hernia
- Metabolic—obesity, control of diabetes mellitus
- Haematological—thrombotic risk, bleeding disorders

Examination

- Examination relevant to condition being treated
- General systemic examination is guided by underlying co-morbidities and the grade of surgery

Investigations

Investigations in healthy people often yield abnormal results that do not change management. Preoperative testing should therefore be selective. NICE has issued guidelines to help focus investigation requests.

General

- **Full blood count** is recommended in all adult women patients and all men >60 years of age. If there is any co-morbidity or surgery of grade 2 or higher is planned, a FBC should be performed. G+S and cross-match is guided by the local blood ordering schedule
- **Renal function** is recommended in all patients over the age of 60 years, in patients with co-morbidity, and those undergoing major surgery
- **Clotting** is indicated in all patients with anticoagulants, bleeding tendency, liver dysfunction, or undergoing grade 4 surgery. It is unnecessary in ASA 1 and 2 patients undergoing surgical grades 1 and 2. Consider in ASA 2 patients with renal impairment and ASA 3 patients with cardiovascular or renal impairment undergoing grade 3 surgery
- **Random serum glucose** is indicated in all patients >40 years undergoing grade 2 and grade 1 surgery in all except ASA 3 with renal impairment
- **Urine analysis** for pH, protein, glucose, ketones, and blood is indicated in all patients
- **ECG** is recommended in all patients >40 years and any patient with cardiovascular co-morbidity
- **Chest radiograph** is indicated in patients with evidence of acute cardiovascular or respiratory disease or chronic disease that has worsened in the past year. Patients at risk of tuberculosis or with malignant disease should also have one unless they have recent imaging
- **Arterial blood gas and lung function tests** are only considered in ASA grade 2 and 3 patients with cardiorespiratory disease undergoing major surgery

Other

- **Pregnancy test** should be performed following informed consent in all female patients of reproductive age. It may be omitted in those with a history of last menstrual period or those who say it is not possible for them to be pregnant
- **Sickle cell test** should be performed following informed consent in all patients with an appropriate ethnic background and unknown sickle status
- **Flexion and extension cervical spine radiographs** are performed in patients with spinal disease that compromises neck movement (e.g. rheumatoid arthritis)

Special

Further special investigations are indicated in patients with other significant co-morbidities and who are undergoing major surgery. These are discussed later in the chapter.

Outcome

Following assessment and investigation patients may need specialist review, further investigations or postponement or even cancellation of surgery. In addition, preoperative assessment should help plan the perioperative care, including thromboprophylaxis, pain management, nutrition, physiotherapy, and level of care (e.g. HDU/ITU).

⚠ Preoperative fasting and medications

Preoperative fasting

Preoperative fasting aims to minimize gastric contents and reduce the risk of pulmonary aspiration. It is usual to fast before GA and RA (in case GA required).

- 6 h—light meal and milky drinks
- 4 h—breast milk
- 2 h—clear fluids
- 1 h—oral medications can be given with a small amount of water

Medications

Most common drugs can be continued in the perioperative period. A few drugs may have to be stopped or altered owing to the anaesthetic or surgery. If in doubt seek advice from an anaesthetist.

Anticoagulation

- Oral anticoagulation with warfarin is managed depending on the indication for warfarinization. Warfarin generally needs to be stopped at least 4 days before a procedure with a risk of bleeding. Patients with prosthetic heart valves need therapeutic LMWH cover but those with AF do not. For patients with a high risk of valve thrombosis or recent arterial thrombosis, consider therapeutic unfractionated heparin cover. Oral anticoagulation can usually be restarted the night following surgery

Psychiatric drugs

- Lithium should be stopped perioperatively. If continued, levels must be within the therapeutic range (0.4–1 mmol/L)
- Monoamine oxidase inhibitors (MAOIs) are no longer stopped perioperatively. Care must be taken to avoid drug interactions

OCP and HRT

For minor surgery there is no indication to stop these drugs. For more major surgery the risk of perioperative thromboembolism may be up to four times greater in patients taking OCP. Consequently for major surgery, the patient should be informed of the increased risk perioperatively and allowed to make their own decision as to whether they wish to stop their medication and take appropriate precautions.

Drugs for diabetes mellitus

Management of type 1 and 2 diabetes mellitus can be complex. It depends on the patient and the planned surgery. (📖 Topic 15.17)

Steroids

Patients who are taking steroids or who have recently stopped may need additional steroids depending on their baseline dose and the planned procedure. (📖 Topic 15.10)

Table 15.7 ASA grading system

Grade	Definition (mortality %)
1	Normal healthy patient (0.05)
2	A patient with mild systemic disease (0.4)
3	A patient with severe systemic disease (4.5)
4	A patient with severe systemic disease that is constantly life-threatening (25)
5	Moribund, not expected to survive 24 h with or without surgery (50)
E	Emergency case

Table 15.8 ET scores for various activities (Duke Activity Status Index)

MET score*	Activity
1–4	Able to care for self, eat, dress, and use toilet unaided Walk indoors around house Walk level ground at 2–3 mph
5–9	Climb one flight of stairs Heavy housework; scrubbing floors, lifting and moving furniture Moderate recreational activities; golf, dancing, mountain walking
>10	Participate in strenuous sport; swimming, tennis, football, bicycling, skiing Heavy professional work

*One MET is the energy expended by a 70 kg man sitting reading a book (3.5 mL O_2/kg/min).

Table 15.9 Elective surgery grades

Grade	Example
1 Minor	Excision of skin lesion
2 Intermediate	Primary inguinal hernia repair, tonsillectomy, knee arthroscopy
3 Major	Total abdominal hysterectomy, transurethral resection of prostate, lumbar discectomy, carotid endarterectomy
4 Major +	Total joint replacement, lung surgery, colonic resection, radical neck dissection

15.6 Acute pain

Pain is defined as an unpleasant sensory and emotional experience resulting from a stimulus causing or likely to cause, tissue damage, or expressed in terms of that potential damage. Analgesia is the reduction or elimination of pain.

In 1990 the World Health Organization (WHO) published an analgesic ladder which has been adopted for all types of pain management (Fig 15.3).

Aetiology

Most surgical interventions cause some degree of discomfort or pain. Procedures leaving a wound in areas that move (e.g. abdominal wall) or highly innervated areas (e.g. hand) often cause disproportionate amounts of pain.

Patients with anxiety, depression or psychological disturbance are more likely to report more severe postoperative pain.

Clinical assessment

The assessment of acute pain is dependent on many individual patient factors, including physical state, age, cognitive function, and cultural background.

Regular self-reporting of pain should be encouraged and is usually an effective method of assessing the level of pain.

Regular use of pain scoring systems can be valuable for monitoring the efficacy of analgesia. They include visual analogue, word descriptor, numerical, or pictorial ranking scales.

Principles of acute pain management

Acute pain management needs to take into account patient factors as well as the underlying aetiology. Different approaches may be required for different patient groups (e.g. children, pregnant women, and the elderly); however, general principles include:

- regular analgesia for baseline pain and analgesia as required for breakthrough pain
- medications for side effects (e.g. antiemetics) and reversal of action (e.g. naloxone for opioids) should be prescribed
- choose appropriate route of administration
- be alert to contraindications and side effects of analgesia
- regular monitoring of pain scores. Patients given strong opioids or epidural analgesia also need routine monitoring of vital signs
- Positive emotional support
- Quiet, private, and comfortable environment

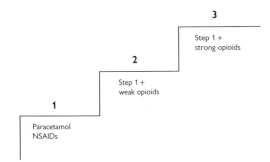

Fig 15.3 WHO analgesic ladder.

Non-opioid analgesics

Paracetamol

Indications

Paracetamol is used in mild to moderate pain and pyrexia. It is also used in compound preparations (see below).

Action

Paracetamol inhibits central prostaglandin synthesis and has a central antipyretic action with minimal peripheral anti-inflammatory effects. There are no gastric irritation or anti-platelet effects as seen with NSAIDs; however, there is a risk of serious hepatotoxicity following overdose.

Contraindications and side effects

Paracetamol is metabolized by conjugation with either a glucuronide or sulphate group within the liver and only a small amount (<1%) of a toxic metabolite is produced. Normally these small quantities are conjugated with glutathione and are excreted from the body.

Paracetamol is very safe in normal doses but in overdose (150+ mg/kg/day) the normal metabolic pathways become saturated, increased quantities of the toxic metabolite are produced, and glutathione stores become depleted.

Hepatocellular damage then occurs and can lead to hepatic failure. Treatment involves early administration of sulphydryl groups in the form of N-acetylcysteine.

Aspirin and non-steroidal anti-inflammatory drugs (NSAIDs)

Indications

NSAIDs have analgesic, antipyretic, anti-inflammatory, and anti-thrombotic effects to varying degrees. They are especially useful in managing inflammatory causes of pain.

Action

They act by inhibiting the cyclo-oxygenase (COX) enzyme system, which catalyses the production of prostanoids from arachidonic acid.

These prostanoids include prostaglandins, prostacyclin, and thromboxanes. There are at least two different isoforms of the COX enzyme. COX-1 is present in all tissues and represents the constitutive form, whereas COX-2 is the inducible form and is produced in high concentrations at sites of inflammation.

Contraindications and side effects

- Contraindicated in the critically ill surgical patient
- Gastrointestinal—evidence of gastric damage is present in approximately 20% of chronic users. They can be combined with gastric protective agents
- Renal—in vulnerable patients renal impairment or even failure can be triggered. This is because prostaglandins have a protective role in maintaining renal blood flow, especially under conditions of physiological stress such as hypovolaemia, and consequently with NSAID treatment this protection is lost
- Respiratory—inhibition of prostaglandin-mediated bronchodilatation causes bronchoconstriction in ~10% of asthmatics
- Antiplatelet effect—platelet aggregation is impaired by thromboxane inhibition and may contribute to intraoperative bleeding

Common drugs

- **Aspirin** is now mainly used for its antiplatelet properties to reduce cardiovascular risk. It is contraindicated in children <16 years owing to increased risk of Reye's syndrome
- **Ibuprofen** has fewer side effects than other non-selective NSAIDs but is weaker. **Naproxen** has similar properties
- **Diclofenac** is slightly stronger and is good for postoperative pain and rheumatic disease
- Selective COX-2 inhibitors (e.g. **celecoxib**) improve gastrointestinal tolerance and antiplatelet complications, but the renal and cardiovascular side effects remain. They are associated with a moderately increased risk of cardiovascular events, and should only be used if specifically indicated

Compound analgesics

Combinations of weak opioids and paracetamol are no better than paracetamol alone if a low dose opioid is used. They also have the disadvantage of opioid side effects.

- **Co-codamol**—paracetamol and codeine phosphate
- **Co-dydramol**—paracetamol and dihydrocodeine

Opioid analgesics

Indications

Opioids are used in moderate to severe pain. They have a wide range of delivery routes, including: oral, buccal, intranasal, subcutaneous, intramuscular, intravenous, epidural, and intrathecal.

Action

Opioids bind to opioid receptors and include both naturally occurring (opiates) and endogenous compounds along with synthetic drugs.

Morphine is metabolized in the liver to morphine-3- and morphine-6-glucuronide; the latter is active. Both are renally excreted and consequently in both renal and hepatic failure, the half-life and effects of morphine will be prolonged.

Contraindications and side effects

A variety of side effects are caused by opioid drugs.

- Respiratory depression
- Drowsiness and sedation
- Nausea and vomiting
- Constipation (especially codeine)
- Pruritis and rash caused by local histamine release
- Miosis
- Hypothermia
- Dependence and withdrawal symptoms with long-term use

Naloxone is an opioid antagonist active on all the receptor subtypes. It can be given to reverse the side effects of opioid drugs,

including sedation, respiratory depression, and pruritus. Unfortunately, it also has side effects and has a shorter half-life than morphine, so repeated dosing or an infusion may be necessary.

Patient-controlled analgesia

Patient-controlled analgesia (PCA) allows the patient a degree of control over their own pain relief. Morphine is most commonly used, but other opioids can be used.

The drug is made up in a syringe pump (morphine sulphate 1 mg/mL in 50 mL normal saline) and attached to a dedicated intravenous cannula.

The patient is given a button which, when depressed, administers a set dose of morphine (1 mg). It is important that this button is only pressed by the patient. Once a dose has been administered the syringe pump is programmed to 'lock out' for a set amount of time, usually 5 min, so that a repeat dose cannot be administered until this time has elapsed.

Safety features include a lockable programme, dedicated IV cannula, and the fact that a drowsy patient will not press the button.

Some pumps have the facility to administer a background infusion with bolus doses superimposed on top. PCA can provide highly effective analgesia, but careful monitoring is needed to avoid respiratory depression or overdose.

Adjunctive drug therapy

These are drugs that can be administered in addition to non-opioid and opioid analgesics, and include steroids (anti-inflammatory effect), anxiolytics, caffeine, antidepressant drugs, antiepileptic drugs, ketamine, and clonidine.

The antidepressant and antiepileptic drugs are commonly used in the treatment of chronic pain. Ketamine is a powerful dissociative anaesthetic and analgesic agent. It can be utilized in nerve blocks as a local anaesthetic adjunct, prolonging the analgesia obtained, as can clonidine.

Inhalational analgesics such as a 50:50 mixture of nitrous oxide and oxygen, known as Entonox, can be administered for analgesia, and have found wide use in the setting of obstetrics and pre-hospital care.

Regional techniques

Local anaesthetic agents targeted at a particular nerve or nerve plexus can provide extremely effective analgesia. In certain cases it may be possible to insert a catheter and give a local anaesthetic infusion. Injection of wounds with long-acting local anaesthesia provides effective postoperative analgesia.

Epidural analgesia can provide the most effective pain relief in the perioperative period and for some patients it may reduce the incidence of perioperative respiratory complications.

Non-pharmacological therapy

There are various non-pharmacological techniques that are mainly used in the chronic pain setting. These include acupuncture, transcutaneous electrical nerve stimulation (TENS), massage, hypnosis, and cognitive behavioural therapy.

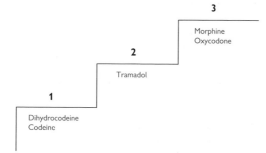

Fig 15.4 Opioid ladder.

Venous thrombosis is the formation of thrombus within the deep venous system. The deep veins of the lower limb are the most common site although it can occur elsewhere.

Deep venous thrombosis (DVT) often results in pulmonary embolization and so the condition is usually considered to be part of the same process as venous thromboembolism (VTE).

DVT can occur within the community but is a common complication among hospital inpatients. It results in increased morbidity and mortality and prolonged admissions.

Aetiology

Patients may have a congenital thrombophilia predisposing them to thrombosis (e.g. Factor V Leiden) or an acquired risk factor (see below).

Major risk factors (relative risk 5–20)
- Age >60 years
- Major abdominal or pelvic surgery
- Hip or knee joint replacement
- Lower limb fracture
- Postoperative intensive care
- Hospitalization and institutional care
- Advanced or metastatic cancer
- Late pregnancy or puerperium
- Varicose veins with associated phlebitis

Minor risk factors (relative risk 2–4)
- Continuous travel >3 h in the 4 weeks before surgery
- Oral contraceptive or hormone replacement therapy
- Prothrombotic disorders (Factor V Leiden, resistance to activated protein C, protein C deficiency, protein S deficiency, antithrombin deficiency, antiphospholipid antibodies, hyper-homocysteineamia)
- Obesity (body mass index ≥30)
- Smoking
- Hypertension
- Congestive cardiac failure

Pathophysiology

Virchow's triad describes three components that may contribute to the development of venous thrombosis. Many of the risk factors for DVT alter one or more of these components.

Virchow's triad
1. Abnormal blood constituents (hypercoagulable state)
2. Abnormal vessel wall (endothelial dysfunction or injury)
3. Abnormal flow (slow or turbulent)

Clinical assessment

Clinical diagnosis is often unreliable as over 50% of patients with DVT are asymptomatic. Only half those suspected of having a DVT actually go on to be diagnosed with one.

A scoring system is used to estimate the clinical probability of a patient having a DVT: unlikely <2 or likely ≥2 (Table 15.10). Alternative diagnoses should always be considered

Differential diagnoses
- Cellulitis
- Ruptured Baker's cyst
- Venous conditions—thrombophlebitis, chronic venous insufficiency, and venous obstruction
- Acute limb ischaemia
- Asymmetrical leg oedema

Investigations
- D-dimers are fibrin degradation products that are specific for thrombus formation but not specific for DVT; they may be elevated in trauma, cancer, infection, and following surgery. A negative D-dimer test in the unlikely group excludes DVT (high negative predictive value), although this may be affected by the assay used (SimpliRED, Vidas, MDA). Patients in the likely or unlikely group with a positive D-dimer need imaging
- Compression duplex ultrasound is the first choice for non-invasive imaging. It is sensitive for proximal DVT, but less accurate for isolated calf DVT
- Venography is the criterion standard but is invasive and has been superseded by colour duplex ultrasound
- Plain chest radiograph, ABG, and ECG should be considered if a PE is also suspected (📖 Topic 15.8)

Management

General
- Avoid excessive mobilization in acute stages (risk of embolization) and elevate leg to reduce oedema
- Maintain good hydration
- Give analgesia as required
- Patient education detailing risks of VTE

Pharmacological treatment
- LMWH rather than unfractionated heparin should be used for initial treatment of DVT as its efficacy is as good and there is a reduced risk of bleeding
- Vitamin K antagonists (warfarin) or LMWH are safe and efficacious for outpatient treatment of DVT
- Anticoagulation is continued for 3–6 months if there are transient risk factors and for >12 months for idiopathic or recurrent DVT
- Graduated compression stockings should be worn for at least 1 year following diagnosis to reduce risk of postthrombotic syndrome affecting the leg

Thrombolysis
The use of thrombolytic agents (e.g. streptokinase or tissue plasminogen activator) or thrombectomy is only indicated for limb salvage in acute venous infarction.

Complications and prognosis

Asymptomatic pulmonary embolism is found in approximately 50% of patients with DVT if they undergo perfusion scanning. The other main complication is chronic venous insufficiency (formerly postthrombotic syndrome), which may develop in up to 25% of patients following DVT. Destruction of the leg vein valves by DVT causes chronic leg pain, dermatitis, and ulceration.

> **➔ Extra**
> - CG46 *Venous Thromboembolism: Reducing the Risk in Surgical Inpatients.* NICE, 2007

◎ Surgical thromboprophylaxis

All surgical inpatients should be individually risk-stratified for VTE before surgery. They should also be given information about VTE, including the signs and symptoms of DVT/PE and the risks and benefits of prophylaxis (see NICE guidelines).

Risk stratification
Both individual patient factors, described earlier, and operation-related factors contribute to risk of VTE. Operative risk increases with the age of the patient, length, and complexity of procedure. Emergency surgery and orthopaedic surgery are particularly high risk.

General measures for all patients
- Consider stopping OCP 4 weeks before elective surgery. There is no evidence for stopping HRT
- Use regional rather than general anaesthesia if possible
- Keep well hydrated
- Give leg exercises to perform whilst immobile
- Encourage early mobilization following surgery

Mechanical measures
- Thigh-length graduated elastic thromboembolism deterrent (TED) stockings should be offered to all patients unless contraindicated (massive leg oedema, dermatitis, PAOD or peripheral neuropathy)
- Knee-length stockings may be used to improve compliance or if thigh-length stockings are impractical
- The stocking compression gradient should be approximately 18 mmHg at the ankle, 14 mmHg at the mid-calf, and 8 mmHg at the upper thigh
- Intermittent pneumatic compression boots intraoperatively and during periods of sedation or immobility should be encouraged as much as possible
- Foot impulse devices are also available

Pharmacological measures
- LMWH is used at a prophylactic dose in all patients with risk factors for VTE and those having orthopaedic surgery. An increased dose is used for very high risk patients
- Fondaparinux is a synthetic pentasaccharide that is a highly selective activated factor Xa inhibitor. It can be used as an alternative to LMWH when indicated
- Heparinoids (e.g. danaparoid) are useful for prophylaxis in patients with heparin-induced thrombocytopenia
- Antiplatelet agents, such as aspirin, provide some thromboembolism protection but are not as effective as prophylactic anticoagulation
- Warfarin is a coumarin derivative and acts as a vitamin K antagonist. Vitamin K is required in the synthesis of active clotting factors II, VII, IX, and XI (as well as the anticoagulant proteins C and S). Warfarin is generally used as a therapeutic oral anticoagulant rather than for VTE prophylaxis

Guidance by surgical speciality

	No risk factors	≥1 risk factors
General	Mechanical	Mechanical **plus** LMWH
Cardiothoracic		
Neurosurgery		
Urological		
Vascular		
Orthopaedic*	Mechanical **plus** LMWH/fondaparinux	Mechanical **plus** LMWH/fondaparinux

*Patients with a hip fracture should have the LMWH continued for 4 weeks. Following hip replacement LMWH is continued for 4 weeks if risk factors are present.

Table 15.10 Pretest probability for DVT*

Clinical feature	Score
Active cancer	1
Paralysis, paresis or recent plaster immobilization of legs	1
Bedbound for >3 days or major surgery within 4 weeks	1
Localized tenderness along deep venous system	1
Entire leg swollen	1
Calf swelling >3 cm compared with asymptomatic leg (measured 10 cm below tibial tuberosity	1
Pitting oedema (worse in symptomatic leg)	1
Collateral superficial veins (non-varicose)	1
Alternative diagnosis as likely as DVT	-2

*Adapted from Wells PS et al. Value of assessment of pre-test probability of deep vein thrombosis in clinical management. *Lancet* 1997; **350:** 1795–8.

15.8 Pulmonary embolism

Pulmonary embolism (PE) is the obstruction of the pulmonary arterial vasculature by emboli which usually arise from the deep veins of the lower limb (venous thromboembolism, VTE). PE is the most common cause of death in the immediate postoperative period.

Aetiology

PE is not an isolated condition and is considered part of the same pathological process of DVT. Risk factors for VTE are discussed in Topic 15.7.

Other emboli that can cause obstruction of the pulmonary vasculature include fat embolism and air embolus.

Pathophysiology

The embolus travels from the venous circulation through the right heart and lodges in the pulmonary vasculature. The size, number, and chronicity determine the extent of obstruction of the pulmonary vasculature.

- Non-massive PE (<50% obstruction) rarely causes pulmonary infarction (10%). It is more likely to occur if the collateral circulation (i.e. bronchial circulation) is inadequate or if there is pre-existing pulmonary or left heart disease
- Massive PE (>50% obstruction) causes haemodynamic instability by obstructing the flow of blood to the left atrium, resulting in reduced cardiac output and shock
- Multiple minor PE will cause a chronic rise in pulmonary vascular resistance, and pulmonary hypertension will result with eventual right heart failure (cor pulmonale)

Clinical assessment

Symptoms and signs depend on the size and location of the emboli and are often non-specific. All patients should have their clinical probability assessed.

Haemodynamically insignificant PE

- Dyspnoea (70%) is the most common symptom but is non-specific
- Pleuritic chest pain (49%)
- Cough (20%) and haemoptysis (7%)
- Multiple small PE cause progressive dyspnoea, intermittent chest pain, pulmonary hypertension, and, eventually, cor pulmonale

Haemodynamically significant PE

- Sudden cardiovascular collapse, engorged neck veins, syncope, and cardiac arrest

Clinical probability

Ask the two questions below. Low = neither; intermediate = either; high = both (follow local guidelines).
1. Is another diagnosis unlikely?
2. Is there a major risk factor? (📖 Topic 15.7)

General investigations

- ECG is usually normal apart from a sinus tachycardia. Atrial arrhythmias may occur, as can right axis deviation, right bundle branch block, and T-wave inversion in leads V1–3. The classical right ventricular strain pattern of S wave in V1, a Q wave, and inverted T wave in lead 3 (S1Q3T3) is rare
- Plain chest radiograph is usually normal: it is helpful to exclude differential diagnoses such as pneumothorax, pneumonia, and pulmonary oedema

- Arterial blood gas—hypoxaemia, hypocapnia, and respiratory alkalosis due to hyperventilation

Diagnostic investigations

- D-dimer is used in low and intermediate probability cases. Patients with a high probability proceed straight to imaging without a D-dimer test. A negative D-dimer excludes PE in patients with low or intermediate clinical probability
- CT pulmonary angiography is now the standard technique for imaging non-massive PE. A good quality negative scan excludes a PE. The lower limbs can also be scanned at the same time, if indicated, to detect a DVT
- Echocardiography will identify acute right heart strain or intrapulmonary/intracardiac thrombus caused by a massive PE. CTPA can also be used
- Compression duplex ultrasound is enough to confirm VTE in patients with a clinical diagnosis of DVT. No further pulmonary imaging is needed

Management

The initial approach is ABC. Massive PE is a medical emergency and is often fatal.

Initial management of massive PE

- Sit up and give high flow oxygen with analgesia PRN
- IV fluids and inotropes may be needed to support the circulation
- Early thrombolysis should follow local guidelines. Alteplase (rt-PA) is often the first line treatment for haemodynamically unstable PE, but is not recommended in non-massive PE. Embolectomy may be considered if thrombolysis is contraindicated or fails

Anticoagulation for PE

📖 Topic 15.7.
- LMWH is given to patients with medium or high probability of PE before imaging
- Oral anticoagulation with target INR 2–3 is started following diagnosis and combined with LMWH until within the therapeutic range (may take 5 days)
- Continue anticoagulation for 3 months for transient risk factors and at least 6 months for idiopathic PE. Longer courses are required for recurrent PE

Inferior vena caval (IVC) filters

Possible indications are listed below. However, there is evidence that they do not improve survival.
- Major haemorrhage precluding anticoagulation
- Recurrent PE despite anticoagulation
- Patients undergoing inpatient surgery with a history of DVT in the last month and contraindications for anticoagulation

Complications and prognosis

The main complication of massive PE is death (50% mortality rate at 30 days). The majority occur within 2 h of the event.

 Extra
- British Thoracic Society Guidelines. www.brit-thoracic. org.uk

A

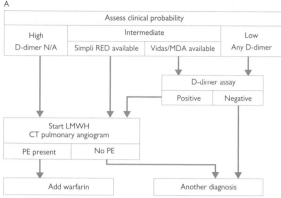

Assess clinical probability			
High D-dimer N/A	Intermediate		Low Any D-dimer
	Simpli RED available	Vidas/MDA available	

D-dimer assay	
Positive	Negative

Start LMWH CT pulmonary angiogram	
PE present	No PE

Add warfarin		Another diagnosis

Fig 15.5 Management of suspected PE with isotope lung scanning unavailable on site (BTS Guidelines, 2003). Reproduced with the kind permission of the BMJ Publishing Group Ltd.

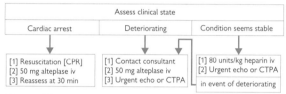

Assess clinical state		
Cardiac arrest	Deteriorating	Condition seems stable
[1] Resuscitation [CPR] [2] 50 mg alteplase iv [3] Reassess at 30 min	[1] Contact consultant [2] 50 mg alteplase iv [3] Urgent echo or CTPA	[1] 80 units/kg heparin iv [2] Urgent echo or CTPA in event of deteriorating

Fig 15.6 Management of probable massive PE (BTS Guidelines, 2003). Reproduced with the kind permission of the BMJ Publishing Group Ltd.

Perfusion

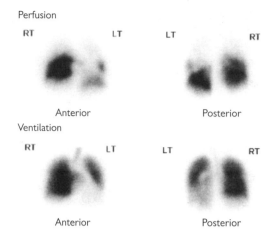

RT   LT   LT   RT

Anterior   Posterior

Ventilation

RT   LT   LT   RT

Anterior   Posterior

Fig 15.7 Ventilation perfusion scan showing multiple segmental and subsegmental perfusion defects in both lungs. The ventilation of these areas appears to be within normal limits. This scan has a high probability for pulmonary embolic disease.

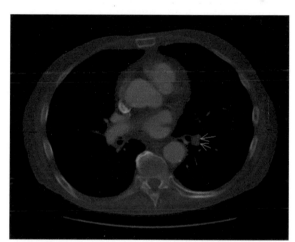

Fig 15.8 CTPA showing thrombus within the left lower lobe pulmonary artery. There was also thrombus in the right upper lobe pulmonary artery.

Respiratory tract infections are the most common infectious condition worldwide. They are usually classified on whether they involve the upper or lower respiratory tract.

Upper respiratory tract infection

Acute upper respiratory tract infections (URTI) are very common. They include rhinitis, rhinosinusitis, nasopharyngitis (common cold), pharyngitis, epiglottitis, laryngitis, and tracheitis. Most are viral.

Clinical assessment

Nasopharyngitis

- Rhinorrhoea, nasal obstruction, and sneezing
- Cough caused by postnasal drip
- Headache
- Fatigue, malaise, and myalgia is more suggestive of influenza

Bacterial pharyngitis

- Sore throat with prominent pharyngeal erythema
- Tender cervical lymphadenopathy
- Rhinorrhoea
- Low grade fever ~38.5°C
- Throat swab—group A streptococcus

Management

Supportive therapy is usually sufficient with good fluid intake and analgesia as required. Antibiotics are not indicated in most cases except in certain patient groups (e.g. COPD) and for streptococcal pharyngitis.

Lower respiratory tract infection

LRTI is generally divided into infections of the large airways (bronchitis) or of the lung (pneumonia). Acute bronchitis is discussed in the COPD topic.

Aetiology

Pneumonia is classified by the environment in which the patient acquired it. A causative organism is identified in approximately 75% of cases.

Hospital-acquired pneumonia (HAP)

Hospital-acquired pneumonia is defined as pneumonia developing at least 48 h after admission. Common organisms include *Streptococcus pneumoniae, Haemophilis influenzae, Staphylococcus aureus,* and sensitive Gram-negative bacteria. Anaerobes are more common in aspiration pneumonia.

Ventilator-associated pneumonia (VAP) is defined as pneumonia developing following at least 48 h of mechanical ventilation. Following recent admission from the community the organisms are likely to be as for community-acquired pneumonia (CAP). Inpatient or long periods of ventilation are more likely to result in Gram-negative bacilli, *Pseudomonas aeruginosa* or MRSA infection.

Community-acquired pneumonia

S. pneumoniae is the commonest bacteria isolated. Others include *H. influenzae,* and *Moraxella catarrhalis.* No bacterial pathogen is identified in over 50% of cases. These may well be viral—influenza, cytomegalovirus, and varicella.

Nursing home-acquired pneumonia falls in between HAP and CAP. *S. pneumoniae* and Gram-negative bacilli are the main organisms.

Pathophysiology

Six mechanisms have been identified in the pathogenesis of pneumonia.

1. Inhalation of microorganisms is commonest route in CAP
2. Aspiration of oropharyngeal or gastric contents is by far the most prevalent mechanism in HAP
3. Haematogenous
4. Invasion from infection in contiguous structures
5. Direct inoculation
6. Reactivation of TB

Once inside the alveoli, the organisms invade, causing inflammation and subsequent debris deposition. Inflammatory cells drawn to the infected area release proteolytic enzymes, altering the bronchial epithelium and ciliary clearance mechanisms, and stimulating excess mucus production which interferes with gas exchange.

Bacterial pneumonia is often classified by the anatomical location of the lung consolidation into lobar and lobular (bronchopneumonia).

Aspiration pneumonitis

Aspiration of oropharyngeal or gastric contents causes a pneumonitis which then predisposes to infection. Risk factors include impaired swallowing, reduced GCS, intubation (nasotracheal, endotracheal, NG), impaired lower oesophageal sphincter function, and gastric stasis.

Clinical assessment

Clinical assessment determines the likely cause of a chest infection and its severity. Postoperative pneumonia generally develops 36–72 h following surgery.

History and examination

Initial presentation is a often with a dry cough, pleuritic chest pain, and fever. Within a few days the cough becomes productive of rusty-coloured sputum (*Streptococcus pneumoniae*). There may also be malaise and acute confusion, especially in elderly patients.

On examination there is tachypnoea, tachycardia, and a fever up to 39.5°C. Consolidated lung results in dullness on percussion. On auscultation there may be reduced air entry and crackles.

Investigations

- Microbiology: sputum for Gram stain, culture, and sensitivities. Blood cultures taken if pyrexial or unwell
- Bloods—FBC, U+Es (renal dysfunction), LFT, CRP
- ABG if SaO_2 <92%
- Plain chest radiograph shows changes in 40% of patients with LRTI signs
- ECG excludes cardiac differential diagnoses

Markers of severe pneumonia

The CURB criteria predict the severity of CAP. The pneumonia is severe if two or more are present. Additional markers of severity are listed below.

1. **C**onfusion of new onset (AMTS 8 or less)
2. **U**rea >7 mmol/L
3. **R**espiratory rate ≥30 per minute
4. **B**P (systolic <90 mmHg or diastolic ≤60 mmHg)
5. Hypoxia PaO_2 ≤8 kPa on room air
6. Age ≥65 years

7. WCC ≤4 or ≥20 x 10⁹/L

8. Co-existing disease (e.g. IHD, CVA, neoplasia)

Management

The initial approach follows ABC guidelines. Antibiotic treatment depends on the severity, likely pathogens, and presence of any co-morbidities. Always follow local guidelines.

- Supplemental oxygen to maintain SaO_2 >92%
- Empirical antibiotic treatment until sensitivities available. Severe cases (CURB ≥2) need IV antibiotics (follow local guidelines)
- Fluid therapy may be needed in severe cases if NBM and pyrexial
- Nebulized saline may reduce sputum retention and nebulized bronchodilators improve bronchospasm
- Chest physiotherapy and adequate analgesia to allow deep cough
- Respiratory support may be required if the patient develops respiratory failure

Complications and prognosis

The majority of patients have a good prognosis. Complications include:

- respiratory and circulatory failure needing support. Non-invasive ventilation may be sufficient initially (e.g. bilevel positive airway pressure; BIPAP)
- ARDS is most common in severe HAP or VAP
- pleural effusion, empyema, and abscess are rare
- Overwhelming sepsis

Mortality rates in HAP are as high as 50%. Preventative measures to reduce aspiration and the need for intubation and mechanical ventilation reduce morbidity and mortality rates from pneumonia.

⚠ Respiratory tract infection

Preoperative

Any patient with an active respiratory tract infection causing a fever and cough with or without chest signs on auscultation should not undergo elective surgery under general anaesthesia owing to the risk of postoperative pulmonary complications.

Adults with viral URTI are at slightly increased risk of laryngospasm perioperatively but are not at increased risk of developing postoperative respiratory complications unless there is pre-existing chronic respiratory disease or they are undergoing major thoracic or abdominal surgery.

Children with ongoing or recent viral URTI are more likely to suffer transient hypoxaemia, which is greater if intubation occurs, and elective surgery should be postponed until the child is well.

Risk factors for pneumonia

- Advanced age
- Obesity
- Smoking
- Reduced level of consciousness
- Diabetes mellitus
- Malignancy
- Gastroparesis and aspiration
- Oropharyngeal colonization with Gram-negative organisms
- Chronic disease
- Endotracheal intubation

Postoperative

Postoperative atelectasis is common, especially after long operations under GA. Hypoventilation results in collapse of alveolar walls which predisposes to pneumonia.

Mucociliary transport is depressed with age, smoking, dehydration, drugs, prior influenza infection, and COPD. This can result in airway obstruction, further contributing to airway collapse.

- Identify patients at risk and optimize their care preoperatively
- Supplemental oxygen as required (keep SaO_2 >92%)
- Good analgesia enables deeper breathing (increased tidal volume) and coughing
- Chest physiotherapy, including incentive spirometry to reduce atelectasis
- Early mobilization

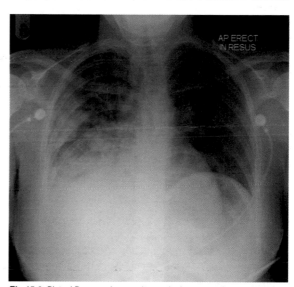

Fig 15.9 Plain AP erect chest radiograph showing right upper, middle, and lower lobe consolidation in an a middle-aged patient who presented with shortness of breath, cough, and fever. This represents a bronchopneumonia as it is causing widespread patchy shadowing in multiple lobes.

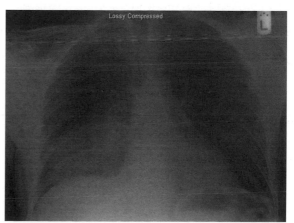

Fig 15.10 Plain AP erect chest radiograph showing dense consolidation in the right midzone. The diaphragm is preserved, as is the right heart border. This is consistent with pneumonia in the apical segment of the lower lobe.

15.10 Asthma

Asthma is a chronic disorder characterized by episodic, reversible airflow obstruction due to bronchoconstriction. It is the commonest chronic respiratory disorder with a rising prevalence (8% of adults and 15–20% of children).

Aetiology

Asthma has a number of causes which can be used to classify the condition, i.e. allergic, non-allergic, occupational, and exercise-induced. Allergic asthma usually develops in childhood and is the commonest form.

Risk factors

- Personal or family history of asthma or atopy
- Maternal smoking
- Premature birth or low birth weight
- Viral URTI in early childhood

Pathophysiology

The underlying pathophysiology is likely to be immunological. Hyperactivity of the bronchial airways can occur in response to a variety of triggers (see below).

Acute airway obstruction is caused by bronchial smooth muscle constriction and inflammation. The inflammation causes mucosal oedema, epithelial damage, hypertrophy, and mucus hypersecretion with plugging.

Triggers

- Respiratory tract infection
- Allergens—cats, house dust mite, and pollen
- Weather—cold and dry air, sudden changes
- Pollution—atmospheric and industrial irritants
- Drugs affecting chemical airway control, e.g. aspirin and beta-adrenergic antagonists

Clinical assessment

History

- Duration and severity of current symptoms, including dyspnoea, cough, wheezing, and chest tightness. Symptoms are often variable, intermittent, and worse at night or provoked by exercise
- Triggering factors
- Frequency and severity of attacks; previous hospital admissions ± ventilatory support
- Drug history and current asthma regime

Examination

The signs depend on the severity of the asthma.

- Level of alertness and GCS
- Assess ability to talk in sentences
- Tachypnoea, wheeze, prolonged expiration, accessory respiratory muscle use
- Severe—incomplete sentences, peak expiratory flow rates (PEFR) <33–50% of expected, HR >110 bpm, RR >25
- Life-threatening—as for severe plus any of PEFR <33%, silent chest, HR <60, systolic BP <100 mmHg, confusion or reduced GCS, silent chest, respiratory failure

Investigations

- Serial PEFR are used for assessment of severity and monitoring in an acute attack. PEFR <50% of predicted normal is severe
- Plain chest radiograph is usually normal or hyperexpanded (exclude pneumonia and pneumothorax)
- Arterial blood gas: low $PaCO_2$ initially. A normal or high $PaCO_2$ is a poor prognostic sign as it suggests reduced alveolar ventilation
- ECG (severe asthma) may show tachycardia but is otherwise normal. Transient right heart strain may be seen in younger patients

Management

Acute asthma attack

Involve anaesthetic team early if concerned.

1. Sit up and give oxygen (40–60%) via a high flow mask, aim for SaO_2 ≥95%
2. High dose inhaled beta-2-agonists via oxygen-driven nebulizer is the first line treatment. Salbutamol is the drug of choice and can be delivered as boluses of 5 mg every 15–30 min or continuously at 5–10 mg/h. Side effects include tachycardia, hypokalaemia, and arrhythmias. Intravenous infusion may be beneficial in ventilated patients or those *in extremis*
3. Corticosteroids should be given in all cases of acute asthma. Oral prednisolone 40–50 mg daily is as effective as IV hydrocortisone 100 mg 6-hourly
4. Nebulized anticholinergics (ipratropium bromide 0.5 mg 4–6-hourly) have good synergy with beta-2-agonists and should be added in severe asthma attacks
5. IV magnesium sulphate (1.2 g over 20 min) is effective in severe and life-threatening asthma with a poor initial response. It bronchodilates by blocking calcium channel-mediated bronchoconstriction and inhibiting parasympathetic acetylcholine release
6. Intravenous aminophylline is unlikely to improve bronchodilatation compared to standard care with inhaled bronchodilators and steroid tablets in acute asthma
7. Antibiotics are only indicated if there is evidence of a bacterial infection

Chronic management

Initial therapy is usually started by the GP; a specialist review is needed if regular additional therapy is needed.

1. Intermittent mild asthma is managed with an inhaled short-acting beta-2-agonist (e.g. salbutamol) as required. Reduce exposure to exacerbating factors
2. Regular preventer therapy is added in if patients are regularly using their bronchodilators, frequently symptomatic or have had acute exacerbations. Inhaled corticosteroid (e.g. beclomethasone, budesonide or fluticasone) is started at an appropriate dose for the severity of asthma
3. Additional therapy may be needed if control remains poor. This may be in the form of a long-acting beta-2-agonist (e.g. salmeterol), leucotriene receptor antagonist or slow release theophylline
4. Persistent poor control may need increased inhaled corticosteroid and the additional therapy as above
5. Frequent or continuous use of high dose oral or inhaled steroids needs regular monitoring

Complications and prognosis

Delayed use of additional asthma therapy is the commonest preventable cause of death in asthmatics. Compliance with treatment and inhaler technique are the two most important factors in delivering effective treatment.

⚠ Asthma

Preoperative assessment

- Patients should preferably have well controlled asthma with peak expiratory flow rates >80% of expected normal prior to elective surgery
- Significant diurnal variation in symptoms or peak flow readings indicates suboptimal control
- Preoperative assessment should elicit an asthma history, including seasonal variation. Try to avoid elective surgery during bad times of the year
- Consider contacting respiratory team for advice

Preoperative management

- Patients should have their usual medications as normal
- If they have a salbutamol inhaler, two puffs on call to theatre or a salbutamol nebulizer immediately preoperatively is helpful
- Prescribe salbutamol nebulizer PRN for all asthmatic patients
- Patients on high dose oral steroids (prednisolone 10 mg daily) in the last 3 months need additional steroid cover for the surgery (Table 15.11)

Table 15.11 Steroid cover for surgery*

Type of surgery	Steroid regimen
Minor (inguinal hernia repair)	Routine preoperative steroid dose or hydrocortisone 25 mg IV at induction
Intermediate (hysterectomy)	Routine preoperative steroid dose plus hydrocortisone 25 mg IV at induction. Post-operatively give hydrocortisone 25 mg 6-hourly for 24 h
Major surgery (cardiac surgery)	Routine preoperative steroid dose plus hydrocortisone 25 mg IV at induction. Post-operatively give hydrocortisone 25 mg 6-hourly for 48–72 h

*Patients with Addison's disease (primary adrenal insufficiency) have a different regime with higher doses of steroids (www.addisons.org.uk).

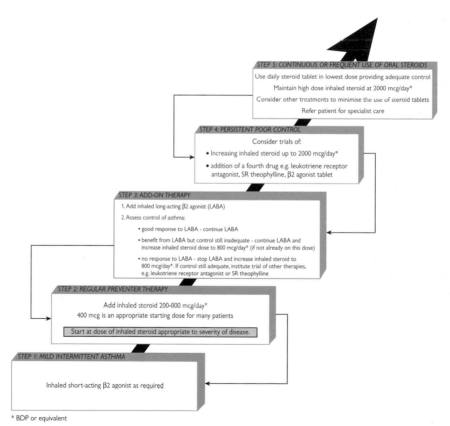

STEP 5: CONTINUOUS OR FREQUENT USE OF ORAL STEROIDS
Use daily steroid tablet in lowest dose providing adequate control
Maintain high dose inhaled steroid at 2000 mcg/day*
Consider other treatments to minimise the use of steroid tablets
Refer patient for specialist care

STEP 4: PERSISTENT POOR CONTROL
Consider trials of:
- Increasing inhaled steroid up to 2000 mcg/day*
- addition of a fourth drug e.g. leukotriene receptor antagonist, SR theophylline, β2 agonist tablet

STEP 3: ADD-ON THERAPY
1. Add inhaled long-acting β2 agonist (LABA)
2. Assess control of asthma:
- good response to LABA - continue LABA
- benefit from LABA but control still inadequate - continue LABA and increase inhaled steroid dose to 800 mcg/day* (if not already on this dose)
- no response to LABA - stop LABA and increase inhaled steroid to 800 mcg/day*. If control still adequate, institute trial of other therapies, e.g. leukotriene receptor antagonist or SR theophylline

STEP 2: REGULAR PREVENTER THERAPY
Add inhaled steroid 200-800 mcg/day*
400 mcg is an appropriate starting dose for many patients
Start at dose of inhaled steroid appropriate to severity of disease.

STEP 1: MILD INTERMITTENT ASTHMA
Inhaled short-acting β2 agonist as required

* BDP or equivalent

Fig 15.11 Summary of stepwise management of chronic asthma in adults. Reproduced with the kind permission of BTS/SIGN Asthma Executive Committee.

Chronic obstructive pulmonary disease (COPD) is a disorder characterized by airflow obstruction, which is usually progressive, not fully reversible, and does not change markedly over several months.

Aetiology

The predominant risk factor for COPD is cigarette smoking. Other factors include air pollution, occupational exposure to dusts and atmospheric pollution, and rarely, alpha-1-antitrypsin deficiency.

Acute exacerbations are usually caused by viral or bacterial infection.

Pathophysiology

All smokers develop a degree of airway inflammation. Around 10–20% will develop an abnormal immune-mediated inflammatory response to the chronic noxious stimuli resulting in COPD. Processes include:

- mucus hypersecretion and ciliary dysfunction (bronchitis)
- airway alveoli destruction (emphysema) resulting in pulmonary hypertension, and increased workload for the right heart. Cor pulmonale is the term used to describe right heart failure secondary to lung disease and is often seen in end-stage COPD
- Inflammation and fibrosis of the small airways (bronchiolitis)

Clinical assessment

COPD results in a variety of clinical presentations. Patients with mild disease often go undiagnosed owing to their vague symptoms and signs.

History

- Dyspnoea, chest tightness, wheeze, productive cough
- Frequent chest infections, mainly in the winter
- Smoking history: number of pack years = (number of cigarettes per day x number of smoking years)/20
- Occupational and environmental exposure
- Medical co-morbidities

Examination

Patients are sometimes described as 'blue bloaters' (chronic bronchitis predominates) or 'pink puffers' (emphysema predominates). In reality, there is usually a mixed picture and this terminology is not used by respiratory physicians.

- 'Blue bloater'—poor respiratory effort, overweight, oedematous, cyanosed with CO_2 retention
- 'Pink puffer'—thin, tachypnoeic, and hypoxic; hypercapnia occurs late
- Wheeze or crepitations on auscultation
- Cor pulmonale is right heart failure owing to chronic lung disease. Features include raised jugular venous pressure, hepatomegaly and peripheral oedema, loud P_2 heart sound, and tricuspid regurgitation

Investigations

- Spirometry is the key and should be performed in all patients with suspected COPD. Airway obstruction is diagnosed if FEV_1 <80% of predicted and FEV_1/FVC ratio <0.7%
- PEFR in COPD can underestimate the degree of airway obstruction and are not used for monitoring

- Sputum culture for MC+S in patients with productive cough with a possible chest infection
- Plain chest radiograph excludes other conditions
- Bloods—FBC (exclude anaemia and polycythaemia secondary to chronic hypoxia)
- ECG and cardiac echo are used to assess cor pulmonale

Management

Smoking cessation and bronchodilators are integral to managing the disease.

Acute exacerbation

- Supplemental oxygen to maintain SaO_2 >90%. Give patients with type II respiratory failure a Venturi mask delivering a fixed FiO_2 (24–28%). Monitor the response with serial ABGs
- Short-acting inhaled bronchodilators: beta-2-agonists and/or anticholinergics
- Short course corticosteroids unless contraindicated
- Antibiotics used in severe exacerbations with purulent sputum; prophylactic use is not recommended
- Physiotherapy prevents atelectasis and sputum retention
- Non-invasive ventilation (e.g. BIPAP) is used in acute exacerbations with persistent hypercapnic ventilatory failure not responding to medical therapy

Chronic management

- Lifestyle advice—stop smoking, weight loss
- Pulmonary rehabilitation programmes with supervision of an intensive breathing exercise regime improves outcomes
- Pneumococcal and influenza vaccinations
- Initial therapy is combined short-acting inhaled bronchodilators as required (e.g. beta-2-agonists and anticholinergics)
- Regular long-acting inhaled bronchodilators replace short-acting drugs if the patient remains symptomatic
- Inhaled corticosteroids are added to the above therapy if FEV_1 ≤50% predicted and ≥two exacerbations per year
- Long-term oxygen therapy and ambulatory oxygen therapy if PaO_2 <7.3 kPa with exercise desaturation

Operative

Patients are usually high risk for surgery. It is reserved for motivated patients with marked restrictions on lifestyle despite maximal medical therapy.

- Bullectomy is indicated for a single large bulla on CT scan, and an FEV_1 <50% predicted
- Lung volume reduction surgery removes segments of emphysematous lung with inefficient gas exchange
- Lung transplantation considered in young patients with advanced disease and a life expectancy of <2 years

Complications and prognosis

COPD is a progressive disease leading to severe breathlessness, causing physical and social limitations. It is the fourth leading cause of death in the UK.

⚠ COPD

Patients with COPD are at high risk of postoperative respiratory complications.

Preoperative

- Assess exercise tolerance
- Optimize medical therapy
- Surgery should not be performed if there is ongoing acute infection and a period of pulmonary rehabilitation prior to surgery is recommended
- Patients should have their inhaled medications changed to nebulized therapy preoperatively and this can continue for a few days postoperatively
- HDU or ITU care may be needed postoperatively

Postoperative

- Mobilize early if possible
- Physiotherapy is important to prevent atelectasis and reduce sputum retention
- Good analgesia is essential to enable deep breathing and coughing postoperatively
- Regular bronchodilator therapy
- Identify and treat chest infections early

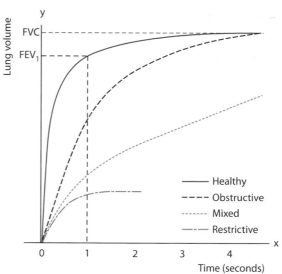

Fig 15.12 Spirometry curves. FVC and FEV_1 are shown for healthy lungs as an example.

- Obstructive conditions have a prolonged expiration of a normal volume. FEV_1 reduced, FVC normal, FEV_1/FVC ratio reduced
- Restrictive conditions have a rapid expiration of a reduced volume. FEV_1 and FVC reduced, FEV_1:FVC ratio normal or increased

Table 15.12 COPD versus asthma

	COPD	Asthma
History of smoking	Nearly all	Possible
Symptoms <35 years	Rare	Common
Cough	Persistent and productive	Intermittent and non-productive
Breathlessness	Persistent and progressive	Intermittent and variable
Night-time waking with breathlessness and/or wheeze	Uncommon	Common
Significant diurnal or day-to-day variability of symptoms	Uncommon	Common

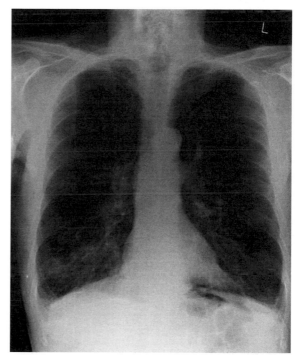

Fig 15.13 Plain PA chest radiograph showing features of COPD, including hyperexpanded lung fields and a flattened diaphragm.

Acute respiratory failure occurs when either the oxygenation or elimination of carbon dioxide no longer meets the metabolic demands of the body. It develops over a period of minutes to hours and can be classified into two types.

Aetiology

- Type I—hypoxic respiratory failure is defined by a low PaO_2 <8 kPa with a normal or low $PaCO_2$. It is caused by most acute lung conditions that reduce gas transfer, e.g. pulmonary oedema, pneumonia, COPD
- Type II—hypercapnic respiratory failure is defined by a high $PaCO_2$ and may be accompanied by low PaO_2. It is caused by impaired ventilation (e.g. neuromuscular failure) and obstructive airway disorders such as asthma and COPD

Pathophysiology

- Ventilation–perfusion mismatch is the most common cause of hypoxic respiratory failure. In normal lungs there is a small mismatch; as a consequence alveolar PO_2 is slightly higher than arterial PO_2. Pathological exaggeration of this leads to respiratory failure.
  Normally ventilated alveoli with poor perfusion act like dead space; conversely, normally perfused but underventilated alveoli act like a shunt
- Ventilatory failure (hypoventilation) results in the retention of carbon dioxide. This usually occurs if a patient's ventilatory capacity is reduced (i.e. muscle fatigue) or exceeded by an increase in demand (retention in COPD)
- Shunting is rare. Venous blood passes from the right side of the heart to the left, avoiding oxygenation. (e.g. congenital heart disease)

Clinical assessment

Clinical assessment and management often run concurrently and should follow the ABC protocol.

History

- Dyspnoea, cough, haemoptysis
- Past medical history (e.g. asthma, COPD, CCF, IHD, neoplasia)

Examination

- Airway
- Breathing—dyspnoea, tachypnoea, accessory muscle use, central cyanosis, lung pathology (oedema, consolidation, asthma/COPD)
- Circulation—tachycardia, fluid overload
- General systems examination—cyanosis

Investigations

- ECG if cardiac cause suspected
- Plain chest radiograph aids diagnosis of underlying cause
- Bloods—FBC (anaemia, polycythaemia), U+Es, LFT
- Arterial blood gas
- Microbiological screening as required

Management of acute respiratory failure

General

- Airway management
- Correct hypoxia—the initial therapy for respiratory failure is the provision of supplemental oxygen. A non-rebreather face mask with reservoir delivers ~80% oxygen concentration at flows of 10–15 L/min. Venturi masks deliver set oxygen concentrations of 24–60%

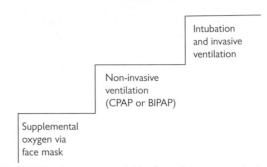

Fig 15.14 Respiratory support ladder. General aims are to maintain PaO_2 >10 kPa, $PaCO_2$ <8 kPa, and respiratory rate 8–25 per min.

- Respiratory support (see below) may be indicated to improve oxygenation and reduce hypercapnia
- Correct fluid overload and pulmonary oedema
- Reverse any bronchoconstriction
- Regular physiotherapy and analgesia
- Secretion clearance with coughing, physiotherapy, and saline nebulizers
- Treat infection and drain any pleural effusions

Indications for intubation

- Airway protection, e.g. in patient with reduced level of consciousness
- Suction of secretions
- To enable sedation and paralysis if indicated
- To overcome upper airway obstruction
- To allow mechanical ventilation

Indications for invasive mechanical ventilation

- Hypoxia
- Hypercarbia
- Respiratory rate >35 per min and exhaustion
- Tidal volume <5 mL/kg or vital capacity <10–15 mL/kg
- Keep under regular review and consider if tiring even with a normal ABG

Respiratory support

Almost all forms of ventilatory support use positive pressure. Negative pressure ventilation in which the patient is enclosed in an airtight tank ('iron lung') is rarely used.

Overview

There are many approaches to understanding ventilatory support. One approach is to consider the:
1. patient's ventilatory effort
2. interface between patient and ventilator, which can be non-invasive via a nasal mask or face mask, or invasive via endotracheal intubation or tracheostomy
3. ventilator modes and the aims of respiratory support

Non-invasive positive pressure ventilation (NIPPV)

For NIPPV the patient must be alert, cooperative, and initiating their own breaths. A NG tube should be placed at the same time. Two commonly used modes are:
- continuous positive airway pressure (CPAP) delivers a constant pressure throughout the respiratory cycle. It helps to keep the alveoli open and so **improves oxygenation.**

It also reduces the work of breathing and the heart and can be useful in pulmonary oedema. It does not improve ventilation (CO_2 excretion)

- bilevel positive airway pressure (BIPAP) allows different inspiratory and expiratory pressures to be set. It **improves ventilation** and so improves both oxygenation and CO_2 excretion

Invasive positive pressure ventilation

In its most basic form mechanical ventilation delivers an intermittent positive pressure 'breath' relying on the natural recoil of the lungs and chest wall for expiration.

Ventilators have many different modes and parameters that can be adjusted (e.g. tidal volume, respiratory rate, inspiratory and expiratory ratio (I:E), and pressure (peak, plateau, and end expiratory pressure).

Ventilatory modes

- Volume-controlled ventilation delivers a set tidal volume and respiratory rate. Pressure-controlled ventilation delivers a set inspiratory pressure and respiratory rate. The tidal volume will vary according to the patient's respiratory compliance. These modes are used in heavily sedated or paralysed patients
- Intermittent mandatory ventilation (IMV) delivers controlled breaths at a certain respiratory rate, tidal volume, and pressure. It is often synchronized with the patient's respiratory effort (SIMV)
- Pressure support ventilation (PSV) or assisted spontaneous breathing (ASB) is initiated by the patient's breathing, and delivers a preset level of positive pressure to support each breath. It is a useful way of weaning a spontaneously breathing patient from ventilatory support

Positive end expiratory pressure (PEEP)

This is used as an adjunct to the various ventilatory modes. It improves functional residual capacity by countering the passive closure of alveolar in expiration and stopping them from collapsing. PEEP is functionally the same as continuous positive airway pressure (CPAP).

Complications and prognosis

Pulmonary complications include pneumonia and acute lung injury. Mechanical ventilation can cause oxygen toxicity, barotrauma, and ventilator-induced lung injury.

Cardiovascular complications include hypotension and haemodynamic instability.

There is significant morbidity and mortality associated with respiratory failure. The mortality rate from ARDS is 40%.

Acute lung injury

Acute lung injury (ALI) and acute respiratory distress syndrome (ARDS) are severe inflammatory disorders of the lung. They are defined by:

- acute respiratory failure
- hypoxaemia (**ALI**-PaO_2/FiO_2 ratio $\leq$300 mmHg; **ARDS**-PaO_2/FiO_2 $\leq$200 mmHg)
- Diffuse bilateral infiltrates on chest radiograph
- No evidence of left atrial hypertension as a cause for pulmonary oedema (pulmonary artery occulsion pressure (PAOP) $\leq$18 mmHg)

Aetiology

Pneumonia and sepsis account for 60% of cases. Causes are either direct (e.g. pneumonia, aspiration pneumonitis, fat embolism, inhalation injury) or indirect (multiple trauma, burns, pancreatitis, drugs, massive blood transfusion).

Pathophysiology

Three stages are described: inflammatory, proliferative, and progressive interstitial fibrosis. This pathological process results in increased secretions and oedema, atelectasis, increased pulmonary vascular resistance, decreased compliance, and increased work of breathing.

Clinical assessment

The condition develops within 24–48 h of injury. Patients become breathless, tachypnoeic, tachycardic, and develop respiratory failure. The diagnosis is confirmed by ABG and chest radiograph.

Management

General

- Treat underlying cause (e.g. pneumonia)
- Treat associated organ failure (e.g. acute renal failure)
- Careful fluid balance to reduce pulmonary oedema whilst maintaining preload
- Prophylaxis for thromboembolism and stress ulceration
- Maintain adequate nutrition, enteral route preferable

Respiratory support

Most patients need endotracheal intubation and mechanical ventilation.

- Lowest FiO_2 to achieve adequate tissue oxygenation
- Low tidal volumes with permissive hypercapnia
- Avoid volume or barotrauma. Limit peak airway pressure and plateau pressure (preferably 30 cmH_2O max.)
- Optimize PEEP to ensure patient on most efficient part of pressure–volume curve (maximal PEEP ~15 cmH_2O)
- Consider inverse ratio ventilation, prone positioning, and inhaled nitric oxide

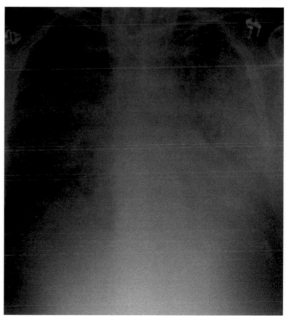

Fig 15.15 Plain AP erect chest radiograph showing acute respiratory distress syndrome. There is widespread bilateral airspace shadowing.

The term IHD is synonymous with coronary artery disease (CAD) and encompasses a range of presentations, from angina pectoris through to acute myocardial infarction (MI). The arterial blood supply of the myocardium is compromised, leading to ischaemia or infarction.

Aetiology

Atherosclerosis (📖 Topic 7.2) is the principal cause of CAD. Coronary artery vasospasm is rare and is occasionally seen following cocaine use.

The metabolic syndrome is an independent risk factor for IHD. It is diagnosed by the presence of three or more of the following five features: enlarged waistline, low HDL-cholesterol, hypertension, increased plasma triglycerides, and fasting plasma glucose of 5.6 mmol/L or more.

Cardiovascular risk

Where possible, all adults over 40 years old with no history of cardiovascular disease (CVD) or diabetes should have their cardiovascular risk assessed in primary care using the Joint British Societies' CVD risk prediction charts. They estimate the risk of CVD (CAD and stroke) over the following 10 years. A total risk of over 20% over 10 years is defined as high risk.

The five key risk factors assessed are:

1. age
2. sex
3. smoking habit
4. systolic blood pressure
5. ratio of total cholesterol to HDL cholesterol

Other identified risk factors for IHD include:

- impaired glucose intolerance, diabetes mellitus
- family history of IHD
- left ventricular hypertrophy irrespective of hypertension
- abdominal obesity
- renal impairment or failure
- environmental stress

Pathophysiology

Atherosclerosis (📖 Topic 7.2) is the underlying pathophysiological mechanism in IHD. The disease leads to narrowing of the coronary arteries and limitation of flow. Plaque erosion or rupture causes acute thrombosis, resulting in worsening myocardial ischaemia or infarction and an acute clinical presentation.

Clinical assessment

Angina pectoris

Angina pectoris refers to chest pain caused by reduced coronary blood flow. Typically it develops during periods of increased myocardial demand, such as on exertion. Progressive narrowing may lead to symptoms at rest, referred to as unstable angina. Beware of atypical presentations of cardiac chest pain (e.g. upper abdominal pain).

Acute coronary syndromes and myocardial infarction

The acute presentation of cardiac chest pain lasting >20 min not relieved by or occurring at rest is referred to as acute coronary syndrome (ACS). The presence or absence of MI is established later based on a troponin test.

ACS is classified as either ST segment elevation (suggesting transmural ischaemia) or non-ST segment elevation (normal or depressed ST segments or T wave inversion). It incorporates unstable angina and MI.

The classic features of acute myocardial ischaemia are below. There is often little to find on examination.

- Crushing substernal chest pain which may radiate to the neck, jaw or arms
- Nausea and vomiting
- Dyspnoea, pallor, and sweating
- Heart failure and acute ischaemic valvular dysfunction (e.g. mitral regurgitation)

Investigations

- 12-lead ECG is the first line investigation. It classifies the ACS and guides management. A normal ECG does not exclude ACS but makes it unlikely
- Elevated cardiac enzymes (troponin I or T) are markers of MI. Check 8–12 h after onset of symptoms to allow for a rise to occur
- Bloods—FBC, U+Es, fasting lipid profile, and glucose
- Plain chest radiograph—pulmonary oedema if left ventricular dysfunction present

Management

Acute coronary syndrome

- Aspirin 300 mg po
- Oxygen
- Nitroglycerine as sublingual glyceryl trinitrate spray or tablet
- Morphine and antiemetic
- Anticoagulation—therapeutic LMWH
- Beta-blocker (contraindications—bradycardia, LVF, inferior MI)
- ACE inhibitor should be considered

ST elevation MI

Patients with ST elevation MI need revascularization. This is achieved with either thrombolytic drugs or percutaneous intervention.

Non-ST elevation MI

- Antiplatelet agents—combined aspirin +/- clopidogrel
- Coronary angiography +/- intervention

Secondary prevention

Secondary prevention is crucial in reducing mortality rates following MI. This includes lifestyle changes, cardiac rehabilitation, and drug therapy.

Lifestyle advice

- Regular physical exercise to improve exercise capacity (20–30 min a day to point of slight breathlessness)
- Quit smoking
- Mediterranean-style diet (increase bread, fruit, vegetables, and fish) and increase intake of omega-3 fatty acids
- Moderate alcohol intake
- Maintain healthy weight (BMI 20–25)

Drug therapy

All non-ST elevation. Most patients should be started on an ACE inhibitor, aspirin, beta-blocker, and statin. Clopidogrel is recommended in addition to aspirin in non-ST elevation MI for a year.

Complications and prognosis

The main complication of IHD is MI and death. Acute MI can cause cardiogenic shock, arrhythmias, and ventricular rupture.

⚠ Cardiac risk in non-cardiac surgery

The current recommendations for the preoperative cardiac risk stratification of patients are based on three elements.

1. Clinical cardiac risk factors are established for each individual. The Revised Cardiac Risk Index (Lee et al) is based on six factors (Fig 15.16)
2. Identification of surgical risk includes both the type of surgery and the haemodynamic stress involved
3. Functional capacity or exercise tolerance can be quantified by the graded metabolic equivalents (MET) scale as defined by the Duke Activity Status Index (Table 15.8). Patients that can achieve activities of ≥4 MET represent a low perioperative risk

Non-invasive cardiac imaging

- Dobutamine stress echocardiography is as good as radio-nuclide stress testing at identifying ischaemic myocardium and regional wall motion abnormalities. It can also be used to identify those patients who may benefit from angiography and percutaneous intervention
- Resting echocardiography has the same indications as for non-surgical patients, i.e. to evaluate left ventricular function and valvulopathies

Non-invasive cardiac stress testing

- Exercise treadmill testing is a positive predictor of risk in intermediate and high risk patients
- Ambulatory ECG (Holter monitoring) may demonstrate silent myocardial ischaemia or episodes of arrhythmia but is not very sensitive or specific

Percutaneous coronary intervention

- Coronary angiography is the criterion standard for assessing CAD. In non-cardiac surgery patients it is indicated in those undergoing intermediate or high risk surgery with equivocal non-invasive results, those with unstable symptoms, and those who meet the usual elective criteria (e.g. left main stem disease or proximal three-vessel disease with left ventricular impairment)

Perioperative management of antiplatelet agents

The continued use of antiplatelet agents has to balance the risk of bleeding against the risk of thrombosis. The bleeding risk is particularly important in neurosurgery, ophthalmology, and some urological surgery (e.g. TURP).

Following percutaneous coronary stenting with a bare metal stent, antiplatelet therapy should be continued for 2 months and for 12 months following a drug-eluting stent. It is imperative that antiplatelet agents are not stopped without prior cardiological consultation, as the risk of in-stent stenosis may be very high, with devastating morbidity and mortality rates. Elective surgery should be delayed but more urgent surgery should be discussed with a cardiologist.

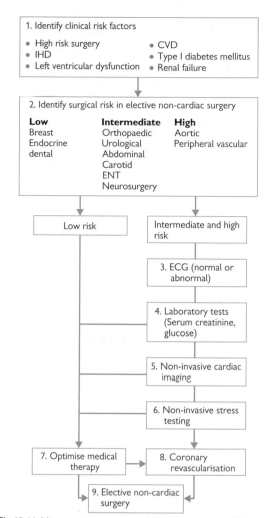

Fig 15.16 Nine steps to assessing and optimizing cardiac risk in non-cardiac surgery (Reproduced with permission from Schouten *et al.* *Heart* 2006; 92: 1866–72).

15.14 Heart failure

Heart failure (HF) is a result of structural or functional impairment of the heart, making it unable to produce a cardiac output that meets the metabolic demands of the body. It is the endpoint of all cardiac disease.

Aetiology

In developed countries, IHD and hypertension are the main causes.

- Cardiac dysfunction—myocardial ischaemia or infarction, hypertension, and cardiomyopathy (dilated, restrictive or obstructive)
- Valvular (atrial and mitral) and congenital heart disease (atrial and ventricular septal defects)
- Arrhythmias, e.g. atrial fibrillation
- Alcohol and drugs, e.g. beta-blockers, certain calcium channel blockers, and anti-arrhythmics
- 'High output' states—anaemia, thyrotoxicosis
- Pericardial disease—constrictive pericarditis, effusion
- Right heart failure—pulmonary hypertension, tricuspid and pulmonary valve dysfunction

Pathophysiology

In non-valvular heart disease the initial precipitating factor is left ventricular dysfunction and reduced cardiac output. The body responds by attempting to use normal physiological mechanisms to improve cardiac output. However, in the failing heart these processes lead to increased myocardial wall stress and oxygen demand, creating a vicious cycle of failure.

- Increased sympathetic stimulation leads to increased heart rate, increased contractility, peripheral vasoconstriction, and stimulation of the renin–angiotensin–aldosterone system (RAAS)
- RAAS is stimulated by both the sympathetic system and reduced renal perfusion; this leads to increased vasoconstriction (angiotensin II) and increased blood volume (sodium and water retention)
- Increased neurohumoral activity includes release of natriuretic peptides (atrial, brain, and C-type), cytokines, and endothelin. ANP and BNP lead to increased sodium and water excretion
- Neurohormonal activity in response to reduced cardiac contractility can lead to eccentric hypertrophy of normal myocardium, with associated thinning and dilatation of any infarcted regions (cardiac remodelling)

Clinical assessment

Right heart failure

- Fatigue, breathlessness, anorexia, and loss of lean body mass (i.e. excluding pulmonary oedema)
- Signs are prominent and include raised jugular venous pressure, hepatomegaly, ascites, and peripheral oedema

Left heart failure

- Dyspnoea and orthopnoea
- Paroxysmal nocturnal dyspnoea and nocturnal cough
- Fatigue and limited exercise tolerance
- Signs are often late but include a gallop rhythm (third heart sound and tachycardia), displaced sustained apex beat due to cardiomegay, mitral regurgitation, and basal crackles and wheeze on auscultation owing to pulmonary oedema

Biventricular failure (congestive cardiac failure)

This term is used to describe cases in which right heart failure is a result of left ventricular failure. The presentation has a combination of symptoms and signs already described.

Acute pulmonary oedema

- Acute breathlessness and tachypnoea
- Anxiety, tachycardia, and sweating
- Cardiogenic shock in severe cases

Investigations

- Serum natriuretic peptides (BNP) and 12-lead ECG (ischaemia, arrhythmias, left ventricular hypertrophy) may exclude HF if normal
- If either are abnormal, echocardiography is used to assess left ventricular systolic (ejection fraction) and diastolic function, and exclude valvular heart disease and intracardiac shunts
- Bloods—FBC, U+Es, LFT, TFT, fasting glucose, and lipid profile
- Plain chest radiograph—pulmonary oedema (Fig 15.17)

Management

Acute pulmonary oedema

- Sit up and give high flow oxygen via a mask with reservoir bag
- IV furosemide causes immediate vasodilatation and delayed diuresis. Monitor fluid balance
- IV morphine or diamorphine (with antiemetic) reduces anxiety and produces transient venodilatation
- Nitrates venodilate and reduce preload. Initially use sublingual GTN but a continuous infusion may be needed
- Advanced management includes inotropes, CPAP, and circulatory assist devices

Long-term management of chronic heart failure

- General advice to reduce salt and fluid intake, stop smoking, reduce alcohol, and increase exercise
- Refer to heart failure specialist nurse
- Beta-blockers are indicated in patients with symptomatic left ventricular dysfunction
- Most patients receive ACE inhibitors (or angiotensin-II receptor antagonists if not tolerated)
- Oral anticoagulation indicated in patients with AF
- Digoxin is considered in worsening or severe HF with sinus rhythm and those patients with atrial fibrillation
- Loop diuretics are used for symptom control to reduce fluid retention. They do not improve mortality rates
- Cardiac resynchronization therapy includes biventricular pacemaker. This improves coordinated contraction and increases cardiac output
- Invasive management includes coronary revascularization, valve repair/replacement, automatic implantable cardioverter-defibrillators, ventricular assist devices, and, rarely, cardiac transplantation.

Complications and prognosis

Complications include cardiac arrhythmias, thromboembolism, hepatic dysfunction, malabsorption, muscle wasting, and pulmonary congestion. The overall 5-year mortality rate for patients with HF is approximately 50%.

⚠ Heart failure

In all the major cardiac risk indices (📖 Topic 15.13), heart failure carries a high score as it is an important predictor of adverse events perioperatively. It is important to assess patients fully and optimize their cardiovascular status preoperatively.

- Full cardiac risk assessment
- Optimize medical therapy
- Ejection fraction >50% is usually sufficient for major surgery
- Ejection fraction <35% predicts adverse cardiac outcome. Consider postponing or modifying surgery and improving medical therapy. Discuss optimization with cardiologist
- Perioperative ICU care should be planned for any patient undergoing major surgery with a low ejection fraction.

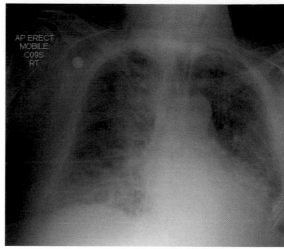

Fig 15.17 Plain AP erect chest radiograph showing pulmonary oedema as a result of left ventricular dysfunction. Features include upper lobe blood diversion, Kerley B lines, 'bat's wings' hila, and alveolar shadowing.

A cardiac arrhythmia is any cardiac rhythm other than sinus rhythm. They can be classified as either a bradycardia (HR <60 beats/min) or a tachycardia (HR >100 beats/min) and by the site from which they originate.

Aetiology

The causes of arrhythmias are many and varied. Cardiothoracic surgery has a much higher incidence of postoperative arrhythmias than non-cardiac surgery. The majority of arrhythmias are supraventricular, with atrial fibrillation (AF) being the most common. Causes include:

- sepsis
- myocardial ischaemia or infarction
- electrolyte disturbance (e.g. hyperkalaemia)
- pulmonary embolus
- cardiac conditions—valvular heart disease, congenital heart disease, cardiomyopathy
- drugs and alcohol

Pathophysiology

Arrhythmias arising following cardiac surgery are likely to be caused by direct irritation of the myocardium or pericardium. Following non-cardiac surgery this irritation is more likely to be caused by the stress response or inflammatory mediators related to the surgery and associated conditions.

Classification

Tachyarrhythmia

Supraventricular

SVTs can originate from the sinoatrial node, atrial tissue or the atrioventricular (AV) node (junctional).

- AF—rapid, disorganized impulses from the sinoatrial node are intermittently conducted by the atrioventricular node, resulting in an irregularly irregular pulse. The fibrillating atria lead to stasis, reduced cardiac output, and an increased risk of intracardiac thrombus formation. It is a tachycardia when associated with a fast ventricular response
- Atrial flutter is a re-entrant rhythm. The flutter rate varies, with only some being conducted by the AV node
- Junctional tachycardia is usually regular with narrow complexes

Ventricular

- Ventricular tachycardia (VT) and ventricular fibrillation (VF)
- Ventricular ectopic beats (extrasystoles, premature beats)

Bradyarrhythmia

Sinus node dysfunction

- Sick sinus syndrome—sinus bradycardia, sinoatrial block or sinus arrest but alternate with paroxysmal atrial fibrillation, flutter or re-entrant tachycardias

Atrioventricular disease

- First degree heart block is caused by delayed conduction through the AV node
- Second degree heart block is caused by failure of conduction of some of the atrial pulses. It is classified as Mobitz type 1 (Wenkebach), in which there is gradual prolongation of the PR interval before a beat is dropped, and Mobitz type 2, in which there is intermittent failure to conduction, usually in a set ratio, i.e. 2:1, 3:1
- Third degree (complete) heart block, in which there is complete dissociation between the atrial and ventricular rhythms

Clinical assessment

In non-cardiac surgery patients, haemodynamic compromise with arrhythmia is uncommon. However, the initial approach should always follow ALS guidelines. If the patient is not acutely unwell, a more detailed assessment includes the following.

History

- Ongoing chest pain, dyspnoea, palpitations
- Syncope, dizziness, and collapse
- Past medical history and pre-existing heart disease
- Drug history

Examination

- Cardiovascular—pulse rate, rhythm, volume, blood pressure
- Low cardiac output—pallor, sweating, cold, clammy, hypotensive, reduced GCS
- Excessive tachycardia >150 beats/min or bradycardia may not be tolerated if poor cardiac reserve
- Signs of acute heart failure (📖 Topic 15.14)
- Systems examination to identify underlying cause

Investigations

- 12-lead ECG identifies arrhythmia and ischaemia. Request continuous monitoring/telemetry
- Bloods—FBC (anaemia), U+Es (K$^+$, Mg^{2+}), TFT (altered thyroid status), LFT
- Arterial blood gas (quick approximation of Hb, electrolytes, acid–base balance and oxygenation)
- Plain chest radiograph—cardiomegaly, pulmonary oedema, infection
- Transthoracic echocardiography—LV dysfunction, valve lesions, evidence of old infarction

Management

Immediate

- Follow ALS guidelines—ABCDE
- Wide bore IV access and fluids if hypotensive
- Antiarrhythmic drugs, electrical cardioversion or cardiac pacing are further options in the immediate management of arrhythmias

Postoperative acute onset atrial fibrillation

This occurs in up to 10% of non-cardiac surgery patients and over 30% following cardiac surgery.

- Correct electrolyte disturbance (potassium and magnesium)
- Synchronized direct current cardioversion is the criterion standard in treating acute AF with or without life-threatening haemodynamic instability
- Control ventricular response with digoxin, calcium channel blockers, beta-blockers or amiodarone
- In patients with known AF with haemodynamic instability owing to poorly controlled ventricular rate (fast AF), urgent pharmacological rate control is indicated with either beta-blockers, rate-limiting calcium antagonists or amiodarone if these are contraindicated or ineffective

Complications and prognosis

The majority of new onset arrhythmias seen in non-cardiothoracic surgery patients revert to sinus rhythm before discharge.

However, there is still a high associated morbidity and mortality owing to the underlying conditions.

⚠ Arrhythmias

Patients with a history of arrhythmia or recent onset of one need a thorough cardiovascular assessment which may include a cardiology referral. All patients should have a 12-lead ECG as a minimum, although others may need further investigations.

Atrial arrhythmias

New onset AF needs to be referred to a cardiologist for consideration of electrical cardioversion. Chronic AF is classified as permanent, persistent or paroxysmal. The aims are rate and rhythm control (beta-blockers, digoxin), and anticoagulation should be considered. Digoxin should be continued during the perioperative period but warfarin is usually stopped and covered with alternative therapy.

Patients with a history of junctional tachycardia are usually controlled with AV node blocking agents or other anti-arrhythmic agents. AF with an accessory pathway is dangerous as it has potential to convert to VF. Symptomatic patients with an abnormal ECG should be referred for further investigations. Radiofrequency catheter ablation of the aberrant pathway is often considered as an alternative to chronic drug therapy.

Ventricular arrhythmias

Ventricular premature beats ('ventricular ectopics') are common and the incidence increases with age. They are usually benign although they may signal an underlying structural heart abnormality. Echocardiography is recommended.

Bradycardia

Patients with a history of syncope related to possible bradycardia need 24 h ECG monitoring (Holter monitoring).

Patients with heart block are at risk of cardiac standstill when under GA. First degree heart block is usually benign. Second and third degree heart block are usually treated with a pacemaker (see below). In an emergency situation new onset heart block may need a temporary pacing wire. Bundle branch blocks do not normally need pacing.

Pacemakers

Patients with a pacemaker should have a cardiology review to ensure it is working correctly.

During surgery it is preferable to use bipolar diathermy. If monopolar diathermy is used, the indifferent pole (plate) should be placed so that the current does not flow through the chest and diathermy use should be limited to short bursts.

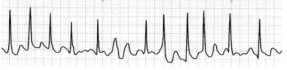

Fig 15.18 Atrial fibrillation. There is an irregular rhythm with a rate of 100–160 bpm. The QRS complexes are normal but there is an absence of P waves; these are replaced with an undulating baseline caused by disorganized atrial activity.

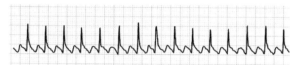

Fig 15.19 Atrial flutter showing a regular rhythm with a ventricular rate of 150 bpm and regular flutter P waves (sawtooth baseline) at a rate of 300 bpm. The QRS complexes are normal. The AV node has a 2:1 block.

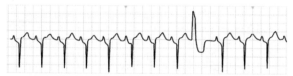

Fig 15.20 Ventricular premature beat with underlying sinus rhythm at a rate of 70 bpm.

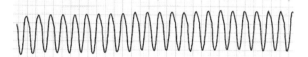

Fig 15.21 Ventricular tachycardia with a regular rhythm, QRS rate 110–250 bpm, widened QRS morphology (>0.12 s). Beware of SVT with abnormal conduction (i.e. LBBB or RBBB) as it will resemble VT.

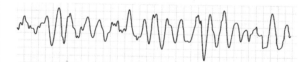

Fig 15.22 Ventricular fibrillation with a grossly irregular rhythm and undulating baseline with no definable QRS complexes.

Hypertension is a major risk factor for cardiovascular disease. It is defined as a persistent blood pressure above 140/90 mmHg on two separate occasions (130/80 mmHg in patients with diabetes). Isolated systolic hypertension is a systolic BP ≥140 mmHg but with a diastolic BP <90 mmHg. The incidence of hypertension in the population older than 35 years is approximately 35% and this increases with age.

Aetiology
Over 90% of hypertension is primary (essential). Secondary hypertension may be caused by:

- renovascular disease—renal artery stenosis, diabetic nephropathy, infection, reflux, connective tissue disorders, obstructive nephropathy
- drugs—corticosteroids, sympathomimetics, OCP
- adrenal disease—phaeochromocytoma, Cushing's disease, Conn's syndrome, congenital adrenal hyperplasia
- other—pre-eclampsia in pregnancy, aortic coarctation

Risk factors for primary hypertension
- Smoking
- Family history
- Diet—high in salt, saturated fat, alcohol, and caffeine
- Obesity and reduced physical activity
- Environmental stress (e.g. surgical career!)

Pathophysiology
Increased peripheral vascular resistance is the primary haemodynamic fault with vascular hypertrophy, resulting in the perpetuation of hypertension. The pathological hallmark of uncontrolled hypertension is accelerated atherosclerosis. If untreated, 50% die of coronary artery disease or congestive failure, 33% of stroke, and 10–15% of renal failure.

Clinical assessment
History
A history suggestive of secondary hypertension should be excluded. Hypertension *per se* is usually asymptomatic, unless malignant. Clinical features are due to end-organ damage. All patients should have estimation of their 10-year risk of cardiovascular disease.

Examination
Markers of end organ damage include:

- renal impairment, e.g. oedema, pigmentation of skin, pruritus, anaemia
- left ventricular hypertrophy, causing left ventricular heave and displaced apex beat
- hypertensive retinopathy—grade 1, narrowing and/or thickening of the arteriolar wall; grade 2, arteriovenous nicking; grade 3, haemorrhage and exudates; grade 4, papilloedema
- cerebral—carotid bruits, altered mini-mental test score (MMTS) (multi-infarct dementia)

Investigations
Further assessment is targeted at assessing cardiovascular risk, secondary causes, and complications.

- Urinalysis—look for protein and blood
- Bloods—U+Es, fasting blood glucose, and lipid profile
- ECG—LVH, ischaemia, arrhythmias

Management
Acute hypertension
Acute hypertension in the postoperative surgical patient is often a stress response to pain or because of omission of their usual antihypertensives. A full clinical assessment should be performed and any obvious underlying causes corrected. Persistent systolic BP >200 mmHg needs treating.

- Exclude underlying cause
- Check drug chart
- Evidence of acute complications is an indication for urgent reduction in BP, otherwise oral therapy can be started

Hypertension in primary care
Patients with primary hypertension need secondary prevention (lifestyle and drugs). Those with secondary hypertension need specialist referral for further investigation and management.

Lifestyle modification
All patients with high normal or borderline hypertension should be offered lifestyle advice.

- Maintain normal BMI
- Increase exercise (30 min moderate activity per day)
- Improve diet (reduced salt, caffeine, and alcohol intake)
- Smoking cessation

Drug therapy
Initiate antihypertensive drug therapy if blood pressure remains high despite lifestyle modification (systolic BP ≥160 mmHg or sustained diastolic BP ≥100 mmHg). Therapy may be initiated at lower blood pressures in diabetic patients and those with evidence of cardiovascular or other target organ damage.

- Target blood pressure is systolic BP <140 mmHg and diastolic BP <85 mmHg
- Target blood pressure in patients with diabetes mellitus is systolic BP <130 mmHg and diastolic BP <80 mmHg
- Aspirin and statin therapy should be considered

Complications and prognosis
- Cardiac—diastolic then systolic left ventricular dysfunction, left ventricular hypertrophy (LVH), heart failure, coronary artery disease
- Extracardiac vascular disease—aneurysmal disease, PAOD
- Renal—microalbuminuria, nephrosclerosis, renal insufficiency, chronic renal failure
- Cerebral—multi-infarct dementia, brain atrophy, ischaemic stroke, intracerebral haemorrhage
- Ophthalmic—hypertensive retinopathy

⚠ Hypertension

Preoperative care

Patients with uncontrolled grade 3 hypertension (isolated SBP (iSBP) ≥180 mmHg and diastolic BP ≥110 mmHg) have been shown to be at increased risk of perioperative cardio-vascular events and should have their blood pressure better controlled before elective surgery.

At lower levels of hypertension, no increased risk has been consistently shown in the absence of end-organ damage. Patients should continue their usual antihypertensive medications during the perioperative period unless they become hypotensive.

Hypertensive crisis

Less than 1% of patients with primary hypertension progress to the accelerated malignant phase. Clinically, diastolic BP is usually ≥140 mmHg, and the signs and symptoms include headache, confusion, seizures, coma, dyspnoea (from congestive cardiac failure), visual loss, nausea, and vomiting.

Immediate aggressive therapy to lower blood pressure is indicated. If there are signs of encephalopathy, then pressures should be lowered using intravenous agents. Speak to the cardiologist on call.

Diabetes mellitus (DM) is a chronic disease of abnormal metabolism caused by reduced circulating insulin or resistance to insulin. There are two main types.

- Type 1 DM (~10%) is caused by pancreatic beta-cell destruction and usually results in absolute insulin deficiency. It is more common in men and has a peak onset at ~12 years
- Type 2 DM (~90%) is caused by beta-cell dysfunction leading to relative insulin deficiency as well as insulin resistance, and increased glucagon levels leading to accelerated hepatic glucose production. It is also more common in men and has a peak incidence over 40 years although it is increasingly seen in a younger population

Glucose metabolism

Insulin is an anabolic hormone responsible for glucose homeostasis and the balanced release of other catabolic hormones. Insulin deficiency, relative or absolute, is the fundamental problem in diabetes mellitus. It results in unopposed catabolism and hyperglycaemia.

Aetiology and pathophysiology

Type 1

Type 1 DM is thought to be caused by infectious or environmental agents triggering a cell-mediated autoimmune attack against pancreatic beta cells. Genetic susceptibility is likely to play a role and there is an increased incidence in patients with other autoimmune diseases. Patients need replacement insulin to sustain life.

Type 2

Type 2 DM is characterized by hyperglycaemia caused by both insulin resistance and inadequate insulin production. There appears to be a strong genetic component which probably interacts with a diabetogenic lifestyle to cause DM.

Metabolic syndrome is primarily caused by insulin resistance but also includes hyperinsulinaemia, hypertension, dyslipidaemia, and obesity.

Clinical assessment

Type 1

Initial presentation is often of symptoms and signs of hyperglycaemia such as polyuria, polydipsia, tiredness, weight loss, and blurred vision. A very acute presentation may be with diabetic ketoacidosis (see box).

Type 2

Patients with type 2 diabetes are often asymptomatic for years. They present with a more insidious onset of symptoms or with complications of related conditions. They are not prone to ketosis but may develop hyperosmotic non-ketotic acidosis.

Investigations

- Diagnosis is based on a fasting plasma glucose >7.0 mmol/L or abnormal glucose tolerance test with serum glucose >11.1 mmol/L 2 h after ingestion of 75 g of glucose. At least two abnormal blood tests on separate occasions are required to make the diagnosis
- Glycosylated haemoglobin (HbA1c) is not used for diagnosis but is the criterion standard for long-term monitoring of glycaemic control (normal level: 3.8–6.4%)
- Other bloods—FBC, U+Es (estimate GFR), fasting lipid profile

- Urinalysis—ketones, protein, glucose. Microalbinuria is a good indicator of renal damage and future renal failure
- ECG—ischaemia, cardiomyopathy

Management

The general aims are to reduce diabetic-related symptoms and reduce the risk of future complications.

General risk reduction

- Lifestyle changes—dietary advice, exercise, weight loss, and reduced alcohol intake
- Microvascular complications are very closely linked to control of blood glucose and blood pressure. Long-term glycaemic target is HbA1c <7%
- Macrovascular complications—control of lipids and blood pressure, smoking cessation, and antiplatelet therapy
- Specialist follow-up and complications monitoring (eye examination, urinalysis, and foot examination)

Type 1

- Subcutaneous human insulin injections are the mainstay of therapy. Different regimens use short-, intermediate-, and long-acting insulin
- A common regimen is to divide the total insulin dose into four, with an injection of short-acting insulin before each meal and long-acting insulin at bedtime
- Regular self-monitoring of blood glucose enables tighter control
- Composition, size, timing, and frequency of meals is important in planning the insulin regimen to reduce preprandial hypoglycaemia and postprandial hyperglycaemia

Type 2

Initially, patients may have high circulating insulin in response to peripheral resistance. Eventually they may become insulopaenic and need insulin therapy.

- Diet control (low fat, high fibre)
- Drug therapy usually starts with one agent such as metformin or a sulphonylurea. If this fails, further agents can be added in. Broad classes of drugs include:
  —sulphonylureas (e.g. glibenclamide, glipazide) stimulate remaining beta cells but cause weight gain
  —biguanides (e.g. metformin) increase glucose uptake and reduce production in the liver
  —glitazones (e.g. rosiglitazone) reduce peripheral insulin resistance

Complications and prognosis

Acute complications include hypoglycaemia and hyperglycaemia (diabetic ketoacidosis and hyperosmolar non-ketotic state).

Chronic complications increase with the duration of the condition and poor glycaemic control. Genetic predisposition and lifestyle also play a role. They include macroangiopathy caused by atherosclerosis (ischaemic heart disease, PAOD, stroke), microangiopathy (nephropathy, neuropathy, retinopathy), infection, cardiac dysfunction (cardiomyopathy and arrhythmias), gastric paresis, and necrobiosis lipoidica.

Patient education is important to enable patients to recognize complications and understand the benefits of long-term management.

⚠ Diabetes mellitus

It is estimated that over 10% of the hospital population suffers from DM. Patients with diabetes undergoing surgery have increased morbidity and mortality rates.

Intercurrent illness and surgery both lead to a stress response, with an increased release of catecholamines, glucagon, and cortisol. In non-diabetic patients, glucose homeostasis is maintained by a rise in insulin but this compensation is impaired or lost in diabetics.

The key aim in the perioperative period is to maintain tight glycaemic control (4–8 mmol/L).

Preoperative

Many patients, especially those with type 2 DM, are undiagnosed. Therefore all patients should be screened for symptoms and signs of DM and undergo routine screening with urinalysis or blood tests if they are at high risk.

Known diabetic patients need a full evaluation of their glycaemic control and to prepare their perioperative management. Try to place diabetic patients at the start of the operating list

Diet- or oral hypoglycaemic-controlled diabetic

Minor and intermediate surgery
Omit morning dose of oral hypoglycaemic agent, and monitor blood glucose 2-hourly.

Restart oral medication postoperatively once stable and eating and drinking normally (usually first meal).

Major surgery
Omit oral hypoglycaemic medication and start an intravenous insulin sliding scale and dextrose infusion before surgery. Carry out BM 2-hourly and adjust insulin infusion rate accordingly. Monitor serum potassium and replace as necessary.

Restart oral medication postoperatively once stable and eating and drinking normally.

Insulin-controlled diabetic

Minor and intermediate surgery
Monitor BM 2-hourly and if BG <7 mmol/L omit normal insulin dose; if ≥7 mmol/L give half normal insulin dose. Restart normal insulin dose postoperatively once stable and eating and drinking normally (usually first meal).

Major surgery
If the patient is taking long-acting insulin it may be safer to change to a short- or intermediate-acting form perioperatively.

Start an IV insulin sliding scale and 5% dextrose infusion with potassium before surgery. Monitor blood glucose 2-hourly.

Restart insulin regimen postoperatively once stable and eating and drinking with BMG 4-hourly.

Insulin sliding scale

- Prescribe 50 units Actrapid in 50 mL 0.9% saline IV to follow sliding scale
- Prescribe 1000 mL 5% dextrose to run with the sliding scale
- Follow local guidelines. Example of sliding scale is below:

BM (mmol/L)	Rate (mL/h)
<4	Stop infusion. Call doctor
4–7	1
7.1–11	2
11.1–20	4
>20	7 Call doctor

⊙ Hypoglycaemia

Hypoglycaemia (blood glucose <3.5 mmol/L) is a complication of diabetic treatment and can result from inadequate caloric intake, insulin overdose or oral hypoglycaemic overdose (sulphonylureas), or excessive exercise.

Hypoglycaemia should always be excluded in any patient with reduced conscious level or abnormal neurology.

Clinical assessment

- Early symptoms include hunger, sweating, and trembling. Signs include pallor, altered GCS, and, eventually, coma and fitting
- Diagnosis is suspected if bedside monitoring of blood glucose (BMG) is <3.9 mmol/L. A venous blood sample should be sent for confirmation but should not delay treatment

Management

- ABC
- Treatment should be initiated straight away. If the patient is conscious and cooperative, oral fast-acting dextrose gel can be given, e.g. Glucogel©
- Other options include 1 mg glucagon SC, IM or IV or 50 mL of 50% dextrose IV with a saline flush
- Normal GCS is expected within 10 min. Continuing disability with a serum glucose >7 mmol/L suggests another cause

⊙ Hyperglycaemia

Diabetic ketoacidosis (DKA) is a common first presentation of type 1 DM and can also occur at any time but rarely in type 2 DM. Hyperosmotic non-ketotic acidosis (HONK) occurs in type 2 DM, especially elderly patients.

Absent or reduced insulin levels with raised catabolic hormones result in hyperglycaemia, lipolysis, and gluconeogenesis. The hyperglycaemia leads to an osmotic diuresis, with loss of water and electrolytes. Oxidation of the products of lipolysis produces ketone bodies and results in a metabolic acidosis. Ketosis is absent in HONK because there is enough circulating insulin to prevent lipolysis.

Clinical assessment

Symptomatic hyperglycaemia develops quickly over a day or two in DKA but has a more insidious onset in HONK. Features include:
- tiredness and lethargy; altered consciousness is a late sign
- polydipsia and polyuria. As it progresses they develop abdominal pain and vomiting
- 'fruity' acetone smell on breath in DKA
- rapid deep breaths (Küssmaul breathing) is respiratory compensation of the metabolic acidosis
- hypotension and tachycardia
- acidosis (pH <7.1 or HCO_3^- <16 mmol/L)
- Urinalysis—ketones +++ in DKA

Management of DKA

- ABC
- Supplemental oxygen
- Initial fluid resuscitation with normal saline and potassium supplementation if K^+ <5.5 mmol/L. 1000 mL over the first 30 min and then titrate to clinical response
- Regular serum K^+ measurements
- Insulin is used to reverse the ketosis and has a secondary effect of reducing serum glucose
- Urinary catheter and NG tube (reduce aspiration due to gastroparesis)
- Call for senior help. HDU/ITU care may be indicated

Acute renal failure (ARF) is rapid deterioration in kidney function, leading to accumulation of nitrogenous waste, abnormal water and electrolyte homeostasis, and altered acid–base balance. Acute renal failure occurs in 1% of hospital admissions and a third of these patients need ITU admission.

Renal failure is now defined in terms of the RIFLE classification (Table 15.13).

Aetiology

Classically ARF is divided into prerenal, renal, and postrenal causes. Prerenal is by far the most common cause seen in surgical patients.

Prerenal (hypoperfusion)

It arises in an otherwise healthy kidney owing to reduced perfusion. If the systemic cause is corrected, then renal function should recover.

Renal (intrinsic renal damage)

In the acute setting this is most commonly caused by acute tubular necrosis (ATN).

- Trauma, sepsis, burns, and cardiopulmonary bypass
- Glomerulonephritis
- Nephrotoxins (radiocontrast media, aminoglycosides, NSAIDs)
- Chronic renal dysfunction owing to heart failure, hypertension, diabetes mellitus, and atherosclerosis
- Renovascular disease
- Interstitial nephritis
- Liver disease and obstructive jaundice
- Rhabdomyolysis as a result of muscle breakdown has many causes, including trauma, drugs, and acute limb ischaemia

Postrenal (obstruction)

Obstructive nephropathy is relatively uncommon. It is most common in the elderly population. Obstruction can occur anywhere along the urinary tract and may be intrinsic or extrinsic. Causes include malignancy, renal calculi, urethral stricture, and prostatic disease.

Chronic renal failure

CRF is usually caused by intrinsic renal disease. Diabetes and hypertension account for two-thirds of cases. Other causes include glomerulonephritis, polycystic kidney disease, analgesic drugs (NSAIDs), reflux, and obstructive nephropathy.

Pathophysiology

Activation of the renin–angiotensin and sympathetic vasoconstrictor mechanisms, inhibition of prostaglandin-induced vasodilatation, and the intrinsic vascular injury seen in sepsis all interact to compromise renal perfusion during a period of shock.

Certain nephrotoxins are clearly associated with ARF by various mechanisms, including reduced GFR, direct tubular damage, hypovolaemia, catabolism, and hyperuricaemia, but the reason for the unpredictable nature of the damage is less clear. Several mechanisms have been proposed to explain the almost complete loss of renal function seen in ATN; tubular injury may affect function primarily, or glomerular function may be initially affected and secondarily impair tubular function.

The end result of these various mechanisms is a reduction in renal function made apparent by retention of the waste products of metabolism. The rate of accumulation of these products is dependent on the severity of renal failure and the rate at which they are being produced. Consequently the severely catabolic patient is at increased risk.

Clinical assessment

History

Evidence of renal dysfunction in the perioperative setting is usually indicated by a decreased urine output and rising serum creatinine. A precipitating factor is often identified.

Examination

Late signs include confusion or coma, arrhythmias (hyperkalaemia), myocardial dysfunction (metabolic acidosis), pulmonary and peripheral oedema (fluid overload).

- Assess patient fluid status, including fluid balance charts and urine output (UO)
- Palpate bladder and check catheter not blocked by flushing with 50 mL of water

Estimation of renal function

- Glomerular filtration rate (GFR) can be defined as the volume of plasma cleared of an ideal substance per unit of time (usually mL/min). The ideal substance is one that is freely filtered at the glomerulus and neither secreted nor reabsorbed by the renal tubules
- GFR can be estimated by measuring creatinine clearance. However, many factors influence the measurement, including age, sex, and muscle mass, and it only becomes abnormal when >50% of GFR is lost

  Creatinine clearance = (urine creatinine x volume*)/serum creatinine
  *collected over 24 h
- Serum urea is less accurate, as many variables unrelated to the glomerulus affect its levels (e.g. GI bleed, tissue breakdown and steroids)

Investigations

- Urinalysis for blood and protein (inflammatory condition); urine microscopy for cells, casts, and crystals. Red cell casts are diagnostic of glomerulonephritis
- Bloods—FBC (anaemia), U+Es (K^+), clotting (DIC)
- ABG—ARF causes metabolic acidosis
- Renal USS is usually normal in ARF but will identify a change in renal size and is used to exclude obstruction
- ECG—arrhythmias and signs of hyperkalaemia
- Plain chest radiograph—pulmonary oedema

Management

Immediate management of ARF is to correct life-threatening complications such as hyperkalaemia (see box), pulmonary oedema, and metabolic acidosis as well as life-threatening causes such as haemorrhage and shock.

- Supplemental oxygen as required
- Support ventilation and cardiac output
- Treat underlying cause and exclude urinary obstruction
- Consider renal replacement therapy (see box)
- Ensure good nutritional support

Complications and prognosis

The mortality rate from ARF is approximately 15% and this rises significantly in patients needing renal replacement therapy. There is no good evidence for drugs in improving the outcomes from ARF.

⊕ Renal replacement therapy in ARF

Acute renal failure is often reversible. Various techniques, such as continuous veno–veno haemofiltration (CVVHF) and haemodiafiltration (CVVHDF), may be used to support the kidneys and manage the hyperkalaemia, hypervolaemia, and metabolic acidosis.

These methods may be needed until renal function recovers or as a bridge to a renal replacement programme involving peritoneal dialysis or intermittent haemodialysis.

Indications

Renal replacement therapy (RRT) is indicated if two of the following are present and should be consider if one factor is present.

- Anuria (no urine output for >6 h)
- Oliguria (urine output <200 mL/12 h)
- Fluid overload with pulmonary dysfunction
- Uncompensated metabolic acidosis (pH <7.1)
- Hyperkalaemia (K^+ >6.5 mmol/L or rapidly rising)
- Uraemia (urea >28 mmol/L or creatinine >265 µmol/L)
- Abnormal temperature control
- Sepsis
- Acute poisoning with toxin that can be dialysed (e.g. lithium)

Continuous renal replacement

Intermittent haemodialysis and peritoneal dialysis are not generally indicated in the acute setting. Continuous renal replacement therapy (CRRT) is favoured and is either:

- CVVHF, in which there is spontaneous generation of an ultrafiltrate with post-filter addition of a replacement fluid
- CVVHDF, in which there is a countercurrent flow of dialysate fluid. The dialysate is pump-controlled so that the spent dialysate outflow is just 100–200 mL/h (as needed to maintain fluid balance) above the dialysate inflow

⊙ Hyperkalaemia (K^+ >6.5 mmol/L)

Clinical assessment

- Nausea, diarrhoea, and vomiting
- ECG—tented T waves, reduced or absent P waves, widened QRS, and eventually ventricular fibrillation and cardiac arrest
- Repeat serum K^+ measurement as haemolysis may give a false high result

Management

- ABC
- Cardioprotection—IV 10 mL of 10% calcium gluconate
- Increased cellular uptake of K^+—IV insulin and inhaled or IV beta-2-agonist (e.g. salbutamol)
- Increased gastrointestinal excretion: oral or rectal calcium resonium 15 g 6-hourly
- Sodium bicarbonate is effective in cases of metabolic acidosis. It stimulates the exchange of cellular H^+ for Na^+ and stimulation of Na^+–K^+ ATPase
- Poor response or severe cases need dialysis
- Reduce dietary intake and stop any medications that increase potassium levels

Table 15.13 RIFLE classification of ARF

RIFLE	GFR criteria	UO criteria
Risk	Increased Cr x 1.5 or decreased GFR <25%	UO <0.5 mL/kg/h for 6 h
Injury	Increased Cr x 2 or decreased GFR > 50%	UO <0.5 mL/kg/h for 12 h
Failure	Increased Cr x 3 decreased GFR 75% or Cr ≥4 mg/dL or acute rise ≥ 0.5mg/dL	UO <0.3 mL/kg/h for 24 h or anuria for 12 h
Loss	Persistent ARF Complete loss of kidney function >4 weeks	
ESKD	End-stage kidney disease	

GFR, Glomerular filtration rate; UO, urine output; Cr, serum creatinine; ARF, acute renal failure.

15.19 Stroke

A stroke is a sudden loss of blood supply to an area of brain associated with a neurological deficit. It is classified as ischaemic (85%) or haemorrhagic. Subarachnoid haemorrhage is discussed elsewhere (📖 Table 10.4). It is the third most common cause of death in developed countries and its incidence increases with age.

Definitions

- Stroke is a focal neurological deficit caused by a vascular lesion that lasts longer than 24 h
- Transient ischaemic attack is a focal neurological deficit caused by a vascular lesion that lasts less than 24 h (usually <1 h) with a complete clinical recovery

Aetiology

Cerebral infarction (70%)

- Cerebral thrombosis within the cerebral circulation forms in areas of reduced blood flow around atheromatous plaques and has the potential to occlude the vessel completely, narrow the vessel, or embolize. Lacunar infarcts are occlusion of the smallest vessels
- Cerebral embolism—emboli may arise from atheromatous plaques in extracranial arteries (e.g. carotid arteries), calcified valve fragments, bacterial vegetations or tumour fragments or cardiac thrombus

Intracerebral haemorrhage (30%)

Uncontrolled hypertension is the most common cause. Others include intracranial tumours, bleeding disorders, and anticoagulation.

Pathophysiology

Cerebral infarction

Vessel occlusion causes hypoxic neuronal injury, although this ischaemia may be reversed with rapid restoration of blood flow.

Intracerebral haemorrhage

Intracerebral haemorrhage is usually caused by rupture of microaneurysms in the brain parenchyma caused by hypertension or a bleed into a previous infarct. Neuronal injury is caused by the blood, local pressure effects, and vasospasm.

Subarachnoid haemorrhage is usually due to rupture of a saccular aneurysm. The blood is mainly in the subarachnoid space rather than the brain parenchyma.

Clinical assessment

Stroke usually presents with a sudden onset of neurological dysfunction. Infarction and haemorrhage are clinically indistinguishable.

Acute cerebrovascular accident (CVA) (stroke, brain attack)

- Cerebral infarction—neurological deficit, symptoms dependent on artery involved
- Intracerebral haemorrhage—sudden onset of neurological deficit, usually with absence of prodromal symptoms, headache, and meningism

Examination

- Neurological deficit with site and extent of damage
- Unilateral numbness, weakness or paralysis
- Receptive/expressive dysphasia
- Visual field defect
- Reduced conscious level
- Hypertension is a common finding. It is a protective response to maintain cerebral perfusion pressure

Investigations

- Urinalysis—DM, UTI
- Bloods—FBC, U+Es, clotting, fasting lipid profile, and troponin I
- ECG—arrhythmias, myocardial ischaemia/infarction
- CT brain should be performed within 24 h or more urgently if the patient has a reduced or fluctuating GCS, a bleeding tendency or is on anticoagulation, or a severe headache. MRI is considered if the CT is equivocal
  CT scan excludes intracerebral haemorrhage and other underlying brain conditions. Infarction is usually only detectable after a couple of hours to days.
- Echocardiography—excludes intracardiac site of embolus
- Carotid duplex ultrasound or CTA is used to assess extracranial arterial disease

Management

The initial approach is ABC. Early imaging with CT and referral to specialist stroke service improves outcomes.

Immediate

- ABC (make NBM)
- Supplemental oxygen to maintain SaO_2 >95%
- Monitoring—routine observations, neurological status, and cardiac rhythm
- Careful fluid and electrolyte balance. Avoid haemoconcentration and hyponatraemia
- Aspirin 300 mg (only cerebral infarction)

Cerebral infarction

- Thrombolysis with alteplase within 3 h of onset of the cerebral infarction reduces morbidity and mortality rates although does carry a risk of bleeding
- Blood pressure control needs specialist input
- Patients with carotid artery stenosis may benefit from carotid endarterectomy (📖 Topic 7.6)

Intracerebral haemorrhage

Acute management is generally the same as for ischaemic stroke, although thrombolysis, antiplatelet agents, and anticoagulation are contraindicated. Large haematomas causing a mass effect and raised ICP may need neurosurgical evacuation.

Prevention of complications and rehabilitation

- Referral to specialist stroke rehabilitation service
- Speech and language therapy (SALT) assessment
- Nutrition—high risk of aspiration; a nasogastric tube may be needed initially
- Maintain stable blood glucose level <10 mmol/L
- Avoid pyrexia which can hasten neuronal damage
- Prophylaxis and treatment of complications such as peptic ulceration, DVT, pressure sores, and seizures
- Secondary prevention of cardiovascular disease and management of atrial fibrillation if present

Complications and prognosis

Transient ischaemic attack is an important prognostic indicator. Within 5 years 40% of patients will have had a stroke and 25% will be dead because of a cardiovascular event.

Complications of stroke include dysphagia, seizures, nosocomial infections, and peptic ulceration.

⚠ Stroke

Any patient with known cerebrovascular disease must be investigated prior to elective major surgery. A carotid duplex ultrasound can identify patients who may benefit from carotid endarterectomy prior to surgery.

Good control of hypertension is vital, and other risk modifications should be encouraged. Optimal medical therapy, including antiplatelet and statin therapy, will decrease the risk of a perioperative cerebrovascular event.

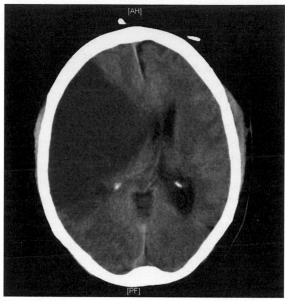

Fig 15.23 CT brain showing a cerebral infarct in the territory of the right middle cerebral artery. This was a repeat scan after 48 h when the patient dropped their GCS to 9. The infarcted area appears hypodense. There is generalized right-sided cerebral swelling and midline shift. No acute haemorrhage is seen.

Acute confusion is a symptom characterized by reversible disorientation in time and place, associated with impaired short-term memory. It is common, occurring in 10–20% of all hospital admissions. Postoperative acute confusion is associated with worse outcomes and prolonged hospitalization.

Definitions

- **Delirium** is acute confusion with the addition of disordered perception, e.g. hallucinations (auditory, visual, or olfactory) or illusions
- **Psychosis** is hallucinations and illusions without confusion
- **Dementia** is a chronic deficit in thinking, memory, and/or personality

Aetiology

There are many causes of acute confusional state (ACS), some factors may co-exist:

- hypoxia
- infection—urinary tract, respiratory tract, wound, peripheral or central line
- fluid or electrolyte disturbance—dehydration, hyponatraemia
- myocardial ischaemia
- organ failure
- metabolic—hyperglycaemia or hypoglycaemia, electrolyte disturbance, vitamin deficiency (thiamine, B_{12}), hypercalcaemia
- Endocrine—thyroid, adrenal or pituitary
- Drug toxicity—benzodiazepines, opiates, anticholinergics, steroids, psychotropic medication or withdrawal
- Alcohol intoxication/withdrawal
- Neurological—raised ICP, dementia, TIA/CVA, head injury, post-ictal, malignancy
- Urinary retention and faecal impaction

Risk factors

- Advanced age
- Poor eyesight and deafness
- Pre-existing cognitive impairment
- Depression
- Drugs or withdrawal
- Alcohol abuse
- Co-morbidities
- Previous episode of acute confusion

Clinical assessment

History

- Ask about hallucinations or illusions
- Attempt to gain an idea of usual mental state and functional capacity from family, friends, carers, and nursing staff
- Review medical notes and observations
- Review current and recent medication
- Alcohol and substance history

Examination

- General behaviour and alertness
- Systems examination to identify acute illness
- Examine for focal neurological signs
- Abbreviated mental test score (Table 15.14)
- Observations—temperature, HR, BP, RR, O_2 saturations, GCS

Investigations

- Urinalysis—DM, UTI
- Bloods—FBC, U+Es, LFT, TFT, serum glucose, bone profile (including Ca^{2+}), haematinics, troponin, CRP
- Microbiology screen—urine, sputum, and blood cultures
- Plain chest radiograph—LRTI, malignancy
- ECG—ischaemia, arrhythmias
- CT scan head if focal neurology or unresolving confusion with no clear aetiology

Management

Acute confusion can be frightening for both the patient and staff. Underlying causes need to be identified and treated promptly.

Immediate

- Treat emergencies, e.g. hypoxia, hypoglycaemia, sepsis
- Protect patient from self-harm and staff from injury
- Try to offer calm reassurance. Avoid confrontation
- Emergency sedation may be indicated if a patient is very agitated or aggressive and a danger to themselves or others. This can be done with restraint.
  Lorazepam 2 mg (1 mg in the elderly or those with renal failure) po/IM/IV or haloperidol 4 mg (2 mg in the elderly) po/IM/IV can be used. Following administration, the patient should have regular 15 min observations. Repeat after 45 min as required
- Drugs may need to be reversed—naloxone for opiates and flumazenil for benzodiazepines

General

- Nurse in a quiet environment with moderate light levels even at night
- Provide necessary sensory aids, e.g. hearing aid and spectacles
- Encourage visits by familiar people
- Maintain continuity of care
- Verbal and visual reminders of time, place, and person
- May need specialist psychiatric or one-to-one nursing provision
- Continuity of care personnel

Complications and prognosis

Complications and outcomes are quite variable and relate to the reversibility of the underlying cause. Postoperative patients often have reversible causes, such as hypoxia or pain, and tend to do well.

Patients with serious underlying causes of their confusion need rapid treatment, without which there may be deterioration leading to death.

⊙ Alcohol

The recommended maximum weekly alcohol consumption is 21 units per week for men and 14 units for women. This should not be consumed all at once nor every day.

Problem drinking is when chronic heavy drinking results in alcohol-related complications. Features of the alcohol dependence syndrome include primacy of drinking over other activities, awareness of a compulsion to drink, and difficulty controlling the amount drunk, increased tolerance to alcohol, and relief or avoidance of withdrawal symptoms by further drinking.

Alcohol dependence usually has a complex, often multifactorial aetiology. Some features predisposing individuals to alcohol abuse include jobs with access to alcohol, stress, personality traits, and psychiatric disorders.

Clinical assessment

Ask about pattern of intake and number of units consumed weekly. Also ask about the symptoms of alcohol-related medical complications, withdrawal symptoms or previous seizures.

Consider performing a mini-mental test and screen with CAGE questionnaire.

- Have you ever felt you should **C**ut down on your drinking?
- Have people **A**nnoyed you criticising your drinking?
- Have you ever felt **G**uilty about your drinking?
- Have you ever had an **E**ye-opener, i.e. a drink first thing in the morning to steady your nerves or get rid of a hangover?

Signs of liver disease include jaundice, bruising, spider naevi, palmar erythema, ascites, hepatomegaly (cirrhotic liver is usually small), caput medusae, and other signs of portal hypertension, peripheral oedema.

Routine blood tests may show deranged LFT (high gamma GT and AST, low albumin) and clotting.

Alcohol withdrawal

If a patient has been identified as having a high alcohol intake, withdrawal symptoms must be anticipated and this period can be smoothed pharmacologically with gradually reducing doses of a benzodiazepine. In cases of severe agitation, a neuroleptic, such as haloperidol, may be indicated in addition to a benzodiazepine.

- Prevent seizures with benzodiazepines
- Give thiamine, folic acid, B12, and multivitamins
- Good nutrition
- Referral to psychiatry once medically well for alcohol withdrawal programme

Delirium tremens

Delirium tremens is a potentially fatal form of acute alcohol withdrawal, with a mortality rate of 5%.

Chronic alcohol intake downregulates GABA receptors and antagonizes N-methyl-D-aspartate receptors; consequently, acute withdrawal leads to central nervous system excitation and catecholamine release.

Clinical presentation includes tremor, irritability, nausea and vomiting, confusion, visual hallucinations, and delusions. Severe cases lead to seizures, hypertension, and cardiovascular collapse.

Symptoms may begin a few hours after cessation of alcohol intake and peak at 48–72 h.

⚠ Acute confusion

ACS and delirium are relatively common after surgery, especially in patients over 65 years old.

Preoperative

- Identify risk factors
- Identify visual or hearing impairment
- Document mental state using mini-mental state examination (MMSE)
- Planned withdrawal of medications and alcohol needs to be in advance of admission

Postoperative

- General measures to maintain the patient orientated in time, place, and person
- Good analgesia but be aware of potential to worsen confusion, i.e. tramadol and codeine
- Poly-pharmacy should be avoided where possible. Interactions between drugs and the prescription of night sedation, anxiolytics, and analgesics warrants careful consideration
- Routine observations and BMs
- Monitor fluid and electrolyte balance
- Maintain adequate nutrition

Table 15.14 Abbreviated mental test score

Each answer carries one point. Maximum score is ten. Normal elderly patient should score eight or above.

1. Patient's age
2. Patient's date of birth
3. Current time to the nearest hour
4. Year
5. Name of institution or current location
6. Repeat 42 West Street (no score until recall)
7. Recognition of two people (e.g. doctor and nurse)
8. Year that World War Two ended
9. Name the monarch
10. Count backwards from twenty to one
11. Recall 42 West Street

15.21 Haematological conditions

Anaemia

Anaemia is caused by reduced numbers of red blood cells and/or low haemoglobin concentration expected for a person's age and sex. Anaemia leads to reduced oxygen-carrying capacity of the blood. It is important to note that different types of anaemia may co-exist.

Aetiology and pathophysiology

Reduced production or abnormal maturation

The most common cause of anaemia worldwide is iron deficiency. This may be caused by blood loss (e.g. menstruation), increased demand for iron (e.g. pregnancy) or poor diet or GI absorption.

Other causes of reduced RBC production include vitamin B12 or folate deficiency and bone marrow failure.

Increased destruction or loss

The life span of a RBC is approximately 120 days. Haemolysis is the premature breakdown of RBC. It is classified as congenital (e.g. thalassaemia, hereditary spherocytosis) or acquired. Acquired causes are either immune-mediated (rare) or non-immune (e.g. drugs, mechanical valves, malaria).

Clinical assessment

Anaemia is often asymptomatic. A slowly falling haemoglobin level is compensated for by enhanced oxygen-carrying capacity of the blood.

- Acute blood loss can present with the features associated with cardiovascular collapse and shock
- Chronic anaemia is more insidious and presents with fatigue, faintness, weakness, and pallor. There may also be exacerbation of angina and intermittent claudication on exertion and evidence of heart failure
- Some types have specific signs—koilonychia in iron deficiency; jaundice in haemolytic anaemia

Investigations

- FBC—low haemoglobin for age and sex of patient. White cell count, platelet count, mean corpuscular volume (MCV), mean corpuscular haemoglobin (MCH), haematocrit
- Total iron-binding capacity and serum iron
- Peripheral blood film identifies abnormal red cell morphology and presence of reticulocytes (immature RBC)
- Further tests such as GI endoscopy and bone marrow biopsy may be indicated

Management

Management depends on the underlying cause and severity. Acute blood loss will need resuscitation with fluid or blood. Generally, use of blood products should be avoided in the treatment of chronic anaemia.

Iron-deficiency anaemia is rare in non-menstruating adults and an underlying cause should be identified and treated (e.g. GI bleeding). Oral iron supplements, such as ferrous sulphate, are used to replace losses.

Anaemia of chronic disease, such as chronic renal failure, is often treated with recombinant erythropoietin which stimulates red cell production.

Haemoglobin abnormalities

Sickle syndromes

Sickle syndromes are the commonest haemoglobin abnormality. They are endemic in Africa, the Mediterranean, Middle East, and India.

Sickle cell haemoglobin results from a single substitution of valine for glutamine on the beta-globin chain. The normal genetic state is HbAA. In the homozygous form (sickle cell anaemia) both genes are abnormal (HbSS). Sickle haemoglobin distorts the shape of RBCs, causing them to become sickle-shaped. These sickle RBCs have a shortened life span and reduced deformability. They stick to vascular endothelium more easily, causing reduced blood flow and vascular obstruction which results in vaso-occlusive crises.

Patients develop both haemolytic anaemia and vasculopathy with ongoing organ damage. Manifestations of sickle cell anaemia do not become apparent until 3–4 months of age.

The heterozygous form (sickle cell trait) has one abnormal gene (HbAS). These patients usually have no clinical abnormality, with sickling only occurring with extreme hypoxia. Another form of sickle cell disease is sickle-haemoglobin C disease, HbSC, which has a less severe course than HbSS. Sickle cell anaemia may co-exist with thalassaemia.

Thalassaemia

Thalassaemia is the absent or deficient synthesis of the alpha- or beta-globin chains of haemoglobin, leading to an imbalance in their production. It is prevalent in those of Mediterranean, North African, and Asian descent.

Beta-thalassaemia is most common. There is a lack of beta chains, resulting in an excess of alpha chains which precipitate in mature RBCs, leading to haemolysis. There are minor, intermediate, and major forms. Patients with the minor form are usually asymptomatic; those with the major form are transfusion-dependent (with administration of the iron-chelating agent desferrioxamine).

Complications of thalassaemia major include iron overload, infection, high output congestive cardiac failure, liver disease, and endocrine abnormalities.

Platelet and vascular disorders

Thrombocytopenia (low platelet count) is caused by either reduced production (e.g. marrow failure), reduced platelet survival (e.g. drugs) or increased consumption (e.g. disseminated intravascular coagulation). It results in purpura and bleeding. Platelet dysfunction occurs in liver and renal impairment and as a consequence of antiplatelet therapy.

Vascular disorders (non-thrombocytopaenic purpuras) lead to bleeding and bruising owing to abnormal vessel characteristics. Blood constituents and coagulation studies are normal. Acquired causes include sepsis, steroid therapy, and allergic conditions such as Henoch–Schönlein purpura; hereditary haemorrhagic telangiectasia is a rare congenital cause.

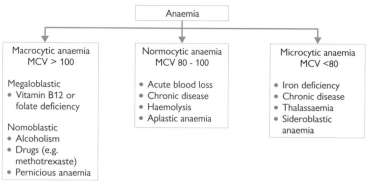

Fig 15.24 Classification of anaemia based on mean corpuscle volume (MCV).

⚠ Haematological conditions

Anaemia

- FBC is performed following NICE guidelines and in any patient at risk of anaemia, with cardiorespiratory disease or undergoing major surgery
- Haemoglobin lower limit is 13 g/dL for men and 12 g/dL for women although over 10 g/dL is often acceptable for elective surgery
- Low haemoglobin discovered before elective surgery needs further investigation and treatment
- Blood transfusions in elective or emergency surgery may be indicated. G&S and cross-match are discussed in Topic 8.5

Sickle cell syndromes

- Full blood count and haemoglobin electrophoresis on all patients with at-risk ethnicity. In sickle cell trait the haemoglobin and blood film are usually normal
- Exchange transfusion—HbS level <30% prior to major surgery in patients with sickle cell anaemia
- Avoid triggers to sickle crisis such as dehydration
- Tourniquets should only be used with extreme caution and the limb must be fully exsanguinated prior to cuff inflation

Haemophilia

- Discuss perioperative care with a haematologist
- Desmopressin (DDAVP®) and antifibrinolytics, e.g. tranexamic acid, aprotonin, and aminocaproic acid, have a role in the patient with mild haemophilia A for minor surgery
- A course of recombinant factor will need to be planned in advance for the majority of haemophiliacs
- The use of topical agents is often helpful, e.g. fibrin sealants
- Avoid IM injections and NSAID use

Disseminated intravascular coagulation

DIC is the most commonly encountered postoperative coagulopathy. It is discussed further in Topic 7.1.

♂ Sickle cell crisis

Precipitants of sickle crisis include dehydration, hypoxia, cold, alcohol, infection, vascular stasis, and acidosis. Types of sickle cell crisis include:

- **aplastic**—depression of erythropoiesis secondary to infection, especially parvovirus B19 and/or folate deficiency
- **infarctive**—vaso-occlusive episodes which can cause a dramatic presentation with acute abdomen, acute chest syndrome, cerebrovascular accident, or priapism, but can occur in the spine or long bones
- **sequestration**—results from massive pooling of red cells within the spleen and is especially common in children and those with HbSC disease
- **haemolytic**—usually accompanies an infarctive crisis. Chronic haemolysis leads to gallstones in virtually all patients with SCA

Management of sickle crisis is with supplemental oxygen, fluid replacement, and strong analgesia. Infection needs to be identified and treated with the appropriate antibiotics. If refractory, consider exchange transfusion (aim for HbS <30%) and steroids.

Case 1

You see a 74-year-old man in the pre-admission clinic. He is due to undergo elective repair of an abdominal aortic aneurysm. It was diagnosed incidentally on an ultrasound scan of his renal tract. He has type 2 diabetes mellitus, hypertension, and ischaemic heart disease.

- What is your approach to pre-assessment of this patient?
- What investigations do you request?
- How do you assess his surgical risk?
- Describe the aetiology and pathophysiology of atherosclerosis

He was first diagnosed with type 2 diabetes mellitus 14 years ago. He believes he is well controlled on glibenclamide and metformin. He has impaired renal function which is being routinely monitored. He has also been recently investigated for haematuria (now resolved), hence the renal ultrasound.

Hb	9.9 g/dL	Ca (total)	2.08
WC	6.9×10^9	Ca (ionized)	1.01
Plts	220×10^9	Phosphate	1.0
MCV	70 fl	Total cholesterol	8.8
Glucose	8.2 mmol/L	VLDL	0.7
HbA1C	6.6%	LDL	5.0
Na^+	133 mmol/L	HDL	0.7
K^+	5.2 mmol/L		
Urea	14.1 mmol/L		
Creatinine	220 mmol/L		

- Discuss his preoperative blood results
- Are there any management improvements that could be made on the basis of these results?
- What specific signs will you look for on the ECG?
- What might you see on his chest radiograph?

The ECG shows significant Q waves in leads aVL, II, and III. The S wave in V1 is 45 mm in depth and there is evidence of left ventricular strain. The chest radiograph reveals cardiomegaly but no pulmonary congestion.

- What can you conclude from this ECG? Does he need further investigation?

Discussion

He has a microcytic anaemia which needs further investigation. More information is needed about the haematuria and whether he has had any GI blood loss. Iron supplementation may be indicated.

He has renal impairment but the results should be compared with his baseline. His diabetes seems to be adequately controlled but he has a raised lipid profile. The ECG suggests an old anterolateral myocardial infarction and left ventricular hypertrophy. He would benefit from a cardiology referral for further cardiac investigations and optimization of his cardiovascular medications.

Case 2

You are called by a nurse to come and urgently review a 77-year-old man who is 5 h postop following a right hemicolectomy. He has become progressively more anxious, breathless, and tachycardic over the last hour.

- What do you ask her to do before you get to the ward?
- When you arrive, what is your approach to initial assessment and management?

He has a history of IHD and you suspect he has gone into acute pulmonary oedema. He starts to complain of left-sided chest pain.

- What is your approach to cardiac chest pain in a postoperative patient?
- What investigations do you arrange?

Your acute management stabilizes him and he is waiting for a medical review. The biochemistry results are phoned through to the ward. He is in acute renal failure and has a serum potassium of 6.7 mmol/L.

- How do you manage hyperkalaemia?
- What are common causes of renal failure in surgical patients and how is the severity of renal dysfunction classified?

Case 3

You are called to see an 82-year-old woman who is 4 days postop following abdominal surgery. She has developed a fever and shortness of breath over night.

- What is your initial assessment and management?
- What is your differential diagnosis?

She has a productive cough and, on examination, you suspect she has right lower lobe consolidation consistent with an infection.

- How are you going to investigate and treat her provisional diagnosis of pneumonia?
- How would you assess her risk for pulmonary embolism?

Later on you are called back to see her as she has become confused and is complaining of chest pain. You fully assess her and the ECG shows fast atrial fibrillation.

- What might the ECG look like?
- How would you manage new onset fast AF in this situation?

Index

Please note that page references to Figures or Tables are in *italic* print

425